SECOND EDITION

HPE-ASU

Physical Activity & Health

An Interactive Approach

DAVID Q. THOMAS
Illinois State University
Normal, Illinois

JEROME E. KOTECKI
Ball State University
Muncie, Indiana

JONES AND BARTLETT PUBLISHERS
Sudbury, Massachusetts
BOSTON   TORONTO   LONDON   SINGAPORE

World Headquarters
Jones and Bartlett Publishers
40 Tall Pine Drive
Sudbury, MA 01776
978-443-5000
info@jbpub.com
www.jbpub.com

Jones and Bartlett Publishers
Canada
6339 Ormindale Way
Mississauga, Ontario L5V 1J2
CANADA

Jones and Bartlett Publishers
International
Barb House, Barb Mews
London W6 7PA
UK

Jones and Bartlett's books and products are available through most bookstores and online booksellers. To contact Jones and Bartlett Publishers directly, call 800-832-0034, fax 978-443-8000, or visit our website, www.jbpub.com.

Substantial discounts on bulk quantities of Jones and Bartlett's publications are available to corporations, professional associations, and other qualified organizations. For details and specific discount information, contact the special sales department at Jones and Bartlett via the above contact information or send an email to specialsales@jbpub.com.

Production Credits
Chief Executive Officer: Clayton Jones
Chief Operating Officer: Don W. Jones, Jr.
President, Higher Education and Professional Publishing: Robert W. Holland, Jr.
V.P., Design and Production: Anne Spencer
V.P., Manufacturing and Inventory Control: Therese Connell
V.P., Sales and Marketing: William J. Kane
Acquisitions Editor: Jacqueline Mark-Geraci
Senior Production Editor: Julie Champagne Bolduc
Associate Editor: Patrice K. Andrews
Editorial Assistant: Amy L. Flagg
Production Assistant: Jennifer M. Ryan
Associate Marketing Manager: Wendy Thayer
Cover Design: Kristin E. Ohlin
Interior Design: Anne Spencer
Cover Image: © Peter Hurley Studio/Chicago
Printing and Binding: Courier Companies
Cover Printing: Courier Companies

Library of Congress Cataloging-in-Publication Data
Thomas, David Q.
  Physical activity and health / David Q. Thomas, Jerome E. Kotecki. -- 2nd ed.
     p. cm.
  Rev. ed. of: Physical activity and health / Kelli McCormack Brown, David Q. Thomas, Jerome E. Kotecki. c2002.
  ISBN-13: 978-0-7637-4150-1 (alk. paper)
  1. Exercise. 2. Physical fitness. 3. Heath. I. Kotecki, Jerome Edward. II. Brown, Kelli McCormack. Physical activity and health. III. Title.
  RA781.K763 2006
  613.7'1--dc22
                              2006022975
6048

Printed in the United States of America
10 09 08 07 06   10 9 8 7 6 5 4 3 2 1

Brief Contents

Chapter 1   The Physical Activity and Health Connection   2

Chapter 2   Foundations of Physical Activity   20

Chapter 3   Understanding and Enhancing Health Behaviors   46

Chapter 4   The Heart of Physical Activity: Cardiovascular Health   64

Chapter 5   Physical Inactivity and Cardiovascular Disease   78

Chapter 6   The Role of Physical Activity in Preventing Diabetes and Cancer   92

Chapter 7   Optimal Nutrition for an Active Lifestyle   106

Chapter 8   Metabolic Health   150

Chapter 9   Achieving and Maintaining a Healthy Weight   168

Chapter 10   Achieving Optimal Bone Health   206

Chapter 11   Muscular Strength and Endurance   226

Chapter 12   Stretching and Flexibility   254

Chapter 13   Understanding Mental Health, Stress, and Physical Activity   276

Chapter 14   Making Informed Decisions About Substance Use   298

Chapter 15   Exercise Consumerism   330

Chapter 16   Developing Healthy Sexual and Intimate Relationships   350

Chapter 17   Preventing Sexually Transmitted Diseases   366

Contents

Preface xi

This Book's Features xiv

About the Authors xix

UNIT 1   ACHIEVING HEALTH THROUGH PHYSICAL ACTIVITY

Chapter 1   The Physical Activity and Health Connection 2

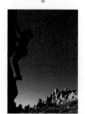

Introduction 4
Physical Activity and Health 4
Health, Wellness, and Lifestyle 6
Physical Activity, Exercise, and Physical Fitness 10
Physical Activity Recommendations for Health 11
Why We Live Sedentary Lives 14
A Lifestyle Approach to Physical Activity 14
Investing in Your Health 15
Physical Activity and Health Connection 16

Chapter 2   Foundations of Physical Activity 20

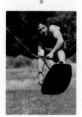

Introduction 22
Your Body Was Meant to Move 22
Prescreening, Medical History, and Self-Assessment 24
Health Benefits and Optimal Fitness 26
Personalizing Your Physical Activity Program 28
How Do I Get Started? 32
Program Design 34
Components of Health-Related Fitness 36
The Principles of Training 37
Becoming Independently Active 38
Overcoming Barriers to Physical Activity 38
Exercise Program Adherence 40
Strategies to Increase Adherence 41
Physical Activity and Intrinsic Motivation 41
Safety and Effectiveness 42
Physical Activity and Health Connection 43

Chapter 3 Understanding and Enhancing Health Behaviors 46

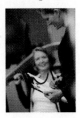

Introduction 48

Health Habits 48

Self-Change Approach 49

A Step-by-Step Approach to Behavior Change 49

Making a Behavioral Change Plan 59

Physical Activity and Health Connection 60

UNIT 2 **PROMOTING HEART HEALTH AND PREVENTING CHRONIC DISEASE**

Chapter 4 The Heart of Physical Activity: Cardiovascular Health 64

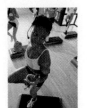

Introduction 66

Cardiovascular Health 70

Designing Your Cardiorespiratory Fitness Program 71

Physical Activity and Health Connection 75

Chapter 5 Physical Inactivity and Cardiovascular Disease 78

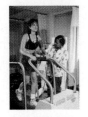

Introduction 80

Understanding Cardiovascular Diseases 81

Risk Factors for Cardiovascular Disease 85

Physical Activity and Health Connection 89

Chapter 6 The Role of Physical Activity in Preventing Diabetes and Cancer 92

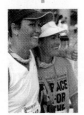

Introduction 94

Understanding Diabetes Mellitus 94

What Is Cancer? 96

Understanding Cancer 96

Common Cancers 99

Taking Responsibility for Your Health 101

Physical Activity and Health Connection 102

UNIT 3   ENERGIZING YOUR BODY

Chapter 7   Optimal Nutrition for an Active Lifestyle 106

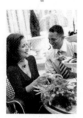

Introduction 108

Nutrition Basics 109

Classes of Nutrients 112

Planning a Nutritious Diet 126

Nutrition and Physical Activity 144

Physical Activity and Health Connection 146

Chapter 8   Metabolic Health 150

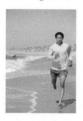

Introduction 152

Energy Balance, Transfer, and Storage 152

First Law of Thermodynamics 152

Anaerobic Metabolism 157

Aerobic Metabolism 157

Physical Activity and Metabolism 157

Inactivity and Metabolism 159

Metabolic Abnormalities 159

An Obesity Epidemic 164

Physical Activity and Health Connection 165

Chapter 9   Achieving and Maintaining a Healthy Weight 168

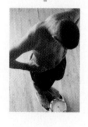

Introduction 170

Overweight and Obesity and Health Risk 173

Maintaining a Healthy Body Weight 186

A Lifestyle Approach to Achieving and Maintaining a Healthy Weight 193

Body Image and Weight 198

Physical Activity and Health Connection 202

UNIT 4   **BUILDING A STRONG BODY**

Chapter 10   Achieving Optimal Bone Health 206

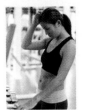

Introduction 208
Understanding Bone Physiology 208
Nutrition and Physical Activity for Bone Health 210
Osteoporosis 215
Physical Activity and Health Connection 222

Chapter 11   Muscular Strength and Endurance 226

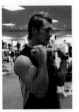

Introduction 228
Muscular Anatomy and Physiology 228
Getting Stronger, Building Size, Toning Up 232
Resistance Training Guidelines 235
Resistance Training Across the Life Span 250
Physical Activity and Health Connection 251

Chapter 12   Stretching and Flexibility 254

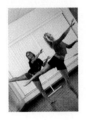

Introduction 256
Muscle Spindles and Golgi Tendon Organs 258
Muscle Elasticity and Compliance 258
Types of Stretching Exercises 258
Passive and Active Stretching 259
Flexibility Guidelines 260
Common Stretching Exercises 261
Changes in Flexibility with Age 270
Role of Flexibility in Injury Prevention 270
Physical Activity and Health Connection 272

UNIT 5   **MAKING HEALTHY DECISIONS**

Chapter 13   Understanding Mental Health, Stress, and Physical Activity 276

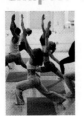

Introduction 278
Mind-Body Relationship 280
Understanding Stress 282
Stress Management 289
The Mental Health Benefits of Physical Activity 292
Quick Relaxation Techniques 293
Physical Activity and Health Connection 295

Chapter 14   Making Informed Decisions About Substance Use 298

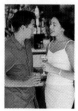

Introduction 300

Drug Terminology 300

Chronic Drug Use 304

Making Substance Use Decisions 306

Commonly Used and Misused Psychoactive Drugs 306

Alcohol and Society 307

Tobacco Use: An Enduring Health Threat 319

Physical Activity and Health Connection 326

Chapter 15   Exercise Consumerism 330

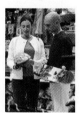

Introduction 332

Facts, Fads, and Fallacies 352

Sources of Information 338

Selecting a Physical Activity Program 339

Selecting a Physical Activity and Fitness Facility 340

Examples of Misleading Products 340

Seeking Redress 343

Physical Activity and Health Connection 346

UNIT 6   **BUILDING HEALTHY RELATIONSHIPS**

Chapter 16   Developing Healthy Sexual and Intimate Relationships 350

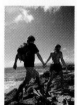

Introduction 352

Defining Sex and Sexuality 352

Gender Identity and Gender Role 354

Sexual Biology 354

Sexual Response Cycle 358

Developing Positive Intimate Relationships 359

Communicating in Intimate Relationships 362

Physical Activity and Health Connection 364

Chapter 17   Preventing Sexually Transmitted Diseases 366

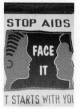

Introduction 368

STD Statistics 368

STD Risk Factors 368

Reactions to STDs 370

Common STDs 370

Preventing Sexually Transmitted Diseases 377

Physical Activity and Health Connection 379

Appendix A Injury Prevention 383

Appendix B Caloric Cost of Selected Activities 387

Appendix C Nutrition and Health for Canadians 393

Appendix D Calculations and Conversions 407

Glossary 413

Photo Credits 423

Index 425

Preface

A physical activity course is one of the most important and exciting classes a college student will take. Physical activity courses can affect students' health not only in the here and now, but also for the rest of their lives. Our goal with *Physical Activity and Health: An Interactive Approach* is to present scientific evidence on the relationship between physical activity and health to today's students in an interesting, purposeful, and motivating manner. Simply stated, we want to help students make physical activity a priority today and throughout their lives.

The value of *Physical Activity and Health* lies in its unique capability to expand students' knowledge of the interconnectedness of physical activity and other related health topics. Traditional fitness books provide multiple chapters on exercise and only one or two chapters about health. Traditional health books provide you with multiple chapters on health and only a brief mention of fitness. *Physical Activity and Health* is designed to be a hybrid of the two, with every chapter and section reinforcing the connection between physical activity and health.

Physical Activity and Health uses a distinctive interactive approach to convey the message that physical activity is an essential lifestyle behavior in promoting well-being. This interactive approach supports our beliefs that each individual must take an active role in achieving a healthy lifestyle. Therefore, self-responsibility is a central focus of this book. We arm each reader with the information, skills, and practical know-how to gain control of his or her health and determine what to do and how and when to do it.

Physical Activity and Health offers expert knowledge based on the latest scientific findings from health research along with a variety of pedagogical elements that assist and encourage readers in developing a personalized physical activity and health plan. We know that if the student reads the chapters carefully and makes an honest effort to complete the various activities and assessments provided in the accompanying manual, they will gain the competence and confidence to make informed decisions to improve their well-being.

A Text for All Students

Physical Activity and Health is written for college students in a wide variety of settings, from community colleges to large four-year universities. The content is carefully constructed to be meaningful to students from all academic disciplines. This book is designed to meet the needs of a course that goes beyond the basics of physical activity and fitness to encompass the interconnectedness of important health topics facing today's college students. It is an adaptable book that fits nicely into a lecture/physical activity format and that easily accommodates a variety of physical activity, fitness, wellness, and health courses.

> *No less than two hours a day should be devoted to exercise.*
> **THOMAS JEFFERSON**
> **(1743–1826)**
>
> *If the man who wrote the Declaration of Independence, was Secretary of State, and twice President could give it two hours, our children can give it ten or fifteen minutes.*
> **JOHN F. KENNEDY**
> **(1917–1963)**

Reviewers

Throughout the preparation of *Physical Activity and Health: An Interactive Approach*, many people have contributed support and guidance. This book has benefited greatly from their comments, opinions, thoughtful critiques, expert knowledge, and constructive suggestions. We are most appreciative for their participation in this project.

We would like to express our appreciation to the following professionals whose insights and suggestions helped make this new edition even stronger:

Mark Casselman, MS, Humber College, Toronto, Canada
Elaine Craig, PhD, Humber Institute of Technology and Advanced Learning, Toronto, Canada
Jeffrey T. Godin, PhD, CSCS, HFPD, Fitchburg State College
Donna M. Kanary, EdS, Christopher Newport University; Longwood University
Marcus Kilpatrick, PhD, CHES, University of South Florida
Roland Lamarine, HSD, California State University, Chico
Susan Massad, HSD, RD, Framingham State College
Michelle K. Miller, MS, Indiana University
Jennifer Musick, MPH, Long Beach City College
Crystal Wilson, BS, MS, St. Louis Community College

We would also like to recognize the reviewers of the first edition of *Physical Activity and Health*. They include:

Phillip G. Bogle, PhD, Eastern Michigan University
L. Jerome Brandon, PhD, FACSM, Georgia State University
Cheryl J. Cohen, PhD, FACSM, Western Illinois University
Mitchell A. Collins, EdD, MEd, Kennesaw State University
Anita M. D'Angelo, MEd, Florida Atlantic University
Teresa C. Fitts, DPE, Westfield State College
Kara I. Gallagher, MS, PhD, Eastern Michigan University
Kathie C. Garbe, PhD, CHES, Kennesaw State University
Bernie Goldfine, PhD, Kennesaw State University
Walter S. Hamerslough, EdD, La Sierra University
Ron Holloway, MA, Kennesaw State University
Gary Ladd, MS, MSEd, Southwestern Illinois College
Kristen M. Lagally, PhD, Illinois State University
Kevin Lorson, BA, MA, Ohio State University
Susan J. Massad, HSD, Framingham State College
Christine M. Miskec, MA, Minnesota State University–Mankato
Beverly F. Mitchell, PhD, MA, Kennesaw State University
Diana Mozen, PhD, Georgia College and State University
David C. Nieman, DrPH, Appalachian State University
Debra Ann Pace, BS, MEd, Ohio State University
Jane A. Petrillo, EdD, MS, Kennesaw State University
Stephen W. Sansone, EdM, Chemeketa Community College
Susan T. Saylor, EdD, RD, Shelton State Community College
Andrew L. Shim, MA, Southwestern College
Douglas W. Strange, MA, HFI, CSCS, Lehigh University
Patricia A. Sullivan, EdD, George Washington University
Frederick C. Surgent, EdD, Frostburg State University
Eileen Udry, PhD, Indiana University-Purdue University–Indianapolis
Jin Wang, MEd, PhD, Kennesaw State University
William H. Zimmerli, EdD, Fort Valley State University

Acknowledgments

The authors' writing is only one portion of the work that goes into the development and production of a textbook. Many other people work long hours with a shared goal: to produce a visually appealing, error-free, up-to-date, high-quality textbook for students. We would like to acknowledge the dedication and hard work of these individuals, for without them this project never would have been realized.

First, for this edition of *Physical Activity and Health*, we brought Michelle K. Miller, MS, Fitness Specialist Coordinator in the Department of Kinesiology at Indiana University, onto the writing team as a contributing author. Michelle took on the task of revising and updating Chapter 10, Achieving Optimal Bone Health. Her expertise and never-ending enthusiasm was deeply valued. We thank Michelle for her professional dedication to the book and her personal commitment to the health of the college students with whom she works on a daily basis.

Second, this book could not have been published without the efforts of the health team at Jones and Bartlett Publishers. We would like to extend our sincere appreciation to Jacqueline Mark-Geraci, Acquisitions Editor, Julie Bolduc, Senior Production Editor, Amy Flagg, Editorial Assistant, Jennifer Ryan, Production Assistant, Wendy Thayer, Associate Marketing Manager, and Anne Spencer, Vice President of Production and Design. They did an extraordinary job of keeping the revision process on schedule by providing constant technical support and encouragement throughout. Furthermore, they helped us remain focused on the needs of our audience.

Third, we would like to thank our colleague and friend, Dr. Kelli McCormack Brown, Professor of Public Health at the University of South Florida. Dr. McCormack Brown was one of the original authors of the first edition of *Physical Activity and Health* and was responsible for encouraging us to take on this project.

Special Acknowledgments

I would like to dedicate this edition to my recently deceased father, Richard. His guidance throughout life has made me much of what I am today. I would also like to acknowledge the support of my mother, Loretta, and my wife, Nancy, who keep me grounded and focused. Finally, I would like to acknowledge my students and colleagues over the years from whom I have learned much. —*Dave Thomas*

I am fortunate to work with administrators who maintain that a well-written textbook based on expert knowledge reflects an important faculty contribution when it comes to the scholarship of teaching and learning. I appreciate the support of Dr. Michael Maggiotto, Dean of the College of Sciences and Humanities, Dr. Terry King, Provost and Vice President for Academic Affairs, and Dr. Jo Ann Gora, President at Ball State University. Finally, I am deeply indebted to those who continue to teach me on a daily basis: my students. —*Jerome Kotecki*

This Book's Features

Physical Activity and Health: An Interactive Approach incorporates a variety of pedagogical features that assist and encourage students to better comprehend intricate issues related to health.

Each chapter starts with What's the Connection? This short scenario profiles a college student who wants to change a specific behavior that is relevant to that chapter's content. At the end of the chapter, Making the Connection shows what the student has learned about the behavior he or she wants to change and the action or actions that should be taken to change that behavior.

what's the connection?

Julie is a sophomore in college and is concerned about her skeletal health. Her biggest concern is developing osteoporosis, a chronic metabolic disease that causes excessive skeletal weakness and increases her chance for developing bone fractures later in life. Julie watched her grandmother suffer from a broken hip as a result of osteoporosis and therefore is quite aware of its crippling effects. Julie pays close attention to her diet, making sure to fulfill her daily requirements of calcium and vitamin D. Moreover, she has recently been reading about the importance of physical activity and its role in preventing osteoporosis. Julie is interested in "making the connection" by beginning a safe and effective physical activity program to build and maintain a strong skeletal system.

making the connection

Julie now knows that, while her bones may seem to be rigid and unchanging, they are actually more like muscles, capable of strengthening with use or weakening without use. Each time a bone is moved, it bends ever so slightly, just enough to stimulate electrical and biochemical changes that stimulate bone formation. The more force, the greater the bending, the greater the stimulus for new bone formation (up to a point). In addition to maintaining the Recommended Daily Intake (RDI) for calcium, Julie knows that a regular physical activity program keeps the density of bone constant or contributes to increased bone mass. Julie now understands that the threat of osteoporosis doesn't just come from a low calcium intake, but from a sedentary lifestyle. She is encouraged to know that by monitoring her dietary habits and participating in a regular weight-bearing physical activity program, she now has the right tools to live strong and live well.

The concepts list identifies the content and skills that should be mastered through reading the chapters. Students should review the concepts before reading the chapter in order to use the concepts effectively.

concepts

1. A self-change approach assumes that we can manage and control our own lives.

2. The transtheoretical model of behavior change is a change model that is based on a time or temporal dimension (*trans*) using well-established psychological theories (*theoretical*) of behavior change.

3. The stages of change are a variable process that is organized in a continuum according to the decision-making process that is required to effect change.

4. Understanding or predicting when change occurs related to a specific behavior can largely be explained by decisional balance and self-efficacy.

5. The processes of change represent the mechanisms through which different techniques influence a change.

4

Understanding or predicting when change occurs related to a specific behavior can largely be explained by decisional balance and self-efficacy.

These key concepts are referenced in the chapter with a numbered icon—this helps the student quickly find the information when reviewing the chapter.

At the end of each chapter, the concepts are reinforced with a brief narrative following each original concept. This reinforces what the student has learned by carefully reading the chapter and provides an excellent chapter review tool.

concept connections

1. **Many factors influence the amount of flexibility you have at a joint.** Many factors can influence range of motion, including anatomical structure of the joint (how the bones are aligned), muscle temperature, disease status, muscle and tendon elasticity and compliance, age, sex, activity status, and tissue interference. Several of these factors are beyond our control (anatomical structure, age, sex); however, we do have the ability to manipulate other factors, such as activity status, muscle temperature, disease status, muscle and tendon elasticity and compliance, and tissue interference.

2. **Sense receptors located in your muscles and tendons play an important role in developing good flexibility.** Muscle spindles and Golgi tendon organs are sense receptors that play an important role in muscle function. They control response to rapid movement. Muscle spindles cause muscles to contract in response to rapid forceful stretching. Golgi tendon organs cause muscles to relax in response to rapid forceful contractions.

3. **Three common categories of flexibility exercises are static, ballistic, and PNF.** *Static* stretching involves putting a muscle into a stretched position and holding that position for 10 to 30 seconds. *Ballistic* stretching involves using pulsing or bouncing movements to stretch a muscle. *PNF* involves the use of sense receptors and forceful agonist and antagonist contractions to stretch a muscle.

4. **Guidelines for improving flexibility suggest stretching a muscle and holding the position for 10 to 30 seconds.** Static stretches held for 10 to 30 seconds provide a safe and effective way to enhance your flexibility. Perform each stretch four times for optimal benefit.

5. **Good flexibility protects against injury, enhances your ability to be physically active, and helps maintain an independent lifestyle.** Maintaining a good range of motion decreases the likelihood of injury, reduces the risk of low-back pain, and enhances physical performance. Sore, inflexible muscles decrease your ability to move efficiently and increase the risk of muscle strain.

6. **Most low-back pain is caused by poor muscular fitness.** Low-back pain is most commonly the result of poor flexibility in the hamstrings, hip flexors, and back extensors. Poor muscular strength and endurance of the abdominal muscles are contributing factors. By regularly performing stretching activities that focus on the lower back, you can reduce your risk for developing low-back pain.

The Physical Activity and Health Connection section reinforces and summarizes the connection between physical activity and health at the end of each chapter.

Physical Activity and Health Connection

Healthy weight management includes a lifelong commitment to a healthy lifestyle. Two elements involved in attaining and maintaining a healthy body weight are eating a nutritious diet and performing regular physical activity. Adequate nutrition and decreased calorie intake are important goals of diet modification for decreasing body fatness. Sufficient physical activity is equally important because it expends excessive fat storage and enhances lean body mass. Moreover, physical activity offsets the harmful effects of a number of morbid conditions that are attributed to excessive body fat storage. The goals of physical activity related to achieving and maintaining a healthy body weight should be based on activities that are enjoyable and can be performed consistently.

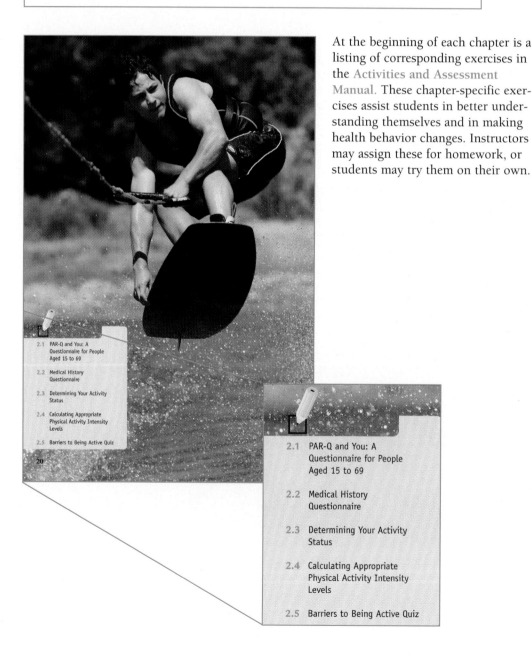

2.1 PAR-Q and You: A Questionnaire for People Aged 15 to 69

2.2 Medical History Questionnaire

2.3 Determining Your Activity Status

2.4 Calculating Appropriate Physical Activity Intensity Levels

2.5 Barriers to Being Active Quiz

20

At the beginning of each chapter is a listing of corresponding exercises in the Activities and Assessment Manual. These chapter-specific exercises assist students in better understanding themselves and in making health behavior changes. Instructors may assign these for homework, or students may try them on their own.

2.1 PAR-Q and You: A Questionnaire for People Aged 15 to 69

2.2 Medical History Questionnaire

2.3 Determining Your Activity Status

2.4 Calculating Appropriate Physical Activity Intensity Levels

2.5 Barriers to Being Active Quiz

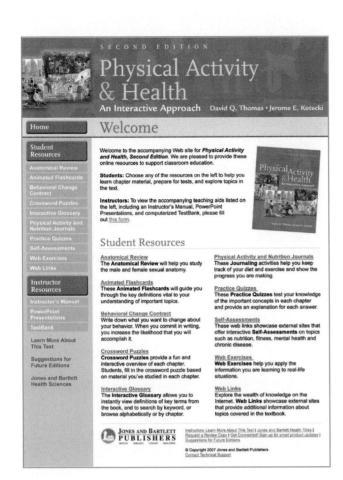

This book has a web site (http://physicalactivity.jbpub.com) that offers animated flashcards, an anatomy review, and much more. Bookmark this Web site for use throughout the course.

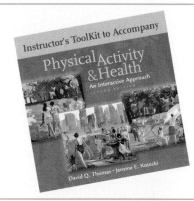

Instructor's ToolKit CD-ROM
Includes Instructor's Manual, computerized testbank, PowerPoint Presentations, and an image and table bank.
(ISBN: 0-7637-4506-5)

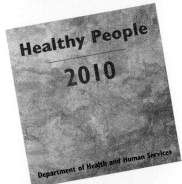

Healthy People 2010 CD-ROM
Written by the U.S. Department of Health and Human Services, Healthy People 2010 sets broad public health goals for the next decade.
(ISBN: 0-7637-1701-0)

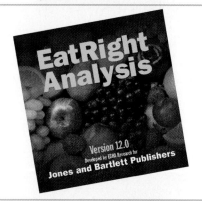

EatRight Analysis Software Version 12.0
Developed by ESHA Research, this innovative software, including more than 20,000 food choices, MyPyramid, and the *2005 Dietary Guidelines,* allows students to analyze their diets by RDAs/DRIs and goal percentages.
(ISBN: 0-7637-4685-1)

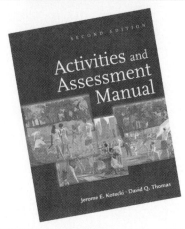

Activities and Assessment Manual
This easy-to-use manual offers activities and self-assessments that motivate students to improve and enhance their health and well-being through physical activity. Students will learn to apply the techniques they are reading about in the text, examine their attitudes toward physical activity, and assess their readiness to change behaviors.
(ISBN: 0-7637-4507-3)

About the Authors

DAVID Q. THOMAS is a Professor and Interim-Director of the School of Kinesiology and Recreation at Illinois State University. He holds doctorate and master's degrees in physical education (emphasis in exercise science) from Arizona State University. His area of expertise is in applied aspects of physical activity and fitness. Dr. Thomas is a Fellow of the American College of Sports Medicine and a Fellow of the Research Consortium of the American Alliance for Health, Physical Education, Recreation, and Dance. He has served as the chairperson of the Physical Fitness Council of the Association for Active Lifestyles and Fitness, and as President of both the Massachusetts and Illinois AHPERDs. He is devoted to physical activity and enjoys jogging, weight lifting, and recreational sports.

JEROME E. KOTECKI is a Professor of Health Science in the Department of Physiology and Health Science at Ball State University. Dr. Kotecki earned his doctorate in health science and his master's degree in exercise science from Indiana University. Professor Kotecki has published more than 30 scientific articles and is co-author of the best-selling textbook *An Introduction to Community Health*. Dr. Kotecki's current research is focused on the impact of lifestyle medicine on chronic diseases. He is the lead scientist on several large healthy lifestyle studies focusing on the role of health-care professionals in physical activity counseling. His previous experience includes serving as a fitness consultant and personal trainer for individuals in the entertainment industry in Los Angeles. He is an avid fitness participant and enjoys weight training, cycling, running, tennis, and yoga.

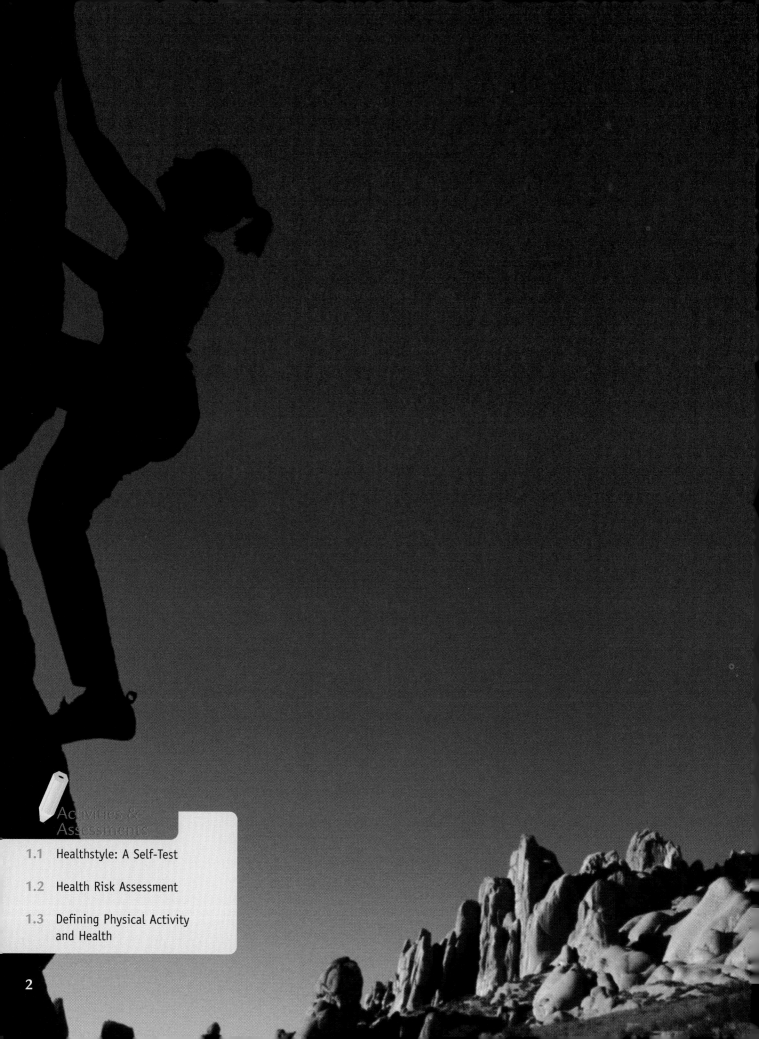

1.1   Healthstyle: A Self-Test

1.2   Health Risk Assessment

1.3   Defining Physical Activity
      and Health

The Physical Activity and Health Connection

what's the connection?

Finding her way to classes. Learning to schedule time for studying. Meeting new people and making friends. These are just a few of Sally's experiences during the first weeks of her freshman year at college. Sally spends lots of time in the library, and when she isn't studying or going to classes she is working as a part-time receptionist at the university bookstore. With all these commitments, Sally is finding it difficult to stay physically active; as a matter of fact, her daily routine requires very little physical activity. In high school, Sally was physically active in club sports and either walked or rode her bike to school every day. As the semester continues, Sally notices that she feels more and more sluggish—she is not as energetic as she used to be. Sally attributes these feelings to being away from home, to the change in environment, and to studying a lot.

concepts

1. Almost everyone wants to enjoy good health now and in the future so that they can live to enjoy what they have.

2. There is no medicinal treatment in current or prospective use that holds as much promise for sustained health as a regular program of physical activity.

3. Health is multidimensional and positive.

4. Wellness is a dynamic process of change and growth that is largely determined by the decisions one makes about how to live one's life.

5. A healthy lifestyle is a recurring pattern of health-promoting and disease-preventing behaviors undertaken to achieve wellness.

6. A self-help approach assumes that human beings can manage their lifestyle change and learn to control environmental factors that are detrimental to health.

http://physicalactivity.jbpub.com

The Web site for this book is a great source for supplementary physical health information for both students and instructors. Visit **http://physicalactivity.jbpub.com** to find a variety of useful tools for learning, thinking, and teaching.

3

The first wealth is health.

—Ralph Waldo Emerson

Introduction

People go to college for many reasons. Perhaps your reason is to find a career that will compensate you fairly and allow for advancement. For example, it is well documented that every bit of education you get after high school increases the chances you'll earn better pay and enhance your future social mobility (Porter, 2005). You may also value the present benefits of a postsecondary education, such as gaining a core education and an appreciation for different ideas, taking part in new opportunities to explore your interests, meeting new people, and experiencing academic success. In the same manner, good health can be viewed as a means to an end, rather than an end in itself, because it allows us to pursue our immediate and future goals.

Good health is one of our most prized possessions; one that is often taken for granted until it is lost. Almost everyone wants to enjoy good health now and in the future so that they can live to enjoy what they have. Nationwide polls indicate that we place great value on our health as a source of happiness. The answer to the question "Why be healthy?" seems obvious; however, the actions of many of us do not produce the good health we desire. As a college student, you face many health choices—choices that can affect you in the here and now and for the rest of your life. You are responsible for learning and implementing the best choices regarding your health. It is a responsibility only you can own. By opening this book, you have taken an important step toward becoming more informed about your health. This book provides you with the information, skills, and practical know-how to develop and maintain a healthy lifestyle.

Physical Activity and Health

Imagine picking up the daily newspaper and seeing the following front-page headline: Miraculous New Health Pill Discovered. You read quickly through the article, which reports that this miracle drug can make you look younger, provide better weight control, give you more energy, a brighter mental outlook, relieve stress and anxiety, make you fit and flexible, and decrease your risk of serious diseases such as heart disease, cancer, diabetes, hypertension, and osteoporosis. All of this with virtually no side effects. You would probably hurry to your physician to get a prescription for a supply of this remarkable new medication. Of course, this pill has not yet been discovered, and despite the miracles of modern medical research, it is not likely to happen any time soon. However, there is a prescription already available to every one of us that can provide all of these benefits and many more. It's physical activity! In fact, there is no medicinal treatment in current or prospective use that holds as much promise for sustained health as a regular program of physical activity (TABLE 1.1). We firmly believe that if physical activity could be packaged in a pill it would be the most widely prescribed pill the world's ever seen.

Unfortunately, nearly two of three U.S. adults (60 percent) are not getting enough leisure time physical activity to benefit their health (Centers for Disease Control and Prevention [CDC], 2005). Furthermore, approximately one in four U.S. adults is completely sedentary or a genuine couch potato. Leading a sedentary lifestyle is not restricted

Almost everyone wants to enjoy good health now and in the future so that they can live to enjoy what they have.

There is no medicinal treatment in current or prospective use that holds as much promise for sustained health as a regular program of physical activity.

Regular physical activity is an essential lifestyle behavior when it comes to promoting health.

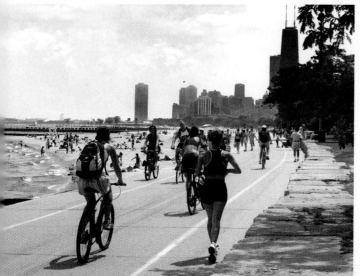

TABLE 1.1	The Health Benefits of Physical Activity

The table is based on a total physical activity program that includes activities and exercises to improve cardiovascular endurance, muscular strength and endurance, flexibility, and body composition.

Physical Activity Benefit	Evidence	Physical Activity Benefit	Evidence
Physical Fitness		**Mental Health**	
Improves cardiorespiratory endurance	+++	Reduces stress symptoms	++
Improves muscular strength	+++	Reduces anxiety symptoms	++
Improves muscular endurance	+++	Reduces depression symptoms	++
Improves flexibility	+++	Enhances memory and learning	++
Decreases body fat percentage	+++	Enhances mood and self-esteem	++
Cardiovascular Disease		**Joint Health**	
Coronary artery disease prevention	+++	Prevents low-back pain	+
Stroke prevention	++	Prevents arthritis	+
Reduces atherosclerosis	++	Treatment for arthritis	+
Treatment for heart disease	++	Strengthens joint structure and functioning	+
High Blood Pressure		**Immune System**	
Prevents high blood pressure	+++	Improves overall immunity	++
Treats high blood pressure	+++	Prevention of common cold	+
High Blood Lipids (Fats)		**Elderly**	
Lowers triglycerides	++	Increases years of healthy life	++
Lowers total cholesterol	++	Increases life-expectancy	+
Lowers LDL-cholesterol	++	Better able to move about without falling	+
Raises HDL-cholesterol	++	Reduces risk of Alzheimer's and dementia	+
Diabetes		**Bone Health**	
Prevents or delays type 2 diabetes	+++	Helps build bone density	+++
Treatment for type 2 diabetes	+++	Prevents osteoporosis	++
Treatment for type 1 diabetes	+	Treats osteoporosis	++
Healthy Weight Management		**Occupational Health**	
Prevents fat gain	+++	Increases productivity	+
Maintains fat loss	++	Reduces short-term sick leave	+
Treatment for obesity	++	Reduces health insurance premiums	+
Cancer		**Pregnancy Benefits**	
Reduces risk of colon cancer	+++	Greater resistance to fatigue	+
Reduces risk of breast cancer	+	Improved posture and stronger back muscles	+
Reduces risk of prostate cancer	+	May lead to easier labor and faster recovery	+
Treatment of cancers	+	Faster return to pre-pregnancy weight	+
Medical Care Expenditures		**Mortality Rates**	
Lower annual direct medical care costs	+	Lower rates for older and younger adults	++
Fewer hospital stays	+	Lower premature death rates	++
Fewer physician visits	+		
Use less medications	+		

+++ Strong data support

++ Data supportive, but more research needed

+ Some data, but much more research needed

SOURCE: Kotecki, J.E. (2006). Updating the evidence that physical activity is good for health: An epidemiological review. A presentation delivered to the College of Pharmacy and Health Sciences, Butler University on May 31, 2006, Indianapolis, Indiana. Manuscript in progress.

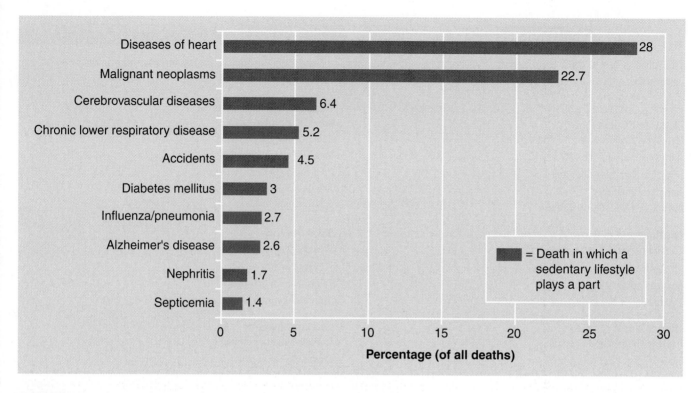

FIGURE 1.1 **Leading Causes of Death in the United States.**
Source: Hoyert, D.L., Heron, M., Murphy, S.L., Kung, H.C. (2006). Deaths: Final data for 2003. Health E-Stats. Online: http://www.cdc.gov.

Chronic diseases Illnesses that can develop early in life and last a long period of time.

Health A state of complete physical, mental, and social well-being and not merely the absence of disease or infirmity.

Health is multidimensional and positive.

to the United States—60 percent of the global population also does not get the recommended amount of physical activity to promote health (World Health Organization [WHO], 2004). We will explain how we got this way later in the chapter. Right now, these enduring rates begin to help us understand why some public health experts have declared that physical inactivity has become the biggest health problem in the 21st century (Blair, 2005). This declaration of crisis is based on decades of research by the finest scientists worldwide, who have revealed that sedentary living is a leading cause of **chronic diseases**—illnesses that can develop early in life and last a long period of time—poor quality of life, disability, and premature death in the United States, Canada, and many other developed countries (**FIGURE 1.1**). Such information shapes the case for current recommendations and guidelines from many national health organizations and expert panels that advise encouraging physical activity as the first-line approach in preventing this unnecessary health crisis. Simply put, their end purpose in recommending physical activity is the promotion of health and wellness. Although many of us use the terms *health* and *wellness* almost unconsciously, few people understand the broad scope of these terms or what they really mean.

Health, Wellness, and Lifestyle

The word *health* is derived from *hal* or *hale*, which means "whole, sound, or well." Health has been defined in a number of different ways. The most notable and widely accepted definition of health comes from the constitution of the World Health Organization, published in 1948. That definition states that **health** "is a state of complete physical, mental, and social well-being and not merely the absence of disease or infirmity" (WHO, 1948). This definition is important in that it recognizes that any meaningful description of health must include the multidimensional aspects of human life and that health is positive (i.e., not merely the absence of illness). In the next section, we examine seven interrelated dimensions of health.

Dimensions of Health

- *Physical health* refers to the overall condition of the organ systems of the body (cardiovascular, respiratory, skeletal, muscular, digestive, nervous, endocrine, immune, reproductive, urinary, and integumentary). Separate chapters in this text are committed to many of these organ systems, with an emphasis on certain health-related outcomes that can be obtained from physical activity: cardiorespiratory endurance, muscular strength and endurance, flexibility, and body composition.

- *Intellectual health* refers to the use of one's mental capacities. The characteristics include having a mind that is open to new ideas and concepts. Intellectual health includes expanding one's decision-making capacity and then being willing to take action. This can be accomplished by processing information using higher-order thinking skills through synthesizing, analyzing, applying, and evaluating information.

- *Emotional health* is the ability to express feelings appropriately. Thoughts cause feelings. We can look at the same event in different ways, optimistic or pessimistic. People who manage their own feelings well and deal with them effectively are more likely to live content and productive lives. These people generally manifest the qualities of optimism, self-esteem, and trust. They feel capable, courageous, worthy, respected, appreciated, and loved.

- *Social health* refers to having the ability to interact effectively with other people. Socially healthy people behave in a way to help others. They accomplish this by understanding and respecting differences in various social groups based on their age, ethnicity, personality characteristics, beliefs, education, religion, and sexual orientation.

- *Spiritual health* pertains to the soul or spirit. Soul or spirit can be defined as the inspiring principle or dominating influence in one's life. Spiritual health is the belief that one is a part of a larger scheme of life and that one's life has purpose. Spirituality provides meaning and direction in life. Selflessness, compassion, a passion for living, faith, a sense of right and wrong, ethics, and morals are important components of spiritual health. It is an awareness and appreciation of the life force that moves us.

- *Career or occupational health* pertains to one's chosen vocation in life. People spend most of their life at work. It is therefore essential that one choose work that is satisfying intrinsically and extrinsically. It means choosing the kind of work that makes the best use of one's abilities and gives accomplishment. It includes being able to earn a living and contribute to society.

- *Environmental health* refers to everything around us, and includes the impact of natural and human-made environments on one's health. It includes working to preserve ecosystems and the biodiversity of our planet. It also means adapting one's human-made environment to reduce the risk of suffering from intentional and unintentional injuries and communicable and noncommunicable diseases.

These seven dimensions, or component parts, of health, all interacting in a synergistic way, allow us to assume higher levels of functioning that can lead to more productive and satisfying lives. To achieve greater levels of health, one has to make a deliberate choice to assume personal responsibility for the process. When a person makes a conscious decision to work toward these enhanced aspects of health, well-being or wellness is identified. Halbert Dunn first wrote about the upper limits of health in his book *High Level Wellness* (Dunn, 1967). Dunn saw **wellness** as a dynamic process of change and growth that was largely determined by the decisions one makes about how to live one's life.

There are as many degrees of health as there are degrees of disease. These points can be viewed on a continuum (FIGURE 1.2). Moving from the neutral

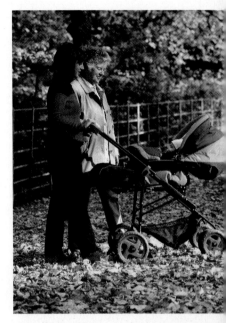

Walks through the park can be relaxing and physically beneficial.

Wellness is a dynamic process of change and growth that is largely determined by the decisions one makes about how to live one's life.

Wellness A dynamic process of change and growth that is determined by the decisions one makes about how to live one's life.

FIGURE 1.2 **The Dimensions of Health and Wellness Continuum.** The continuum allows you to visualize the difference between the wellness and medical approaches to health.

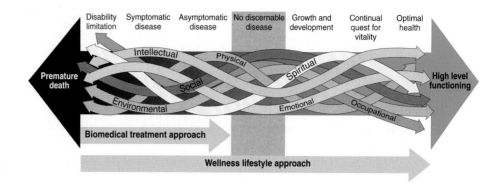

A healthy lifestyle is a recurring pattern of health-promoting and disease-preventing behaviors undertaken to achieve wellness.

point, or center, to the left indicates a progressive worsening of health due to inappropriate and undesirable adaptation by the body or *dis-eases* of maladaptation. Moving to the right of the neutral point indicates not only an absence of disease, but also increasing levels of health and optimal functioning. The continuum includes the seven interrelated dimensions of health. No matter where a person is located on the continuum, he or she has some degree of health.

The biomedical treatment approach to health attempts to bring you to the neutral point where signs, symptoms, and disability are alleviated. The biomedical treatment approach to health, however, is not designed to take you past the neutral point to higher levels of growth and functioning. Only you can decide to do that. Additionally, the wellness lifestyle approach to health can be utilized at any point on the continuum including for individuals with differing degrees of disease or disability. The motivation to improve quality of life within the framework of one's own unique capabilities is important to achieving wellness.

It is important to recognize that the wellness approach to health is not intended to replace the biomedical treatment approach, but to work in combination with it. Modern biomedical treatment is a great thing, but there is a problem with it: people expect too much from it. Many people have the attitude, "Here I am, doctor, with all my worn-out parts; fix me up." Even as scientists explore the frontiers of biomedicine, they keep confirming the truism that health is easier to preserve than it is to repair. Promoting healthy lifestyles has become increasingly important in recent years as the evidence of the association between behavior and disease has continued to grow (Schoenborn et al., 2004).

Unhealthy lifestyles are major contributing factors to many chronic medical conditions, including cardiovascular disease, cancer, diabetes mellitus, obesity, high blood pressure, and high blood lipids (CDC, 2004). These diseases are generally not cured by medication, nor do they just disappear (Kotecki & Clayton, 2003). Despite the major advances made in biomedical research, this progress has not been able to fully restore us to health. These advances merely help us cope better with serious and often debilitating conditions. So, while we continue to be in awe at the advances in medical technology, we need to recognize that this is not *restorative* health care. Only the human body, when it is kept fit, has its own restorative capacities.

We describe a **healthy lifestyle** as a recurring pattern of health-promoting and disease-preventing behaviors undertaken to achieve wellness. It is a way of life based on the idea that our chances of self-fulfillment are increased or decreased directly by our level of health. Further, it can decrease significantly the risk of disease and increase the chances of living healthfully into the later decades of life. Or as we sometimes like to say, "It is to allow us to die young as late as possible."

It should be mentioned that a person can do only so much to promote longevity since people do not have complete control over all factors influencing their health. Other factors that play a key role in premature death include heredity

Healthy lifestyle A recurring pattern of health-promoting and disease-preventing behaviors undertaken to achieve wellness.

and human biology, a person's environment, and medical care. Heredity refers to the transfer of biological characteristics from our natural parents. Environment refers to everything around us, with a primary focus on our human-made environment. Medical care refers to limited or inadequate services from the health care system. **FIGURE 1.3** shows the extent to which our longevity is affected by these factors along with our lifestyle decisions.

An old military tactic says "Know your enemy." Because we are in a war when it comes to increasing our years of healthy life, it is important to know who that enemy is. At least half of our nation's premature deaths are attributable to personal behavior and health habits such as tobacco use, lack of physical activity, alcohol and drug misuse, and risky sexual practices (Mokdad, Marks, Stroup, & Gerberding, 2004). Our lifestyle choices are also linked to higher ambulatory care and hospitalization costs, with preventable illness accounting for as much as 70 percent of all medical care spending (U.S. Department of Health and Human Services [USDHHS], 2003).

"We have met the enemy, and he is us" is the famous and most frequently quoted phrase of cartoonist Walt Kelly and is applicable here. As protectors of our own health, it is no secret that we are frequently our own worst enemy. We harm ourselves repeatedly in many ways. What is worse, we seldom realize it. We can be our own best friend, too, but more commonly, we are our own worst enemy. After honest self-reflection, we are likely to see some ill-fated lifestyle choices we have made. Identifying these choices and evaluating their consequences is the first step toward being responsible for our health.

Studies show that most Americans desperately want to live healthy lives, yet it's an elusive dream for so many because health is lost before it's valued and before its maintenance is understood. Choosing to participate in a healthy lifestyle requires self-responsibility and a self-help approach. You cannot blame someone else, make excuses, or avoid personal accountability. Taking responsibility for your health is recognizing that your daily choices affect your total well-being. This includes being physically active, eating sensibly, maintaining a healthy weight, managing stress effectively, avoiding tobacco, following sensible drinking habits, and being safety conscious. Your challenge is to make smart decisions. Halbert Dunn (1967) states it simply: "We cannot take high-level wellness like a pill out of a bottle. It will come only to those who work at following its precepts."

A self-help approach assumes that human beings can manage their lifestyle change and learn to control environmental factors that are detrimental to health. It puts you in control of your health and permits you to determine what to do and how and when to do it. A self-help approach requires planning and takes time, effort, and most importantly, the development of special lifestyle skills. We have devoted Chapter 3 to discussing a self-help approach that implements a multistep process used by thousands of successful self-changers.

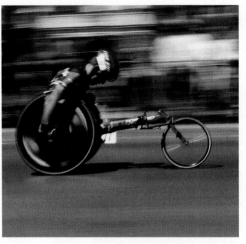

A wellness lifestyle approach to health can be utilized at any point on the health continuum, including for individuals with differing degrees of disability or disease. In such cases the goal is to move above physical or mental limitations to live richer, fuller lives.

A self-help approach assumes that human beings can manage their lifestyle change and learn to control environmental factors that are detrimental to health.

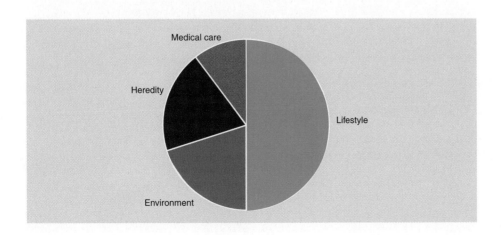

FIGURE 1.3 **Factors Influencing Premature Death or Longevity.** Lifestyle is the single most important and modifiable factor influencing health and disease.

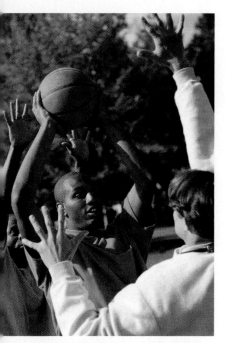

Recreational activities like playing basketball can be an enjoyable way to exercise.

Physical activity All energy expended by skeletal muscular movement.

Exercise A subset of physical activity that is a planned, structured, repetitive, and purposeful attempt to improve or maintain physical fitness.

Physical fitness A set of health-related attributes a person has, such as cardiorespiratory endurance, muscular strength and endurance, flexibility, and body composition, that contribute to one's capacity to do physical activity.

Different fitness levels are the result of our levels of physical activity.

Throughout this book, we emphasize that physical activity is an essential lifestyle behavior when it comes to promoting health and preventing many major chronic diseases. It provides health benefits that cannot be obtained in any other way. Not only does it contribute directly to the physical health dimension, but it also contributes indirectly to the other six dimensions of health. It is important to establish what we mean by *physical activity* and its related term, *exercise*, when it comes to health.

Physical Activity, Exercise, and Physical Fitness

Physical activity refers to all energy expended by skeletal muscular movement. The major contributors to this form of energy expenditure usually come from everyday activities that involve moving your body around, such as walking or riding your bike to class, taking the stairs instead of the elevator, or performing domestic duties such as shopping, sweeping floors, dusting your furniture, and cutting the lawn, with much of it occurring as an incidental part of our daily routines. **Exercise**, on the other hand, refers to a subset of physical activity that is a planned, structured, repetitive, and purposeful attempt to improve or maintain physical fitness. It might include leisure-time activities such as distance running, swimming, aerobic dancing, mountain biking, and weight lifting and sporting activities such as basketball, racquetball, and tennis. These activities generally require considerably more effort and energy than walking to class or other routine daily activities.

Unlike physical activity and exercise, which are behavioral processes, **physical fitness** is a set of health-related attributes a person has, such as cardiorespiratory endurance, muscular strength and endurance, flexibility, and body composition, which contribute to one's capacity to do physical activity. Different fitness levels are mainly a result of our levels of physical activity, and exercise programs can be devised to improve various aspects of fitness. These physical fitness attributes can be attained through exercising at the frequency (days per week), intensity (how hard; for example, light, moderate, vigorous), time (amount for each session or day), and type of activity (e.g., running, weight training) prescribed by the American College of Sports Medicine (ACSM, 2006).

Our physical fitness levels, however, are also partly a result of our genetic endowment. There is no question that some individuals have a higher natural capacity to excel at various exercises or sports because of their genetic makeup. Scientific evidence, however, suggests that it is regular participation in physical activity rather than our inherited component of fitness that is related to health (Hein, Suadicini, & Gyntelberg, 1992). Those who feel they cannot benefit from

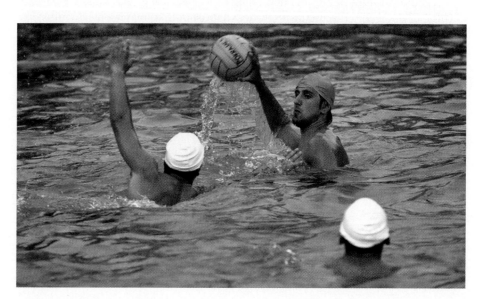

physical activity because they have not been dealt genetic cards allowing them to obtain elite fitness levels are mistaken. Physical activity is required to make use of the genetic makeup of any individual. Sedentary individuals differ in their health-related fitness level because of physical inactivity and not genetic capabilities. Although we cannot choose our parents, we can choose how we live our lives. The human body is clearly designed for physical activity, so perhaps we should not be surprised that in a chronic sedentary state it shows signs of breakdown.

Physical Activity Recommendations for Health

The Centers for Disease Control and Prevention (CDC) and the American College of Sports Medicine (ACSM) recommend "adults should engage in moderate-intensity physical activity for at least 30 minutes or more on 5 or more days of the week" or "vigorous-intensity physical activity 3 or more days per week for 20 or more minutes per occasion" during recreational or leisure-time activities (i.e., not work related) (CDC, 2005). This recommendation translates into a goal of expending at least 150 calories a day, or about 1000 calories a week, in physical activity (**FIGURE 1.4**).

You will note there are differences in the duration and intensity of physical activity needed to obtain and maintain health in this recommendation. Time depends on intensity. The intensity of physical activity, or how hard your body is working, is usually categorized as light, moderate, or vigorous based on the

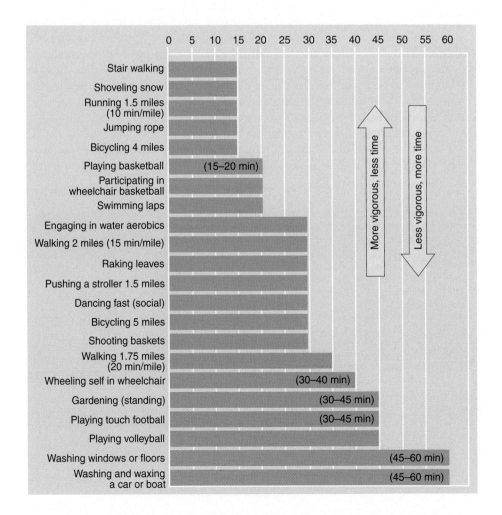

FIGURE 1.4 **Number of Minutes Required to Burn 150 Calories.**
SOURCE: Centers for Disease Control and Prevention, National Center for Chronic Disease Prevention and Health Promotion. (2005). Physical activity for everyone: Recommendations. Online: http://www.cdc.gov/nccdphp/dnpa/physical/recommendations/.

FIGURE 1.5 **Duration and Intensity of Physical Activity to Stay Healthy.** SOURCE: Handbook for Canada's Physical Activity Guide to Healthy Active Living, Public Health Agency of Canada. (1998). © Reproduced with the permission of the Minister of Public Works and Government Services Canada, 2006.

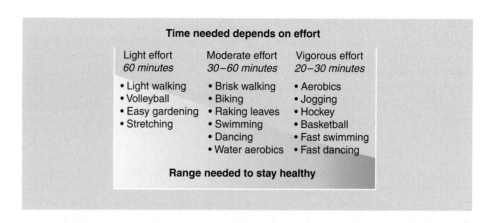

amount of effort or energy you expend in performing the activity (**FIGURE 1.5**). Light-intensity activities require more time than moderate-intensity activities, and moderate-intensity activities require more time than high-intensity activities. Light-intensity activities include walking slowly, easy gardening, and stretching. Moderate-intensity activities are those that require you to exert some effort but not to push yourself as hard as more vigorous-intensity activities—for example, brisk walking (15 to 20 minutes per mile) as compared with running (8 to 12 minutes per mile).

Although both moderate- and vigorous-intensity activities have important health implications, one needs to understand that physical activity does not have to be strenuous to provide health-promoting benefits. In fact, the greatest proportional benefit to health is obtained from changing from inactivity or a sedentary state (not engaging in any regular pattern of physical activity beyond normal daily functioning) to a regular pattern of moderate-intensity physical activity (**FIGURE 1.6**). Furthermore, both accumulated and continuous bouts of moderate-intensity activity can provide health benefits. The 30 minutes of daily moderate-intensity activities do not have to be done all at once. If you don't have a 30-minute block of time during the day, you can break up your physical activity into five 6-minute, three 10-minute, or two 15-minute intervals to accumulate the recommended 30 minutes throughout the day.

Physical activity is one of the 10 leading health indicators established by Healthy People 2010 that are being used to measure the health of the nation. Each

FIGURE 1.6 **Health Benefits and Activity Levels.** Moving from the sedentary category to the moderately active category provides the greatest improvement in health benefits, although additional gains may be achieved by becoming vigorously active.

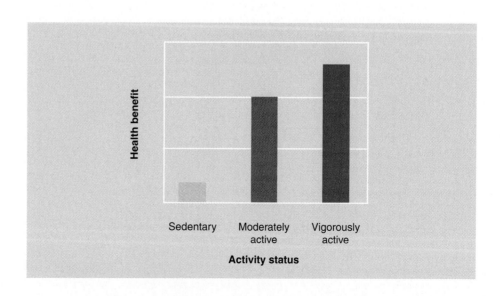

of the 10 leading health indicators has one or more objectives associated with it. There are currently 15 physical activity and fitness objectives stated in Healthy People 2010 that have the overall goal of improving health, fitness, and quality of life through daily physical activity (TABLE 1.2). Healthy People 2010 is a national health promotion and disease prevention initiative that brings together national, state, and local government agencies; nonprofit, voluntary, and professional organizations; businesses; communities; and individuals to promote two overall goals: increasing quality of life and years of healthy life and eliminating health disparities (USDHHS, 2000). The Healthy People initiative, currently in its third decade, provides a set of 10-year

TABLE 1.2	Healthy People 2010 Physical Activity and Fitness Objectives
Physical activity in adults	1. Reduce the proportion of adults who engage in no leisure-time physical activity.
	2. Increase the proportion of adults who engage regularly, preferably daily, in moderate physical activity for at least 30 minutes per day.
	3. Increase the proportion of adults who engage in vigorous physical activity that promotes the development and maintenance of cardiorespiratory fitness 3 or more days per week for 20 or more minutes per occasion.
Muscular strength/ endurance and flexibility	4. Increase the proportion of adults who perform physical activities that enhance and maintain muscular strength and endurance.
	5. Increase the proportion of adults who perform physical activities that enhance and maintain flexibility.
Physical activity in children and adolescents	6. Increase the proportion of adolescents who engaged in moderate physical activity for at least 30 minutes on 5 or more of the previous 7 days.
	7. Increase the proportion of adolescents who engage in vigorous physical activity that promotes cardiorespiratory fitness 3 or more days per week for 20 or more minutes per occasion.
	8. Increase the proportion of the nation's public and private schools that require daily physical education for all students.
	9. Increase the proportion of adolescents who participate in daily school physical education.
	10. Increase the proportion of adolescents who spend at least 50 percent of school physical education class time being physically active.
	11. Increase the proportion of children and adolescents who view television 2 or fewer hours on a school day.
Access	12. Increase the proportion of the nation's public and private schools that provide access to their physical activity spaces and facilities for all persons outside normal school hours (i.e., before and after the school day, on weekends, and during summer and other vacations).
	13. Increase the proportion of work sites offering employer-sponsored physical activity and fitness programs.
	14. Increase the proportion of trips made by walking.
	15. Increase the proportion of trips made by bicycling.

SOURCE: U.S. Department of Health and Human Services. (2000). Healthy People 2010. (PHS 017-001-00550-9). Pittsburgh, PA: U.S. Government Printing Office. Online: http://health.gov/healthypeople/.

objectives that is a road map for improving the health of all people in the United States. In addition to physical activity, the other major indicators are overweight and obesity, tobacco use, substance abuse, responsible sexual behavior, mental health, injury and violence, environmental quality, immunization, and access to health care. As a group, the leading health indicators reflect the major health concerns in the United States at the beginning of the 21st century.

Why We Live Sedentary Lives

There has been a drastic decrease in our physical activity levels over the last half-century due to changes in society and in the economy. Among the major factors contributing to this decrease are technological changes in the workplace leading to a decline in physically active occupations, widespread use of the automobile as the major form of transport, the introduction of laborsaving devices for the home, and increases in sedentary activities such as watching television and playing computer and video games during one's spare time. The last factor is notable from our perspective because TVs and computers provide highly entertaining things to do in a sedentary position. It is hard to compete with 200 stations on your satellite dish, great video games, and other choices on your computer. In fact, television watching has become America's most popular leisure-time activity. According to Nielsen Media Research, Americans watch an average of more than 4 hours of television a day, or 2 full months a year (Nielsen Media Research, 2005). However, almost anything uses more energy than watching television.

In addition to the increases in low-activity occupations, conveniences that make our lives easier, and the increase in sedentary activities during our spare time, there are many personal variables, including our underlying thoughts and feelings, that make us resistant to being physically active. The most common reasons we hear from our students is that they lack time, they're too exhausted by their other commitments, they don't like to sweat, they don't like to go to the gym, or they are afraid they will make a fool of themselves. In Chapter 2, we discuss how to overcome each of these barriers to physical activity.

A Lifestyle Approach to Physical Activity

Most national goals address leisure time rather than occupational physical activity because people have more personal control over how they spend their leisure time and because most people do not have jobs that require regular physical activity. Furthermore, the use of laborsaving devices such as washing machines, dishwashers, garage door openers, and riding lawnmowers makes our lives easier and leaves us with more free time.

Earlier you read about the good news related to the scientific evidence that shows that physical activity done at moderate intensity can produce important health benefits. That's right—you really do not have to suffer. Furthermore, it's not necessary to carve out one 30-minute block of time from your busy schedule. The cumulative effect of your physical activity throughout the day is what counts, and many types of activity can help.

College students usually have very busy schedules and often place exercise at the bottom of their list of priorities. It is easy to spend an entire day sitting in classes and meetings, studying in the library, and completing assignments using a computer. Some of you even have jobs and family commitments on top of your educational responsibilities. And of course you must allow for some social time with your friends and classmates. What most of these pursuits have in common is that they are sedentary activities.

Even with all of the commitments you have as a college student, it is essential that you make time for moderate-intensity physical activity. For example, did you know that fitting regular and moderate-intensity physical activity into your daily routine will likely help you better accomplish your educational goals for the day, such as studying and being attentive in class? Because regular moderate-intensity physical activity can increase your concentration, mental well-being, stamina, and energy, you are more likely to be more proficient when it comes to learning. Fitting moderate-intensity physical activity into your daily routine may be easier than you might think if you follow a lifestyle approach.

We define a lifestyle approach to physical activity as accumulating at least 30 minutes of self-selected activities, which can include leisure, occupational, or domestic activities (either intentional or unintentional) that are at least moderate in their intensity and are part of your everyday life. You may not even have to adjust your schedule. For instance, walk briskly to class, the library, or the campus dining hall. Include marching in place, jumping jacks, stretching, or walking around in your study breaks. These activities can be done in short intervals several times a day, as long as they add up to at least a half-hour each day. The health benefits will accumulate without having to take an hour and half out to go to the gym or some of the other things you may have a hard time fitting into your schedule.

Of course, you may intend to add an exercise program to your schedule and take advantage of the exercise facilities (e.g., weight room, track, basketball and tennis courts) that your college offers. This is also a very good idea. Although participating in a regular exercise program can provide a higher intensity that can offer greater health benefits, it is imperative to remember that there are plenty of other ways to obtain the daily recommended amount of physical activity to accumulate the health benefits.

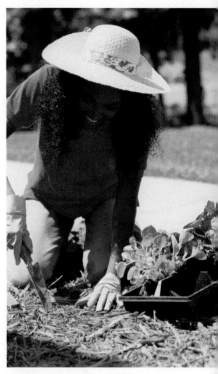
Gardening is enjoyable and expends energy.

Investing in Your Health

If good health came with a guarantee, we bet most of you would pay any price asked. Obviously, that will never happen. However, you can invest in an insurance policy of sorts in the form of physical activity. Since physical activity is one of the most effective ways you can safeguard yourself from developing a number of major chronic degenerative diseases, it's really a major investment in minimizing the risks of developing debilitating conditions. You can also add years to your life and life to your years from this investment. As you have already learned, a little can go a long way, and it doesn't take as much of an investment to begin collecting quickly on the many benefits of physical activity.

If you are currently physically active, we want to commend you for including this as part of your healthy lifestyle. You may already be aware of the many dividends you are reaping from this choice. Furthermore, you will learn about additional benefits that will reinforce this choice as well as add extra protection against you becoming inactive later on in life. It is important to remember that the benefits of physical activity last only as long as they are enjoyed. Based on large population studies, the level of physical activity currently decreases throughout the entire human lifespan due largely to societal factors. No one is immune from becoming inactive. The most significant decline occurs in young people as they enter adolescence and young adulthood. This decrease generally continues throughout college and beyond.

As you proceed through the remaining chapters, you will clearly see the role that physical activity plays in your overall health and well-being. This connection between physical activity and health is one that is inseparable.

Physical Activity and Health Connection

Physical activity is an essential lifestyle behavior when it comes to promoting health and preventing many major chronic disease killers. It provides health benefits that cannot be obtained in any other way. It can assist with every other aspect of a healthy lifestyle and is central to wellness.

One of the most important things you can do to promote well-being is to become knowledgeable enough to take responsibility for your own health. To achieve this level of understanding, you need to make every effort to read the chapters and participate in the activities provided in this book. As a college student, you are beginning to develop a personal lifestyle, which, with slight modifications, you will likely follow for the rest of your life. Practicing positive health behaviors, with systematic reinforcement and follow-up, throughout your college years will provide you with the best opportunity for achieving wellness as well as preventing the development of dangerous and health-threatening behaviors that lead to serious diseases during the middle and later years of life.

concept connections

1. **Almost everyone wants to enjoy good health now and in the future so that they can live to enjoy what they have.** By opening this book, you have taken an important step toward becoming more informed about your health. This book provides you with the information, skills, and practical know-how to develop and maintain a healthy lifestyle.

2. **There is no medicinal treatment in current or prospective use that holds as much promise for sustained health as a regular program of physical activity.** Regular physical activity can make you look younger, provide better weight control, give you more energy and a brighter mental outlook, relieve stress and anxiety, make you fit and flexible, and decrease your risk of serious diseases such as heart disease, cancer, diabetes, hypertension, and osteoporosis.

3. **Health is multidimensional and positive.** The seven component parts of health, all interacting in a synergistic way, allow us to assume higher levels of functioning that can lead to more productive and satisfying lives. To achieve greater levels of health, one has to make a deliberate choice to assume personal responsibility for the process.

4. **Wellness is a dynamic process of change and growth that is largely determined by the decisions one makes about how to live one's life.** There are as many degrees of health as there are degrees of disease. These points can be viewed on a continuum. The wellness approach to health is not intended to replace the biomedical treatment approach, but to work in combination with it.

5. **A healthy lifestyle is a recurring pattern of health-promoting and disease-preventing behaviors undertaken to achieve wellness.** It is a way of life based on the idea that our chances of self-fulfillment are increased or decreased directly by our level of health. Further, it can decrease significantly the risk of disease and increase the chances of living healthfully into the later decades of life.

6. **A self-help approach assumes that human beings can manage their lifestyle change and learn to control environmental factors that are detrimental to health.** It puts you in control of your health and permits you to determine what to do and how and when to do it. A self-help approach requires planning and takes time, effort, and most importantly, the development of special lifestyle skills.

Terms

Chronic diseases, 6
Health, 6
Wellness, 7

Healthy lifestyle, 8
Physical activity, 10
Exercise, 10

Physical fitness, 10

making the connection

Sally realizes that she is in college to learn and do well academically. Her mid-term grades are fine, but she doesn't like feeling tired all the time. After reading Chapter 1, Sally realizes that she must take more responsibility for how she is feeling. She surmises that the lack of physical activity in her life may be contributing to her worn-out feeling and begins to think of ways she can find time to become more physically active while still maintaining other positive aspects of college life.

Critical Thinking

1. Are you feeling lethargic and tired, like Sally? Could it be because of lack of physical activity? If so, what physical activity are you currently doing? If not, what can you do to increase your physical activity? Develop a list of campus events or organizations that involve physical activity (hiking club, co-ed intramural volleyball, walking club, kick boxing). Investigate several of them to see which one best fits your needs and schedule. Begin adding this activity into your daily or weekly college routine.

2. Using the seven dimensions of health, identify two behaviors you do that would be an example of enhancing each dimension.

3. The morning newspaper headline is "Scientific studies indicate physical activity is important to health and quality of life." The article mentions studies from the "Prestigious International Health & Medicine Journal." Later that day you hear a local radio report suggesting that too much physical activity can lead to an instant heart attack, maybe even death. We are bombarded with health messages daily. What is your major source of health information? Television? If so, which shows in particular? Magazines? School? Friends? How carefully do you analyze health information? Do you believe most of what you read about health, or does it depend on the source?

References

American College of Sports Medicine. (2006). *ACSM's Guidelines for Exercise Testing and Prescription*, 7th ed. Baltimore: Williams & Wilkins.

Blair, S. (2005, January). Physical inactivity: The biggest public health problem of the 21st century. A presentation delivered to the University of Alberta, Alberta, Canada. Online: http://www.centre4activeliving.ca/Research/2005StevenBlair.pdf.

Centers for Disease Control and Prevention, National Center for Chronic Disease Prevention and Health Promotion. (2004). The burden of chronic diseases and their risk factors: National and state perspectives 2004. Online:

http://www.cdc.gov/nccdphp/burdenbook2004/index.htm.

Centers for Disease Control and Prevention, National Center for Chronic Disease Prevention and Health Promotion. (2005). Physical activity for everyone: Recommendations. Online: http://www.cdc.gov/nccdphp/dnpa/physical/recommendations/.

Dunn, H. (1967). *High Level Wellness*. Arlington, VA: Charles B. Slack.

Hein, H.O., Suadicini, P., & Gyntelberg, F. (1992). Physical fitness or physical activity as a predictor of ischaemic heart disease? A 17-year follow up in the Copenhagen Male Study. *Journal of Internal Medicine* 232:471–479.

Kotecki, J.E., & Clayton, B.C. (2003). Educating pharmacy students about nutrition and physical activity counseling. *American Journal of Health Education* 34(1):28–34.

Mokdad, A.H., Marks, J.S., Stroup, D.F., & Gerberding, J.L. (2004). Actual causes of death in the United States, 2000. *Journal of the American Medical Association* 291:1238—1245.

Nielsen Media Research. (2005). Nielsen reports Americans watch television at record levels. Online: http://www.nielsenmedia.com/.

Porter, K. (2005). *The Value of a College Degree* (ED70038). Washington, DC: ERIC Clearinghouse on Higher Education.

Schoenborn, C.A., Adams, P.F., Barnes, P.M., Vikerie, J.L., & Schiller, J.S. (2004). Health behavior of adults, 1999–2001. *Vital Health Statistics* 10(219):1–89.

United States Department of Health and Human Services. (2000). *Healthy People 2010: Understanding and Improving Health*, 2nd ed. Washington, DC: U.S. Government Printing Office.

United States Department of Health and Human Services. (2003). Prevention makes common "cents." Online: http://aspe.hhs.gov/health/prevention/prevention.pdf.

World Health Organization. (2004). Global strategy on diet, physical activity and health. World Health Assembly resolution WHA57.17. Online: http://www.who.int/dietphysicalactivity/goals/en/.

World Health Organization. (1948). *Constitution of the World Health Organization.* Geneva, Switzerland: Author.

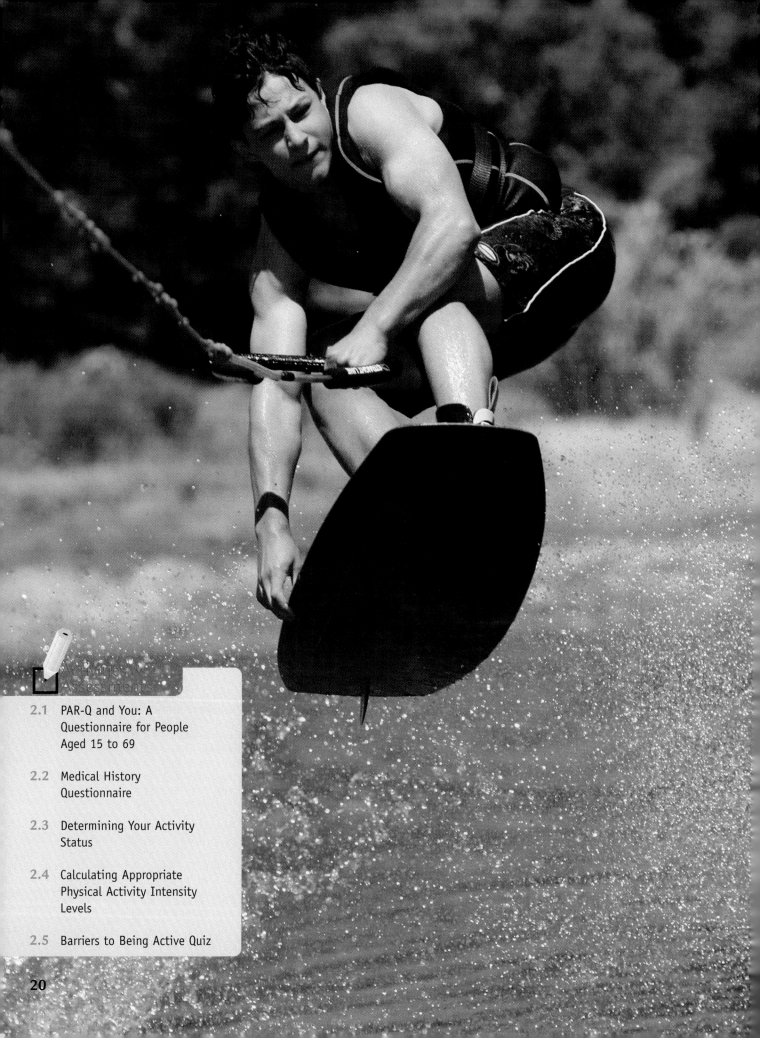

2.1   PAR-Q and You: A Questionnaire for People Aged 15 to 69

2.2   Medical History Questionnaire

2.3   Determining Your Activity Status

2.4   Calculating Appropriate Physical Activity Intensity Levels

2.5   Barriers to Being Active Quiz

Foundations of Physical Activity

what's the connection?

Bob is planning to start a regular physical activity program. He has never participated in one before. He is not pleased that he feels out of shape and has gained nearly 10 pounds over the last year. His time schedule has been hectic, with classes most of the day and a part-time job in the evenings. However, Bob's grandfather had a heart attack last month and the doctor attributed some of its origin to a sedentary lifestyle. This experience made Bob realize that maybe he should begin taking better care of himself, especially when it comes to being physically active. Bob is not altogether sure about the benefits of physical activity, and even less sure about how to get started and exactly which activities would be best for him.

concepts

1. Being physically active provides many health benefits.

2. A safe and effective physical activity program requires proper preparation.

3. How much activity you need is dependent on your goals, interests, and fitness level.

4. Optimize your benefits by individualizing your program.

5. A flexible approach is important in overcoming obstacles to physical activity.

6. Adhering to your program ensures an active lifestyle.

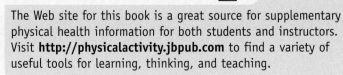

http://physicalactivity.jbpub.com

The Web site for this book is a great source for supplementary physical health information for both students and instructors. Visit **http://physicalactivity.jbpub.com** to find a variety of useful tools for learning, thinking, and teaching.

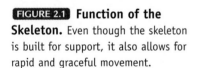
Being physically active provides many health benefits.

Introduction

Why should people be concerned about their physical activity patterns? What benefits are there to being physically active? What is the difference between physical activity and exercise? How does someone begin a physical activity program? If you have ever asked yourself any of these questions, then this chapter is designed for you. We start off with a discussion of the importance and benefits associated with being physically active. We then present the basic principles that underlie a regular physical activity program. Then we will help you determine if your body is ready for physical activity and explain how to select appropriate activities based on your needs and objectives. Overall, we show you how to establish a regular physical activity routine and how to achieve positive results while ensuring safety and effectiveness.

Your Body Was Meant to Move

The human body was built for movement. Our skeletal system provides us with a lightweight framework on which our muscles can act to produce motion. The structure of our skeleton is designed to provide stability and shock absorption, while remaining light enough to allow for rapid movement. We can withstand daily compressive forces many times our body weight, yet still move gracefully. As further proof that our bodies need movement, our bones actually become stronger over time when we are active (**FIGURE 2.1**).

However, it's not just our skeletal system that benefits from regular movement. Our cardiorespiratory system provides us with an efficient means of delivering needed fuels and oxygen while simultaneously removing waste products. The functional capacity of our cardiorespiratory system can be enhanced through regular physical activity (see Chapter 4). By making the heart and blood vessels function under the physical stress of being active, the cardiac and smooth muscles

FIGURE 2.1 **Function of the Skeleton.** Even though the skeleton is built for support, it also allows for rapid and graceful movement.

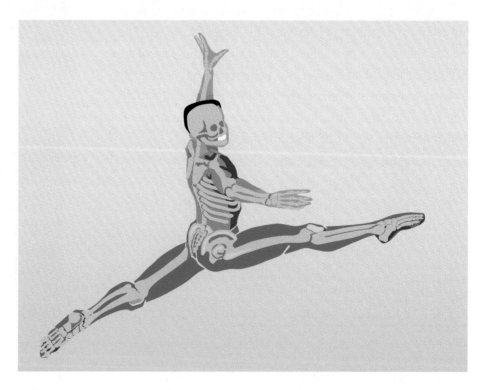

found in these systems become stronger. In fact, all systems of the body respond best to regular exposure of moderate levels of physiological stress.

We also know that an inactive body shows symptoms of **degeneration**. Inactive muscle **atrophies**, becoming weak and flabby. We put on extra fat (e.g., the old beer bicep, spare tire, or saddle bags) when we expend fewer calories than we consume. Sores may even result when inactivity leads to being in one position for an extended period of time.

We need to remember to pay attention to our bodies; they will remind us of the need to move. If we resist being physically active, we will feel tired and lack energy. We may feel weak and stiff, our joints may ache, and we may start getting soft and flabby. This chapter offers tips on how you can get started and achieve the most from your physical activity program.

Response and Adaptation to Physical Activity

Physical activity acts as a stimulus on the human body. Applied in appropriate doses, it can bring about positive changes in the way your body functions. A short-term change in an **organ system** is termed a **response**. A long-term change is termed an **adaptation**. With respect to physical activity, organ system response and adaptation typically determine the fitness level of the body. For example, when you first start to move, there is almost an immediate change in your heart rate. With increasing workloads, the heart rate increases rapidly. Such a change would be an example of a response of the cardiovascular system to the body's increasing demand for greater blood flow. If the body is regularly exposed to a stimulus that brings about this response, an adaptation will occur. For example, regular exposure to physical activity will result in a lowering of the resting heart rate. The change in resting heart rate is due to an adaptation in the cardiac muscle. This adaptation takes place in reaction to being regularly stressed by physical activity. The heart muscle becomes capable of contracting with greater force, thereby increasing the stroke volume, or the amount of blood forced out of the heart, with each contraction. If more blood can be ejected with each contraction, the heart does not have to beat as often to circulate the same amount of blood.

All systems of the body that are affected by the stress of physical activity will undergo response and adaptation. It should be noted that these changes are not always positive. For instance, if a joint is exposed to physical stress far beyond its normal functional capacity, the response may be swelling and pain to prevent further activity from potentially damaging the joint. With this in mind, the need to apply the correct amount of physical stress to the organ systems of the body becomes evident. Too much can cause damage, whereas just the right amount results in positive adaptation.

Benefits Associated with Regular Physical Activity

We know that physical activity has numerous beneficial physiological effects. The organ systems most affected are the cardiovascular and musculoskeletal systems, but benefits in the function of metabolic (including increasing your metabolic or energy utilization rate), endocrine (including the secretion of hormones that cause improved bone density, increased fat utilization, and greater muscle building), and immune (disease prevention) systems are also considerable (U.S. Department of Health and Human Services [USDHHS], 1996a).

We know that many of the beneficial effects of exercise training diminish within 2 weeks if physical activity is substantially reduced, and benefits completely disappear within 2 to 8 months if physical activity is not resumed (USDHHS, 1996a).

Degeneration A gradual decrease in function.

Atrophy Decrease in cell size, usually in reference to muscle or fat.

Organ system A collection of specialized tissues that provide an important body function (musculoskeletal, cardiovascular).

Response A short-term change in reaction to a stimulus (e.g., increased breathing rate after moving from inactive to active state).

Adaptation A long-term change in reaction to regular exposure to a stimulus (e.g., lower resting heart rate with increased fitness).

Physical Activity and Women's Health

As more and more women become physically active, it is important to take a look at what is currently known about women and physical activity. More than 60 percent of U.S. women do not engage in the recommended amount of physical activity (USDHHS, 1996b), with more than 25 percent of U.S. women not active at all.

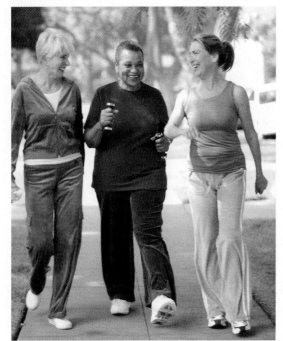

Physical activity plays an important role in women's health.

As a group, girls and women are less active than boys and men are, with women of color the least active (USDHHS, 2005). Additionally, participation rates for physical activity start to decline during the middle school years when social pressures against being active are highest.

There is strong observational and experimental evidence that physical inactivity plays a significant role in the development of cardiovascular disease in women, and that habitual physical activity and at least a moderate level of cardiorespiratory fitness offers protection from these diseases in women as well as in men (American Heart Association, 2005). Although there is less research available, it seems clear that regular physical activity reduces the risk of hypertension in women and is a primary preventive measure against stroke (AHA, 2005). Physical activity may also enhance the effect of estrogen replacement therapy and help decrease bone loss after menopause (USDHHS, 1996b). Research shows that lifetime physical activity appears to reduce the risk of colon cancer and breast cancer in women (American Cancer Society [ACS], 2005).

Title IX has helped women and girls gain more opportunity for participation in sport and physical activity. Social support from family and friends has been consistently and positively related to regular physical activity (USDHHS, 1996b). There is no physiologic reason for a healthy woman not to be physically active.

Prescreening, Medical History, and Self-Assessment

A safe and effective physical activity program requires proper preparation.

It is very important to make sure that your body is ready for physical activity before starting any activity program, and prescreening is the first step in ensuring safety and effectiveness. Several parts of the prescreening process can be completed on your own. Others require a visit to your physician.

The United States Public Health Service (USPHS) and the Surgeon General's Office suggest that all individuals consult with a physician, regardless of their age, before beginning a new physical activity program (USDHHS, 1996a). Consulting with a physician is especially important for people with chronic diseases, such as cardiovascular disease and diabetes mellitus, or for those who are at high risk for these diseases. Men over 45 years of age and women over age 55 are advised to consult a physician before beginning a vigorous activity program.

Prescreening and Medical History

According to Heyward (2002), the key components of a comprehensive pre-exercise health evaluation are as follows:

1. A physical activity readiness questionnaire (PAR-Q) to determine one's readiness for physical activity.
2. A determination of any signs or symptoms of disease to identify an individual in need of medical referral.
3. A coronary risk factor analysis to determine the number of coronary heart disease risk factors.

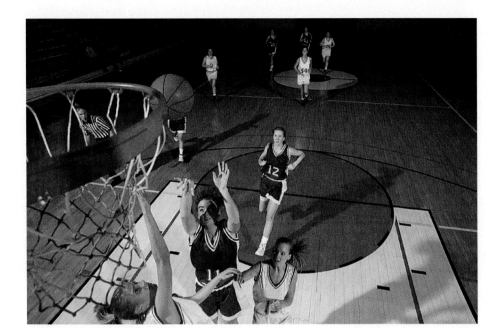

Title IX has increased opportunities for women and girls.

4. A disease risk classification to categorize yourself as apparently healthy, at increased risk, or with known disease.

5. A medical history to review your past and present personal and family health histories, focusing on conditions requiring medical referral and clearance.

6. A physical examination to detect signs and symptoms of disease.

7. Medical clearance indicating physician approval for exercise testing and participation.

8. Laboratory tests (including triglyceride levels) to provide a more thorough assessment of your health status, particularly if you have known disease.

9. Cholesterol and lipoprotein (high-density lipoprotein [HDL], low-density lipoprotein [LDL], and very low density lipoprotein [VLDL]) profiling to determine if you have hyperlipidemia (high blood lipids or fats) and to aid in determining coronary risk status. High HDL levels protect you against heart disease. High LDL or VLDL levels place you at greater risk for heart disease.

10. Blood pressure assessment to determine if you are hypertensive (have high blood pressure) and to aid in determining coronary risk status.

11. Measurement of your resting heart rate and a 12-lead ECG (an electrocardiogram that traces the electrical activity of your heart) to help evaluate cardiac function and detect cardiac abnormalities that would exclude you from participating in an exercise program.

12. A graded exercise test to assess aerobic fitness capacity and to detect cardiac abnormalities due to exercise stress.

Self-Assessment

Self-assessment plays an important role in allowing you to take responsibility for your own physical activity program. By testing yourself, you learn how much progress you are making, gain a better understanding of the aspect of fitness you are working on, and understand when to make adjustments to your physical activity program.

How much activity you need is dependent on your goals, interests, and fitness level.

FIGURE 2.2 **Disease Risk Versus Activity Status.** Moving from the sedentary category to the moderately active category provides the greatest decrease in health risk, although additional reductions may be achieved by becoming vigorously active.

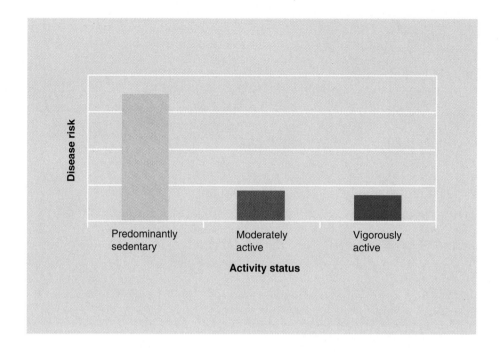

Hypokinetic diseases Diseases associated with an inactive lifestyle (cardiovascular disease, obesity, diabetes).

People can be classified as belonging to one of three physical activity categories. The first includes those individuals who are predominantly sedentary. Participation in physical activity is not a regular component of their lifestyles. In the United States, these individuals constitute the largest segment of our society. They are at the greatest risk for developing **hypokinetic diseases.** Examples of hypokinetic diseases include cardiovascular disease, obesity, diabetes, stroke, and some forms of cancer.

The second group includes those individuals who are moderately active on most if not all days of the week. They may be participating in a wide variety of physical activities such as walking, yard work, or recreational sport. We now know that moving from the first category to the second provides a great deal of protection against hypokinetic disease.

The smallest segment of our society falls into the category of those who are vigorously active on a regular basis. This category would include athletes in training and individuals seeking maximal fitness and health benefits. These individuals receive the highest degree of protection from hypokinetic disease (**FIGURE 2.2**).

Health Benefits and Optimal Fitness

Although we have known for some time that an active body is a healthy body, evidence supporting this fact has gained increasing attention in the last decade. Where it was once thought that activity had to be extremely stressful to bring about improvements in fitness, it is now recognized that physical activity of lower intensities is also beneficial. In fact, we now know that recreational and leisure activities of low to moderate intensity offer significant improvements in health status (USDHHS, 1996a).

However, because we can obtain some benefit from low- to moderate-intensity activity, we should not take this to mean that more intensive exercise is not beneficial. For those who are already active, and for those wishing to achieve optimal health and fitness benefits, vigorous exercise offers benefits beyond those available through moderate-intensity physical activity (USDHHS, 1996a). It is wise for pre-

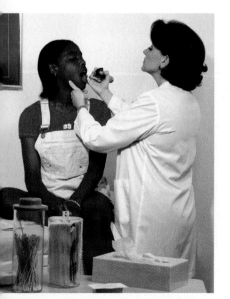

Check with your physician before starting a physical activity program.

viously sedentary people who are embarking on a physical activity program to start with short-duration, low- to moderate-intensity activity and gradually increase the duration or intensity or both until their goals are reached (USDHHS, 1996a).

One of the keys to achieving health benefits from physical activity is consistency. Physical activity should be performed on most, if not all, days of the week. It is the regularity of physical activity that is responsible for the long-term adaptations that bring about protection from hypokinetic diseases (USDHHS, 1996a). However, if your activity pattern becomes temporarily disrupted, don't panic. Just pick back up again when possible, making modifications as necessary.

Different Guidelines for Different Outcomes

The American College of Sports Medicine (ACSM) has established guidelines for physical activity programs that are designed to meet the diverse needs of the general public (ACSM, 2006). Based on the best research available to date, the ACSM recognizes that there are at least two sets of guidelines that you might follow depending on desired outcomes. For those interested solely in obtaining basic health benefits (lowered risk of developing degenerative disease, for example), the guidelines suggest adults should engage in moderate-intensity physical activity for at least 30 minutes or more on 5 or more days of the week or vigorous-intensity physical activity 3 or more days per week for 20 or more minutes per occasion during recreational or leisure-time activities (i.e., not work related) (Center for Disease Control and Prevention [CDC], 2005). This recommendation translates into a goal of expending at least 150 calories a day or about 1000 calories a week in physical activity.

For those wishing to obtain optimal fitness and health benefits, the guidelines just outlined may be built upon to include exercise that is performed 3 to 5 days per week, at moderate to vigorous intensity (50 to 85 percent of aerobic capacity) for 20 to 60 minutes, while utilizing the larger muscle masses of the body. This means performing activities that primarily use the arms, legs, and trunk muscles.

The bottom line is that some physical activity is better than none, while more (to a certain extent) is better than some. Significant improvements in fitness and health will result in moving from a sedentary lifestyle into a regularly active lifestyle. These benefits can be extended further for those interested in the attainment of optimal function, by moving from the category of regularly active to a category that includes exposure to vigorous exercise on a regular basis.

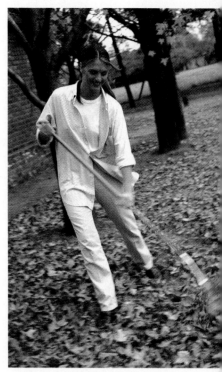

Physical activity includes many forms of movement, even yard work.

How Much Physical Activity Is Enough?

As stated earlier, some physical activity is better than none. However, based on the most current research, to obtain basic health benefits, adults should engage in moderate-intensity physical activities for at least 30 minutes on 5 or more days of the week during recreational or leisure-time activities (i.e., not work related) (CDC, 2005). These guidelines allow for flexibility in the types of activities you may select and even allow you to break your activity session into multiple segments. For instance, activities such as yard work, walking, or cycling will meet the basic health benefit goal, and you may break a 30-minute session down into two 15-minute segments or three 10-minute sessions.

There is, however, a minimal level of activity that must be consistently maintained. Being active fewer than 2 days per week, at less than 40 to 50 percent of aerobic capacity, and for less than 10 minutes, is generally not a sufficient stimulus for developing and maintaining fitness in healthy adults (ACSM, 1998).

Make physical activity a family affair.

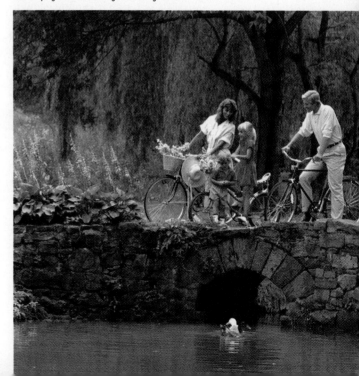

For those interested in more health benefit, and who wish to obtain higher levels of fitness, more vigorous guidelines are suggested. The following section contains a spectrum of activity recommendations that may be followed based on your desired outcomes.

Personalizing Your Physical Activity Program

Optimize your benefits by individualizing your program.

Physical activity programs must be tailored to meet the needs of the individual. Choose activities that are fun for you and that you think you would like to continue for some time. Be aware that by alternating activities, you are less likely to become bored and more likely to make physical activity a regular part of your lifestyle. TABLE 2.1 presents suggested activities that you may find enjoyable.

Choosing Activities

Your activity program needs to relate specifically to the outcomes you wish to obtain. Franks (1997) recommends activities based on your current activity status and your goals and objectives:

1. **Activities everyone should do as part of their daily routine.** Activities should be of the type that can be done as part of an individual's routine at home, work, and during leisure. To increase physical activity as part of your daily life, you need to walk rather than ride when possible; climb stairs rather than take the elevator or escalator; park farther away from the store, school, or office for a short walk to and from the car; and get off the bus or train one stop earlier and walk the rest of the way to the office, store, school, or home. You need to emphasize weight-bearing activities to use more energy and enhance bone health. Include a daily routine of stretching to prevent low-back problems.

2. **Advice for sedentary individuals starting a physical activity program.** Some physical activity is better than none at all. Sedentary (inactive) individuals should strive to incorporate activity in their daily routine. Learn to appreciate small improvements in lifestyle. Start slowly with modest goals and then enhance them.

   Recommended activities for sedentary individuals include walking, yard work, cycling, slow dancing, and low-impact exercise to music. The activity can be broken into two to four segments: for example, take two 10-minute exercise breaks during the workday, add another exercise break in the morning or at night during the week, and add a 30-minute walk on the weekend. You also

TABLE 2.1	Physical Activities		
Backpacking	Cricket	Kayaking	Snowboarding
Baseball	Equestrian sports	Racquetball	Soccer
Basketball	Fishing	Roller blading	Squash
Bicycling	Football	Rowing	Swimming
Boating	Golf	Rugby	Tennis
Bowling	Handball	Skating	Walking
Bungee jumping	Hang gliding	Skateboarding	Water skiing
Camping	Hiking	Skiing	Weight training
Canoeing	Jogging	Snorkling	Windsurfing

need to include weight-bearing activities, without being overly concerned with trying to maintain a moderate-to-high intensity level. Learn to appreciate how small adjustments in your daily routine can contribute to accumulating 30 minutes of moderate-intensity physical activity. Be patient while expecting results. Accept minor improvements as the pathway leading to further improvements.

3. **Activities for moderately active people focusing on health goals.**   Individuals who have specific health goals should perform all of the previous recommendations plus the activities in ⌐TABLE 2.2⌐ based on the health goal desired.

4. **Activities for moderately active people with fitness goals.**   Individuals seeking fitness goals should perform all of the previous recommendations and consult ⌐TABLE 2.3⌐ to achieve the desired fitness goal.

TABLE 2.2	Physical Activity for Specific Health Goals

Health Goal	Recommendations
Cardiovascular health	• Do at least 30 minutes of daily moderate-intensity physical activity. • Include longer-duration and/or higher-intensity activities, as you become accustomed to being active.
Bone health	• Choose weight-bearing activities like walking. • Perform resistance exercises such as weight lifting.
Low-back health	• Perform static stretching in the mid-trunk and thigh regions. • Include abdominal curl-ups.
Psychological health	• Select enjoyable activities performed in a fun environment.

SOURCE: Franks, B.D. (1997). Personalizing physical activity prescription. *President's Council on Physical Fitness and Sports Research Digest* 2(9):1–8.

TABLE 2.3	Physical Activity for Fitness Goals

Fitness Goal	Recommendations
Aerobic fitness	• Perform 20–60 minutes of vigorous-intensity activity, 3–5 days per week.
Relative leanness	
Too little fat	• Eat more calories, especially carbohydrates. • Include resistance exercise to build muscle.
Too much fat	• Reduce caloric consumption, especially fat. • Increase duration of aerobic activity to increase caloric expenditure. • Include resistance exercise to maintain muscle.
Muscular strength/endurance	• Include resistance exercise, 8–10 exercises, 1–2 sets, 10–15 repetitions involving each major muscle group, 2–3 days per week.
Flexibility	• Perform daily static stretching. Hold each stretch for 10–30 sec and perform each stretch 2–3 times.

SOURCE: Franks, B.D. (1997). Personalizing physical activity prescription. *President's Council on Physical Fitness and Sports Research Digest* 2(9):1–8.

| TABLE 2.4 | **Physical Activity for Performance Goals** |

Performance Goal	Recommendations
Sport or physical task	• Develop and/or maintain fitness levels.
	• Perform interval training (high-intensity activity interspersed with low- to moderate-intensity activity).
	• Practice motor tasks related to performance.
	• Target specific skills related to performance.
	• Prepare strategy and become mentally ready.

SOURCE: Franks, B.D. (1997). Personalizing physical activity prescription. *President's Council on Physical Fitness and Sports Research Digest* 2(9):1–8.

5. **Activities for vigorously active individuals with performance goals.** People interested in vigorous activity, or those who have performance goals, should fulfill all of the previous recommendations and check TABLE 2.4 for additional suggestions.

Determining Activity Status

It is important to remember that activity recommendations should be based on an individual's activity status. The goal is to get each person involved in a daily routine that is active in nature and to supplement that routine with 30 minutes of moderate-intensity activity. After an individual is engaging in the daily activities on a regular basis and not experiencing any problems, discomfort, or fatigue, activities for the development of greater health and fitness goals may be included. After daily physical activity and fitness activities have been included as part of a person's lifestyle, then a variety of performance goals, based on personal interests, can be considered (Franks, 1997). There are numerous ways to calculate the appropriate intensity level for optimal fitness (see Chapter 4).

Guidelines for Those Seeking Optimal Fitness

The following guidelines (ACSM, 1998) are designed for the middle to higher end of the physical activity continuum. They particularly target those seeking optimal fitness and maximal health benefit. For optimal cardiorespiratory fitness and body composition, it is recommended that you:

1. Exercise at a frequency (F) of 3 to 5 days per week. Exercising less than 3 days per week will not bring about maximal fitness benefit. Exercising more than 5 days per week at these higher intensities will bring about marginal fitness improvements and increase the risk of injury dramatically. It is recommended that you remain active on the two "off" days by performing activities of low to moderate intensity.

2. Depending on the method selected to determine aerobic capacity, the intensity (I) should fall between 50 and 85 percent of your aerobic capacity. Exercising at an intensity beyond the recommended levels shifts you from **aerobic** exercise back into **anaerobic** exercise. Aerobic exercise is best for improvements in cardiovascular fitness (FIGURE 2.3).

Aerobic Metabolic process that relies on oxygen. For aerobic metabolism to take place, exercise intensity must be low to moderate.

Anaerobic Metabolic process that does not rely on oxygen. Anaerobic metabolism occurs at the start of physical activity and when intensity is very high.

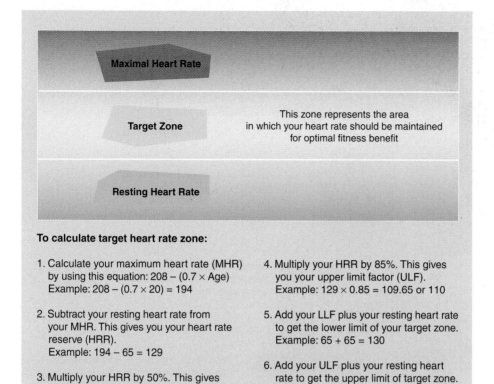

FIGURE 2.3 **Calculating Your Target Heart Rate Zone.** To improve your fitness, try to keep your heart rate in your target zone.

To calculate target heart rate zone:

1. Calculate your maximum heart rate (MHR) by using this equation: $208 - (0.7 \times \text{Age})$
   Example: $208 - (0.7 \times 20) = 194$

2. Subtract your resting heart rate from your MHR. This gives you your heart rate reserve (HRR).
   Example: $194 - 65 = 129$

3. Multiply your HRR by 50%. This gives you your lower limit factor (LLF).
   Example: $129 \times 0.50 = 64.5$ or 65

4. Multiply your HRR by 85%. This gives you your upper limit factor (ULF).
   Example: $129 \times 0.85 = 109.65$ or 110

5. Add your LLF plus your resting heart rate to get the lower limit of your target zone.
   Example: $65 + 65 = 130$

6. Add your ULF plus your resting heart rate to get the upper limit of target zone.
   Example: $110 = 65 = 175$

7. You should exercise at a heart rate that falls between 130 and 175 bpm for optimal fitness.

3. The duration (T) of each exercise session should be established at 20 to 60 minutes of continuous or intermittent (minimum of 10-minute bouts accumulated throughout the day) aerobic activity. The duration is dependent on the intensity of the activity. Thus, lower-intensity activity should be conducted over a longer period of time (30 minutes or more).

   Moderate-intensity activity of longer duration is recommended for adults not training for athletic competition. This recommendation is made because of the importance of "total fitness," which is more readily attained with exercise sessions of longer duration, and because of the potential health and adherence hazards associated with high-intensity activity.

4. For the mode (S), or type of activity, you can select any activity that uses the large-muscle groups, which can be maintained continuously and is rhythmical and aerobic in nature. Examples would include walking/hiking, running/jogging, cycling/bicycling, cross-country skiing, aerobic dance/group exercise, rope skipping, rowing, stair climbing, swimming, skating, and various endurance game activities or some combination thereof.

   An additional source of information on how much activity to perform is the exercise and physical activity pyramid (**FIGURE 2.4**):

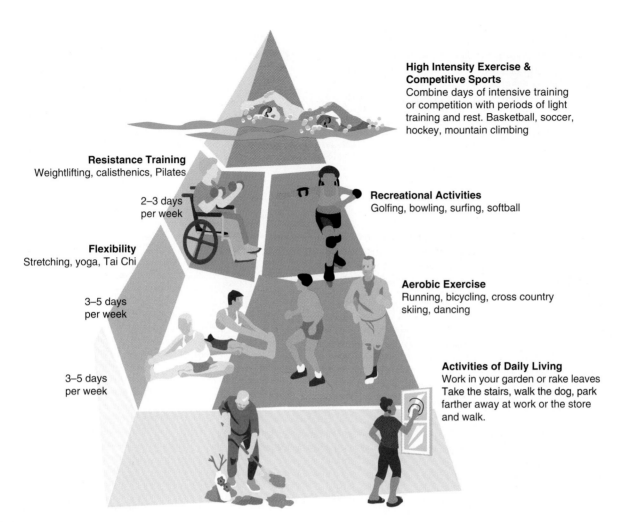

**High Intensity Exercise &
Competitive Sports**
Combine days of intensive training
or competition with periods of light
training and rest. Basketball, soccer,
hockey, mountain climbing

Resistance Training
Weightlifting, calisthenics, Pilates

2–3 days
per week

Recreational Activities
Golfing, bowling, surfing, softball

Flexibility
Stretching, yoga, Tai Chi

3–5 days
per week

Aerobic Exercise
Running, bicycling, cross country
skiing, dancing

3–5 days
per week

Activities of Daily Living
Work in your garden or rake leaves
Take the stairs, walk the dog, park
farther away at work or the store
and walk.

FIGURE 2.4 **The Exercise and Physical Activity Pyramid.** An active lifestyle can involve many different activities. SOURCE: Adapted from *Exercise and Activity Pyramid,* Metropolitan Life Insurance Company, 1995.

How Do I Get Started?

When starting a physical activity program, the first step should always be to determine your goals and objectives. People are active for a variety of reasons. To optimize the benefits associated with being regularly active, you must have a clear idea of what you wish to obtain from your activity program. Some people start activity programs to obtain health benefits; others are interested in improving their overall fitness levels; still others are simply interested in looking and feeling better.

Setting Goals

Whatever your reasons for wanting to start a physical activity program, you need to develop a clear idea of where you are going in order to get there efficiently. In contemplating your reasons for becoming active, remember to be realistic when you define your goals and objectives. Goals and objectives should be attainable, adjustable, and allow for individual need. Remember that the overriding factors that must be incorporated in any physical activity program are *safety* and *effectiveness*. You want to make sure that you don't injure yourself, and you want to make sure that your goals are achieved. Planning a safe and effective program should influence your goal setting by encouraging you to think in terms of both short-term and long-term goals.

We are all born with different genetic blueprints. In terms of our responses and adaptations to physical activity, this difference means that we all will respond and adapt at different physiological rates and magnitudes. Some people will see rapid changes in response to exercise, whereas others will see measurable change only over an extended period of time. Certain individuals will see their body function improve to an extent not achievable by other individuals, who might be working just as hard or harder. Taking the variation in improvement rate into consideration, programs must be **individualized** to bring about optimal benefit based on individual need and response. Not everyone should be performing the same activities at the same intensities for the same period of time. You need to find the activities that are best suited to meet your individual needs.

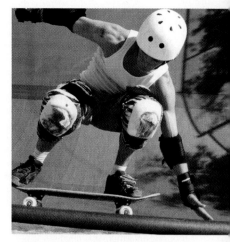

Safety is an important factor to consider when participating in physical activity.

Confirming Your Health Status

All individuals should consult with their physician before starting or making major adjustments to any physical activity program. For most healthy individuals, this step may only reinforce what appears to be obvious: you are healthy. However, many underlying health conditions do not have overt signs and symptoms and are only detectable through a medical exam. Activity, though safe in almost all instances, can trigger life-threatening events if performed improperly and without knowledge of underlying disease.

Building Slowly

When beginning an activity program it is wise to start gradually, build slowly, and maintain consistency. A common mistake made by beginners is to try to do too much, too soon. Relying on what others are doing to determine how much you should do is not wise. Remember that fitness is individual in nature. What may appear to be a low-intensity warm-up for one person may be an exhaustive workout for another. It is far better to delay the acquisition of benefits to some degree rather than to do too much, become sore or injured, and set your program back significantly—or, worse, stop completely. Chapter 3 provides more information on strategies to use when changing your behavior.

> **Individualized** Based on differing needs of different people.
> **Variability** The differences among people.
> **Heritability** The amount genetics determines the differences between people.

Heredity and Health-Related Fitness

We know that our genetics will affect the extent and rate at which we will benefit in response to being physically active. The best estimates tell us that genetics accounts for about 25 percent of the **variability** we see in people's body fatness levels (Bouchard, 1993). Approximately 20 to 40 percent of the variability for muscle fitness, and 10 to 25 percent for cardiovascular fitness, is inherited (Bouchard, 1993; Beunen & Thomis, 2004). For example, the **heritability** for body fatness (25 percent) tells us that factors (environment, diet, activity status) other than genetics account for 75 percent of the variability we see when we compare different people. Therefore, the majority of variation in body fatness is due to lifestyle factors: food consumption and physical activity levels. Twenty-five percent is due directly to our genetics.

Not only do people differ in fitness based on heredity, but people of different genetic backgrounds respond differently to training. In other words, two people of different genetic backgrounds could do the same exercise program and get quite different benefits. Some people may get as much as ten times the benefit from activity as others who do the same program (Bouchard, 1993).

The genetic influence on how we respond to being physically active makes recognizing individual differences even more important. Assumptions about a person's fitness are not always good indicators of their current activity levels. Bouchard (1993) also suggests that different people

Genetic variation affects our response and adaptation to physical activity.

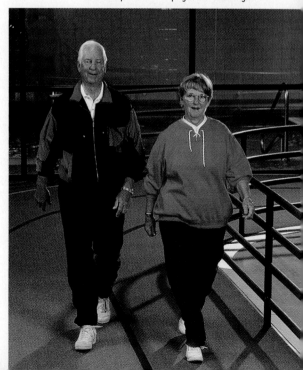

respond differently to each component of fitness. So, while some people may respond well to strength training, they may not respond as well to cardiorespiratory training. Typically, we see a three- to tenfold difference between low responders (people who don't show much change) and high responders (people who show a good deal of change) on the same standardized physical activity regimen if performed for a period of 15 to 20 weeks (Bouchard, 1993). The magnitude of the difference is somewhat dependent on the component of fitness considered.

Program Design

There are several factors that must be considered when developing a physical activity program. The amount of time you are willing to set aside for activity, your access to exercise equipment, your motivation, the activities you enjoy, and your current state of conditioning will all play important roles in designing a regular physical activity program.

The Three Stages of Conditioning

There are three recognized stages of conditioning programs (Heyward, 2002). The **initial stage** defines the early portion of a program, in which you become accustomed to making physical activity a regular portion of your life. During this phase, you should be exposed to a wide variety of activities, learn the proper techniques of various activities, experience the fastest rate of improvement, and determine a schedule to accommodate physical activity in your lifestyle.

In the second stage, the **progression stage**, you continue to apply the principles of conditioning to develop greater levels of fitness and more health benefit. This stage is usually short because of the high level of stress it can apply to the body. It is, however, during this stage that optimal levels of fitness and health are obtained.

The **maintenance stage** is the stage in which most active people spend the majority of their time. During the maintenance stage, you have established a regular physical activity routine and participate frequently to maintain your current level of fitness and health. This stage allows for the consolidation of gains and for recovery from the progression stage. Occasionally, people in the maintenance stage shift back into the progression stage to move their fitness and health to a higher level. They then shift back to the maintenance stage to hold onto the gains they have just achieved.

Components of an Activity Session

All exercise and physical activity sessions should follow a similar format. This format allows you to optimize gains while minimizing the risk of injury. Depending on the type of physical activity you are going to perform, you may need to modify these instructions slightly.

PREPARATION   The first stage is to prepare the body for physical activity. Make sure you are in appropriate attire and using safe equipment that is designed for the activity to follow (see Chapter 15). If you are preparing for a walking program, make sure you are in comfortable clothes and have good walking shoes; if you are about to perform yard work, make sure you have on clothes suited for the activity and the weather.

Preparing your body is best accomplished by gradually shifting the body from an inactive state to an active state. Low-intensity aerobic activity (slow walking) and slow stretching usually characterize this portion of an exercise routine. The purpose of this is to increase blood flow to the muscles, increase the temperature of the muscles, and ease into the cardiorespiratory adjustments required for the

Initial stage Early portion of a program in which you become accustomed to making physical activity a regular part of your life.

Progression stage Stage in which you stress your body so as to develop greater levels of conditioning and fitness. This stage is short due to high levels of stress on the body. Optimal levels of fitness are obtained.

Maintenance stage Stage of established regular physical activity designed to maintain current levels of fitness and health. Consolidation of gains and recovery from the progression stage.

Stretching exercises help to improve flexibility.

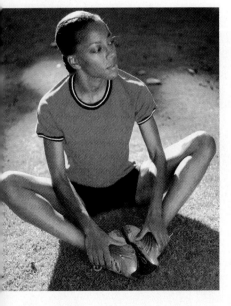

more intensive activity to follow. Though you may be performing an activity that is not traditionally "exercise," you still need to warm up. Muscle strains and low-back injuries can occur when a person performs a sudden movement for which the body is not prepared. You don't have to be "exercising" for this to happen.

TRANSITION   The second phase is one of transition, in which you move gradually into the focal point of the activity you will be performing. It is necessary to move gradually during this phase, increasing intensity as the body indicates that it has adjusted to the physiological demands of the activity. You will begin to loosen up and your body temperature will start to increase. You may also notice that you start to perspire during this transitional phase.

ACTIVITY   The third phase is that in which you focus on the activity in which you are participating for its health benefit or for improvement of fitness. The intensity and duration of activity will be determined by your goals, fitness level, access to facilities and equipment, and allotted time.

COOLDOWN   The fourth and final phase is a combination cooldown/flexibility enhancement phase. During this portion of an activity routine, you gradually bring the intensity down toward resting values. Reducing the intensity is important in keeping blood from pooling in the legs and aiding the flow of blood back to the heart for recirculation. Breathing rate, heart rate, and temperature are all brought back to baseline levels. The speed with which you return to pre-activity levels can be a good indicator of your fitness level. Fit people return to resting levels more rapidly than people who are less fit. It is important to perform stretching exercises during the cooldown because it is during the cooldown that the muscles are their warmest. Warm muscles are more pliable muscles, so the stretching exercises will have their greatest impact on improving your flexibility or range of motion.

Variety of Experiences and Cross Training

Exposure to a wide range of activities is important for individuals starting physical activity programs. Boredom can be one of the major obstacles to being regularly active. We all know that variety is the spice of life, and if we have a range of activities to select from we are more likely to find something we like and to adhere to our activity program. **FIGURE 2.5** shows several combinations of activities that one may choose.

FIGURE 2.5 **Cross Training Combinations.** It's best to vary your activity program by combining different types of activities.

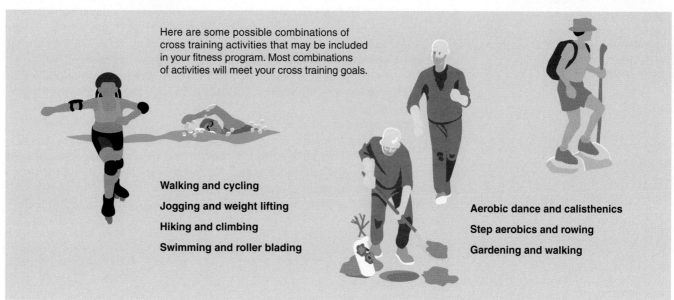

Here are some possible combinations of cross training activities that may be included in your fitness program. Most combinations of activities will meet your cross training goals.

Walking and cycling

Jogging and weight lifting

Hiking and climbing

Swimming and roller blading

Aerobic dance and calisthenics

Step aerobics and rowing

Gardening and walking

Cross training involves the incorporation of different activities into your program. Cross training serves the purpose of adding variety to an activity program and making sure that various body systems and muscle groups are included. By using cross training effectively, you also allow one system to recover on what would be an "off" day while stressing another system. Stressing one system while another recovers allows you to meet the surgeon general's suggestion to be active on most if not all days of the week.

Monitoring Your Progress

It is important to check regularly to see if your program is working and if adjustments need to be made. Monitoring is accomplished by performing self-assessment on a regular basis. Another important aspect of monitoring your progress is that it will provide positive motivation as you see that what you are doing is actually producing benefit and moving you closer to the attainment of your goals and objectives. It also allows you to update your objectives so that new ones may be set after initial ones have been achieved.

Components of Health-Related Fitness

Physical activity is a process that produces improvement in health and fitness. Several aspects of fitness directly relate to health and are considered to be components of health-related fitness.

Cardiorespiratory fitness refers to the integration of the pulmonary and cardiovascular systems. Being able to breathe in oxygen and transfer it into the blood, circulate the blood to our muscles, exchange the oxygen and other nutrients at the muscle, and remove carbon dioxide and other waste products is important when it comes to sustaining physical activity (see Chapter 4).

Body composition refers to the major chemical components of the body. The main components under consideration are fat mass, muscle mass, bone density, and water volume (see Chapter 9). If we have too much of one component, or not enough of another, our health will suffer.

Muscular strength is the ability of the muscles to generate force. The larger the cross-sectional area of the muscle, the greater the amount of force it can produce (see Chapter 11). Stronger muscles allow us to do more work, protect our joints from injury, and help to make our bones stronger.

Muscular endurance is the muscle's ability to generate force repeatedly. Improved endurance allows us to repeat a physical activity for a greater number of repetitions or for a longer period of time (see Chapter 11). Good muscular endurance is important in carrying out the activities of daily living and in protecting the back against chronic pain.

Flexibility describes the range of motion available at a joint (see Chapter 12). Several factors affect flexibility, including muscle elasticity, muscle temperature, bony structure, connective tissue integrity, and the points of origin and insertion of the muscles. In physical activity programs, flexibility is enhanced through stretching exercises. When stretching, one attempts to improve muscle elasticity and compliance. Good flexibility helps prevent injury and low-back pain and provides greater mobility.

Cardiorespiratory fitness The integration of the pulmonary and cardiovascular systems. The lungs, heart, and vascular network deliver key nutrients while removing waste products.

Body composition The major chemical components of the body: fat mass, muscle mass, bone density, and water volume.

Muscular strength The ability of the muscles to generate force.

Muscular endurance The muscle's ability to generate force repeatedly.

Flexibility The range of motion available at a joint.

The Principles of Training

There are certain principles that govern how your body will respond to the physical stress of physical activity. Following these principles will ensure the safety and effectiveness of your activity program.

The **overload principle** states that a body system (muscular, skeletal) must be exposed to physical stress beyond the ordinary in order to adapt and improve function. For example, to build stronger muscles you must work against resistance that pushes your muscles to their limits. Over a period of time, your muscles adapt to this new workload and become stronger.

The **principle of progression** states that, to ensure safety and effectiveness, the overload must be applied in a systematic and logical fashion. If too much physical stress is applied too soon, the system will not have time to adapt properly and benefits may be delayed or injury may occur. You need to overload your body gradually so it has time to adjust and improve. If you are sore after exercising, you are doing more than your current level of fitness allows. You should reduce the intensity of your activity and progress more gradually.

The **principle of specificity** states that particular activities must be performed to bring about particular adaptations. For instance, if the goal is to build muscular strength, you need to undertake an activity that overloads the muscles. For example, you must do exercises that physically stress the biceps muscles of the upper arm if strength gain in the biceps is desirable. Stressing the quadriceps muscles of the thigh will not develop strength in the biceps of the arm.

The **principle of reversibility** tells us that any gains we may get through regular physical activity will disappear if we do not continue to be active—thus the maxim "Use it or lose it." If we decrease our activity levels, we will experience some loss in fitness in as little as 2 weeks (Coyle, 1990). This is why it is important to continue our activity program for life (**FIGURE 2.6**).

The **principle of individuality** reinforces the concept that all people have different genetic blueprints, and activity programs must be designed with this in mind. Determine what you wish to achieve, find activities that will bring about those results, and set out to obtain your desired outcomes.

Overload principle A body system (muscular, skeletal, cardiovascular) must be exposed to physical stress beyond that which is ordinary in order to adapt and improve function.

Principle of progression The logical and systematic application of the overload principle.

Principle of specificity You must target activities to specific systems to improve their particular function.

Principle of reversibility All benefits gained through participation in a physical activity program will be lost if the activity is not continued.

Principle of individuality All people are different genetically and have different levels of potential physical development.

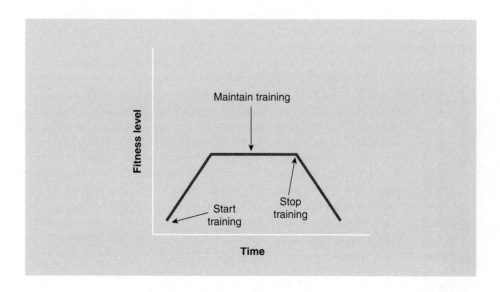

FIGURE 2.6 **Principle of Reversibility.** If you don't continue to do the things that drive up your fitness level, it will degrade and return to previous levels.

Principle of recovery An adequate rest period must be allowed for your body to adapt and become stronger.

A flexible approach is important in overcoming obstacles to physical activity.

The **principle of recovery** reminds us that our bodies take time to adjust to the physical stress of being active. We must allow adequate time for adaptation to take place. It is generally recommended that we allow 48 to 72 hours between exhaustive activity sessions that are similar in nature. This doesn't mean that we shouldn't be active at all for this period of time. It does mean that we should vary our activities so that one system is allowed time to adjust before it is stressed again.

Becoming Independently Active

To maintain an active lifestyle successfully, you must learn the knowledge and skills associated with becoming independently active. A lifestyle of physical activity requires that you select activities that are enjoyable, meaningful, and designed with your needs in mind. The most effective way to increase adherence to an activity program is to make sure the program meets your goals and objectives. Responsibility for this lies with the person developing and executing the activity program. You must learn to gather information on how to become physically active, discern what is of use for your particular needs, and develop a program structured to meet those needs. Dependence on someone else for your activity program limits your ability to obtain optimal benefit and satisfaction.

Overcoming Barriers to Physical Activity

Barriers to physical activity may be psychological or physical. The number and strength of these perceived barriers are consistently related to participation rates in physical activity for both adults and adolescents. The more barriers you perceive, or the stronger those barriers, the less likely it is that you will continue to participate in a physical activity program (Sallis, 1994).

Time

Physical activity can be performed in three 10-minute segments to fit a busy schedule.

The most common barrier is a perceived lack of time. When this explanation is presented as the reason for being inactive, it usually means that participation in physical activity is not high enough on your priority list. Physical activity must be considered as important to your body as eating, sleeping, and breathing. Physical activity does not take long intervals of time, and the benefits you receive will bring you a longer life that is of a higher quality. By preventing many of the diseases that rob us of a healthy life, physical activity actually provides us with additional free time. Once you have determined that physical activity is important to you, you can begin to overcome potential barriers to activity. Physical activity is an essential part of our daily lives, not just something we do if we have extra time.

If limited time is a concern, recent information demonstrates that we can benefit from activity without having to participate in exercise of long duration. We now know that activity sessions broken down into multiple intervals over the course of a day provide significant health benefits. In other words, instead of having to schedule a continuous 30-minute exercise period into your day, you can obtain similar benefits by accumulating the 30 minutes in three 10-minute sessions.

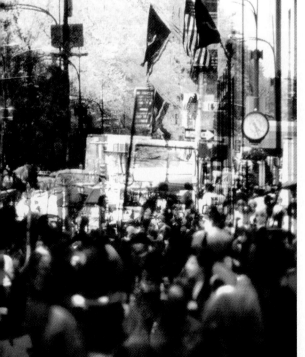

You could take 10-minute walks in the morning, at lunch, and in the evening to achieve this goal.

No Pain, No Gain

A second barrier to being regularly active involves thinking that activity has to be unpleasant to be effective. The perception that activity must be unpleasant usually derives from previous negative experiences with physical activity. Unfortunately, some physical educators and coaches have used exercise and activity as punishment. Using exercise as punishment teaches us to avoid exercise. Being active should be an enjoyable experience. Don't let past negative experiences prevent you from finding activities that you may enjoy.

If we perform activities improperly, or try to perform beyond our level of competence and fitness, any resultant soreness and injury could develop into another barrier to physical activity. We need to realize that if we hurt while being active, our body is telling us that we are doing something wrong. Forget the old adage "No pain, no gain." Pain brought on by physical activity is equivalent to injury. *There will be no gain without effort or without fatiguing our muscles, but we shouldn't look to hurt ourselves in an attempt to improve our fitness or health.*

Skill

To make physical activity a part of your lifestyle, you must choose activities that you find enjoyable and interesting. However, confidence in your ability to perform the activity increases the likelihood that you will enjoy what you are doing. To increase your skill in various activities, it is recommended that you receive instruction from an expert and then practice the activity on a regular basis. See the websites on professional organizations and sources of information on physical activity for more on finding expert advice.

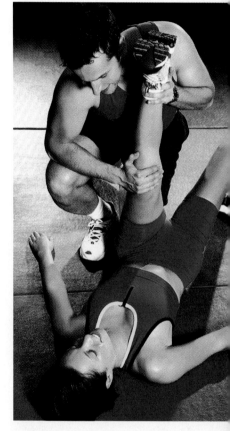

Qualified instruction can enhance your physical activity experience.

Psychological Factors

A number of psychological factors appear to influence participation in physical activity among adults (Sallis, 1994). Your personal beliefs about your physical abilities are usually related to your participation in physical activity. If you have a strong self-image and confidence regarding your ability to be regularly active, you are more likely to continue participating in physical activity. We know that both adults and children must enjoy physical activity if they are to continue it. One of the main determinants of whether a person enjoys an activity is the degree of exertion required by that activity (Sallis, 1994). Not surprisingly, children and adults usually prefer activities with lower levels of exertion. Dropout rates are significantly higher from vigorous activities than from moderate-intensity activities. Examples of lower-intensity activities include walking and gardening. More vigorous activities include running, heavy weight lifting, or rock climbing. Chapter 3 contains more information on psychological barriers to physical activity.

Social and Environmental Factors

The social and physical environment in which you live may also supply barriers to physical activity. These barriers could be community based, or they may be individual in nature. If you live in a community that does not provide adequate outlets for being physically active, this may be a barrier to your participation. Some communities have developed centers to provide facilities for recreational sport and exercise options; others have built walking, cycling, or roller blading trails to provide another outlet for being physically active.

Support from friends, coworkers, or family members affects individual adherence to activity programs (Sallis, 1994). Another societal factor, important to some parents, is the availability of child care. For adolescents, the influence of peers is extremely important. The younger the child, the more influential parents are. Parents can be supportive by being a role model, providing encouragement, and directly helping children to be active through participating in activities with them, organizing activities, or transporting children to places where they can be active.

Climate and weather, sedentary leisure activities, and the availability of labor-saving devices may also prove to be barriers to physical activity (Sallis, 1994). We must counter these barriers by providing safe and attractive space for outdoor activities, and access to exercise equipment, facilities, and programs.

Other Barriers

Other barriers to physical activity include age, gender, previous injury, genetics, cultural environment, biological factors such as weight and age, educational level, and economic status (Sallis, 1994). Activity tends to decrease across the age span, with the decline starting with entry into school. Women and girls have been traditionally less active than men and boys at virtually all ages. A partial explanation for this may relate to the different socialization processes boys and girls experience. Another factor that may prove to be a barrier to physical activity is a previous history of injury. Once a person has been injured, the likelihood of continuing to be active diminishes. We also know that people with higher educational levels and a more secure financial status participate in physical activity programs at higher rates than others, so educational and socioeconomic barriers must be considered. Individuals who understand the benefits of being active, who can afford the time, and who have greater opportunity for exposure to a variety of activities are more active.

Contrary to popular belief, activity levels in childhood are not always reliable predictors of becoming a physically active adult (Sallis, 1994). One potential explanation for this might be that many children are taught activities like team sports that are difficult to carry over to adulthood (Sallis, 1994). We must ensure that children are exposed to individual activities if we wish to have a carryover effect into adulthood.

Exercise Program Adherence

Many factors affect program adherence. Perhaps the most important is establishing regular physical activity as a priority in your life. Once activity becomes self-motivated, adherence is no longer a problem. Several categories of factors are related to exercise program adherence (Heyward, 2002). The first category includes **biological factors** such as being overweight. Sometimes people who are overweight, or who have a high proportion of fat to muscle, find activity difficult to perform because of the mechanical stresses placed upon the body. They may also feel uncomfortable exercising around others, or be dissatisfied with their own appearance when dressed in exercise attire.

The second category includes **psychological factors** such as self-motivation, self-efficacy, the attainment of exercise goals, and depression/anxiety/introversion. These factors all relate to how you perceive yourself. You need to ask yourself, are you confident in your ability to perform certain activities properly? Do you feel good about yourself?

Adhering to your program ensures an active lifestyle.

Biological factors Factors related to your biology that affect your adherence to an activity program.

Psychological factors Factors related to your state of mind that affect your adherence to an activity program.

The third category includes **social factors** such as family support, family problems, exercise/job conflicts, and income and education levels. Are the social aspects of your life conducive to your participation in a physical activity program?

The fourth category includes **behavioral factors** such as smoking, leisure time availability and use, and Type A behavior. Do negative lifestyle behaviors interfere with your ability to get the most out of yourself physically?

The final category includes **program factors** such as social support (group vs. individual exercise), location and convenience of an activity facility, activity leadership and supervision, initial activity intensity, variety of activity options, and program costs. Is it easy for you to be active?

> **Social factors** Factors from your social environment that affect your adherence to an activity program.
>
> **Behavioral factors** Factors related to your behavior patterns that affect your adherence to an activity program.
>
> **Program factors** Factors related to your physical activity program that affect your adherence to that program.

Strategies to Increase Adherence

The best strategies for increasing adherence include individualizing your program, finding activities you like, and scheduling the activities into your lifestyle. The importance of scheduling the activity is that you ensure having the time to be physically active (make it a priority), you develop a sense of consistency, and you reinforce its importance in your life.

Exercising with others has been shown to be effective for some people. Knowing that someone else is depending on them to show up for an exercise session will make some people show up those days even when they don't feel like exercising for themselves. Others prefer to exercise alone.

The following strategies can increase physical activity program adherence (Heyward, 2002). In developing your activity program, incorporate both group and individual activities; select times and locations that are convenient for you; select a variety of exercise and fitness activities; monitor your progress toward your goals; set realistic short-term and long-term goals; educate yourself about exercise, physical fitness, and health benefits; reward yourself for maintaining a regular activity program; and encourage social support.

If you prefer to exercise under the direction of an exercise leader, choose one who is a positive role model, shows interest in participants (follow-up phone calls when you have several unexplained absences, for example), exhibits enthusiasm, develops good rapport with program participants (learns their names), rewards accomplishments of participants, motivates and encourages participants to make a long-term commitment to exercise, and attends to orthopedic and musculoskeletal problems of participants.

According to the National Institutes of Health (1995), physical activity is more likely to be initiated and maintained if the individual perceives a net benefit, chooses an enjoyable activity, feels competent doing the activity, feels safe doing the activity, can easily access the activity on a regular basis, can fit the activity into the daily schedule, feels that the activity does not generate undue financial or social costs, experiences a minimum of negative consequences (injury, loss of time, negative peer pressure, problems with self-identity), is able to address issues of competing time demands, and recognizes the need to balance the use of laborsaving devices and sedentary activities with activities that involve a higher level of physical exertion.

Group activities are preferred by some people.

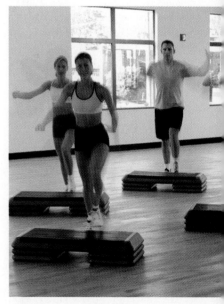

Physical Activity and Intrinsic Motivation

To enhance **intrinsic motivation**, Whitehead (1993) suggests that we do emphasize individual mastery; don't overemphasize peer comparisons of performance; do promote perceptions of choice; don't undermine an intrinsic focus by misusing extrinsic rewards; do promote the intrinsic fun and excitement of exercise; don't turn

> **Intrinsic motivation** Performing a behavior (being active) because you want to rather than because some outside influence is motivating you to do it.

exercise into a bore or a chore; do promote a sense of purpose by teaching the value of physical activity to health, optimal function, and quality of life; and don't create a motivation by spreading fitness misinformation. Rather than relying on a bland repetitive "diet" of a physical activity, we should think of a "menu" in which taste is enhanced by new "recipes," and the "sugar and spice" of fun, excitement, and thrills are added in (Whitehead, 1993).

Safety and Effectiveness

The cornerstones of any physical activity program are safety and effectiveness. If you get hurt when physically active, the point of the activity is lost. Remember that we are physically active to improve our health, to look better, and to feel better. Injury is counterproductive to these outcomes. Many people make physical activity unsafe by trying to rush results. Patience is crucial to reducing the risk of injury.

An effective activity program is one that allows you to reach your goals and objectives and one that makes you wish to continue to be physically active. By following the suggestions outlined in this book, an effective program is ensured.

Overtraining and Overuse Syndrome

Physical activity can provide wonderful benefits to those who participate regularly. However, too much physical activity can be harmful. Remember that what constitutes too much activity for one may be nothing more than a warm-up for another. In other words, too much exercise is relative to your state of fitness.

If you exercise at a level well beyond your current state of fitness (overtrain), you may develop a condition called **overuse syndrome**. Overuse syndrome may involve symptoms of fatigue, lethargy, depression, more frequent colds and illnesses, muscular strain, joint soreness, and feelings of being overwhelmed. Overuse syndrome may be caused by a variety of factors, including an inadequate warm-up, poor conditioning, ill-fitting or worn-out shoes, biomechanical abnormalities, rushing results, or differences in activity surfaces. The best way to prevent overuse syndrome is to plan carefully, follow the plan, progress gradually, and listen to your body. If you start to feel that your body is not responding the way it should be, you need to reassess what you are doing.

Overuse syndrome Condition in which too much exercise or physical activity causes the body to start to break down (symptoms: increased risk of injury, lethargy, loss of appetite, irritability, decreased motivation).

Injuries

The *Surgeon General's Report on Physical Activity and Health* (USDHHS, 1996a) suggests that being active may increase your risk for getting injured. However, most musculoskeletal injuries related to physical activity are believed to be preventable if you gradually work up to a desired level of activity and avoid excess. Serious cardiovascular events can occur with physical exertion, but the net effect of regular physical activity is a lower risk of mortality from cardiovascular disease. Shephard (1994) explains that a big fear is that an activity program will provoke a fatal heart attack. However, the risk that vigorous physical activity will provoke a cardiac emergency is low—about one death per 400,000 hours of jogging—and this risk is even lower in those who are regularly active (Shephard, 1994).

Proper prescreening will further lower this risk. The American College of Sports Medicine (2006) outlines factors to be considered in prescreening subjects, including the age of the subject (males over 45, females over 55), the proposed intensity of effort, and associated symptoms or major cardiac risk factors. A common rule to follow in beginning an activity program is that it is better to progress slowly and possibly delay benefits than to rush into activities for which your body is not prepared and risk injury.

A variety of injuries may be related to improper exercise. These include muscular strains, ligamentous sprains, and more serious injuries such as heart attack or stroke. By planning carefully and following directions properly, we know that the risk of injury is lessened. If an injury occurs, it is best to seek professional medical advice.

Being active can also play an important role in the recovery from an injury. Injured muscles lose strength and fitness. Being active is the best way to regain these lost attributes. Remember that just because you have an injury in one part of your body, you should not neglect using other parts of your body. Water-based activity is a therapeutic modality that allows you to stress healthy portions of your body while protecting injured areas. It is best to seek your physician's advice on what you can and cannot do when injured. For more information on injuries, see Appendix A.

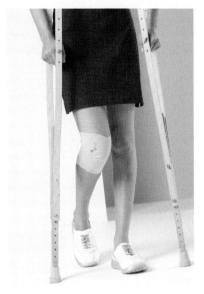

Too much activity for your level of fitness can lead to injury.

Physical Activity and Health Connection

Regular participation in a physical activity program provides many health benefits, including the prevention of hypokinetic diseases. Physical activity improves the function of the heart, lungs, muscles, and bones, leading to better health and lowered risk for injury. Being active has also been shown to improve immune function, decreasing the likelihood of catching colds, and allowing you to recover faster. Recent evidence indicates that physical activity is an important factor in the health of women. Activity increases bone mass and reduces the risk for osteoporosis. We now know that we don't have to torture ourselves with exhaustive exercise to obtain health benefits. In fact, regular participation in low- to moderate-intensity physical activity for 30 minutes on most days of the week provides significant health benefit. Physical activity and health are interconnected. You cannot have good health without being physically active.

concept connections

1. **Being physically active provides many health benefits.** An active lifestyle has been shown to provide physical and mental health benefits. You do not need to exercise vigorously to obtain these benefits. Simple daily activity can help you to live longer and with a higher quality of life.

2. **A safe and effective physical activity program requires proper preparation.** To obtain optimal benefit from a physical activity program, you need to make sure you are prepared to be active, you need to know if there are any medical limitations to your being active, you need to be aware of how much activity you can handle safely, and you need to make sure that your body is prepared to participate in the activity you have selected.

3. **How much activity you need is dependent on your goals, interests, and fitness level.** There are two recommended guidelines for physical activity. The first focuses solely on health benefit. These goals require that you accumulate 30 minutes of moderate-intensity physical activity on most if not all days of the week. The second set of goals is for the attainment of the optimal health and fitness benefit. These guidelines require that you exercise at moderate to vigorous intensities, 3 to 5 days per week, for 20 to 60 minutes. These guidelines should be met in addition to the first set of guidelines.

Optimize your benefits by individualizing your program. To achieve optimal health and fitness benefits and to make sure that the physical activity program you start is one that you will adhere to, be certain the program is developed with your particular likes and dislikes taken into consideration. The program must be enjoyable and help lead you to meet your individual goals and objectives. Your physical activity program should reflect your personality and lifestyle.

 A flexible approach is important in overcoming obstacles to physical activity. There are many factors that may interfere with your desires to be more active. You need to deal with these factors by developing a physical activity program that meets your needs within the limitations of your lifestyle. Being flexible in developing your program will allow you to find activities that you can fit into your daily routine and provide the health benefits you desire. An important first step is to give being active a higher priority. Second, make sure you are active because you desire to be active and not because someone else is forcing you to be active.

 Adhering to your program ensures an active lifestyle. The benefits of being physically active are transient. Any benefits you achieve will disappear over a period of time if you do not continue to be active. Adhering to a physical activity program is therefore crucial if you wish to live a life that is both long and of high quality.

Terms

Degeneration, 23
Atrophy, 23
Organ system, 23
Response, 23
Adaptation, 23
Hypokinetic diseases, 26
Aerobic, 30
Anaerobic, 30
Individualized, 33
Variability, 33
Heritability, 33

Initial stage, 34
Progression stage, 34
Maintenance stage, 34
Cardiorespiratory fitness, 36
Body composition, 36
Muscular strength, 36
Muscular endurance, 36
Flexibility, 36
Overload principle, 37
Principle of progression, 37
Principle of specificity, 37

Principle of reversibility, 37
Principle of individuality, 37
Principle of recovery, 38
Biological factors, 40
Psychological factors, 40
Social factors, 41
Behavioral factors, 41
Program factors, 41
Intrinsic motivation, 41
Overuse syndrome, 42

making the connection

Bob has learned that regular physical activity has numerous beneficial physiological effects, especially when it comes to the cardiovascular and musculoskeletal systems. He has also learned that participating in a prescreening program is an essential step toward ensuring safety and effectiveness. Finally, he has learned the basic principles that govern how the body responds to the physical stress of physical activity.

Critical Thinking

1. Unfortunately, sometimes it takes an incident (Bob's grandfather having a heart attack) to motivate our change of behavior. However, based on what Bob has learned, he is beginning to make a physical activity plan for himself. You can do the same. One step in the planning process is overcoming barriers to physical activity (page 39). Identify the barriers *you* have for participating in regular physical activity. Make sure you consider time and skill, as well as psychological, social, and environmental fac-

tors. Review the barriers you have listed, ask yourself *why* they are barriers, and list several ways you might begin overcoming each one.

2. Physical activities, like your nutrition habits, need to have variety. To maintain a physically active lifestyle, you will want to have a variety of activities to participate in; otherwise, you will get bored doing the same activity all the time. List five activities in which you would enjoy participating (e.g., hiking, basketball, jogging, biking). For each activity, find someone (social support) who also likes to do the activity, or find a university, college, or community club that supports the activity. Begin making plans to participate in different activities, to add spice to your life!

3. "I just don't have time!" This is commonly heard when referring to physical activity. What you need to do is examine *how* you spend your time and determine how you can make time for physical activity. Keep a diary of what you do daily. Include when you get up, classes you attend, breakfast, lunch, dinner, work schedule, study time, time spent with friends, and time spent watching TV. Look at your daily patterns. When can you make time for physical activity? If there isn't an hour block of time, do you have two 30-minute blocks? Can't find 30 minutes? How about 15 minutes? As your daily diary builds, you will be able to see when you can fit physical activity in your daily routine, and soon you'll be saying "I make time to be physically active!"

References

American Cancer Society. (2005). *Breast Cancer* (Publication 3002.02). Atlanta, GA: Author.

American College of Sports Medicine. (1998). Position stand: The recommended quantity and quality of exercise for developing and maintaining cardiorespiratory and muscular fitness, and flexibility in healthy adults. *Medicine and Science in Sports and Exercise* 30(6):975–991.

American College of Sports Medicine. (2006). *ACSM's Guidelines for Exercise Testing and Prescription*, 7th ed. Baltimore: Lippincott, Williams & Wilkins.

American Heart Association. (2005). http://www.americanheart.org.

Beunen, G., & Thomis, M. (2004). Gene powered? Where to go from heritability (h^2) in muscle strength and power. *Exercise and Sport Science Reviews* 32(4):148–154.

Bouchard, C. (1993). Heredity and health-related fitness. *President's Council on Physical Fitness and Sports Research Digest* 1(4):1–8.

Centers for Disease Control and Prevention, National Center for Chronic Disease Prevention and Health Promotion. (2005). Physical activity for everyone: Recommendations. Online: http://www.cdc.gov/nccdphp/dnpa/physical/recommendations/.

Coyle, E.F. (1990). Detraining and retention of training-induced adaptations. *Sports Science Exchange* 2(23).

Franks, B.D. (1997). Personalizing physical activity prescription. *President's Council on Physical Fitness and Sports Research Digest* 2(9):1–8.

Heyward, V.H. (2002). *Advanced Fitness Assessment and Exercise Prescription*, 4th ed. Champaign, IL: Human Kinetics.

National Institutes of Health. (1995). *Physical Activity and Cardiovascular Health: NIH Consensus Statement*. Kensington, MD: NIH Consensus Program Information Center.

Sallis, J.F. (1994). Influences on physical activity of children, adolescents, and adults, or determinants of active living. *President's Council on Physical Fitness and Sports Research Digest* 1(7):1–8.

Shephard, R.J. (1994). Readiness for physical activity. *President's Council on Physical Fitness and Sports Research Digest* 1(5):1–8.

United States Department of Health and Human Services. (1996a). *Physical Activity and Health: A Report of the Surgeon General. Executive Summary*. Washington, DC: Author.

United States Department of Health and Human Services. (1996b). *A Report of the Surgeon General: Physical Activity and Health, Women*. Washington, DC: Author.

United States Department of Health and Human Services. (2005). *Women's Health USA 2005*. Rockville, MD: Author. Online: http://mchb.hrsa.gov/whusa_05/pages/0402pa.htm.

Whitehead, J.R. (1993). Physical activity and intrinsic motivation. *President's Council on Physical Fitness and Sports Research Digest* 1(2):1–9.

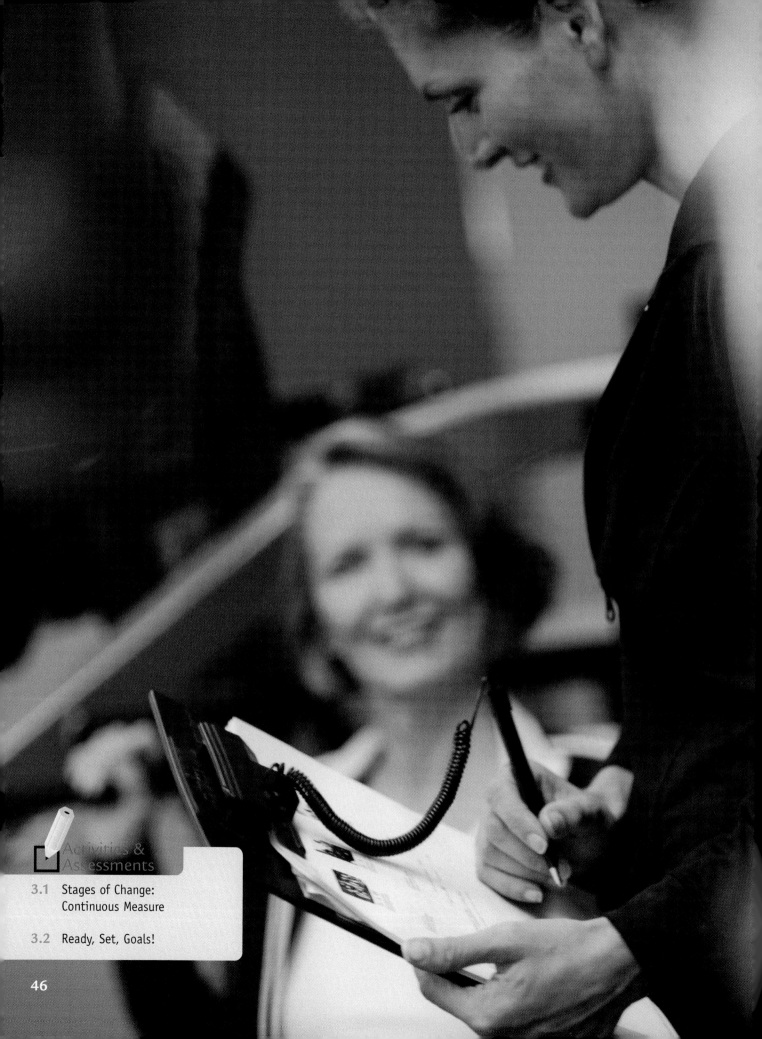

Activities & Assessments

3.1   Stages of Change:
      Continuous Measure

3.2   Ready, Set, Goals!

Understanding and Enhancing Health Behaviors

what's the connection?

John is 20 years old, a college sophomore majoring in telecommunications and earning mostly A's. John is well liked by his classmates and is socially active in his fraternity. When he experienced low-back pain and visited the college health center, the attending physician noted that he was overweight with slightly elevated blood pressure. Questioned about physical activity, John said he doesn't exercise at all. "Exercise involves a lot of discomfort and requires too much effort. The idea of participating in an activity whose mantra is 'No pain, no gain' just doesn't appeal to me," he explained. "Besides," he continued, "I'm way too busy and don't have time to exercise. I'm here to receive treatment for low-back pain, not to start a physical activity program."

concepts

1. A self-change approach assumes that we can manage and control our own lives.

2. The transtheoretical model of behavior change is a change model that is based on a time or temporal dimension (*trans*) using well-established psychological theories (*theoretical*) of behavior change.

3. The stages of change are a variable process that is organized in a continuum according to the decision-making process that is required to effect change.

4. Understanding or predicting when change occurs related to a specific behavior can largely be explained by decisional balance and self-efficacy.

5. The processes of change represent the mechanisms through which different techniques influence a change.

6. Successful behavior change requires a careful assessment of exactly what it is that you want to change.

http://physicalactivity.jbpub.com

The Web site for this book is a great source for supplementary physical health information for both students and instructors. Visit **http://physicalactivity.jbpub.com** to find a variety of useful tools for learning, thinking, and teaching.

Introduction

Lifestyle is the single most important and modifiable factor influencing health and disease today (see Figure 1.3). We described a healthy lifestyle as a recurring pattern of health-promoting and disease-preventing behaviors undertaken to achieve wellness (Chapter 1). Reducing risky behaviors is important in disease prevention. Risky behaviors eventually translate into disease, disability, and premature death. Focusing on risky behaviors rather than specific diseases is crucial because one risk factor can result in or worsen several major diseases and conditions. For example, physical inactivity plays a major role in cardiovascular disease, diabetes, high blood pressure, obesity, and osteoporosis. Alcohol misuse and abuse contributes to dementia (neurological damage and memory loss), cirrhosis, cancer of the liver, and injuries and death due to accidents and violence. Unsafe sexual practices can lead to HIV/AIDS, other sexually transmitted infections, and unwanted pregnancies. These practices and other similar preventive actions constitute **primary prevention**—actions that keep the disease process or health condition from becoming established in the first place by eliminating causes of disease or increasing resistance to disease.

There are two additional types or levels of interventions valuable in disease prevention. **Secondary prevention** aims at early detection of asymptomatic disease through preventive screenings and tests. Routine screenings can identify a previously undiagnosed condition or potential risk of a condition early in the disease process before it becomes symptomatic. For example, screening for high blood pressure or high blood lipids is important in identifying individuals who may be at risk for cardiovascular disease. This allows primary care medical professionals to intervene early with treatments to control the disease before it progresses. When coupled with lifestyle changes, these treatments are much more effective. Unfortunately, many Americans do not routinely follow some basic health screening recommendations.

Tertiary prevention is treatment after a person is already ill and is typically offered by medical specialists. Examples are bypass surgery or angioplasty to treat coronary artery disease. The methods are designed to limit the physical and social consequences of disease or injury *after* it has occurred or become symptomatic. However, these methods are extremely expensive and, more often than not, fail to restore people to the same health status they enjoyed before acquiring the disease.

> **Primary prevention** Actions that keep the disease process or health condition from becoming established in the first place by eliminating causes of disease or increasing resistance to disease.
>
> **Secondary prevention** Aims at early detection of asymptomatic disease through preventive screenings and tests.
>
> **Tertiary prevention** Treatment after a person is already ill; typically offered by medical specialists.

Health Habits

Pursuing healthy habits related to chronic disease prevention now may not seem important. Take the example of brushing your teeth, however: it prevents a lot of pain later from a dentist needing to use a high-speed drill to remove the decay (cavity) and prepare the tooth for a filling. Clean teeth look better too, and fresh breath is much more appealing. Similarly, healthy habits not only prevent or delay the onset of many chronic killers, but also add sparkle and vitality to our lives. You may be thinking that lifestyle-related chronic diseases are not likely to affect you at your age, and hopefully you are right. However, that does not mean that your current lifestyle is not contributing to the development of many disease processes, many of which may be currently without symptoms. Seven of the 10 leading causes of death each year are the result of degenerative chronic diseases (Centers for Disease Control and Prevention [CDC], 2004). The underlying causes of these deaths are common health habits that can be successfully modified years before they ultimately contribute to morbidity and needless suffering (Cifuentes et al., 2005; Kotecki et al., 2004). In fact, some health experts believe that today's youth and young adults are on their way to becoming the

As a college student you are developing a personal health lifestyle, which, with slight modifications, you will likely follow for the rest of your life.

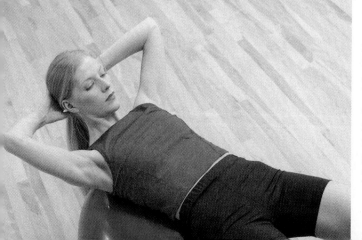

first generation in modern times who will have a shorter life expectancy than their parents due to their poor health habits (Olshansky et al., 2005). Therefore, it has become more important than ever to practice good health behaviors and eliminate detrimental ones as early in life as possible.

As a college student you are developing a personal health lifestyle, which, with slight modifications, you will likely follow for the rest your life. Every action you choose sets into motion a behavior that may become a health habit. A **health habit** is a health-related behavior that is firmly established and often performed automatically, without thought. Although the habit may have developed because it was reinforced by specific positive outcomes, eventually it becomes independent of the reinforcement process and is maintained by the environmental factors with which it is customarily associated (Hunt, Matarazzo, Weiss, & Gentry, 1979). As such, the habit can be highly resistant to change. The good news is that there are comprehensive self-change strategies available for modifying deeply rooted harmful behaviors.

Self-Change Approach

When you think about it, there is something truly remarkable in the fact that practically all of us want to be better than we are. Life continually presents us with opportunities for achieving what we desire. Most of us strive to be **self-changers.** A *self-change* approach assumes that we can manage and control our own lives. Self-change means that our behavior is under our control—that when it is necessary to change, we can do it. We want to be able to control our behavior so that we can change in a desired way, increasing physical activity if we are sedentary, and managing stress more effectively if we are feeling overwhelmed. Self-change means recognizing the changes you want and being able to actualize your own values. When it comes to an unhealthy lifestyle behavior, it can be a difficult task to change, however, because the thoughts we have fed our behavior for so long are deeply ingrained in our mind, and the habit of thought is hard to break. Many times our good intentions result in an unsuccessful attempt at behavior change. These failed attempts may occur because we pursue things the wrong way. Instead, we must learn to adequately prepare or ready ourselves for our eventual change.

Making important lifestyle changes—such as quitting smoking, becoming physically active, switching from junk food to nutritious food, or managing stress—requires that we go through a series of stages to adequately prepare or ready ourselves for that eventual change. Behavioral research suggests that you will more likely succeed if you think of change as a journey. It helps to have a map and to know where you are heading, the best ways to get there, and the ways to travel without getting lost or running into detours. There exists such a map and we will discuss it next. This map will keep you from getting lost and repeating errors that caused your previous good intentions to result in failures. It charts the path that successful self-changers have followed. The approach is simple to understand and makes a lot of sense when it comes to modifying problem behaviors and adding new, healthier behaviors.

A Step-by-Step Approach to Behavior Change

The **transtheoretical model of behavior change (TTM)** is a change model that is based on a time or temporal dimension (*trans*) using well-established psychological theories (*theoretical*) of behavior change (Prochaska, Norcross, & DiClemente, 1994). Contrary to its long name, the TTM is a user-friendly model of change that is unique in four ways. First, it is evidence based—that means that the conclusions

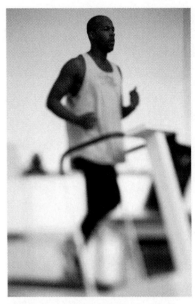
Physical activity increases the likelihood of enjoying a more satisfying life.

A self-change approach assumes that we can manage and control our own lives.

Health habit A health-related behavior that is firmly established and often performed automatically, without thought.
Self-changers Individuals who can manage and control their own lives.
Transtheoretical model of behavior change (TTM) A change model that is based on a time or temporal dimension (*trans*) using well-established psychological theories (*theoretical*) of behavior change.

The transtheoretical model of behavior change is a change model that is based on a time or temporal dimension (*trans*) using well-established psychological theories (*theoretical*) of behavior change.

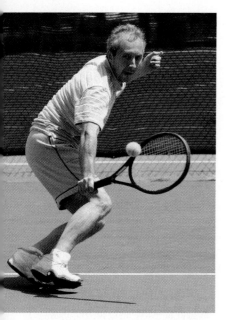

Physically active people are likely to be healthier and more vigorous later in life.

Stages of change A variable process that is organized in a continuum according to the decision-making process that is required to effect change.

have come out of many scientific studies of various individuals. By studying thousands of successful self-changers, scientists were able to describe how these individuals followed a commanding and controllable course to change a wide range of problem behaviors.

Second, the model conceptualizes change in *stages*, or as points on a motivational continuum that essentially begins with a firm conviction to maintain the status quo by never changing (precontemplation) and proceeds through the conditions of intending to change someday (contemplation), soon (preparation), now (action), and forever (maintenance). The basic premise is that behavior change is a process and not an event, and that individuals are found at varying levels of motivation, or readiness, to change. They change their behavior incrementally or in a stepwise fashion.

Third, the model depicts change as a cycle as opposed to a linear progression. Typically, people move back and forth along the readiness continuum. It is not reasonable to expect everyone to be able to modify a habit perfectly without any slips. This cyclical nature of change is a normal part of the change process, indicating that it may take several trips through the various stages to make lasting change. Fourth, each stage requires its own unique set of *processes*, or things people must think about or do, in order to be successful in moving through the stages. Let's look at these distinctive features more closely.

Stages of Change or Motivational Readiness

The TTM has identified five **stages of change** that people go through along their way to eliminating problem behaviors or adopting new healthy habits. The stages of change are a variable process that is organized in a continuum according to the decision-making process that is required to effect change.

Precontemplation is the stage during which individuals are not intending to make a long-term lifestyle change in the foreseeable future (usually the next 6

Successful self-changers recognize that behavioral change is a process.

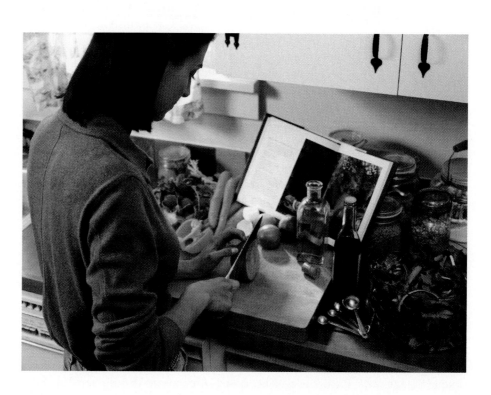

months); this is the "I won't" stage. Individuals in this stage are either unaware, unwilling, or too discouraged to change. They may be unaware of the risks associated with their behaviors. Or they may think, "It can't happen to me" or "It's not that serious." Or, they may want to change but do not intend to take action because they may have become discouraged as a result of being unsuccessful in previous attempts to change. A precontemplator may feel safe because he or she can't fail in this stage.

Having read Chapters 1 and 2, you hopefully have discarded any lingering skepticism about the importance of regular physical activity. It should be perfectly clear that your regular participation in physical activity is vital for your health and well-being, especially as you move further through adulthood.

The **contemplation** stage begins when the individual starts to think seriously about intending to make a long-term change in the near future (within 6 months); this is the "I might" stage. In this stage, individuals are more open to information and want to learn more. They have become more aware of the problem behavior, but have not yet made a commitment to act. Contemplators are not completely convinced that the effort to change is worth it and have indefinite plans to take action. It is easy to be stuck in this stage for a very long time.

Since you are reading this book, you are at least considering beginning a regular physical activity program even if it has been some time since you previously engaged in this important health behavior. You may now be thinking about getting in better shape, and specifically about how and where you might begin in the near future.

The **preparation** stage is when the individual intends to take action in the immediate future (usually in the next month); this is the "I will" stage. People in this stage realize that the behavior change is an important part of who they are. Preparers believe the effort to change is worth it and begin figuring out the best way to go about taking behavioral action. Although they have made a firm commitment to change, no consistent action has taken place.

In this stage, you feel certain that you will begin a regular exercise program soon. You might have already checked out various exercise facilities (e.g., weight room, track, basketball and tennis courts) that your college offers, signed up for an aerobics class, or talked to a friend about walking or running with you on a regular basis. Additionally, as you continue to read the ensuing chapters you will have a better understanding of what types of activities are right for you.

In the **action** stage, the desired level of the new behavior has been reached, and it is consistently adhered to although the individual has been doing it for less than 6 months; this is the "I am" stage. The individual has made significant effort to change and, more important, has achieved some degree of success with the change. Action takers need to be recognized and their new behaviors reinforced so that they continue their new behavior. Some encouragement and social support is essential because the risk for relapse in this stage is relatively high.

Have you started exercising with the intention of continuing on a regular basis? If so, you are in the action stage. In the past, you may have found it hard to adhere to an exercise program for more than a month or two. If this is the case, you will find many suggestions in this and subsequent chapters to help sustain you.

The **maintenance** stage is when the behavioral practice is becoming habit; this is the "I have" stage. People in this stage are strongly committed to their changed behavior and have maintained the desired level for more than 6 months. Maintainers have a much lower risk of relapse than action takers. Generally, the maintenance stage lasts for up to about 5 years for many health behaviors. As the maintenance of the desired behavior becomes lengthened, heightened resistance to relapse develops over time; individuals could theoretically exit the stages of change and find themselves in the termination stage.

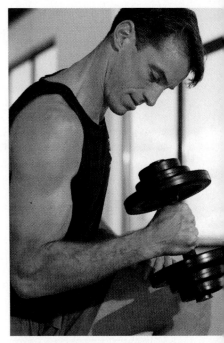

Weight lifting is an excellent form of physical activity.

The stages of change are a variable process that is organized in a continuum according to the decision-making process that is required to effect change.

Precontemplation Stage of change during which individuals are not intending to make a long-term lifestyle change in the foreseeable future (usually the next 6 months).

Contemplation Stage of change that begins when the individual starts to think seriously about intending to make a long-term change in the near future (within 6 months).

Preparation Stage of change in which the individual intends to take action in the immediate future (usually in the next month).

Action Stage of change in which the desired level of the new behavior has been reached and is consistently adhered to, although the individual has been doing it for less than 6 months.

Maintenance Stage of change in which the behavioral practice is becoming habit.

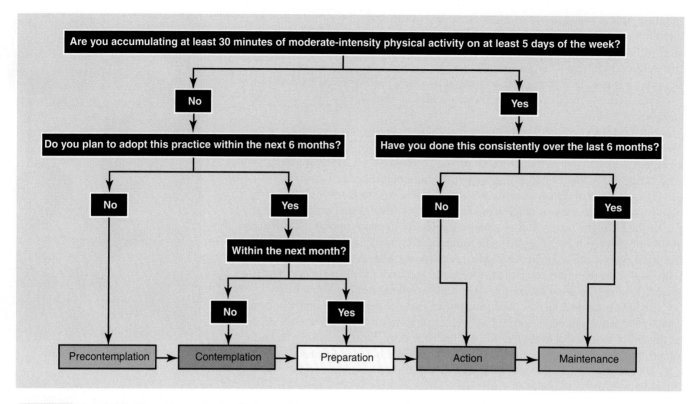

FIGURE 3.1 Assessing Your Stage or Readiness to Change.

Termination Stage of change in which the individual's former problem behavior represents no threat or temptation; it denotes the concept of exiting the stages of change or the cycle of change.

Spiral model of change A relapse model that demonstrates that individuals move back and forth along the change continuum a number of times before attaining their behavioral goal and therefore views setbacks as positive because changers are learning something new every time they change.

The **termination** stage is when the individual's former problem behavior represents no threat or temptation. People in this stage have complete confidence that they will cope without fear of relapse. They no longer are in the stages of change as it relates to a problem behavior. Termination is not a practical reality for most health behaviors, and is alluded to here solely to denote the concept of exiting the stages of change or the cycle of change.

Look at the flowchart in **FIGURE 3.1**. This is a useful visual aid for understanding the stages of change. By answering each question, you can identify your current stage or degree of intention for meeting the current recommendation for obtaining moderate-intensity physical activity. You can also substitute a number of other lifestyle questions in place of physical activity in the flowchart. It is common to be at various stages of change for different behaviors.

Understanding Relapse: The Spiral Model of Change

Linear progression through each of the five stages is a possible but relatively rare occurrence. Typically, individuals move back and forth along the change continuum a number of times before attaining their behavioral goal. Thus, the stages of change are better conceptualized as *spiraling* rather than linear (Prochaska, Norcross, & DiClemente, 1994) (**FIGURE 3.2**). In the **spiral model of change**, the good news is that all of your setbacks can be viewed positively because the path you are taking is always spiraling upward. Looking at relapse or a slip in this manner means that you are learning something new every time you change.

Despite our best efforts, relapses remain the rule rather than the exception when it comes to solving most of our health behavior problems. We make mistakes because we are human; we are imperfect. It is normal at the time of our relapse to be conscious of our incompetencies while lacking awareness of our abilities. The

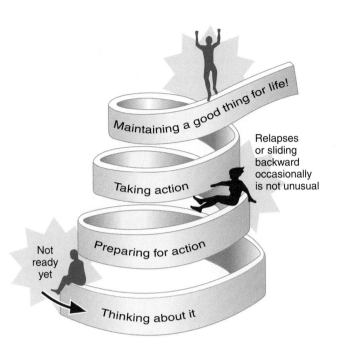

FIGURE 3.2 **The Spiral Model of Change.** These stages represent a spiral path to adopting healthy behaviors. SOURCE: Centers for Disease Control and Prevention, National Center for Chronic Disease Prevention and Health Promotion. (2005). Physical activity for everyone: Getting started. Online: http://www.cdc.gov/nccdphp/dnpa/physical/starting/index.htm.

feelings and beliefs evoked by relapse are not pleasant. You may feel that you have completely failed, which may lead to guilt or embarrassment. You may begin to believe all of your efforts were wasted. A couple of setbacks in succession may trigger your wanting to give up completely on changing the problem behavior, so you slide from the action or maintenance stage back to contemplation or precontemplation and decide that you have gained nothing from your attempts. This is where you are dead wrong!

Changing unfavorable behavior patterns or adopting favorable health-enhancing ones usually requires a number of attempts. For example, even though you intend to remain an ex-smoker when you quit, you may slip up and smoke a cigarette. Slips often occur with any behavior change. Do not think about yourself as a failure; instead, think about a slip as a learning experience. Most people are not completely successful in their first couple of attempts of health behavior change. Mark Twain summed it up this way: "Quitting smoking is easy. I've done it a thousand times." Regression or relapse may occur at any part of the change sequence, but most often it happens in the action stage. For example, more than half of the individuals who begin an exercise program quit within the first 6 months, and most people need four attempts or more before they finally can quit smoking permanently.

With the stages of change, the good news is that all your setbacks are positive because you are learning new things every time you try. We can always rechart our steps and, armed with experience, make some corrections. Corrections triggered by our relapses lead to increased learning and can be responsible for improved outcomes. Never is a task completed without some modifications along the way. In fact, relapses may be thought of as necessary to focus on our health behavior change. We need to dwell not on the relapse but on the remedy. You have to have a relapse plan ready for just such a time. You need to have strategies in place that will help you get back on track, such as the support of family and friends, or a membership to a gym, or the presence of a store near you that carries fresh fruits and vegetables. You have to keep renewing your commitment to change even when it seems hardest.

One of the major reasons for relapse is that we rush through stages too quickly. When changing health habits, it is better to make one small change at a time than a series of sudden and dramatic changes. The latter are likely to be short-lived and you are likely to regress to your old habits very quickly. The likelihood of successfully changing problem behaviors improves when you make slow but sure changes, which give you time to unlearn negative patterns and substitute positive ones. Again, we quote Mark Twain: "Habit is habit and not to be flung out the window by man, but coaxed downstairs a step at a time."

When and Why People Change

Understanding or predicting when change occurs related to a specific behavior can largely be explained by decisional balance and self-efficacy.

Understanding or predicting when change occurs related to a specific behavior can largely be explained by two measures: decisional balance and self-efficacy (Prochaska & Velicer, 1997). **Decisional balance** reflects the individual's relative weighing of the pros and cons of changing (Janis & Mann, 1977). The *pros* represent the positive aspects of changing, or the benefits of change. In contrast, the *cons* are the negative aspects of changing, or the costs of change. During the precontemplation stage, the cons far outweigh the pros. In the contemplation stage, the pros and cons are balanced evenly. In the preparation stage, the balance has shifted and the pros outweigh the cons. In the advanced stages of action and maintenance, the pros continue to mount.

Listing the pros and cons as you contemplate a specific health behavior change is essential. However, many people do not correctly weigh the health and lifestyle pros and cons regarding participating or not participating in specific behaviors. For example, people who lead a sedentary lifestyle may want to spend their spare time relaxing after work by watching television or playing computer games. They may believe that exercising instead would take too much time away from their favorite activity. They are confusing what they want with what they need regarding their health. Our cultural environment further contributes to this confusion of what we want and what we need. For instance, advertisers send the messages that alcohol drinking and cigarette smoking are pleasurable and that fattening fast foods are good tasting, all of which promise immediate positive experiences. We pride ourselves on our intelligence and know that many of these products lead to harmful effects. In spite of this, we are not particularly good at weighing the short-term benefits versus the long-term risks (Cloninger, 1987). This will lead many of us to engage in a risky behavior and opt for short-term pleasure over long-term benefits.

So slow down the decision-making process when you are listing your pros and cons and carefully consider the results of your specific behavior in both the short term and the long term. Become more familiar with the immediate short-term benefits associated with many health-promoting behaviors. In the previous example, people believed that participating in physical activity during their leisure time would cut into their relaxation time, as well as their television viewing time. Instead, they could relish the immediate reduction in mental and muscular tension that comes from taking a brisk 15-minute walk.

The other factor that greatly enhances motivation for change is self-efficacy. **Self-efficacy** is the confidence you have in your ability to perform specific behaviors in specific situations (Bandura, 1986). Self-efficacy assesses your belief that you can perform the behavior in order to achieve the desired outcome; it is your perceived confidence that you can change and maintain your behavior across a variety of difficult situations. Numerous research studies have substantiated what most people knew all along: people who strongly believe that they can initiate and adhere to a behavior change, do. What's more, they exert an elevated level of effort to accomplish this goal, persisting in the face of the difficulties that inevitably rise. Similarly, people who believe they will fail usually do. In other words, there is truth to the adage "Whether you believe you can, or whether you believe you can't, you are probably right."

Decisional balance An individual's relative weighing of the pros and cons of changing.

Self-efficacy The confidence one has in one's ability to perform specific behaviors in specific situations.

In studies that have measured the self-efficacy of people in different stages of change, self-efficacy has been found to increase steadily from precontemplation to contemplation to preparation, but rises significantly in the action and maintenance stages, when actual performance attainment is most evident and convincing. High self-efficacious persons invest more effort and persist longer to accomplish a specific behavior than those low in self-efficacy. Self-efficacy is specific to each behavior. A person who feels confident about exercising after work every day may have less belief in his or her ability to reduce saturated fat from his or her diet on a regular basis.

ENHANCING SELF-EFFICACY   According to Bandura (1986), there are four important ways that you can enhance self-efficacy: performance attainment, vicarious experience, verbal persuasion, and physiological states. *Performance attainments* are the most convincing because they are based on personal success experiences. Having swum on the high school swimming team will no doubt enhance your belief that you can choose swimming as part of your college physical activity program. *Vicarious experience* increases self-efficacy through observing the effective performances of others. If you are a nonswimmer, watching your friends swim may convince you that you can learn to swim. *Verbal persuasion*, or counseling, is thought to be less effective than vicarious experience, but it can be useful nevertheless to have a good friend talk you through the swim experience. Finally, *physiological states* may inform individuals (correctly or not) as to whether they are capable of performing a given action. You may feel a bit anxious about getting into the pool, but your friend reminds you that this is normal.

How People Change

The stages of change call attention to particular shifts that occur in intention and behavior. This part of the TTM describes nine processes that people engage in when they attempt to modify their behaviors (Prochaska, Norcross, & DiClemente, 1994). The processes were identified by asking people how they changed, what helped, and what made change more difficult. The **processes of change** represent the mechanisms through which different techniques influence a change. The processes are divided into two categories: cognitive/emotional (involving thinking, attitudes, and feelings) and behavioral (involving actions). Cognitive/emotional processes include (1) increasing knowledge, (2) experiencing negative emotions, (3) caring about others, (4) comprehending personal benefits, and (5) committing yourself; behavioral processes include (1) rewarding yourself, (2) eliciting social support, (3) substituting alternatives, and (4) reminding yourself.

    Furthermore, each stage requires its own unique set of processes, or things people must think about or do, in order to move successfully to the next stage (FIGURE 3.3). In summary, these processes are any activities you initiate to help modify your thinking, feelings, or behaviors to progress through the stages of change. Following is a brief description of the nine major processes of change, along with a single technique, that may be used to mediate change. It is important to remember that for each process there are a myriad of techniques that can be employed.

INCREASING KNOWLEDGE   This process requires assimilating accurate and detailed information so that you can have an advanced understanding of the behavior. For example, not only do you know that a sedentary lifestyle and unhealthy eating habits are harmful to your health, but you know that they are

The processes of change represent the mechanisms through which different techniques influence a change.

Processes of change The mechanisms through which different techniques influence a person's behavior change.

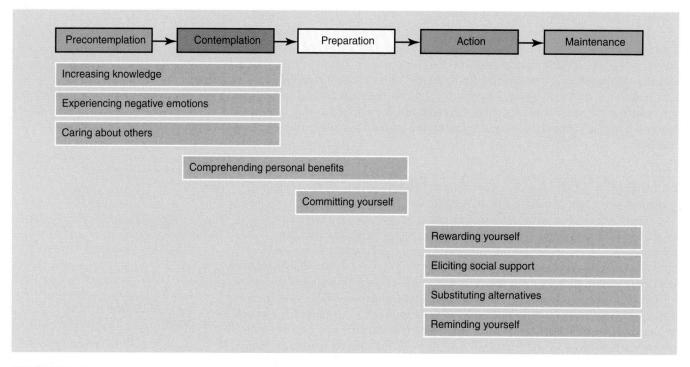

FIGURE 3.3 **The Process of Change, or How Change Occurs.**

linked to an increased risk of more than 20 physical ailments, as well as a number of psychological problems. One way to increase your knowledge or awareness related to your lifestyle is to measure what you are doing now. In the activities and assessments manual, we have provided paper-and-pencil assessments on the various topics covered in each chapter. The completion of each assessment assists you in determining which aspects of your personal behavior and habits can be left as they are and which need to be changed. By the time you have completed all of the assessments in this manual, you will have a better overall picture of the adequate and inadequate aspects of your current lifestyle.

EXPERIENCING NEGATIVE EMOTIONS   This process relates to a deeper way of increasing awareness by seeing when and how your problem behavior conflicts with your personal values. You begin to become afraid or fear the consequences of not participating in a particular health behavior. For example, how do you perceive yourself as a sedentary person? To express your emotions about it, try the following rational emotive technique recommended by Ellis and Harper (1971). Using a journal:

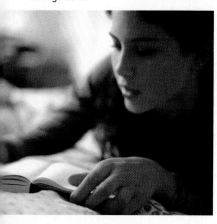

A daily planner is a helpful behavior change tool.

1. Record the events as they occurred at the time you felt emotionally uneasy about becoming physically active. Be objective and avoid judgments.
2. Next, write down your subjective assumptions, worries, and beliefs related to your emotions about becoming physically active.
3. Then, write down your emotions about physical activity, stating both appropriate and inappropriate emotions.
4. Finally, list your beliefs about why you had the right to be upset by the events and to respond the way you did. Is there support or truth for any of your beliefs? Explore appropriate alternative thoughts, emotions, and actions.

CARING FOR OTHERS   This process requires that you recognize the harmful effects of how participating in a problem behavior affects your family, friends, and others around you. A way to see if this is the case is to use a self-monitoring record-keeping technique. Record each of the times you practiced a problem behavior during the past 2 weeks. Next to each, write down whether you felt you were a poor role model for those around you or whether your problem behavior negatively affected others. For example, if you are a cigarette smoker, did children or young adults see you light up a cigarette or did others around you have to inhale the smoke from your cigarette?

COMPREHENDING PERSONAL BENEFITS   This process requires a thoughtful appraisal of what our self-concept or self-identity is like while continuing a problem behavior and what it would be after changing it. Several of the successes and failures that we experience in many areas of life are closely related to the ways that we have learned to view ourselves and our relationships with others. Some people tend to focus on their weaknesses rather than their strengths. For example, when it comes to exercise, they may see themselves as uncoordinated, too slow, or nonathletic. These are all self-limiting thoughts. Self-talk phrased in the negative regarding something positive is processed by the mind as a punishment and wastes valuable energy.

Instead, you could use positive affirmations or self-talk and thereby increase your self-concept regarding exercise. An *affirmation* is a statement that claims characteristics of the ideal self. Focus on your strengths rather than your weaknesses. Changing your statements to yourself to "I like to take brisk walks" or "I feel more confident when I exercise" or "I feel better about myself when I exercise" allows you to use energy as a positive search for ways that will eventually lead to your goal. Remember, your self-concept reflects years of experience and self-evaluation. It will take a few days to get to know and record the internal critic. Challenging or shutting up the critic may take weeks. Continually increase the number of positive affirmations you make about exercise. Self-talk, when positive, cultivates a healthy self-concept—one that offers security. Taking charge of the messages we send ourselves is an option that is always available to us.

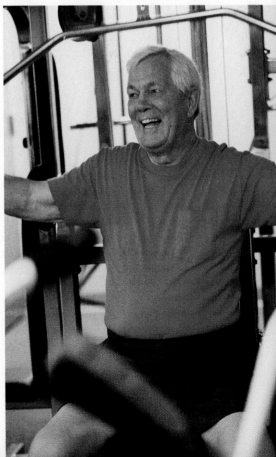

Repeated successful performances increase your confidence in your ability to perform the desired activity.

COMMITTING YOURSELF   This process is related to the belief that one can change and the commitment to act on that belief. Making a self-contract is a very helpful technique in this process. Try making a physical activity contract with yourself. This interpersonal agreement to act should be consistent with your physically active self-image. You must understand what motivates you to be physically active and write it down. Research shows that goals are more likely to be accomplished when they are written down. Don't just think it, ink it. Be as specific as possible in detailing your goal of physical activity (**FIGURE 3.4**). When you commit in writing what you want to accomplish, you increase the likelihood that you will act accordingly within a certain period of time. Eliciting this type of personal commitment has been shown to be one of the most important aspects of health behavior change, especially when you share this self-contract with others close to you.

REWARDING YOURSELF   This process is based on the fact that a response followed promptly by an effective reward (reinforcement) will be more likely to occur again. This is called the *law of effect*; it is the basis of operant conditioning and the major means of changing voluntary behavior. Periodically check your goals and reward yourself for your progress toward specific goals. Internal reinforcement is generally better than external.

FIGURE 3.4 **Self-Contract.** When you commit in writing what you want to accomplish, you increase the likelihood that you will act accordingly within a certain period of time.

Self-Contract

I _____ commit to begin a physical activity program.

Goal Type (Circle one)   Short-term   Mid-term   Long-term

Goal: _____

Date goal set: _____

Date you'd like to accomplish goal: _____

Date goal accomplished: _____

Plan of attack for accomplishing my goal: _____

_____

_____

Goal re-evaluation and change from first writing: _____

_____

_____

However, we recommend both. An internal reinforcement occurs when your own experience or perception of an event has value. For example, when you finish your run for the day, you feel a sense of enjoyment or accomplishment. Relive your positive experiences by stating aloud to yourself and others that you are proud of your recent accomplishments: "I feel good about myself after running 2 miles." Remember, positive self-talk allows a flow of positive energy that not only makes a goal obtainable but also can significantly assist in maintaining it. An external reinforcement would be providing yourself with a special treat, such as buying a new outfit when a short-term weight goal has been reached.

ELICITING SOCIAL SUPPORT   One of the most important external resources is the availability of social support. This process is defined as information from others that one is loved, cared for, valued, and esteemed. It is much easier to maintain your habit of regular physical activity if you are encouraged by others. Share your goals with your friends and family. Obtaining encouragement and support from significant people in your life is a powerful reinforcement for keeping you on your physical activity program. Social support can be obtained by signing up for an exercise class at your college or university or organizing your own physical activity group that meets regularly.

SUBSTITUTING ALTERNATIVES   The basic idea with this process is that you substitute an alternative healthy behavior for those behavior traits that lead to the problem behavior. Since all of our behavior is conditional, it becomes important to anticipate the trigger situations and then counter the urges you know are coming by substituting a healthier alternative. For example, if you know that around 8:00 p.m. every evening you start craving sweets, eat a piece of fruit—a snack that's low-calorie, nutritious, and somewhat sweet. Alternatively, substitute a brisk walk in place of eating the sweets. Physical activity reduces cravings as effectively as sweets and expends calories rather than accumulating them. Furthermore, even something like a short, brisk walk can enhance your mood and relieve stress as well as remove you physically from the temptation.

REMINDING YOURSELF   This process is similar to substituting alternatives in that it is action-oriented; however, cravings or temptations are eliminated by restructuring the environment to eliminate the stimulus. For example, try having cut-up fruit and vegetables ready to eat in the refrigerator rather than sweets like soda and ice cream. If you are a smoker, remove the ashtrays from the house. Other techniques include using reminder systems. Place positive reminders throughout your environment to prompt you. These reminders can take the form of notes left in places where you will see them, like your daily planner or the front of the refrigerator or television.

Making a Behavioral Change Plan

What one thing do you most want to change about your health this semester? It may be much too early to answer this question since you have not had the opportunity to read the remaining chapters of the book or complete the accompanying activities and assessments in the manual. Successful behavior change requires a careful assessment of exactly what it is that you want to change. Having a long laundry list of items only serves to discourage you, scatter your focus, and slow significant progress toward accomplishing even one goal. For instance, did you place becoming physically active at the top of the list and then follow that with four other items of equal importance? This may set the stage for failure. After assessing yourself, focus on one change; commit to it, and the rest may very well be addressed along the way. A resolution to achieve a healthy lifestyle, one goal at a time, opens the door to daily success.

If you are in the early cognitive stages of change—that is, thinking about whether the pros outweigh the cons of making the change (decisional balance) or making decisions about whether you have the skills and resources to make the necessary changes (self-efficacy), you may not be ready for behavioral action. However, if you have committed to changing one specific behavior, your motivation is high enough to begin to set actual behavioral goals (preparation stage).

Successful behavior change requires a careful assessment of exactly what it is that you want to change.

Setting SMART Goals

To properly set a goal, we recommend that you follow a set of standard guidelines. An effective expression of these guidelines is that you should set SMART goals. SMART stands for specific, measurable, attainable, relevant, and trackable.

- *Specific.* A specific goal has a much greater chance of being accomplished than a general goal. With a specific goal, you can clearly see what it is you want to achieve, and you have specific standards for that achievement. A general goal would be "get some physical activity." But a specific goal would be "I am going to make brisk walking part of my physical activity program."

- *Measurable.* A measurable goal establishes concrete criteria for quantifying progress. The goal needs to have a yardstick for measuring outcomes. It should take into account the principle of a specific goal as well. For example, "I am going to walk briskly for 30 minutes on Monday, Wednesday, and Friday."

- *Attainable.* A goal needs to stretch you slightly so you feel you can do it, and it will need a real commitment from you. Although it is important to set goals just out of our reach, it is imperative not to set goals that are so high that they are unattainable. If your goal is not attainable, chances are you will give up hope trying to reach it and quit. You may even want to break down your goal into different measured parts by setting short-term goals as well as long-term goals. Short-term goals are ones that you will achieve in the near future (e.g., in a day, within a week, or within a few months). Long-term goals are ones that you will achieve over a longer period of time (e.g., one semester, 1 year, 5 years, or 20 years).

- *Relevant.* Make sure the goal is consistent with other goals you have established for yourself and that it fits into your immediate and long-term plans. In other words, your goal should be important to you, rather than simply done as an assignment for class.

- *Trackable.* Trackable goals allow you to monitor your progress. By monitoring your progress, you will be able to see what you have achieved. Monitoring your progress is simply a case of writing down everything you did related to accomplishing your goal. For example, you may want to use the daily physical activity training logs in the activities and assessment manual to record your physical activity sessions or the food intake logs to monitor your diet.

The self-change worksheets in the activities and assessment manual are adapted to fit the stages of change. Using the flowchart in Figure 3.1, you will be able to assess your level of readiness for a number of health behaviors. Depending on your stage of readiness, your goals will be different. You will learn to write SMART goals.

Physical Activity and Health Connection

The path to obtaining a high quality of life, or a wellness lifestyle, lies in our behaviors. Our choices and subsequent actions make our lives what they are. They *do* make an enormous difference. With respect to overall health, no behaviors are more essential than performing regular stimulating physical activity and eating nutritious food. The human body is clearly designed for physical activity. If you want to remain healthy, regular physical activity should be part of your lifestyle.

In today's world, physical activity is a unique health behavior that encompasses a complex and dynamic range of behavioral demands. Planning for physical activity, its initial adoption, and your continued participation and maintenance involve different factors and justify different self-change techniques. In the first two chapters of this book we touted the many benefits of regular physical activity. As college instructors, we know that informing our students about the many benefits of physical activity is important, but not necessarily enough to get our students to do it regularly. To become and stay physically active takes time, effort, and, most importantly, the development of special self-change skills. This chapter provided you with a state-of-the-art, step-by-step approach to behavior change that utilized various skill-building strategies for building regular physical activity into your life. It concluded with ways to properly set a goal.

concept connections

1. **A self-change approach assumes that we can manage and control our own lives.** We want to be able to control our behavior so that we can change in a desired way, increasing physical activity if we are sedentary, and managing stress more effectively if we are feeling overwhelmed. Self-change means recognizing the changes you want and being able to actualize your own values.

2. **The transtheoretical model of behavior change is a change model that is based on a time or temporal dimension (*trans*) using well-established psychological theories (*theoretical*) of behavior change.** Behavioral research suggests that you will more likely succeed if you think of change as a journey. It helps to have a map and to know where you are heading, the best ways to get there, and the ways to travel without getting lost or running into detours. The transtheoretical model is such a map.

3. **The stages of change are a variable process that is organized in a continuum according to the decision-making process that is required to effect change.** This process begins with a firm conviction of maintaining the status quo by never changing (precontemplation), and proceeds through the conditions of intending to change someday (contemplation), soon (preparation), now (action), and forever (maintenance). The basic premise is that behavior change is a process and not an event, and that individuals are found at varying levels of motivation, or readiness to change.

4. **Understanding or predicting when change occurs related to a specific behavior can largely be explained by decisional balance and self-efficacy.** Decisional balance reflects the individual's relative weighing of the pros and cons of changing. The *pros* represent the positive aspects of changing, or the benefits of change. In contrast, the *cons* are the negative aspects of changing, or the costs of change. Self-efficacy assesses your belief that you can perform the behavior in order to achieve the desired outcome; it is your perceived confidence that you can change and maintain your behavior across a variety of difficult situations.

5. **The processes of change represent the mechanisms through which different techniques influence a change.** The processes are divided into two categories: cognitive/emotional (involving thinking, attitudes, and feelings) and behavioral (involving actions). Cognitive/emotional processes include (1) increasing knowledge, (2) experiencing negative emotions, (3) caring about others, (4) comprehending personal benefits, and (5) committing yourself; behavioral processes include (1) rewarding yourself, (2) eliciting social support, (3) substituting alternatives, and (4) reminding yourself.

6. **Successful behavior change requires a careful assessment of exactly what it is that you want to change.** To properly set a goal, you should follow a set of standard guidelines. An effective expression of these guidelines is that you should set SMART goals. SMART stands for specific, measurable, attainable, relevant, and trackable.

Terms

Primary prevention, 48	Stages of change, 50	Spiral model of change, 52
Secondary prevention, 48	Precontemplation, 51	Decisional balance, 54
Tertiary prevention, 48	Contemplation, 51	Self-efficacy, 54
Health habit, 49	Preparation, 51	Processes of change, 55
Self-changer, 49	Action, 51	
Transtheoretical model of behavior change (TTM), 49	Maintenance, 51	
	Termination, 52	

making the connection

Based on what you have read in this chapter about the stages of change, John would be considered to be in the precontemplation stage. John is not ready to begin a physical activity program at this time. He may need to increase his knowledge about the benefits of participating in a regular physical activity program. In addition, John may want to acknowledge his feelings related to participating in regular physical activity by using the rational emotive technique described in this chapter (see the section "How People Change").

Critical Thinking

1. Often, like John, we are not ready to make a health behavior change, especially if we think our effort will be greater than the benefit of the behavior. List 10 reasons people begin a physical activity program (benefits) and 10 reasons people do not begin a physical activity program (barriers). Put an "L" next to the benefits that are long term, and a "B" next to those that are short term. Turning to the barriers, indicate which you have control over and which you do not. Do the barriers seem to outweigh the benefits? This time focus on short-term benefits and on barriers over which you have control. Does this change the picture?

2. As a friend, housemate, fraternity brother, or sorority sister, what role(s) can you play in supporting someone who is beginning a physical activity program? In analyzing your role, be aware of things you might do that would deter your friend from beginning or maintaining a physical activity program. Avoid those behaviors.

References

Bandura, A. (1986). *Social Foundations of Thought and Action: A Social Cognitive Theory.* Englewood Cliffs, NJ: Prentice Hall.

Centers for Disease Control and Prevention, National Center for Chronic Disease Prevention and Health Promotion. (2004). The burden of chronic diseases and their risk factors: National and state perspectives 2004. Online: http://www.cdc.gov/nccdphp/burdenbook2004/index.htm.

Cifuentes, M., Fernald, D.H., Green, L.A., Niebauer, L.J., Crabtee, B.F., Stange, K.C., & Hassmiller, S.B. (2005). Prescription for health: Changing primary care practice to foster healthy behaviors. *Annals of Family Medicine* 3(Suppl. 2):4–11.

Cloninger, C.R. (1987). A systematic method for clinical description and classification of personality variants. *Archives of General Psychiatry* 44:573–588.

Ellis, A., & Harper, R. (1971). *A Guide to Rational Living.* Hollywood, CA: Wilshire.

Hunt, W.A., Matarazzo, J.D., Weiss, S.M., & Gentry, W.D. (1979). Associative learning, habit, and health behavior. *Journal of Behavioral Medicine* 2:111–115.

Janis, I.L., & Mann, L. (1977). *Decision Making: A Psychological Analysis of Conflict, Choice and Commitment*. New York: Free Press.

Kotecki, J.E., McKenzie, J.F., Banter, A.E., Bird, J.C., Reece, J.S., & Brown, S.C. (2004). Indiana family physicians: Beliefs and practices regarding health promotion. *Journal of Eta Sigma Gamma* 36(1):13–22.

Olshansky, S.J., Passaro, D.J., Hershow, R.C., Layden, J., Carnes, B.A., Brody, J., Hayflick, L.,

Butler, R.N., Allison, D.B., & Ludwig, D.S. (2005). A potential decline in life expectancy in the United States in the 21st century. *New England Journal of Medicine* 352:1138–1145.

Prochaska, J.O., Norcross, J.C., & DiClemente, C.C. (1994). *Changing for Good*. New York: Avon.

Prochaska, J.O., & Velicer, W.F. (1997). The transtheoretical model of health behavior change. *American Journal of Health Promotion* 12(1):38–48.

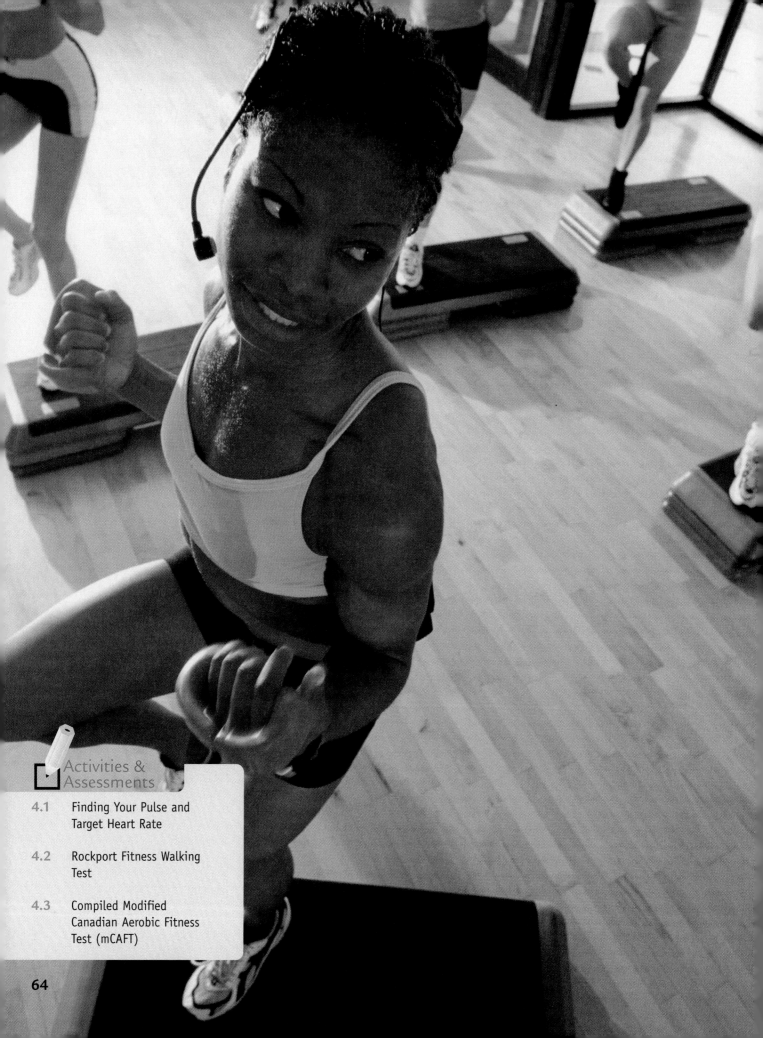

Activities &
Assessments

4.1   Finding Your Pulse and
       Target Heart Rate

4.2   Rockport Fitness Walking
       Test

4.3   Compiled Modified
       Canadian Aerobic Fitness
       Test (mCAFT)

The Heart of Physical Activity: Cardiovascular Health

4

what's the connection?

Mike is a former athlete who is concerned about fitness. He knows that physical activity is good for him, but he has only been performing resistance training since his sporting days ended. Mike has decided to incorporate some aerobic exercise into his daily routine, primarily to help maintain optimal body composition but also to help his endurance. Mike had heard that being active also helps his heart, but he is unsure what type of exercise is necessary to provide the benefits he desires.

concepts

1. The circulatory system consists of the heart and blood vessels—veins, arteries, and capillaries.

2. The heart is a specialized muscle made stronger by regular physical activity.

3. Many different activities may be performed to protect your cardiovascular health.

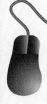

http://physicalactivity.jbpub.com

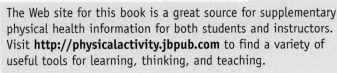

The Web site for this book is a great source for supplementary physical health information for both students and instructors. Visit **http://physicalactivity.jbpub.com** to find a variety of useful tools for learning, thinking, and teaching.

The circulatory system consists of the heart and blood vessels—veins, arteries, and capillaries.

Pericardium Thin, closed outer sac that surrounds the heart.

Myocardium Muscular middle layer that surrounds the heart.

Endocardium Thin, inner layer that lines the heart.

FIGURE 4.1 **The Circulatory System.** The circulatory system includes the heart, arteries, and veins. The heart receives oxygenated blood from the lungs and pumps it to all tissues in the body.

Introduction

Cardiovascular health is an important aspect of one's overall well-being. Physical activity plays an essential role in optimizing cardiovascular health (Hayman et al., 2004; Myers, 2003; Warburton, Nicol, & Bredin, 2006). This chapter explains how to design a program for cardiorespiratory fitness, the component of fitness that develops cardiovascular health. To understand how cardiorespiratory fitness lays the foundation for good cardiovascular health, it helps to have an understanding of how the cardiovascular system works.

The Heart

The cardiovascular system consists of the heart (the pump) and a network of blood vessels that transport the blood throughout the body (**FIGURE 4.1**). The heart's primary function is to pump blood containing oxygen and nutrients throughout the body. The heart also receives blood filled with waste products (such as carbon dioxide) that need to be eliminated from the body. The heart is a highly specialized muscle about the size of an adult fist that pumps blood throughout the body. The heart pumps slightly more than a gallon of blood per minute through the approximately 50,000 miles of blood vessels in the body. Each day the heart expands and contracts 100,000 times, pumping about 2000 gallons of blood. In a 70-year lifetime, an average human heart beats more than 2.5 billion times. Maintaining a healthy heart and blood vessels is essential for survival. The walls of the heart are composed of three layers: the pericardium, the myocardium, and the endocardium. The **pericardium** is a thin, closed sac that surrounds the heart. The middle layer is the thickest, consists of muscle cells, and is called the **myocardium**. The **endocardium** is the inner layer that lines the heart chambers.

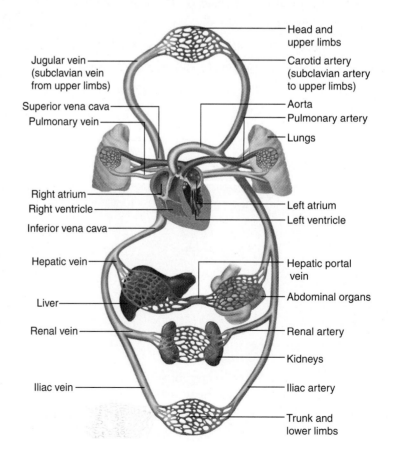

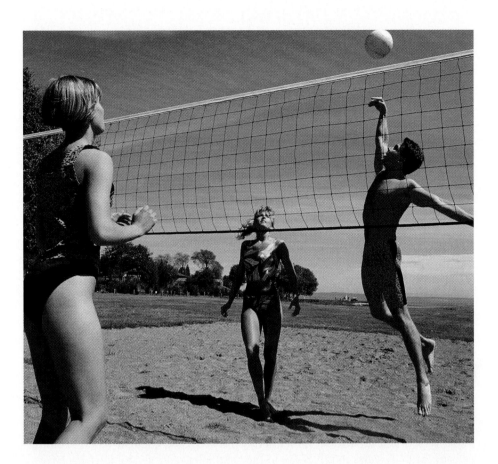

Physical activity improves
cardiovascular function.

The heart contains four separate chambers: the upper two chambers are the
left and right atrium; the lower two chambers are the right and left ventricle
(FIGURE 4.2). The heart also has four valves: the tricuspid valve (located between
the right atrium and right ventricle), the pulmonary valve (between the right ventricle and pulmonary artery), the mitral valve (between the left atrium and left
ventricle), and the aortic valve (between the left ventricle and aorta). To maintain
uniform blood flow in one direction through arteries and veins, the cardiovascular

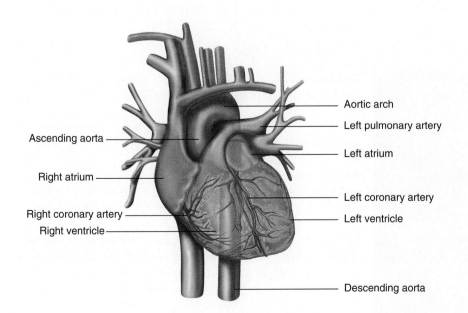

FIGURE 4.2 **The Heart.**
Oxygenated blood is pumped
through the arteries (red), and
oxygen-depleted blood is returned
to the heart via veins (blue).

Aorta Large artery that receives blood from the heart's left ventricle and distributes it to the body.

Deoxygenated blood Blood returned to the heart, to be replenished with oxygen in the lungs.

Oxygenated blood Blood leaving the heart that is oxygen-rich.

Sinoatrial node The natural pacemaker of the heart.

Arteries Blood vessels that carry oxygenated blood from the heart to the body.

Arterioles Small, muscular branches of arteries; when they contract, they increase resistance to blood flow, and blood pressure increases.

Capillaries Tiny blood vessels that circulate blood to all the body's cells.

Veins Blood vessels that return deoxygenated blood to the heart.

Blood pressure The force blood applies to the walls of the blood vessels.

Blood pressure cuff (sphygmomanometer) Instrument that measures blood pressure.

Systolic pressure The highest blood pressure measured in the arteries; occurs as the heart contracts with each heartbeat.

system is equipped with one-way valves, both in the chambers of the heart and in blood vessels. With every heartbeat, the valves in the heart open and close to allow blood to circulate in just one direction.

Blood that is depleted of oxygen returns to the heart via the right atrium and then flows to the right ventricle. From there blood is pumped to the lungs, where it is reoxygenated and returned via the pulmonary artery to the left atrium. Finally, the fresh blood is pumped throughout the body's tissues from the left ventricle through the large artery called the **aorta**. The atria receive blood entering the heart: the right atrium receives **deoxygenated blood** returning from the various cells and muscles of the body, and the left atrium receives **oxygenated blood** from the lungs. The right ventricle pumps deoxygenated blood out to the lungs, while the left ventricle pumps oxygenated blood out to the cells and muscles of the body.

A healthy heart beats rhythmically at a pace initiated by the heart itself. In the right atrium, a region called the **sinoatrial node** (pacemaker) generates an electric signal that causes the heart to contract and pump blood. The pace of the heartbeat is also influenced by electrical signals from the brain, which explains how emotions, excitement, or stress can suddenly change the rhythm of the heartbeat.

The Blood Vessels

There are many different types of blood vessels that carry blood through the body. **Arteries** carry oxygenated blood from the heart to all organs and tissues in the body. The arteries closest to the heart are large; as they move farther from the heart they divide into smaller vessels called **arterioles**. Arterioles lead to **capillaries**, tiny blood vessels that branch out from arteries and veins and circulate blood to all the cells in the body. **Veins** return blood to the heart after oxygen and nutrients have been exchanged for carbon dioxide and waste products. Blood vessels can be damaged by injury or by disease; this damage may obstruct the flow of blood carrying oxygen and nutrients. The blood in the arterial system moves from the heart, which generates a great deal of pressure, into smaller and smaller vessels, which help to maintain a high-pressure outflow. This pressure is referred to as *blood pressure*. Maintaining adequate blood flow is important in the delivery of oxygen and the removal of carbon dioxide. If the blood pressure drops rapidly (for example, if you stand up too quickly), you feel dizzy. This dizziness is caused by diminished blood flow to the brain. Veins and arteries for the most part run side by side throughout the body.

Knowing your blood pressure is vital to your overall health and well-being.

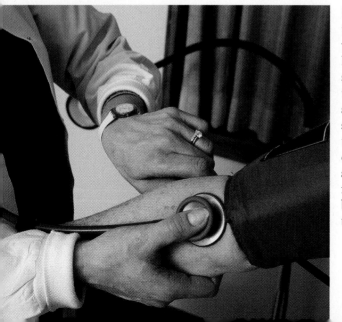

MEASURING BLOOD PRESSURE **Blood pressure** is the force that blood applies to the walls of a blood vessel. Blood pressure varies from time to time, based on our physical activity or stress levels. Blood pressure is measured using a **blood pressure cuff**, or **sphygmomanometer**. The blood pressure cuff is wrapped around the upper part of the arm, and a stethoscope is placed over the artery just below the cuff. Air is pumped into the cuff until pressure stops the flow of blood through the artery. The pressure in the cuff is gradually reduced as the air is released. The measure of the blood's pressure as it starts flowing through the vessel again is known as **systolic pressure**; this is the higher of the two numbers stated in a blood pressure reading. The air continues to be released from the cuff until no pulse is audible, indicating that the blood is flowing normally through the artery; this is known as the **diastolic pressure**. A typical reading for a healthy, young adult is 120/75, although readings may vary from individual to individual.

The Circulation of Blood

When returning to the heart, blood moves from one-cell-thick capillaries into larger venules and then even larger veins. This movement from small vessels into larger vessels accounts for the low-pressure return system of our vascular network. One of the benefits of moving during the cooldown phase of a workout is that muscle contraction aids in **venous return**, making it easier for blood to return to the heart and helping you recover from exercise more rapidly. It will also prevent you from fainting and keeling over from rapid blood pressure fluctuations.

The Function of Blood

The heart (a muscle) is responsible for circulating the blood that nourishes our cells and maintains life. Blood (the fluid circulated by the heart) plays an important role in removing waste products, assisting in *thermoregulation* (temperature control), and delivering hormones. A fluid portion of the blood, called *plasma*, consists primarily of water and thus makes circulation possible. The blood also contains **hemoglobin**, which is responsible for the transportation of oxygen. Oxygen binds to the hemoglobin found in red blood cells. Carbon dioxide is also carried in the blood, primarily in the form of **bicarbonate ions**. The circulatory system functions to deliver oxygen to working muscles and remove carbon dioxide.

This closed system maintains blood pressure and flow. When you start to move, your heart must respond by beating more forcefully and rapidly to deliver the blood that the muscles need. The more fit you are, the easier your heart adjusts to the stress of physical activity.

Neural Control

The heart has its own electrical conduction network, which is regulated by the sinoatrial (SA) node. The SA node is a collection of specialized tissue that sets the neural rhythm regulating cardiac function. This **autoregulation** allows the cardiac muscle to maintain a regular rhythm, or rate of beating, without the brain having to become consciously involved in setting the pace of the heart. The heart also responds to chemical and neural impulses that can alter the force or rate of contraction. When our skeletal muscles send signals that they need more oxygen, the heart responds by beating faster or harder. The electrical activity within the heart can be measured through the use of an electrocardiograph (ECG).

The Pulmonary/Respiratory Link

The **pulmonary system**, like the circulatory system, is important to the delivery of oxygen and the removal of carbon dioxide. In fact, the integration of the circulatory and pulmonary systems is crucial for survival and activity. In terms of physical activity, movements that stress (and improve) the circulatory system also stress (and improve) the functioning of the pulmonary system. We need to be aware that the environment in which we exercise has an impact on pulmonary function. We need to choose locations for physical activity where air quality is optimal. In most instances, unless an individual has a chronic obstructive pulmonary disease (bronchitis, emphysema, asthma), pulmonary function will not be a major limiting factor to activity performance.

Diastolic pressure The lowest blood pressure measured in the arteries; occurs when the heart muscle is relaxed between beats.

Venous return Blood returning through the veins to the heart.

Hemoglobin The oxygen-carrying pigment of the red blood cells.

Bicarbonate ions (HCO_3) As a buffer, they prevent a change in blood pH.

Autoregulation Self-regulation.

Pulmonary system Pertaining to the lungs; includes pulmonary arteries and veins.

The heart is a specialized muscle made stronger by regular physical activity.

Cardiac output The amount of blood ejected from the heart each minute; calculated by multiplying heart rate by stroke volume.

Stroke volume The amount of blood ejected with each contraction of the heart.

Heart rate The frequency at which the heart beats (contracts).

A VO₂max test can be used to assess cardiorespiratory fitness.

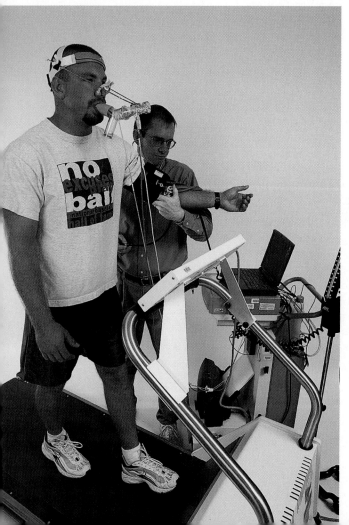

Cardiovascular Health

Physical activity plays an important role in optimizing cardiovascular function. Cardiovascular function responds to physical activity by becoming more efficient, which directly affects the health of the cardiovascular system.

Cardiac Output, Stroke Volume, and Heart Rate

As stated previously, the heart is a special type of muscle (cardiac muscle). Like the other muscles in your body, the heart responds to the stress of physical activity by becoming stronger. One of the best measures of your heart's ability to function is its **cardiac output**. Cardiac output refers to the heart's ability to pump out blood every minute. When analyzing cardiac output, the amount of blood squeezed out of the heart with each contraction (**stroke volume**) is important, but so is the rate at which the blood is squeezed out (**heart rate**). With improved fitness, the force with which the heart can contract increases. Another adaptation to regular exercise is the improved ability of the heart to expand and allow more blood to flow into it. This increased contractile force and greater elasticity allows more blood to be squeezed out with each contraction. If you can squeeze more blood out with each contraction (greater stroke volume) the heart doesn't have to beat as often. Therefore, one way to monitor improvement in cardiovascular fitness is to measure your heart rate. The lower your resting heart rate, the higher your stroke volume and the stronger your heart.

With increasing amounts of work, a fit person's heart rate will be lower than an unfit person's heart rate at any workload. The lower heart rate is due to the fit person's heart being stronger (greater stroke volume), so it doesn't have to beat as often. As the workload continues to increase, the unfit person will fatigue before the fit person. The fit person will be able to continue to be active at higher intensities and for a longer time than the unfit person. The unfit person's weaker heart will reach its maximal rate and will not be able to maintain cardiac output. If cardiac output cannot be maintained, the unfit person fatigues. The fit person will be able to be active longer before reaching maximal heart rate because the stroke volume is greater. Therefore, the fit person will be able to postpone fatigue for a longer time.

Cardiorespiratory fitness was defined as the integration of the pulmonary and cardiovascular systems in Chapter 2. This type of fitness reflects how well your heart and lungs work together to supply oxygen to the body during physical activity and exercise. Improvement in aerobic fitness level is measured by assessing changes in VO₂max, which is the maximal volume of oxygen you can breathe in and deliver to your muscles. It is the best indicator of cardiorespiratory fitness. Increases in VO₂max may range from 5 to 30 percent when starting an aerobic physical activity program. Individuals with low initial levels of aerobic fitness will see the greatest percent increase in VO₂max through aerobic activity. This happens because less fit individuals have more room for improvement. The best way to improve your cardiorespiratory fitness involves an exercise routine that uses large muscle groups, is maintained for long periods, and is rhythmic in nature.

Designing Your Cardiorespiratory Fitness Program

Cardiorespiratory fitness should be the mainstay of any fitness program. For maximum effectiveness and safety, a cardiorespiratory exercise program has specific instructions on the frequency, duration, and intensity. These three important components of cardiorespiratory exercise are needed to understand and implement in your program. The following sections explain each of these components.

Selecting Activities

Recommended forms of activity for improvement of cardiorespiratory fitness and cardiovascular health are usually focused on the larger muscle masses of the body and include such activities as walking, jogging, hiking, gardening, cycling, and swimming (see Chapter 2). Some believe that the greatest benefit comes from large-muscle dynamic or "aerobic" activity that substantially increases cardiac output with rather small increases in mean arterial blood pressure (Haskell, 1995). These activities not only involve the larger muscles of the body but are also rhythmical in nature. The cyclical pumping action of the muscles assists blood flow, keeps blood pressure in healthy zones, and allows for the adequate delivery of oxygen. Activities that involve smaller muscle masses (e.g., arm cranking, heavy-resistance weight lifting) may actually restrict blood flow, elevate blood pressure, and retard the delivery of oxygen.

Activities that require the cardiovascular system to perform at a level above its normal resting state for an extended period of time are best for improving cardiovascular function. Such exercises are frequently referred to as being *aerobic* in nature. Examples include traditional exercises such as walking, jogging, cycling, swimming, roller blading, and cross-country skiing. Other activities that would help you improve your cardiovascular health include house and yard work and physically active recreational pursuits. You can choose any of the activities listed in Table 2.1 when exercising to improve cardiorespiratory fitness. You may wish to engage in several different types of activities to reduce repetitive stress to your bones and joints and to involve a greater number of muscle groups.

Many different activities may be performed to protect your cardiovascular health.

You can select from a variety of activities to improve your cardiorespiratory fitness.

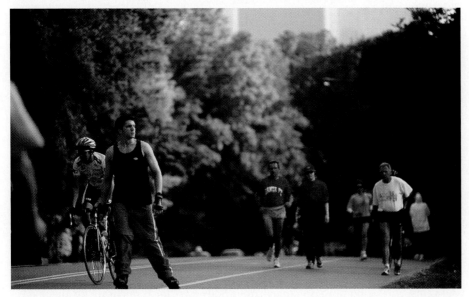

Finding the Right Intensity

As indicated in Chapter 2, the recommended intensity (I) for developing optimal cardiorespiratory fitness is between 55 and 65 percent, up to 90 percent of your maximum heart rate (determined by using the equation $208 - 0.7$ (age)) (American College of Sports Medicine [ACSM], 2006). An alternative way of setting your intensity is to use from between 40 and 50 percent up to 85 percent of your **VO₂ reserve** (VO_2R) or **heart rate reserve** (HRR) (ACSM, 2006). All three of these methods may be used to determine your aerobic capacity. Reserve methods utilize a percentage of the difference between your maximal score and your resting score. Reserve methods are preferred over the heart rate maximum (HR_{max}) method because they include an indirect measure of fitness (the resting score). Exercising at intensities beyond the recommended level shifts you from aerobic exercise into anaerobic exercise. Although this may increase your power, aerobic exercise is best for improvements in cardiorespiratory fitness.

Similar increases in cardiorespiratory endurance may be achieved by a lower-intensity, longer-duration activity as opposed to higher-intensity, shorter-duration activity. The lower-intensity values—that is, 40 to 49 percent of VO_2R or HRR, and 55 to 64 percent of HR_{max}—are most applicable to individuals who are unfit (ACSM, 2006). Higher-intensity, shorter-duration activity is preferred by many people because they can be active for shorter periods of time. The drawback to this type of activity is that you are at greater risk of injury, and it can feel very stressful mentally and physically. Lower-intensity, longer-duration activity will provide the same benefits with a lower risk of injury and less mental and physical stress. The only drawback is that it takes longer to perform.

To reduce the risk of injury and to enhance adherence to your activity program, lower-intensity, shorter-duration activity is typically recommended for beginners. It is also recommended for those with previous injury and those who have no desire for physically challenging activities. However, athletes in training, those of higher fitness levels, and those who enjoy a physical challenge usually perform higher-intensity activities. We also know that the more fit the person, the higher the intensity needs to be to bring about further improvement. For the majority of the healthy adult population, intensities within the range of 70 to 85 percent HR_{max} or 60 to 80 percent of HRR are sufficient to achieve improvements in cardiorespiratory fitness, when combined with an appropriate frequency and duration of training (ACSM, 2006).

Several factors should be considered when determining exercise intensity. These include your level of fitness, any medications you might be taking, your risk for cardiovascular or orthopedic injury, your preference for different types of exercises, and your program objectives (ACSM, 2006). You will learn to modify the intensity of the activity you select to get the best response from your training program.

Monitoring Your Intensity

HEART RATE   There are several ways in which you can monitor your cardiovascular response to physical activity. The most common way is by measuring your heart rate response. This will be most accurate when performing exercise of low to moderate intensities. During this type of exercise there is a linear relationship between heart rate and oxygen consumption. This means that as heart rate increases, oxygen consumption increases at the same rate and magnitude. When exercise intensities go beyond the moderate range, heart rate is not a good indicator of cardiovascular response. This is because as muscles go beyond 60 percent of their force-generating capacity, the muscles spend a longer time compressing the arteries and veins, and blood flow is reduced. Your body tries to compensate for this by having your heart beat more frequently. However, blood flow is still restricted, so heart rate increases at a much faster rate than oxygen delivery. The rise in heart

VO₂ reserve The difference between maximal oxygen uptake (VO_2max) and resting oxygen consumption.

Heart rate reserve The difference between maximum heart rate and resting heart rate.

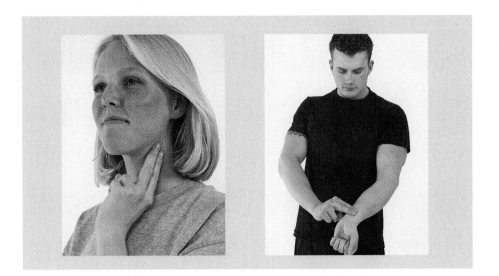

FIGURE 4.3 **How to Find Your Pulse.** The (a) carotid artery and (b) radial artery are frequently used to monitor heart rate response to physical activity.

rate is therefore not a good indicator of oxygen consumption at higher intensities of activity.

    To monitor your exercise response using heart rate, you must first learn how to locate and measure your pulse (**FIGURE 4.3**). The next step involves calculating your target heart rate. Your *target heart rate* represents the zone that your heart rate needs to reach in order to receive optimal results from your activity session (**FIGURE 4.4**).

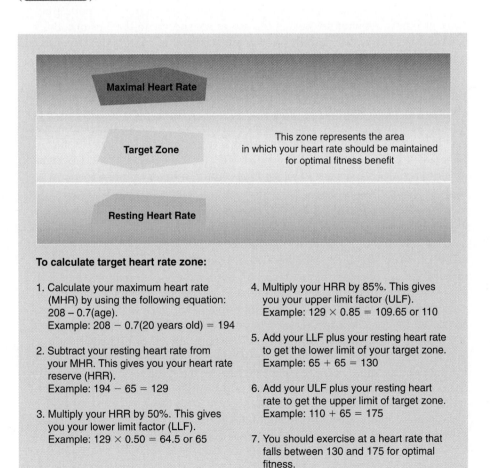

To calculate target heart rate zone:

1. Calculate your maximum heart rate (MHR) by using the following equation: 208 – 0.7(age).
   Example: 208 – 0.7(20 years old) = 194

2. Subtract your resting heart rate from your MHR. This gives you your heart rate reserve (HRR).
   Example: 194 – 65 = 129

3. Multiply your HRR by 50%. This gives you your lower limit factor (LLF).
   Example: 129 × 0.50 = 64.5 or 65

4. Multiply your HRR by 85%. This gives you your upper limit factor (ULF).
   Example: 129 × 0.85 = 109.65 or 110

5. Add your LLF plus your resting heart rate to get the lower limit of your target zone.
   Example: 65 + 65 = 130

6. Add your ULF plus your resting heart rate to get the upper limit of target zone.
   Example: 110 + 65 = 175

7. You should exercise at a heart rate that falls between 130 and 175 for optimal fitness.

FIGURE 4.4 **How to Calculate Your Target Heart Rate.** To improve your fitness, try to keep your heart rate in your target zone.

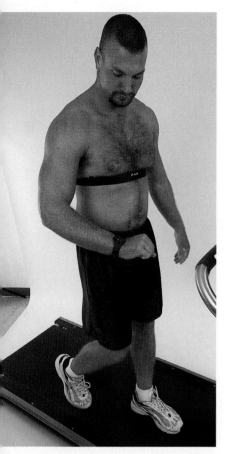

Heart rate can be used to monitor your cardiovascular system's response to physical activity.

Adenosine triphosphate A high-energy phosphate that is the only useable form of energy in the human body.

The American College of Sports Medicine (2006) reminds us that some people prefer to exercise at the low end of the target heart rate range and focus on long-duration activities to achieve their program goals. This may help adherence in certain populations. We must also remember that different activities bring about different heart rate responses (ACSM, 2006). For example, the target heart rate you might choose while cycling would be different from the target heart rate when swimming. This reinforces the importance of selecting a prescreening test that is similar to the type of activity you plan on performing.

RATING OF PERCEIVED EXERTION (RPE) You can also monitor your response to exercise by determining your perceived exertion. Swedish scientist Gunnar Borg developed a rating scale, the *rating of perceived exertion (RPE) scale*, that has since gained widespread acceptance and recognition (Borg, 1998). The original scale was based on a combination of numerical and descriptive associations with feelings of fatigue or exertion. To use the RPE scale, you select a number from the chart that corresponds with your perception of overall fatigue or exertion. The descriptors associated with the numbers (6 to 20) assist you in selecting the appropriate numbers. There tends to be a relatively good relationship between the number on the RPE scale and exercise heart rate. If you multiply the number from the scale by 10, you will find it relates well with your current exercise heart rate. An RPE rating of 12 to 16 ("somewhat hard" to "hard") is considered to be of moderate intensity and recommended for training to improve cardiorespiratory fitness (ACSM, 2006).

The original RPE scale has been modified into a zero-based scale that may also be used to monitor exercise response. The modified scale was developed to present a baseline measure of zero to represent no exertion. It is used in the same way as the original scale. A rating of 5 to 8 is recommended for improvement of cardiovascular fitness. As with heart rate, RPE scores are specific to the type of activity you perform. Remember that the prescreening test you use to set RPE levels should be consistent with the type of activity you will be performing (ACSM, 2006).

METS You may also use *multiples of your resting metabolism*, or METS, to monitor exercise intensity. One MET is equal to your metabolic rate at rest. Its equivalent in VO_2 is 3.5 mL $\times$ kg^{-1} $\times$ min^{-1}. Exercising at 10 METS means that your metabolism is working at a rate 10 times its resting level, or at 35 mL $\times$ kg^{-1} $\times$ min^{-1}. Generally it is recommended that you use MET levels between 50 and 85 percent of your maximal MET capacity for optimal cardiorespiratory fitness benefit in healthy adult populations (ACSM, 2006). Thus, if a person had a MET capacity of 10 METS, we would suggest that he or she exercise at an intensity of 5 to 8.5 METS. This represents 5 to 8.5 times the resting metabolic rate.

CALORIC EXPENDITURE Another way of monitoring exercise intensity is through the use of caloric expenditure. All human movement requires the expenditure of energy. In the human body, this energy takes the form of a molecule called **adenosine triphosphate** (ATP). Monitoring caloric expenditure involves estimating the caloric cost of performing physical activity. The unit of heat produced when energy is expended is called a *calorie* (technically it's called a *kilocalorie [kcal]*, but in our metric-phobic society we tend to drop the *kilo* part). The more work we do, the more energy we expend, and the more calories we use. Several charts have been developed for estimating the caloric expenditure of a number of activities.

Caloric expenditure is dependent on body size and sex. Large people expend more energy than small people doing the same activity. Men usually expend more energy than women do when performing the same activity. Additionally, whether your body weight is supported when performing an activity will affect caloric expenditure. For example, running expends more energy per unit of distance traveled than cycling.

Generally, it is recommended that we expend approximately 150 to 400 kcal per activity session (ACSM, 2006). This would be equivalent to walking 1.5 to 4 miles. A goal to shoot for is a weekly caloric expenditure between 1000 and 2000 kcal, which has been associated with providing protection against cardiovascular disease. You can achieve 2000 kcal by performing activities that expend 400 kcal per session 5 days per week, 500 kcal per session 4 days per week, or any other combination that adds up to 2000 kcal for the week. It is best to spread the 2000 kcal over several days. See Appendix B on caloric cost of various activities to select the activities that will allow you to achieve this recommendation.

Duration of Physical Activity

How long you need to exercise to protect your cardiovascular system will be dependent on the intensity of your activity. The lower the intensity, the longer you need to be active. If you follow the recommendations from the *Surgeon General's Report*, you need to accumulate 30 minutes of moderate-intensity physical activity on most if not all days of the week.

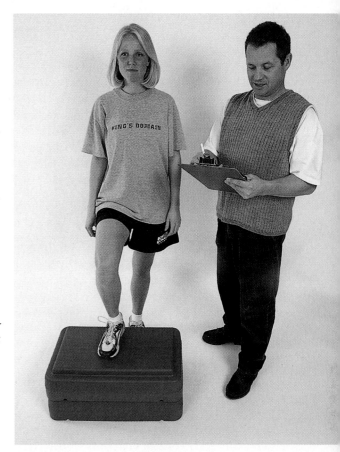

A step test is an easy way to assess your cardiorespiratory fitness.

Progression

As pointed out in Chapter 2, it is very important that you progress gradually whenever you start, or make significant changes to, a physical activity program. You must give your body time to adjust to being physically active. If you do not, you run the risk of injury and dissatisfaction with your program.

Assessing Your Cardiorespiratory Fitness

To modify your exercise intensity optimally, you must have an accurate understanding of your current fitness level. There are many ways in which you can assess your cardiorespiratory fitness. Remember, if you have not been physically active recently, or if you are not "apparently healthy" (see Chapter 2), check with your physician before performing any of the tests.

Physical Activity and Health Connection
....

Regular physical activity has a number of proven, positive health effects, especially on heart health. It strengthens the heart as a pump, making it a larger, more efficient muscle and improving the function of all components of cardiovascular health. Regular exposure to physical activity also benefits the pulmonary system, allowing it to coordinate more efficiently in the exchange of oxygen and carbon dioxide. Together, the enhancement of the cardiovascular and pulmonary systems through regular physical activity enhances one's cardiorespiratory fitness, making one more fit and allowing for more sustained activity during the day.

concept connections

1 **The circulatory system consists of the heart and blood vessels—veins, arteries, and capillaries.** Arteries carry oxygenated blood from the heart to all the organs and tissues, whereas veins return blood to the heart after oxygen and nutrients have been exchanged for carbon dioxide and waste products. Physical activity helps these vessels function properly.

2 **The heart is a specialized muscle made stronger by regular physical activity.** The heart is a specialized muscle that responds to the physical stress of being active by becoming stronger and more enduring. By making your heart stronger and more enduring, not only do you improve your ability to be physically active but you also make the cardiovascular system less susceptible to disease.

3 **Many different activities may be performed to protect your cardiovascular health.** There is no one perfect activity for improving your cardiovascular health. However, there are many different activities that may be selected to achieve this goal. It is best to vary your activities and incorporate several that use the large muscle masses of the body in a rhythmical pattern for extended periods of time (accumulation of 30 minutes).

Terms

Pericardium, 66
Myocardium, 66
Endocardium, 66
Aorta, 68
Deoxygenated blood, 68
Oxygenated blood, 68
Sinoatrial node, 68
Arteries, 68
Arterioles, 68

Capillaries, 68
Veins, 68
Blood pressure, 68
Blood pressure cuff (sphygmo-manometer), 68
Systolic pressure, 68
Diastolic pressure, 69
Venous return, 69
Hemoglobin, 69

Bicarbonate ions (HCO_3), 69
Autoregulation, 69
Pulmonary system, 69
Cardiac output, 70
Stroke volume, 70
Heart rate, 70
VO_2 reserve, 72
Heart rate reserve, 72
Adenosine triphosphate, 74

making the connection

Mike has started a cycling program to supplement his weight workouts. He now knows that the cycling program will provide him with additional protection against cardiovascular disease. Mike has also noticed the added benefit of some fat loss. He thinks this has made his muscles appear bigger.

Critical Thinking

1. In the vignette, Mike added a cycling program to supplement his weight workouts. Why would the addition of aerobic activity help Mike lose fat? How does being physically active reduce Mike's risk for developing CVD?
2. Identify four activities in which you are likely to participate that will enhance your cardiovascular system. Describe how you will incorporate each activity into your daily and weekly routine.
3. You have been invited to speak at a local high school health class about how physical activity affects heart (cardiovascular) health. In 250 words, explain the impact that physical activity has on heart health.

References

American College of Sports Medicine. (2006). *ACSM's Guidelines for Exercise Testing and Prescription*, 7th ed. Philadelphia: Lippincott, Williams & Wilkins.

Borg, G. (1998). *Borg's Perceived Exertion and Pain Scales*. Champaign, IL: Human Kinetics.

Haskell, W.L. (1995). Physical activity in the prevention and management of coronary heart disease. *President's Council on Physical Fitness and Sports Research Digest* 2(1):1–7.

Hayman, L.L., Williams, C.L., Daniels, S.R., Steinberger, I., Paridon, S. Dennison, B.A., & McCrindle, D.W. (2004). Cardiovascular health promotion in schools. *Circulation* 110:2266–2275.

Myers, J. (2003). Exercise and cardiovascular health. *Circulation* 107:e2–e5.

Warburton, D.E.R., Nicol, C.W., & Bredin, S.S.D. (2006). Health benefits of physical activity: The evidence. *Canadian Medical Association Journal* 174(6):801–809.

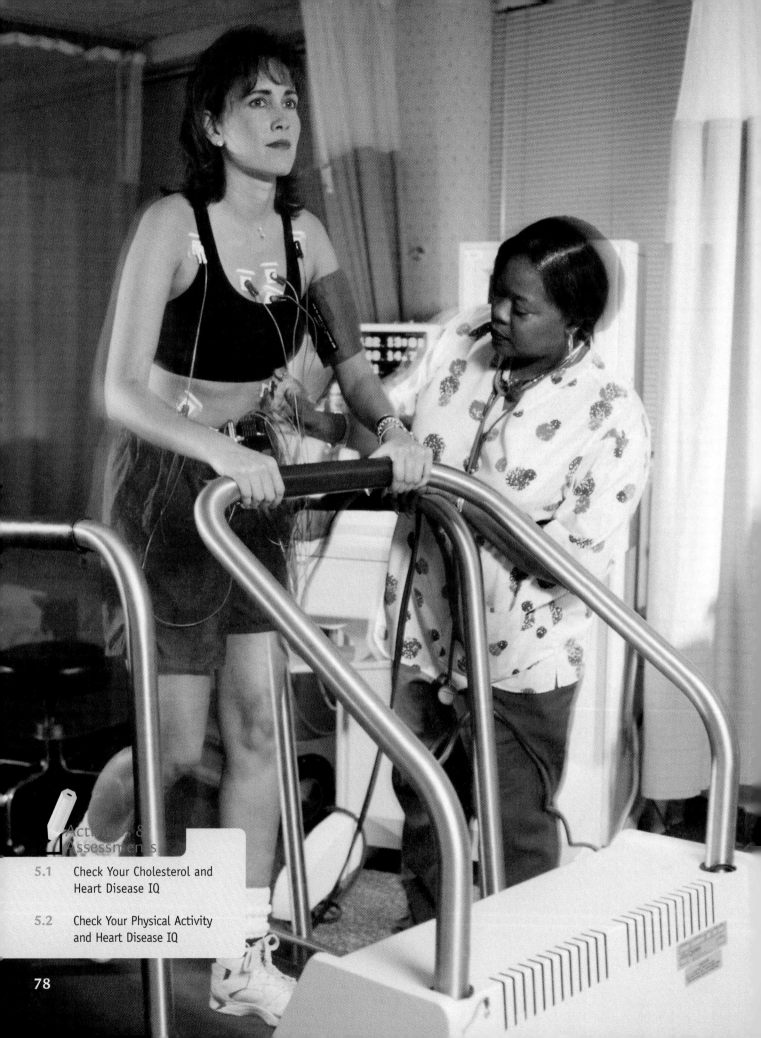

5.1   Check Your Cholesterol and
             Heart Disease IQ

5.2   Check Your Physical Activity
             and Heart Disease IQ

Physical Inactivity and Cardiovascular Disease

what's the connection?

Richard is worried about dying from a heart attack. His father suffered a heart attack at age 45 last year, and both of his grandfathers died of cardiovascular disease. Richard does not intend to follow in their footsteps. He knows that his family history and gender put him at risk, so he focuses on things he can control. He doesn't smoke, and he has his blood pressure and cholesterol levels monitored on a regular basis. Richard is convinced that physical activity is unrelated to his risk of developing cardiovascular disease. He thinks he is doing all he can to reduce his risk of cardiovascular disease. Is Richard correct in believing this? Are there any other factors that Richard should be aware of that could reduce his chances of developing cardiovascular disease?

concepts

1. Physical inactivity is an independent risk factor for cardiovascular disease (CVD).

2. The National Institutes of Health has concluded that being physically active helps prevent heart disease.

3. There are many forms of cardiovascular disease.

4. *Angina pectoris* and *heart attack* are not synonymous terms.

5. Hypertension is a major risk factor for coronary heart disease.

6. Arteriosclerosis and atherosclerosis are key factors in cardiovascular disease.

7. Cerebrovascular accident (CVA), or stroke, is a cardiovascular disease that affects the central nervous system.

8. The three unmodifiable risk factors for CVD are age, family, and gender.

9. The six modifiable CVD risk factors are hypertension, high blood cholesterol, cigarette smoking, diabetes, obesity, and physical inactivity.

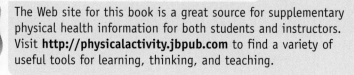

http://physicalactivity.jbpub.com

The Web site for this book is a great source for supplementary physical health information for both students and instructors. Visit **http://physicalactivity.jbpub.com** to find a variety of useful tools for learning, thinking, and teaching.

Physical inactivity is an independent risk factor for cardiovascular disease.

Independent risk factor A disease risk factor that stands alone; by itself, an independent risk factor can cause a disease.

The National Institutes of Health has concluded that being physically active helps prevent heart disease.

Introduction

Cardiovascular disease (CVD) is the leading cause of death in the United States, accounting for approximately 4 in 10 deaths. Extensive scientific research studies have identified several factors that increase the risk of developing cardiovascular disease, many of which can be controlled or modified. One important risk factor is leading a sedentary lifestyle.

Physical Inactivity as an Independent Risk Factor

In the past two decades, several studies have demonstrated that leading a sedentary lifestyle is an **independent risk factor** for the development of cardiovascular disease (Blair et al., 1989; Paffenbarger, Hyde, Wing, & Hsieh, 1986). The term *independent risk factor* means that if all other potential risks for disease were controlled (or eliminated), living a sedentary lifestyle would, by itself, put you at greater risk for developing cardiovascular disease than if you lived an active lifestyle.

We have known for years the risk of cardiovascular disease associated with cigarette smoking, high cholesterol levels, and hypertension (high blood pressure). If we analyze the percentage of people who have these risks and compare those figures to the percentage of people who live predominantly sedentary lifestyles, we can see that, of all the major cardiovascular disease risk factors, physical inactivity affects the largest percentage of the population (**FIGURE 5.1**). If we were to focus on just improving one risk factor, getting more people physically active would have the greatest impact on the health of the population of the United States.

In addition, if we get those people who have other risk factors for CVD to increase their activity levels, their degree of protection against cardiovascular disease will increase significantly.

Evidence of the Protective Effects of Physical Activity

The National Institutes of Health (NIH) Consensus Statement (1995) was developed by a panel of medical, physical activity, and health experts to report on the status of what is known about the relationship between physical activity and cardiovascular disease. The report concluded that physical inactivity is one of the most important factors that we must deal with if the health of the population is to be improved. The major findings of the NIH Consensus Statement are summarized in (TABLE 5.1). These findings support the notion that people need to participate in

FIGURE 5.1 **Disease Distribution and Physical Activity.** Physical inactivity affects the largest segment of our society when compared with the other major causes of disease. SOURCE: Adapted from S.N. Blair, H.W. Kohl III, R.S. Paffenbarger, D.G. Clark, K.H. Cooper, and L.W. Gibbons. (1989). Physical fitness and all-cause mortality. *JAMA*, 262(17):2395–2401.

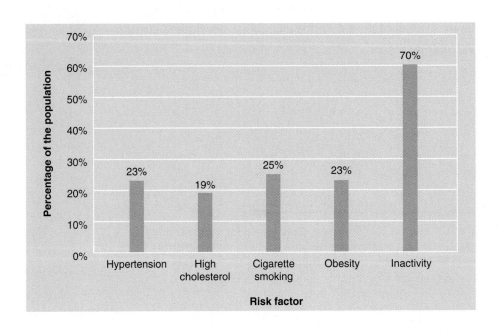

| TABLE 5.1 | **Major Findings of the NIH Consensus Statement** |

- Physical activity protects against the development of CVD and also favorably modifies other CVD risk factors, including high blood pressure, blood lipid levels, insulin resistance, and obesity.
- Physical activity is also important in the treatment of patients with CVD or those who are at increased risk for developing CVD, including patients who have hypertension, stable angina, or peripheral vascular disease, or who have had a prior myocardial infarction or heart failure. Physical activity is an important component of cardiac rehabilitation, and people with CVD can benefit from participation.
- Evidence indicates that physical inactivity and lack of physical fitness are directly associated with increased mortality from CVD. The increase in mortality is not entirely explained by the association with elevated blood pressure, smoking, and blood lipid levels.
- Physical activity increases HDL, normalizes blood pressure, and increases insulin sensitivity. A number of factors that affect thrombotic function—including hematocrit, fibrinogen, platelet function, and fibrinolysis—are related to the risk of CVD. Regular endurance exercise lowers the risk related to these factors.

SOURCE: National Institutes of Health. (1995). Physical activity and cardiovascular health. *NIH Consensus Statement* 13(3):1–33.

physical activity on a regular basis to live longer and to live healthier. It also supports the direct relationship between participating in physical activity and cardiovascular health benefits.

The 1996 Surgeon General's Report suggests that physical activity can help to decrease the risk of cardiovascular disease mortality in general, and coronary heart disease mortality in particular. The report also states that participation in regular physical activity prevents or delays the development of high blood pressure, and that exercise reduces blood pressure in people with hypertension (U.S. Department of Health and Human Services, 1996).

Physical activity can play a role in preventing a first heart attack from occurring and reducing the risk of cardiac events (Haskell, 1995). Physical activity also aids in the recovery of patients following myocardial infarction, coronary artery bypass surgery, or cardiac angioplasty, through cardiac rehabilitation. Active people are at lower risk of CVD, develop less CVD, develop CVD at a later age, and tend to have less severe forms of CVD compared to those who are inactive (Haskell, 1995).

Only moderate activity is necessary for protection against heart disease. The greatest improvement in protection comes from moving from a sedentary lifestyle to one that is moderately active. We also know higher levels of fitness provide more protection from cardiovascular disease.

Understanding Cardiovascular Diseases

Cardiovascular diseases include a variety of diseases of the heart and blood vessels, coronary heart disease, stroke, hypertension, congestive heart failure, and peripheral artery disease. Cardiovascular diseases claimed 930,000 lives in the United States in 2002 (American Heart Association [AHA], 2005) (**FIGURE 5.2**). This is more than 40 percent of all deaths, or 1 of every 2.6 deaths. In 2002, the total cost of CVD was estimated at $330 billion (AHA, 2005). In fact, CVD claims more lives each year than the next seven leading causes of death combined. We will review several types of CVD: coronary heart disease, hypertension, arteriosclerosis, and stroke.

Coronary Heart Disease

Coronary heart disease (CHD) is the most prevalent form of heart disease in the United States (AHA, 2005) (**FIGURE 5.3**). Coronary heart disease occurs when the coronary arteries become occluded with blood fats and other substances that collect on their

There are many forms of cardiovascular disease.

Coronary heart disease Disease of the heart caused by atherosclerotic narrowing of the coronary arteries.

FIGURE 5.2 **Some Facts About Cardiovascular Disease (CVD).**
SOURCE: American Heart Association. 2005.

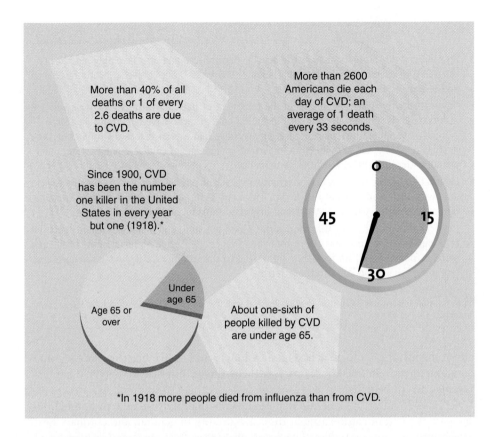

FIGURE 5.3 **Some Facts About Coronary Hearth Disease (CHD).**
SOURCE: American Heart Association. 2005.

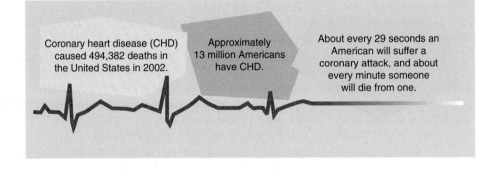

Angina pectoris and *heart attack* are not synonymous terms.

Angina pectoris Chest pain due to coronary heart disease.

Ischemia Decreased blood flow to an organ, usually due to constriction or obstruction of an artery.

Myocardial infarction (MI) Death of, or damage to part of, the heart muscle due to insufficient blood supply. Also known as a *heart attack*.

walls, narrowing the opening through which blood can flow. When the coronary arteries become clogged or narrowed, they cannot supply enough blood to the heart. Coronary heart disease, or coronary artery disease, most often is implicated in causing angina and heart attack.

ANGINA PECTORIS   If not enough oxygen-carrying blood reaches the heart, the heart may respond with pain called **angina pectoris**, or simply *angina*. This pain is usually felt on the left side of the chest or sometimes in the left arm to shoulder. Lack of blood supply is called **ischemia**. Angina can occur when blood circulation to the heart is not sufficient to meet the heart's increased needs during physical activity or emotional excitement. Running up several flight of stairs to class or to a meeting could trigger an angina attack. Angina may be a warning sign for a heart attack.

HEART ATTACK   When the blood supply to the heart is completely cut off, the result is a **myocardial infarction (MI)**, or what is commonly referred to as a *heart attack* (TABLE 5.2). The part of the heart that does not receive oxygen (via the blood) begins to die, and this sometimes causes permanent damage to the heart muscle.

TABLE 5.2	**Heart Attack Warning Signs**

- **Chest discomfort:** Most heart attacks involve discomfort in the center of the chest that lasts for more than a few minutes, or that goes away and comes back. The discomfort can feel like uncomfortable pressure, squeezing, fullness, or pain.
- **Discomfort in other areas of the upper body:** Can include pain or discomfort in one or both arms, the back, neck, jaw, or stomach.
- **Shortness of breath:** Often comes along with chest discomfort. But it can also occur before chest discomfort.
- **Other symptoms:** May include breaking out in a cold sweat, nausea, or light-headedness.

SOURCE: National Heart, Lung, and Blood Institute. (2006). Heart attack warning signs. Online: http://www.nhlbi.nih.gov/actintime/haws/haws.html.

Hypertension

Hypertension, or high blood pressure, is known as the "silent killer" and remains a major risk factor for CHD and stroke. Approximately 65 million adult Americans have high blood pressure, but almost three-fourths of them are unaware of it (AHA, 2005). An acceptable blood pressure for an adult is less than 120/80 mm Hg (AHA, 2005; National Heart, Lung, and Blood Institute, 2005) (TABLE 5.3). If an adult's systolic pressure is equal to or greater than 140 mm Hg and/or the diastolic pressure is equal to or greater than 90 mm Hg, and these readings occur for an extended period of time, that person is said to have hypertension. With high blood pressure, the heart is working harder, resulting in an increased risk of heart attack, stroke, heart failure, kidney and eye problems, and peripheral vascular disease.

The two types of hypertension are primary (or essential) hypertension and secondary hypertension. **Primary hypertension** accounts for more than 90 percent of all hypertension cases. Although the cause of primary hypertension is unknown, we know that arteriosclerosis contributes to the elevation of blood pressure. **Secondary hypertension** refers to cases for which a cause is known, such as a kidney abnormality, tumor of the adrenal gland, or a congenital defect of the aorta.

Hypertension is a major risk factor for coronary heart disease.

Hypertension A chronic increase in blood pressure above its normal range.
Primary hypertension Hypertension where the cause is unknown.
Secondary hypertension Hypertension arising from another physical condition, such as kidney disease.

TABLE 5.3	**Categories for Blood Pressure Levels in Adults***

| Category | Blood Pressure Level (mm Hg) | |
	Systolic	Diastolic
Normal	Below 120	Below 80
Prehypertension	120–139	80–89
High blood pressure		
• Stage 1	140–159	90–99
• Stage 2	160 or above	100 or above

*For those not taking medicine for high blood pressure and not having a short-term illness. These categories are from the National High Blood Pressure Education Program. Adults are those age 18 years and older.

SOURCE: National Heart, Lung, and Blood Institute. (2005). What is high blood pressure? Online: http://www.nhlbi.nih.gov/health/dci/Diseases/Hbp/HBP_Whatis.html.

Arteriosclerosis and atheroscle-rosis are key factors in cardio-vascular disease.

Arteriosclerosis "Hardening of the arteries"; arterial walls thicken and lose elasticity.

Atherosclerosis A form of arteriosclerosis in which the inner layers of the artery become thick and irregular due to fatty deposits called plaque.

Plaque A fatty deposit on the inner lining of the artery wall.

Cerebrovascular accident (CVA), or stroke, is a cardiovascular disease that affects the central nervous system.

Stroke Loss of muscle function, vision, or speech resulting from brain-cell damage caused by insufficient blood supply. Also known as *cerebrovascular accident* (CVA).

Ischemic strokes Strokes caused by clots.

Cerebral thrombosis Blood clot in an artery that supplies the brain.

Cerebral embolism Blood clot formed in one part of the body and then carried by the bloodstream to the brain, where it blocks an artery.

Atherosclerosis

Arteriosclerosis, hardening and thickening of the arteries, includes several conditions that cause the walls of the arteries to thicken and lose their elasticity. The most common form of arteriosclerosis is **atherosclerosis**, which can begin as early as childhood (Ross, 1993). Atherosclerosis is a slow, progressive process that begins with damage to the heart's arteries and leads to formation of fibrous, fatty deposits called **plaque**. These plaque deposits accumulate on the artery walls, causing the arteries to lose their elasticity (ability to expand and contract), and eventually restricting blood flow (**FIGURE 5.4**). The restriction of blood flow also makes the blood more susceptible to forming blood clots. Restriction or obstruction of blood flow to an artery is very serious because heart cells die when deprived of oxygenated blood.

Stroke

When considered separately from other cardiovascular diseases, stroke ranks as the third leading cause of death in the United States, behind diseases of the heart and cancer. **Stroke**, or *cerebrovascular accident* (CVA), is a form of cardiovascular disease that affects the arteries of the central nervous system. A stroke results when the brain doesn't get enough oxygen because the arteries supplying blood to the brain are blocked or damaged. Brain cells die within minutes without oxygen.

There are two broad categories of stroke: ischemic and hemorrhage. **Ischemic strokes** are caused by clots and account for approximately three-fourths of all strokes. The two types of ischemic strokes are cerebral thrombosis and cerebral embolism. **Cerebral thrombosis** is the most common type of stroke; it occurs when a thrombus (blood clot) forms and blocks flow in an artery bringing blood to the brain. A **cerebral embolism** occurs when a wandering clot (embolus) occurs in a blood vessel away from the heart. The embolus is carried through the bloodstream until it lodges in an artery, blocking blood flow to the brain. Arteries damaged by arteriosclerosis are generally present in both types of ischemic strokes.

Hemorrhagic strokes occur when blood seeps from a hole in the wall of a blood vessel. There are two types of hemorrhagic strokes: cerebral hemorrhage and subarachnoid hemorrhage. **Cerebral hemorrhage** occurs when a defective artery in the brain ruptures, flooding the surrounding tissue with blood. A **subarachnoid hemorrhage** occurs when a blood vessel on the surface of the brain ruptures and bleeds into the space between the brain and the skull.

The effects of a stroke vary from person to person, depending on the type of stroke and the area of the brain affected (**FIGURE 5.5**). A stroke can cause paralysis and affect sight, touch, movement, and cognitive abilities.

FIGURE 5.4 **Plaque in an Artery.** Plaque is the buildup of fatty material on the artery wall. The illustration (left) shows the interior of an artery narrowed by plaque. The photo (right) shows an occluded blood vessel that has been entirely blocked by plaque and a blood clot (dark area).

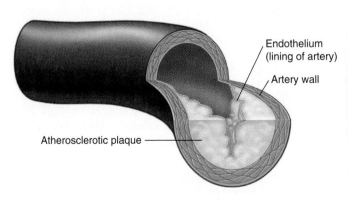
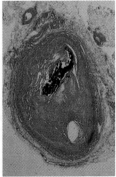

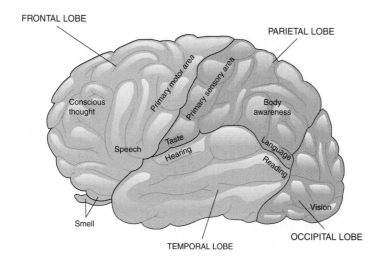

FIGURE 5.5 Areas of the Brain Potentially Impacted by a Stroke.

Risk Factors for Cardiovascular Disease

The answer to the problem of cardiovascular disease is prevention. Over the years, researchers have identified risk factors that can increase your risk for developing heart disease. Some risk factors cannot be changed (age, family history, gender), but some can be changed (high cholesterol, cigarette smoking, diabetes, obesity, hypertension, physical inactivity). Factors that cannot be changed are referred to as *unmodifiable* risk factors, whereas factors that can be changed are referred to as *modifiable* risk factors. *Contributing* risk factors are associated with an increased risk of cardiovascular disease, but their significance has not yet been scientifically measured. These factors include stress and misuse of alcohol.

Unmodifiable Risk Factors

AGE   The risk of cardiovascular disease increases as we get older (Corti, Guralink, & Bicato, 1996). The majority of people who die of a heart attack are 65 or older. Although you can't change your age, you can change your physical activity, diet, and smoking habits.

FAMILY HISTORY   There appears to be a hereditary tendency toward heart disease and atherosclerosis. If you have close relatives who have had a heart attack or a stroke before 50 years of age, you are at increased risk for having a heart attack or stroke. Another significant factor is race—African Americans are two times as likely to have high blood pressure as whites, which increases the risk of cardiovascular disease. Again, despite your genetics, you can choose lifestyle changes to decrease your risk for cardiovascular disease.

GENDER   Men are more likely than women to develop cardiovascular disease, especially before the age of 40. However, after menopause, women's risk of heart disease increases. Current theory speculates that male hormones (androgens) increase risk, whereas female hormones (estrogens) protect against atherosclerosis.

Modifiable Risk Factors

HYPERTENSION   The relationship between high blood pressure and CVD is a complex one (Lembo et al., 1998). High blood pressure increases the heart's workload, causing the heart to weaken over time. Combine high blood pressure with obesity, smoking, high blood cholesterol, or diabetes and the risk of heart attack or stroke increases several times. Lembo and associates (1998) indicate that reducing high blood pressure alone does not entirely remove the risk of developing coronary

Hemorrhagic strokes Strokes caused by blood seeping from a hole in the wall of a blood vessel.

Cerebral hemorrhage Bleeding within the brain that results from a ruptured aneurysm or a head injury.

Subarachnoid hemorrhage Bleeding from a blood vessel on the surface of the brain into the space between the brain and the skull.

The three unmodifiable risk factors for CVD are age, family, and gender.

The six CVD risk factors that can be changed are hypertension, cholesterol level, cigarette smoking, diabetes, obesity, and physical inactivity.

heart disease. Hagberg (1997) suggests that the preventive benefit of exercise is probably underestimated, and that "physical activity and physical fitness also appear to diminish the rate of development of hypertension" (p. 117).

There is a direct relationship between sodium intake and hypertension (He et al., 1999). The more sodium you consume, the higher your blood pressure; this tendency is particularly true for people who are overweight. Obesity causes changes in the sympathetic nervous system and other metabolic pathways that result in enhanced sodium reabsorption and sodium retention in the kidneys. While everyone may want to limit their sodium intake, reducing sodium intake may be more beneficial for overweight persons (He et al., 1999.)

HIGH BLOOD CHOLESTEROL   **Cholesterol** is a fatty, wax-like substance that combines with protein and other lipids called **lipoproteins** and is carried in the blood plasma. There are two types of lipoproteins that carry cholesterol in the blood. **Low-density lipoproteins (LDL)**, or so-called bad cholesterol, transport cholesterol from the bloodstream into cells and promote atherosclerosis by transporting cholesterol into the arterial wall. *High-density lipoproteins* (HDL), or *good* cholesterol, remove cholesterol from the cells and carry it to the liver for removal, thus protecting against atherosclerosis. Our HDL helps prevent cholesterol buildup in blood vessels, while low LDL levels increase heart disease risk. Low-density lipoproteins and other risk factors may contribute synergistically to the incidence of CVD (Chien et al., 1999).

One way LDL cholesterol levels become too high in blood is through eating too much of two nutrients: saturated fat (found mostly in animal products) and cholesterol (found only in animal products). Saturated fat raises LDL levels more than anything else in the diet. Cholesterol levels are determined through a chemical analysis of a blood sample. The National Cholesterol Education program has developed a cholesterol classification (TABLE 5.4).

CIGARETTE SMOKING   Cigarette smoking contributes to heart disease in several ways (**FIGURE 5.6**). First, it speeds up the development of atherosclerosis by potentially damaging the arterial walls and allowing cholesterol to deposit. Smoking also decreases the HDL, or good cholesterol, and may contribute to blood

Cholesterol Waxy substance that circulates naturally in the bloodstream; when levels are too high, it deposits in the walls of blood vessels.

Lipoproteins Lipid (fatty, insoluble substance in blood) surrounded by a protein; the protein makes it soluble in blood.

Low-density lipoproteins (LDL) Carriers of harmful cholesterol in the blood; "bad" cholesterol.

TABLE 5.4	Cholesterol Levels

Cholesterol levels for people over 20 who do not have heart disease*

Desirable blood cholesterol	• Total blood cholesterol is less than 200 mg/dL
	• LDL is lower than 130 mg/dL
	• HDL level is 60 mg/dL or higher
Borderline high cholesterol	• Total blood cholesterol level is between 200 and 239 mg/dL, OR
	• LDL is 130 to 159 mg/dL
High blood cholesterol	• Total blood cholesterol level is greater than 240 mg/dL, OR
	• LDL is 160 mg/dL or higher
	• LDL above 100 is too high for a patient with heart disease
	• HDL level less than 40 mg/dL is considered low and increases risk of heart disease

*Cholesterol levels are measured in milligrams per deciliter (mg/dL).

SOURCE: U.S. Department of Health and Human Services. (2005). *High Blood Cholesterol What You Need to Know* (NIH Publication No. 05-3290). Bethesda, MD: National Institutes of Health.

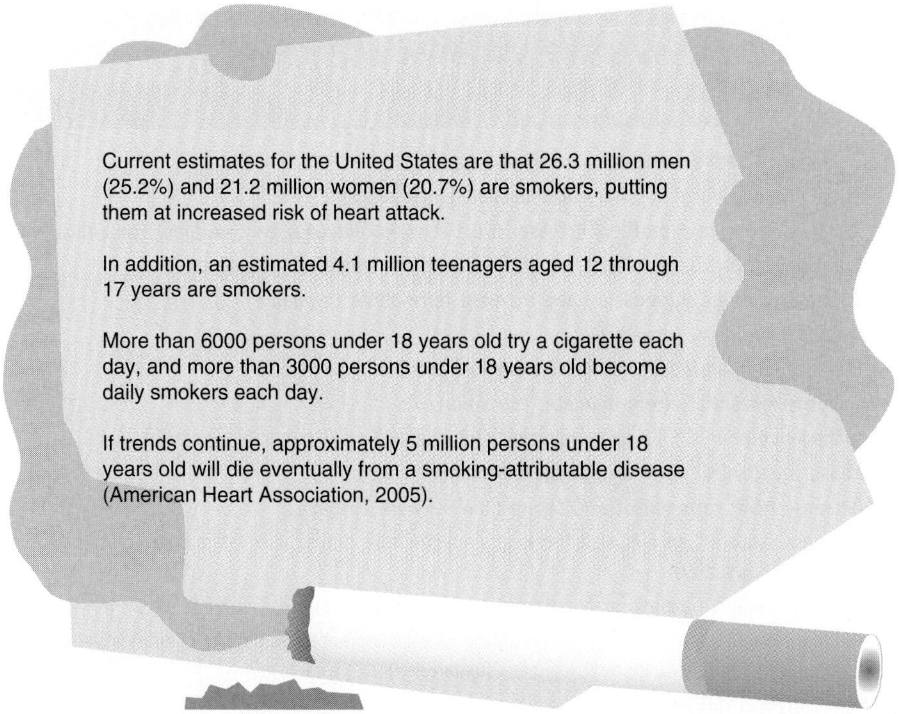

FIGURE 5.6 **Some Facts About Cigarette Smoking.**

Current estimates for the United States are that 26.3 million men (25.2%) and 21.2 million women (20.7%) are smokers, putting them at increased risk of heart attack.

In addition, an estimated 4.1 million teenagers aged 12 through 17 years are smokers.

More than 6000 persons under 18 years old try a cigarette each day, and more than 3000 persons under 18 years old become daily smokers each day.

If trends continue, approximately 5 million persons under 18 years old will die eventually from a smoking-attributable disease (American Heart Association, 2005).

clot formation, which can cause a heart attack if the clot becomes lodged in an atherosclerotic artery.

DIABETES MELLITUS   Diabetes mellitus is a disorder of the endocrine system that interferes with the body's production of insulin. Insulin is needed for the body to metabolize glucose (sugar). Diabetes affects cholesterol and triglyceride levels, which explains why a large number of people with diabetes die from some cardiovascular disease. A good diet, physical activity, weight control—and sometimes a prescription medication—can assist in keeping diabetes in control. See Chapter 6 for further information on diabetes.

OBESITY   Overweight and obesity are increasing globally, with a 25 percent increase noted just over the past three decades (Centers for Disease Control and Prevention, 2005). Obesity is a risk factor for heart disease, even if there are no other risk factors present, because carrying excess weight places a strain on the heart.

PHYSICAL INACTIVITY   Lack of physical activity is a major risk factor for heart disease. Numerous studies have been published during the past 50 years that show people who exercise regularly have better cardiovascular health (Haskell, 1997). Although research results vary from study to study, it is important to note that all studies consistently showed that being physically active does not increase an individual's risk of coronary heart disease. The primary and secondary prevention benefits of physical activity are numerous (TABLE 5.5). See Chapter 4 for more details about physical activity and cardiovascular health.

Other Factors

ALCOHOL MISUSE   Drinking too much alcohol can raise blood pressure, contribute to high levels of triglycerides in the blood and lead to obesity. Each are associated with increased risk for cardiovascular disease. See Chapter 14 for more information on alcohol.

TABLE 5.5	Biological Mechanisms by Which Exercise May Contribute to the Primary and Secondary Prevention of Coronary Heart Disease

Maintain or increase myocardial oxygen supply

- Delay progression of coronary atherosclerosis (possible)
- Improve lipoprotein profile (increase HDL/LDL ratio, decrease triglycerides) (probable)
- Improve carbohydrate metabolism (increase insulin sensitivity) (probable)
- Decrease platelet aggregation and increase fibrinolysis (probable)
- Decrease adiposity (usually)
- Increase coronary collateral vascularization (unlikely)
- Increase epicardial artery diameter (possible)
- Increase coronary blood flow (myocardial perfusion) or distribution (possible)

Decrease myocardial work and oxygen demand

- Decrease heart rate at rest and submaximal exercise (usually)
- Decrease systolic and mean systemic arterial pressure during submaximal exercise (usually) and at rest (usually)
- Decrease cardiac output during submaximal exercise (probable)
- Decrease circulating plasma catecholamine levels (decrease sympathetic tone) at rest (probable) and at submaximal exercise (usually)

Increase myocardial function

- Increase stroke volume at rest and in submaximal and maximal exercise (likely)
- Increase ejection fraction at rest and during exercise (likely)
- Increase intrinsic myocardial contractility (possible)
- Increase myocardial function resulting from decreased "afterload" (probable)
- Increase myocardial hypertrophy (probable); but this may not reduce CHD risk

Increase electrical stability of myocardium

- Decrease regional ischemia or at submaximal exercise (possible)
- Decrease catecholamines in myocardium at rest (possible) and at submaximal exercise (probable)
- Increase ventricular fibrillation threshold due to reduction of cyclic AMP (possible)

Likelihood that effect will occur for an individual participating in endurance-type training—for 16 weeks or longer, at 65 to 80 percent of functional capacity, for 25 min or longer per session (300 kcal), for three or more sessions per week—ranges from unlikely, possible, likely, probable, to usually.

ABBREVIATIONS: HDL = high-density lipoprotein cholesterol; LDL = low-density lipoprotein cholesterol; CHD = coronary heart disease; AMP = adenosine monophosphate.

SOURCE: W.L. Haskell. (March 1995). Physical Activity in the Prevention and Management of Coronary Heart Disease. *Physical Activity and Fitness Research Digest,* 2(1): 8–9. President's Council on Physical Fitness and Sports, Department of Health and Human Services.

Stress may contribute to heart disease.

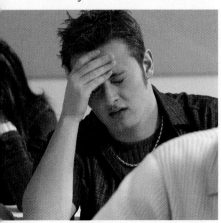

STRESS   Stress is a given in our society today. The ordinary events at home, on the job, and even at leisure can trigger stress responses as we try to maintain ourselves in an increasingly complex set of circumstances. We may not be able to get away from stress, but we can learn to deal with it (see Chapter 13). Research has not yet revealed exactly how stress affects the heart, but there appears to be a relationship between the occurrence of a heart attack, for instance, and the person's stress level, risky behaviors (cigarette smoking, diet), and socioeconomic status. For instance, an individual may develop high blood pressure due to stress, or may respond to stress by overeating or smoking.

Physical Activity and Health Connection

Although cardiovascular disease is the leading cause of death in the United States, it can be prevented through not smoking, maintaining a good diet low in cholesterol, maintaining a normal blood pressure, and participating in regular physical activity. Cardiovascular disease is thought of as a lifestyle disease; however, there are some risk factors over which you have no control (age, gender, family history).

Participation in regular physical activity helps to strengthen the function of all components of your cardiovascular system. This is important not only in terms of cardiovascular efficiency but also in terms of disease protection. Many of the chronic diseases of the cardiovascular system result from disuse. Physical activity stresses the cardiovascular system and makes it more fit. The more fit you are, the easier your cardiovascular system adjusts to the stress of physical exertion. Those who have a fit cardiovascular system are less likely to suffer a heart attack, less likely to die if they have a heart attack, and more likely to recover fully after a heart attack.

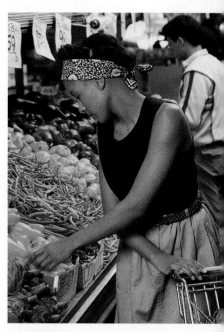

A diet rich in fruits and vegetables may decrease risk for CVD.

concept connections

1. **Physical inactivity is an independent risk factor for cardiovascular disease (CVD).** Physical inactivity, by itself, is a significant risk factor for the development of cardiovascular disease. If all other risk factors for CVD were minimized and you were sedentary, you would still be at increased risk for CVD.

2. **The National Institutes of Health has concluded that being physically active helps prevent heart disease.** Several government agencies, including the NIH, have issued policy statements supporting the importance of participating in regular physical activity. All of these statements have pointed to the role physical activity plays in helping to prevent heart disease.

3. **There are many forms of cardiovascular disease.** Coronary heart disease is the most prevalent form of CVD; it occurs when the coronary arteries become clogged and blood flow is restricted. Heart attack and angina pectoris are most often caused by CVD.

4. **_Angina pectoris_ and _heart attack_ are not synonymous terms.** Angina is caused by reduced blood flow to the heart; a heart attack results from the complete shutdown of blood supply to the heart.

5. **Hypertension is a major risk factor for coronary heart disease.** Hypertension, the "silent killer," is a condition where the blood pressure to and from the heart is above the normal range. When the cause of the hypertension is unknown, it is referred to as _primary hypertension_. _Secondary hypertension_ refers to cases in which the cause is known.

6. **Arteriosclerosis and atherosclerosis are key factors in cardiovascular disease.** _Arteriosclerosis_ is the hardening of the arteries, which causes the walls of the arteries to thicken and lose their elasticity. _Atherosclerosis_ is the most common form of arteriosclerosis and is a slow, progressive disease sometimes beginning in childhood. When the arteries lose their ability to contract and expand, blood flow to the heart is restricted.

Cerebrovascular accident (CVA), or stroke, is a cardiovascular disease that affects the central nervous system. Stroke is a form of CVD that affects the arteries of the central nervous system. There are two types of stroke: ischemic (caused by clots) and hemorrhagic (caused by blood seeping from a hole in the wall of the blood vessel).

 The three unmodifiable risk factors for CVD are age, family, and gender. Three cardiovascular risk factors that cannot be changed are age, gender, and family history.

 The six modifiable CVD risk factors are hypertension, high blood cholesterol, cigarette smoking, diabetes, obesity, and physical inactivity. Choices we make in how we live can profoundly impact our risk for cardiovascular disease.

Terms

Independent risk factor, 80
Coronary heart disease, 81
Angina pectoris, 82
Ischemia, 82
Myocardial infarction (MI), 82
Hypertension, 83
Primary hypertension, 83

Secondary hypertension, 83
Arteriosclerosis, 84
Atherosclerosis, 84
Plaque, 84
Stroke, 84
Ischemic strokes, 84
Cerebral thrombosis, 84

Cerebral embolism, 84
Hemorrhagic strokes, 85
Cerebral hemorrhage, 85
Subarachnoid hemorrhage, 85
Cholesterol, 86
Lipoproteins, 86
Low-density lipoproteins, 86

making the connection

Richard has learned about the biological mechanisms by which physical activity may contribute to the prevention of coronary heart disease. So, in addition to what he was already doing to prevent cardiovascular disease for the past couple years, he has added a 30-minute walk to his daily routine over the past couple months. Not only does Richard feel better physically as a result of his daily walk, but the internal satisfaction of knowing that he is doing even more to lower his risk of developing coronary heart disease is also very rewarding to him.

Critical Thinking

1. Make a list of all the factors that increase your chances of getting CVD. Order the list from the highest to lowest risk. Which risk factors pertain to you? How can you modify or change any of these risk factors?
2. Richard knew that diet, in particular cholesterol, was a factor in lowering his risk for coronary heart disease. Identify three ways in which you can lower your cholesterol.
3. A risk factor of cardiovascular disease is family history. Family history of CVD does not guarantee that you will get the disease,

nor does it cancel out the importance of a healthy lifestyle (good nutritional balance, regular physical activity, and no smoking). A family history of CVD does predispose you to the disease, so it is important for you to determine your family CVD history. Construct a family tree by listing your biological parents, siblings, grandparents (maternal and paternal), and aunts and uncles (paternal and maternal). Next to each name, list the CVD disease and the age at which it was discovered. Your family may be helpful with this activity. After completing your tree, you may want to share it with your family and discuss prevention efforts.

4. Melissa is a 21-year-old college student who is very studious. Because her studies are her number one priority (she wants to go to graduate school), Melissa finds it difficult to make time to maintain a healthy lifestyle, despite knowing how important it is. Although Melissa is not a regular smoker, she has a tendency to smoke when under stress (studying for finals), and frequently eats fast food. Melissa was active in high school sports, but she does not seem to find time for sports now that she is in college. As a matter of fact, she has gained about 15 pounds, although she would not be considered overweight. What can you suggest to help Melissa reduce her risk of cardiovascular disease?

References

American Heart Association. (2005). *Cardiovascular Disease Statistics.* Online: http://www.americanheart.org/presenter.jhtml?identifier=4478.

Blair, S.N., et al. (1989). Physical fitness and all-cause mortality: A prospective study of healthy men and women. *Journal of the American Medical Association* 262(17):2395–2401.

Centers for Disease Control and Prevention. (2005). *Overweight and Obesity.* Online: http://www.cdc.gov/nccdphp/dnpa/obesity/.

Chien, K.L., et al. (1999). Lipoprotein A level in the population in Taiwan: Relationship to sociodemographic and atherosclerotic risk factors. *Atherosclerosis* 143(2):267–273.

Corti, N.C., Guralink, J.M., & Bicato, C. (1996). Coronary heart disease risk factors in older persons. *Aging Clinical Experimental Research* 9:75–79.

Hagberg, J.M. (1997). Physical activity, physical fitness, and blood pressure. In Leon, A.S., ed. *Physical Activity and Cardiovascular Health: A National Consensus.* Champaign, IL: Human Kinetics.

Haskell, W.L. (1995). Physical activity in the prevention and management of coronary heart disease. *President's Council on Physical Fitness and Sports Research Digest* 2(1):1–7.

He, J., Ogdon, L.G., Vupputury, S., Bazzano, L.A., Loria, C., & Whelton, P.K. (1999). Dietary sodium intake and subsequent risk of CVD in overweight adults. *Journal of the American Medical Association* 282(21):2027–2034.

Lembo, G., et al. (1998). Systemic hypertension and coronary artery disease: The link. *American Journal of Cardiology* 82(3A):2H–7H.

National Heart, Lung, and Blood Institute. (2005). What is high blood pressure? Online: http://www.nhlbi.nih.gov/health/dci/Diseases/Hbp/HBP_Whatis.html.

National Institutes of Health. (1995). Physical activity and cardiovascular health. *NIH Consensus Statement* 13(3):1–33.

Paffenbarger, R.S., Jr., Hyde, R.T., Wing, A.L., & Hsieh, C. (1986). Physical activity, all-cause mortality, and longevity of college alumni. *New England Journal of Medicine* 314(10):605–613.

Ross, R. (1993). The pathogenesis of atherosclerosis: A perspective for the 1990s. *Nature* 362:801–810.

Simon, J.A., & Hudes, E.S. (1999). Serum ascorbic acid and cardiovascular disease prevalence in U.S. adults: The Third National Health and Nutrition Examination Survey. Annals of Epidemiology 9(6):358–365.

United States Department of Health and Human Services. (1996). *Physical Activity and Health: A Report of the Surgeon General, Executive Summary.* Washington, DC: U.S. Government Printing Office.

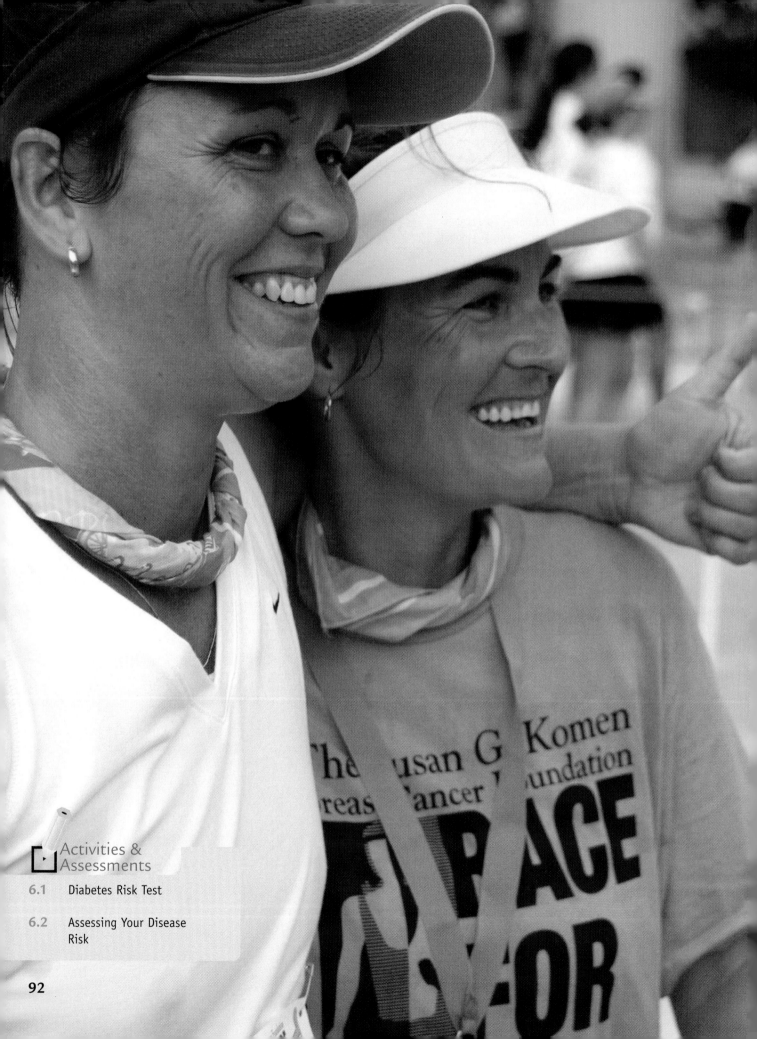

Activities & Assessments

6.1   Diabetes Risk Test

6.2   Assessing Your Disease Risk

The Role of Physical Activity in Preventing Diabetes and Cancer

6

what's the connection?

Monica became aware of the genetic tendency in her family for the development of type 2 diabetes. Monica decided that she wanted to take some positive steps to reduce her risk. She found that in addition to genetics, diabetes mellitus is linked to poor nutrition and physical inactivity. Realizing that she would not be able to alter her genetics, Monica decided she would learn what she could about the role that nutrition and physical activity played in reducing risk for type 2 diabetes. After gathering some information, Monica decided that she would be more careful about consuming refined sugars and would incorporate daily physical activity into her life. In this way, Monica felt that she was taking responsibility for her own health.

concepts

1. The incidence of chronic diseases is steadily increasing.

2. Diabetes mellitus is a condition in which the body is unable to produce and/or properly use insulin.

3. A sedentary lifestyle increases your risk of developing diabetes mellitus.

4. The incidence of diabetes mellitus in children and adolescents is increasing.

5. Cancer is a group of diseases characterized by the uncontrollable growth and spread of abnormal cells.

6. Cancer is the second leading cause of death in the United States.

7. Breast cancer is prevalent among women, and physical activity is thought to be a protective factor.

8. Colorectal cancer and physical activity is the most thoroughly investigated cancer–physical activity relationship.

http://physicalactivity.jbpub.com

The Web site for this book is a great source for supplementary physical health information for both students and instructors. Visit **http://physicalactivity.jbpub.com** to find a variety of useful tools for learning, thinking, and teaching.

The incidence of chronic diseases is steadily increasing.

Incidence The frequency of occurrence of a particular disease, the number of new cases of a disease.

Introduction

The **incidence** of chronic diseases has seen a steady increase over the past century. More than 90 million Americans live with chronic disease (Centers for Disease Control and Prevention [CDC], 2006). Chronic diseases account for more than 70 percent of all deaths in the United States (CDC, 2006). The major chronic disease killers—cardiovascular disease, cancer, diabetes, and chronic obstructive pulmonary disease (COPD)—are basically caused by what people do or do not do; they are thus sometimes referred to as "lifestyle diseases." Not only are the costs in lives overwhelming, but the medical costs due to chronic diseases are also staggering: over $1.275 trillion annually, or more than 75 percent of the total medical care expenditures in the United States (based on data from 2003), is spent on treating chronic diseases (CDC, 2006; USDHHS, 2005).

Cardiovascular disease and obesity receive the most attention as diseases that are heavily influenced by living a sedentary lifestyle. These important topics are dealt with in Chapters 5 and 9. However, two other common diseases linked to physical inactivity are diabetes mellitus and some forms of cancer. This chapter provides an overview of the link between physical inactivity and these two major chronic diseases.

Understanding Diabetes Mellitus

Diabetes mellitus affects approximately 18.2 million people in the United States, and over 5.2 million of these people do not know they have the disease (CDC, 2004). Diabetes has been ranked among the top ten leading causes of death in the United States since 1932 (Bishop, Zimmerman, & Roesler, 1998), and during the last decade it has been the sixth leading cause of death (CDC, 2004) (**FIGURE 6.1**). Despite the fact that diabetes has been known for centuries, and is epidemic in many countries, our knowledge of the nature of diabetes is still incomplete (USDHHS, 2005). More than 9 percent of persons aged 20 years and older and about one-fifth of adults 60 years and older have diabetes, including those with undiagnosed diabetes (USDHHS, 2005). The latest figure (2002) for the estimated

FIGURE 6.1 **Leading Causes of Death, 2002.** SOURCE: U.S. Department of Health and Human Services. (2005). *Health, United States, 2005*. Hyattsville, MD: Author.

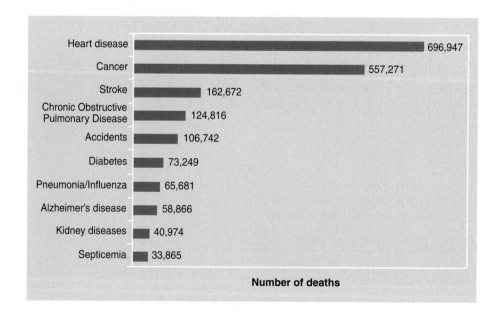

economic impact of diabetes in the United States is $132 billion, with $92 billion in direct medical costs and another $40 billion in indirect costs (CDC, 2004).

Diabetes mellitus includes a group of diseases in which the body is unable to produce and/or properly utilize insulin. Insulin, a hormone secreted by the pancreas, is needed by muscle, fat, and the liver to metabolize glucose. Diabetes is diagnosed by identifying high levels of blood glucose. Not all people who have insulin-regulating difficulties have clinical diabetes. Diabetes is also related to conditions in which glucose regulation is impaired. In pre-diabetes, impaired glucose tolerance (IGT) or impaired fasting glucose (IFG), or both, exists (American Diabetes Association [ADA], 2006). With IFG, blood sugar levels are elevated after an overnight fast, but not to levels high enough to be classified as clinical diabetes (ADA, 2006). With IGT, blood glucose levels are elevated after a glucose tolerance test, but again not at levels high enough to be classified as clinical diabetes (ADA, 2006). It is estimated that 41 million Americans have pre-diabetes (ADA, 2006). For those with pre-diabetes, the best way of preventing this condition from progressing to diabetes is to maintain a healthy weight, follow sound nutritional practices, and increase physical activity levels. Although clinical diabetes alone is a very dangerous disease, there is also an increased risk for cardiovascular disease even with pre-diabetes.

There are four types of clinical diabetes: type 1, type 2, gestational, and other. Type 1, or what used to be referred to as insulin-dependent diabetes mellitus (IDDM), is simply defined as diabetes caused by an inability to produce enough insulin. This form of diabetes has a high genetic component and usually starts in childhood or adolescence. Five to 10 percent of the U.S. population has type 1 diabetes (ADA, 2006). Diabetes is a serious, lifelong condition that can cause heart disease, kidney failure, and blindness.

Type 2 diabetes, or what was once called non-insulin-dependent diabetes mellitus (NIDDM), accounts for 90 to 95 percent of all diagnosed cases of diabetes. Type 2 diabetes is often associated with obesity, poor nutritional habits, and physical inactivity, which may account for recent occurrences of type 2 diabetes among younger people. This type of diabetes allows sufficient production of insulin, but the body is unable to use it effectively. The term **hyperglycemia** describes a condition where there is too much glucose in the blood. Hyperglycemia means that either your pancreas is not producing enough insulin or your body cannot use its own insulin well; both result in an increased amount of glucose in the blood. This is the opposite of **hypoglycemia**, which indicates insufficient glucose in the blood.

Gestational diabetes develops in 2 to 5 percent of all pregnancies and usually disappears when the pregnancy is over. Other types of diabetes result from specific genetic syndromes, drugs, malnutrition, infection, and other illnesses. This type of diabetes accounts for 1 to 2 percent of all diagnosed cases of diabetes.

Type 2 Diabetes and Children

Over the last decade, there has been an increasing **prevalence** of type 2 diabetes in children and adolescents. About 176,500 people under 20 have diabetes (ADA, 2006). This represents 0.22 percent of all people in this age group (ADA, 2006). Approximately one in every 400 to 600 children and adolescents has type 1 diabetes (ADA, 2006). Type 2 diabetes is becoming even more common among Native Americans, African Americans, and Hispanic/Latinos (ADA, 2006; USDHHS, 2005).

Most experts agree that the increasing prevalence of type 2 diabetes in children and adolescents is associated with the increase in overweight and obesity that has paralleled the rise in diabetes. Combined with decreasing levels of physical activity in this population, a continued rise in childhood diabetes is predicted (Eyre et al.,

Diabetes mellitus is a condition in which the body is unable to produce and/or properly use insulin.

A sedentary lifestyle increases your risk of developing diabetes mellitus.

Hyperglycemia Too much blood sugar.

Hypoglycemia Not enough blood sugar.

Prevalence The predominance of a disease, the number of people who have the disease at one given point in time.

The incidence of diabetes mellitus in children and adolescents is increasing.

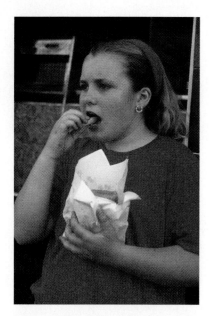

Poor nutrition and a sedentary lifestyle increase risk for childhood diabetes.

Cancer is a group of diseases characterized by the uncontrollable growth and spread of abnormal cells.

Cancer A term for diseases in which abnormal cells divide without control. Cancer cells can invade nearby tissues and spread through the bloodstream and lymphatic system to other parts of the body.

Tumors An abnormal mass of tissue that results from excessive cell division. Tumors perform no useful body function and can be benign or malignant.

Benign Not cancerous; does not invade nearby tissue or spread to other parts of the body.

Malignant Cancerous; a growth with a tendency to invade and destroy nearby tissue and spread to other parts of the body.

Metastasis The spread of cancer from one part of the body to another. Cells in the metastic (secondary) tumor are the same as those in their original (primary) tumor.

2004). The long-term health care costs associated with this trend, both in terms of human and economic factors, will be extraordinary.

Type 2 Diabetes and Physical Activity

There is considerable research supporting the relationship between physical inactivity and type 2 diabetes (USDHHS, 2005). Studies suggest that exercise burns calories, which in turn helps with weight reduction, in turn improving the body's response to insulin (USDHHS, 2005). Physical activity has been shown to play a role in the prevention of type 2 diabetes (Colberg & Swain, 2000).

The mechanism for physical activity's positive impact on diabetes prevention comes from its role in improving insulin sensitivity and reducing the incidence of overweight and obesity. With improved insulin sensitivity, cells in the body do not require as much insulin to regulate blood sugar levels. Physical activity also increases energy expenditure, thereby reducing the likelihood of a positive energy balance occurring, with resultant weight gain. Poor insulin sensitivity and a sedentary lifestyle place one at major risk for the development of type 2 diabetes.

Many people with type 2 diabetes can control their blood glucose by following a careful diet and exercise program, losing excess weight, and taking oral medication. The more physical activity one participates in, the less likelihood there is of developing type 2 diabetes. People with diabetes need to balance their diet and insulin (type 1) with their physical activity regimen. Whether you have type 1 or type 2 diabetes, physical activity is a cornerstone in diabetes therapy.

What Is Cancer?

Cancer is actually a group of more than one hundred diseases characterized by the uncontrollable growth and spread of abnormal cells. In normal body cells, the rate of cell division is controlled; however, when cancer is present, the cells divide rapidly, assuming irregular shapes, and **tumors** develop and invade normal tissue. Tumors can be either benign or malignant. **Benign** tumors grow slowly and remain localized, but a **malignant** tumor grows rapidly and infiltrates surrounding tissues, frequently infiltrating the bloodstream and lymphatic system. When cancer spreads from its primary site to another site, the process is called **metastasis**. The term *cancer* is used to indicate any type of malignant tumor.

Tumors are named according to the type of tissues and cells from which they originate. There are many types of malignant tumors, but they all can be classified into three groups: carcinoma, sarcoma, and leukemia. Like most classification systems, there are exceptions. Although they do not fall into one of the three groups just mentioned, lymphomas and skin tumors have their own separate classifications (TABLE 6.1).

Understanding Cancer

Cancer is the second leading cause of death in the United States (USDHHS, 2005). Approximately one of every two American males and one of every three American females will develop some type of cancer during their lifetimes, and about one person in four will die from cancer. However, the most recent data (2003) indicate that for the first time in more than 70 years, annual cancer death rates in the United States have fallen (USDHHS, 2005). This is most likely related to the decline in cigarette smoking and improved medical practices (USDHHS, 2005). Incidence rates for all cancers combined declined from 1990 to 2002 for males, but not for females. The rates for men experienced a 1 percent drop, whereas women experienced a statistically significant increase of 0.4 percent (USDHHS, 2005).

TABLE 6.1	**Classification of Malignant Tumors**

Classification	Definition	Example(s)
Carcinoma	Any malignant tumor arising from surface, glandular, or parenchymal epithelium.	Squamous cell carcinoma of the esophagus Adenocarcinoma of the pancreas
Sarcoma	A general term referring to a malignant tumor arising from primary tissues other than the surface, glandular, or parenchymal epithelium. Prefixing the term by designating the cell of origin identifies the exact type of sarcoma.	Chondrosarcoma (cartilage) Fibrosarcoma (fibrous tissue) Myosarcoma (muscle) Osteosarcoma (bone)
Leukemia Lymphomas	Any neoplasm of blood-forming tissues. All tumors of lymphoid tissue are lymphomas. Lymphomas are malignant, with rare exception.	Hodgkin's disease
Melanomas	Skin tumors that arise from the keratin-forming cells or pigment-producing cells of the epidermis.	Basal cell carcinoma Squamous cell carcinoma (a more aggressive tumor)

SOURCE: Adapted from L.V. Crowley. (2001). *Introduction to Human Disease*, 5th ed. Sudbury, MA: Jones and Bartlett.

The most frequent cancer sites in males are the prostate, followed by the lung, and then the colon and rectum (USDHHS, 2005). Rates are higher for African American men than for other racial and ethnic groups: 50 percent greater for prostate cancer, 49 percent greater for lung cancer, and 16 percent greater for colon and rectum cancer (USDHHS, 2005).

Breast cancer is the most frequently diagnosed cancer among females (USDHHS, 2005). Rates are higher for non-Hispanic white women than others: 33 percent higher than for African American women, 52 percent higher than for Asian or Pacific Islanders, and 75 percent higher than for Hispanic females (USDHHS, 2005).

Despite the prevalence of cancer, most cancers can be prevented. Several researchers have estimated overall cancer deaths due to various causes or factors. Brownson, Reif, Alavanja, and Bal (1998, p. 340) suggest "priority must be given to eliminating tobacco use, becoming more physically active, and adopting diets that contain less fat and more fresh fruits and vegetables." The American Cancer Society (ACS) contends that about one-third of cancer deaths are related to nutrition and other lifestyle factors and could be prevented through behavioral changes (ACS, 2006). The risk factors for specific types of cancer are provided in TABLE 6.2 .

Evidence is available indicating that physical activity reduces the risk of breast and colon cancers (ACS, 2006; Eyre et al., 2004). Physical activity is thought to affect cancer risk by helping maintain a healthy body weight (ACS, 2006; Eyre et al., 2004). Excess body weight increases the levels of estrogen, androgens, and insulin in the blood that are associated with cell and tumor growth (Eyre et al., 2004). Physical activity can also help to prevent type 2 diabetes, which has been associated with increased risk for a variety of cancers (Eyre et al., 2004).

Regular screenings by health care professionals can result in the early detection of cancers of the breast, colon, rectum, cervix, prostate, testes, oral cavity, and skin. Early detection is important, because the earlier cancer is diagnosed, the more likely it is that treatment will be successful.

The Healthy People 2010 goal for cancer reduction is 158.7 cancer deaths per 100,000 population (USDHHS, 2000), compared with just under 194 cancer deaths per 100,000 population currently (USDHHS, 2005). We are seeing a decline in cancer deaths, in part due to systematic cancer control efforts. These efforts have six key elements: (1) reducing the prevalence of smoking, (2) reducing the percentage of total calories in the diet from fat, (3) increasing the average daily consumption of fiber, (4) increasing the percentage of women who undergo annual

Cancer is the second leading cause of death in the United States.

TABLE 6.2	Risk Factors for Common Cancers
Cancer	**Risk Factors**
Lung cancer	• Cigarette smoking (greatest risk factor)
	• Exposure to industrial substances
	• Some organic chemicals
	• Radon and asbestos
	• Air pollution
	• Tuberculosis
	• Environmental tobacco smoke (in nonsmokers)
Breast cancer	• Age
	• Personal or family history
	• A long menstrual history (menstrual periods starting early in life and ending late in life)
	• Recent use of oral contraceptives or postmenopausal estrogen
	• Never had children or had first child after age 30
	• Consuming two or more drinks of alcohol daily
	• Higher education and socioeconomic status
	• Possible susceptibility genes for breast cancer (BRCA1 and BRCA2)
Prostate cancer	• Age (more than 75% of all prostate cancers are diagnosed in men over age 65)
	• Race (Black Americans have the highest prostate cancer incidence rates in the world)
	• Strong familial disposition
	• Dietary fat
Colorectal cancer	• Personal or family history of colorectal cancer or polyps
	• Low-fat and/or high-fiber diet
	• Physical inactivity
Skin cancer	• Excessive exposure to ultraviolet radiation
	• Fair complexion
	• Occupational exposure to coal tar, pitch, creosote, arsenic compounds, or radium
	• Family history
	• Multiple moles (nevi) or atypical mole

breast cancer screening, (5) increasing the percentage of women who have annual Pap tests, and (6) increasing adoption of state-of-the-art cancer treatments. The majority of these efforts require the individual to take action—to quit smoking, to eat a nutritionally balanced diet, increase physical activity, and to receive annual cancer screening.

Because many of the causes of cancer are known, it is possible to reduce cancer incidence rates. Ames, Gold, and Willett (1995) stated: "Decreases in physical activity and increases in smoking, obesity, and recreational sun exposure have contributed importantly to increases in some cancers in the modern industrial world, whereas improvements in hygiene have reduced cancers related to infection."

Common Cancers

Cancer can strike virtually any part of the body; however, it occurs more commonly in certain areas. Some cancers of particular concern include lung cancer, breast cancer, prostate cancer, colon and rectum cancer, and skin cancer. This chapter focuses on the three most influenced by physical activity: prostate cancer, colorectal cancer, and breast cancer.

Breast Cancer

Breast cancer is the most commonly diagnosed cancer and the leading cause of cancer deaths among women in the United States (USDHHS, 2005). The incidence rate of breast cancer increases with age, with approximately 77 percent of new cases of breast cancer occurring in women over the age of 50.

At the present, early detection through the use of mammography is the most effective method for detecting breast cancer early and before it spreads (USDHHS, 2005). Current estimates indicate that breast cancer mortality can be reduced by between 19 to 30 percent through routine clinical breast examinations and mammography screening for women aged 50 through 74 years (U.S. Preventive Services Task Force, 1996).

Healthy People 2010 set a goal to have 70 percent of women aged 40 years and older screened for breast cancer within the past 2 years (USDHHS, 2000). Despite efforts to reach these goals, breast cancer screening services are still underutilized.

Breast cancer is prevalent among women, and physical activity is thought to be a protective factor.

BREAST CANCER AND PHYSICAL ACTIVITY
Several studies have been published suggesting physical activity is a protective factor against breast cancer (ACS, 2006; USDHHS, 2005). Kavanagh, Singletary, Einhorn, and Depetrillo (1999) reported that women who spent 1 to 3 hours in physical activity per week reduced their risk of breast cancer by 30 percent as compared with inactive women. They also noted that women who exercised at least 4 hours per week reduced their breast cancer risk by 50 percent. Another study evaluated the influence of both work and leisure-time physical activity on the risk of breast cancer in a group of 25,624 pre- and postmenopausal women (Thune, Brenn, Lund, & Gaard, 1997). The researchers concluded that physical activity during leisure time and at work is associated with a reduced risk of breast cancer.

A study conducted by the researchers at the Netherlands Cancer Institute compared the physical activity histories of 918 women aged 20 to 54 who had been diagnosed with invasive breast cancer with those of 918 women who did not have cancer (ACS, 2000b). The researchers found that active women had a 30 percent lower risk of breast cancer than those who were inactive. According to the American Cancer Society, exercising harder and longer may be linked to a reduced risk for breast cancer (ACS, 2006). In fact, the ACS states that the best advice for reducing breast cancer risk is to engage in vigorous physical activity at least 4 hours per week, avoid or limit intake of alcohol to no more than one drink per day, and reduce lifetime weight through the combination of limiting calories and exercising regularly (ACS, 2006).

The mechanism by which exercise reduces the risk for breast cancer is still under investigation. One possible explanation is that vigorous physical activity may decrease the exposure of breast tissue to circulating ovarian hormones (Eyre et al., 2004).

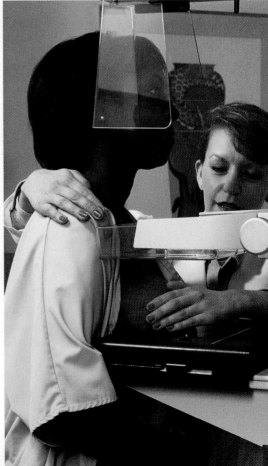

Mammograms are one means of detecting breast cancer early.

Physical activity plays a role in the prevention of breast cancer.

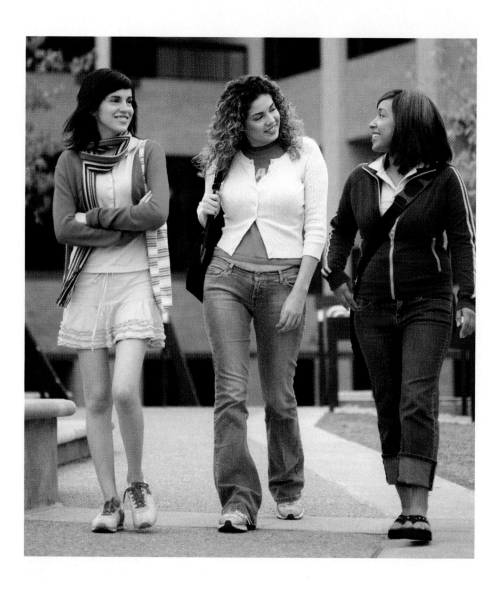

Prostate Cancer

Prostate cancer is a major health problem worldwide and has been described as an epidemiological enigma (Mettlin, 1997), with many different suspected risk factors but few showing consistent or strong associations with the disease. Dramatic increases in prostate cancer occurred in the late 1980s and early 1990s in the United States, with peak incidence in 1992 (Mettlin, 1997; National Cancer Institute [NCI], 1998).

Prostate cancer is the most prevalent cancer among men and the second leading cause of cancer death among men (ACS, 2006). Between 1989 and 1992 the prostate cancer incidence rates increased dramatically; however, between 1992 and 1996, prostate cancer mortality rates declined significantly (ACS, 2000a), and they continued to decline through 2002 (USDHHS, 2005). The increase in incidence rates could be due in part to earlier diagnosis in men without symptoms, increased use of prostate-specific antigen (PSA) blood test screenings, and digital rectal exams. Prostate cancer is rarely diagnosed in men under the age of 50, but the incidence rises faster for every decade after that (NCI, 1999).

PROSTATE CANCER AND PHYSICAL ACTIVITY   The effects of physical activity on prostate cancer have been the most commonly studied second to colorectal cancer (USDHHS, 1996). Data to date reveal inconsistent results with regard to the relationship between physical activity and prostate cancer. Brownson, Chang, Davis, and Smith (1991) investigated the risk of various cancer types, including prostate and testicular cancer, in relation to occupational physical activity. They found an inverse association (the more physical activity on the job, the greater the risk) between occupational physical activity and prostate and testicular cancer, noting that their findings should be considered preliminary and required confirmation from other studies. Apparently nutritional factors such as limiting intake of animal products (especially red meat and high-fat dairy products) and eating five or more servings of vegetables and fruits each day are more important than physical activity in reducing the risk of prostate cancer (ACS, 2006); however, the jury is still out.

Colon and Rectum Cancer

Cancer of the colon and rectum, or colorectal cancer, is the second leading cause of cancer-related deaths in the United States (ACS, 2006) and is the third leading cancer and cause of cancer deaths in both men and women (ACS, 2006). Colorectal cancer mortality is greater for men than women, and higher among blacks than whites (ACS, 2006). Two-thirds of the people who get colorectal cancer are over the age of 50. However, there are people under the age of 50 who get colorectal cancer.

COLORECTAL CANCER AND PHYSICAL ACTIVITY   The relationship between physical activity and colorectal cancer has been the most thoroughly investigated cancer–physical activity relationship (USDHHS, 2005). Increasing evidence indicates that those who are moderately active on a regular basis have a lower risk for colon cancer (ACS, 2006). More vigorous exercise may even further reduce risk (ACS, 2006). The American Cancer Society suggests that the best advice for lowering the risk of colorectal cancer is to increase physical activity, eat more fruits and vegetables, limit intake of red meats, avoid obesity, and avoid excess alcohol (ACS, 2006).

Colorectal cancer and physical activity is the most thoroughly investigated cancer–physical activity relationship.

The mechanism for the protective effect of physical activity on colon cancer is that physical activity causes food to move more quickly through the intestine, reducing the length of time that the bowel lining is exposed to potential carcinogens (Eyre et al., 2004).

The surgeon general's report on physical activity states: "Together, the research on occupational and leisure-time physical activity strongly suggests that physical activity has a protective effect against the risk of developing colon cancer" (USDHHS, 1996, p. 116).

Summary

Many questions regarding the impact of physical activity on cancer risk remain unanswered (Eyre et al., 2004). Further research is necessary to determine the optimal intensity, duration, and frequency needed to affect cancer risk (Eyre et al., 2004). The general recommendations provided in Chapter 2 for appropriate levels of physical activity for basic and optimal health appear to be sufficient to reduce the risk of breast and colon cancers (Eyre et al., 2004).

Taking Responsibility for Your Health

Although you may not be thinking about chronic diseases because you are young and healthy, at some point in your life it is likely that you or someone you care about will be diagnosed with a chronic disease. We now know what we can do today to decrease the chances of getting a chronic disease tomorrow. All the data to date suggest that risk factors for most chronic diseases are factors over which you have control—physical activity, cigarette smoking, and dietary habits. You have the ability to begin to make changes in your lifestyle today that can make a difference for you in the future, especially when you consider that physical activity is a protective factor against breast cancer, colon cancer, and diabetes.

Physical Activity and Health Connection

Chronic diseases are commonly related to lifestyle, and their symptoms may take many years to surface. A lack of physical activity and poor nutrition are major contributors to the increased incidence of such chronic diseases as cardiovascular disease, diabetes, and several forms of cancer. Evidence now demonstrates that by leading a physically active lifestyle and eating a healthy diet, you can reduce your risk for developing hypertension, stroke, heart attack, breast cancer, colorectal cancer, and type 2 diabetes. Physical activity plays its most important role in the prevention of chronic diseases, but in certain circumstances (cardiovascular disease, diabetes), it can also play an important role in the rehabilitation process. The amount of research supporting the preventive role of physical activity and chronic disease varies by disease. Compelling evidence exists regarding the role of physical activity in the prevention of cardiovascular disease, type 2 diabetes, breast cancer, and colorectal cancer. This chapter has illustrated the integral connection between physical activity and health.

concept connections

1. **The incidence of chronic diseases is steadily increasing.** Chronic diseases account for seven of every 10 deaths in the United States. The major chronic disease killers are related to lifestyle or by what people do or do not do.

2. **Diabetes mellitus is a condition in which the body is unable to produce and/or properly use insulin.** Diabetes has been ranked among the top ten leading causes of death in the United States since 1932. Diabetes mellitus is a group of diseases in which the body is unable to produce and/or properly use insulin. Types of diabetes include type 1 (insulin dependent) and type 2 (non-insulin-dependent). The more physical activity you participate in, the less likely it is that you will develop type 2 diabetes.

3. **A sedentary lifestyle increases your risk of developing diabetes mellitus.** Being sedentary can lead to overweight and glucose intolerance, factors that predispose you to diabetes mellitus. Physical activity helps you to maintain a healthy body composition profile and glucose sensitivity.

4. **The incidence of diabetes mellitus in children and adolescents is increasing.** With ever-increasing numbers of children and adolescents living sedentary lifestyles and becoming overweight and obese at earlier ages, the incidence of diabetes in these populations is increasing. These gateway conditions will have a profound impact on health care costs and quality of life.

(5) **Cancer is a group of diseases characterized by the uncontrollable growth and spread of abnormal cells.** Tumors can be benign or malignant. The term *cancer* is used to indicate any type of malignant tumor.

(6) **Cancer is the second leading cause of death in the United States.** Although the incidence of cancer decreased for the first time in 2003, cancer is still the second leading cause of death in the United States. Lung cancer is the number one form of cancer.

(7) **Breast cancer is prevalent among women, and physical activity is thought to be a protective factor.** Breast cancer is the most commonly diagnosed cancer and the second leading cause of cancer deaths among women in the United States. Several recent studies have suggested physical activity as a protective factor against breast cancer.

(8) **Colorectal cancer and physical activity is the most thoroughly investigated cancer–physical activity relationship.** Colorectal cancer is the second leading cause of cancer-related deaths in the United States. Many studies that have measured occupational physical activity and the risk of colon cancer strongly suggest that physical activity has a protective effect against colon cancer.

Terms

Incidence, 94	Prevalence, 95	Benign, 96
Hyperglycemia, 95	Cancer, 96	Malignant, 96
Hypoglycemia, 95	Tumors, 96	Metastasis, 96

making the connection

Monica has learned much about the causes of type 2 diabetes. In so doing, she has gained an appreciation for the ways in which behavioral changes could help her lessen her own risk of developing type 2 diabetes. She understands that she needs to change her sedentary lifestyle. In addition, eating a wide variety of fruits and vegetables will supply her with nutrients that will not only help her obtain optimal health now but will also pave the way for years of health in the future. Eating better and maintaining a physically active lifestyle will help Monica keep her body weight in a healthy zone.

Critical Thinking

1. Poor nutrition, inactivity and being overweight increase your risk for developing type 2 diabetes. Analyze your diabetes risk profile and develop strategies that you can follow to reduce your chances of developing this common disease.

2. A risk factor for cancer is family history. Family history of cancer does not guarantee that you will get the disease, nor does it cancel out the importance of a healthy lifestyle (good nutritional balance, regular physical activity, and no smoking). A family history of cancer does predispose you to the disease; therefore, it is important for you to determine your family cancer history. Construct a family tree by listing your bio-logical parents, siblings, grandparents (maternal and paternal), and aunts and uncles (paternal and maternal). Next to each name, list the type of cancer and the age at which it was discovered. Your family may be helpful with this activity. After completing your tree, you may want to share it with your family and discuss prevention efforts.

3. Make a list of all the factors that increase your chance of getting cancer (review Table 6.2). Order the list from the highest to lowest risk. Which risk factors pertain to you? How can you modify or change any of these risk factors?

References

American Cancer Society. (2000a). *Cancer Facts and Figures, 2000.* Atlanta: Author.

American Cancer Society. (2000b). Regular exercise may lower breast cancer risk. *ACS News Today*, February 23.

American Cancer Society. (2006). The complete guide—nutrition and physical activity. Online: http://www.cancer.org/docroot/PED/content/PED_3_2X_Diet_and_Activity_Factors_That_Affect_Risks.asp.

American Diabetes Association. (2006). Total prevalence of diabetes and pre-diabetes. Online: http://www.diabetes.org/diabetes-statistics/prevalence.jsp.

Ames, B.N., Gold, L.S., & Willett, W.C. (1995). The causes and prevention of cancer. *Proceedings of the National Academy of Science of the United States of America* 92:5258–5265.

Bishop, D.B., Zimmerman, B.R., & Roesler, J.S. (1998). Diabetes. In Brownson, R.C., Remington, P.L., & Davis, J.R., eds. *Chronic Disease Epidemiology and Control*, 2nd ed. Washington, DC: American Public Health Association.

Brownson, R.C., Chang, J.C., Davis, J.R., & Smith, C. (1991). Physical activity on the job and cancer in Missouri. *American Journal of Public Health* 81(5):639–642.

Brownson, R.C., Reif, J.S., Alavanja, M.R.R., & Bal, D.G. (1998). Cancer. In Brownson, R.C., Remington, P.L., & Davis, J.R., eds. *Chronic Disease Epidemiology and Control*, 2nd ed. Washington, DC: American Public Health Association.

Brownson, R.C., Remington, P.L., & Davis, J.R. (1998). *Chronic Disease Epidemiology and Control*, 2nd ed. Washington, DC: American Public Health Association.

Centers for Disease Control and Prevention. (2004). National diabetes fact sheet: General information and national estimates on diabetes in the United States. 2003. Rev. ed. Atlanta, CA: U.S. Department of Health and Human Services, Centers for Disease Control and Prevention.

Centers for Disease Control and Prevention. (2006). Costs of chronic disease. Online: http://www.cdc.gov/nccdphp/overview.htm#2.

Colberg, S.R., & Swain, D.P. (2000). Exercise and diabetes control. *The Physician and Sports Medicine* 28(4):63ff.

Eyre, H., Kahn, R., & Robertson, R.M. (2004). Preventing cancer, cardiovascular disease, and diabetes: A common agenda for the American Cancer Society, the American Diabetes Association, and the American Heart Association. *CA: A Cancer Journal for Clinicians* 54(4):190–207.

Kavanagh, J.J., Singletary, S.E., Einhorn, N., & Depetrillo, A.D. (1999). *Breast Cancer.* New York: Blackwell Science.

Mettlin, C. (1997). Recent developments in the epidemiology of prostate cancer. *European Journal of Cancer* 33(3):340–347.

National Cancer Institute. (1998). Cancer facts—Screening. Questions and answers about early prostate cancer. Online:

http://cancernet.nci.nih.gov/Cancer_Types/ Prostate_Cancer.shtml.

National Cancer Institute. (1999). Screening for prostate cancer. PDQ screenings and prevention: Health professional. Online: http://www.cancer-net.net.nih.gov/clinpdg/screening/Screening_for_ Prostate_Cancer.html.

Omran, A.R. (1971). The epidemiologic transition: A theory of the epidemiology of population change. *Milbank Quarterly* 49:509–538.

Omran, A.R. (1977). A century of epidemiologic transition in the United States. *Preventive Medicine* 6:30–51.

Thune, I., Brenn, T., Lund, E., & Gaard, M. (1997). Physical activity and the risk of breast cancer. *New England Journal of Medicine* 336(18):1269–1275.

United States Department of Health and Human Services. (1996). *Physical Activity and Health: A Report of the Surgeon General*. Atlanta: U.S. Department of Health and Human Services, Centers for Disease Control and Prevention.

United States Department of Health and Human Services. (2000). *Healthy People 2010: Conference Edition—Cancer* [CD-ROM]. Washington, DC: Author.

United States Department of Health and Human Services. (2005). *Health, United States, 2005*. Hyattsville, MD: Author.

United States Preventive Services Task Force. (1996). Screening for breast cancer. In *Guide to Clinical Preventive Services*, 2nd ed. Baltimore: Williams & Wilkins, 73–87.

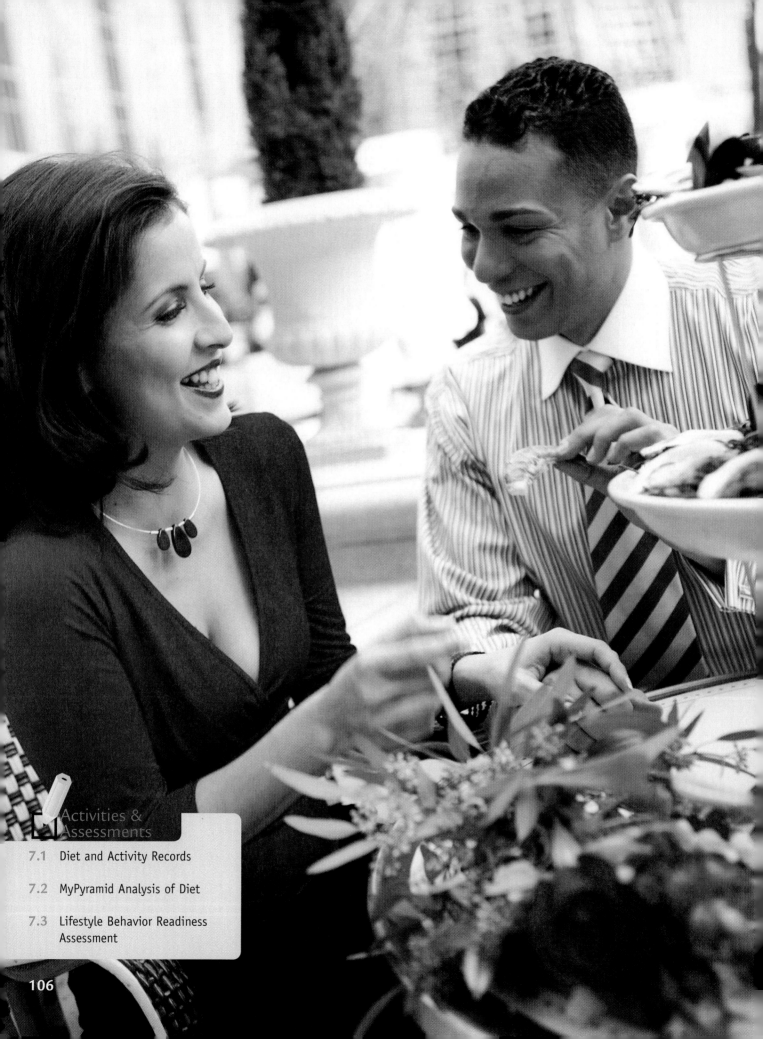

Activities & Assessments

7.1   Diet and Activity Records

7.2   MyPyramid Analysis of Diet

7.3   Lifestyle Behavior Readiness
      Assessment

Optimal Nutrition for an Active Lifestyle

7

what's the connection?

Mary is a junior in college and is extremely attentive to her physical health. She began her weekly running program as a freshman and is now very fit. She runs approximately 20 miles a week and lifts weights twice a week. Mary adheres strictly to the MyPyramid food guidance system when selecting foods for her daily diet. In addition, she closely follows the recommended number of servings from each food group, selecting the most nutrient-dense foods from each group. Recently, a number of friends with whom Mary exercises have recommended that she take special vitamin and mineral supplements because she is physically active. Mary is uncertain about whether she needs to supplement her diet. Besides, dietary supplements can be expensive and she is on a tight budget. Mary schedules a meeting with the nutritionist at the university health center. The nutritionist asks Mary to record her food intake for a week so they can analyze Mary's diet.

concepts

1. Nutrition plays a major role in our overall health.

2. Nutrients provide energy, regulate body processes, and nourish tissues.

3. Food can be divided into six classes and each class plays a different role.

4. The *Dietary Guidelines for Americans* provides general recommendations that focus attention on the association between diet and chronic diseases.

5. The MyPyramid food guidance system provides a wealth of information for you to apply in developing a nutritious diet and a physically active lifestyle.

6. The diet recommended for the person who participates in physical exercise differs little in nutrient composition from the diet advised for any healthy individual.

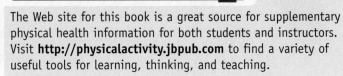

http://physicalactivity.jbpub.com

The Web site for this book is a great source for supplementary physical health information for both students and instructors. Visit **http://physicalactivity.jbpub.com** to find a variety of useful tools for learning, thinking, and teaching.

Nutrition plays a major role in our overall health.

Introduction

Good nutrition is vital to your good health—both in the present and in the distant future. Hippocrates, an ancient Greek physician, commonly regarded as one of the most outstanding figures in medicine of all time and known as the "father of medicine," recognized the value of diet and nutrition to enhance health and declared, "Let food be your medicine and medicine be your food." Hippocrates said this more than two thousand years ago, and it is still meaningful today, as the preventive and therapeutic health values of food relative to the development of chronic diseases are unraveled. Today, scientific studies indicate that diet and nutrition often play a crucial role in the development and progression of chronic diseases that are the major killers of adults: cardiovascular disease, stroke, high blood pressure, diabetes, and some types of cancer (see Chapters 5 and 6). Obesity and osteoporosis also have been associated with faulty nutrition (see Chapters 9 and 10). Consequently, sensible lifelong eating habits play an important role in maintaining good health and preventing chronic disease (FIGURE 7.1).

We define *healthy eating* as the practice of making choices about what one eats with the intention of improving or maintaining good health. Typically this means following the recommendations of "experts" regarding a nutritional diet. Regrettably, there are many misconceptions and misunderstandings as to what constitutes a good, nutritional diet. This is seen by the many different diets available, the articles written in popular magazines and books, and the eating patterns of people. What is needed are very clear science-based dietary guidelines that you can follow in selecting your nutritional plan. As you increase your knowledge about nutrition and gain a better understanding of your eating habits, you improve your chances of enjoying good health now and later in life.

This chapter highlights the nutrients, their major food sources and roles in the body, and their recommended dietary allowances. It introduces you to science-based guidelines that you can use to design a healthy diet plan as well as several practical tools designed to help guide you in making healthy food selections. The information in this chapter, along with the accompanying activities and assessments, will assist you in evaluating the nutritional adequacy of your diet and plan-

FIGURE 7.1 **Nutrition and Your Health.** Many health conditions are related to diet. For example, consuming fruits and vegetables can be helpful to your heart, whereas eating too much saturated fat can be harmful to your heart; drinking too much alcohol can lead to cirrhosis of the liver; and an adequate amount of calcium is important for strong bones.

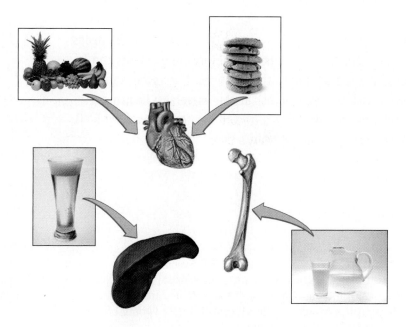

ning nutritious menus. Finally, information about nutrition should always be linked to information about physical activity because the health benefits of each support those of the other.

Nutrition Basics

Nutrition is all about the study of food and how our bodies use food as fuel for growth and daily activities. The Council on Food and Nutrition of the American Medical Association (AMA) defines *nutrition* as "the science of food, the nutrients and the substances therein, their action, interaction, and balance in relation to health and disease, and the process by which the organism ingests, digests, absorbs, transports, utilizes, and excretes food substances" (AMA, 1999). This definition stresses the biochemical or physiological functions of food we eat, but public health experts note that nutrition may be interpreted in a broader sense and be affected by our behavior and environment as it relates to these functions (Bush, 2005).

Most people know that nutrients in food nourish the body and are essential for promoting health. Nevertheless, most people choose foods for reasons other than their nutrient content. Instead, people's food choices tend to be influenced by a variety of personal factors, including pleasure or preference, emotional comfort, values, attitudes, social pressure, image, habit, ethnic and cultural background, availability, convenience, and cost (Bush, 2005). In principle, eating well is not difficult. Yet to master that principle and put it into practice can be challenging because of the powerful preferences just noted. Simply put, even though people may know about nutritious foods, that doesn't mean they actually eat such foods all the time. Although our food selection and nutritional status is greatly influenced by these personal factors, it is in every person's best interest to understand optimal nourishment first; therefore, we will begin with the primary purpose of why we must eat food—for the nutrients themselves.

Nutrient Needs

The principal purpose of eating is to provide our body with **nutrients**. Nutrients perform three major functions in the body that are essential for life: (1) provide energy, (2) help regulate body processes, and (3) build and repair tissues.

ENERGY   All biological and physiological body functions require energy. The human body must be supplied continuously with its own form of energy to perform its many complex functions. The nutrients contained in food provide the energy necessary to maintain bodily functions both at rest and during various forms of physical activity. The most obvious example of our body's need for energy is the mechanical work generated by muscle contraction. Our muscles must be provided with chemical energy from food to accomplish this mechanical work. Your physical functioning related to jogging, swimming, aerobic dancing, and weight lifting is considerably influenced by your capacity to extract energy from food nutrients and deliver it to the skeletal muscles (see Chapter 8).

In addition to the energy required for physical activity, the body requires considerable energy for absorption and assimilation of food nutrients during **digestion**, a series of complex mechanical and chemical reactions. **FIGURE 7.2** depicts the digestive system and its major organs. The raw fuel for both biological and mechanical energy requirements comes in the form of three **macronutrients**: carbohydrates, fats, and proteins. These energy-yielding nutrients continuously replenish the energy you expend daily from biological and mechanical work.

Nutrients provide energy, regulate body processes, and nourish tissues.

Nutrients Elements in foods that are required for energy, growth, and repair of tissues and regulation of body processes.

Digestion Metabolizing of food through a series of complex mechanical and chemical reactions.

Macronutrients Raw fuel, in the form of protein, carbohydrates, and fats, for biological and mechanical energy requirements.

FIGURE 7.2 **The Human Digestive System.** Teeth and glandular secretions in the mouth help break up food, which the esophagus transports to the stomach. The stomach breaks down some of the food molecules and passes the food to the rest of the digestive tube: the duodenum, jejunum, ileum, colon, and rectum. The pancreas secretes enzymes and fluid into the duodenum to help the digestive process. The liver controls release of absorbed nutrients into the body. Undigested material is eliminated from the body at the anus.

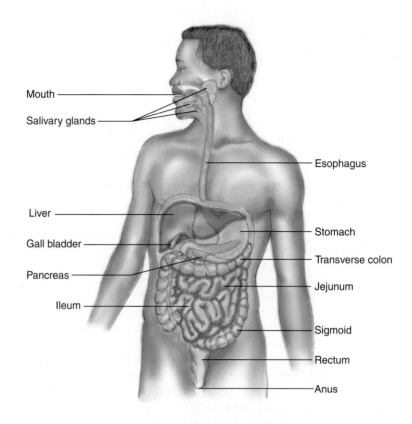

Mouth

Salivary glands

Esophagus

Liver

Stomach

Gall bladder

Transverse colon

Pancreas

Jejunum

Ileum

Sigmoid

Rectum

Anus

Calorie Amount of heat it takes to raise the temperature of 1 gram of water 1 degree Celsius.

There are a variety of ways to express the energy value of food. The term used and understood by most people is "calorie." A **calorie** is the amount of heat it takes to raise the temperature of 1 gram of water 1 degree Celsius. Calories are such small units of measurement that nutrition scientists find it easier to express food energy in 1000-calorie units called *kilocalories* (abbreviated kcalories, or kcal). When you see the term *calorie* on a food label, or when you calculate your energy expenditure in calories, you are actually using kilocalories, but since the term *calorie* is commonly used in everyday life we will use it here.

The energy in a particular food depends on how much carbohydrate, protein, and fat the food contains. Carbohydrate and protein yield 4 calories of energy from each gram, and fat yields 9 calories per gram (TABLE 7.1). Once you know the number of grams of each of these substances contained by a certain food, you can derive the number of calories available in that food. Simply multiple the carbohydrate grams times 4, the protein grams times 4, and the fat grams times 9, and add all three together.

Calories are a highly desirable feature of food since they are used to do the body's physiological work or to exercise the muscles. Without calories, we would not survive. A constant flow of energy is so vital to life that other functions are sacrificed to maintain it. The average adult requires about 2000 calories per day to meet energy needs. The "evil" reputation of calories relates to energy storage in the body and is not deserved. If your body doesn't use all the energy-yielding nutrients to fuel its requirements, it rearranges them into storage compounds, primarily body fat, and puts them away for later use (see Chapter 9). This connection with excess body weight is the way many people think about calories, but it is a distortion of their true value.

TABLE 7.1	Classes of Nutrients	
Nutrient	**Function**	**Major Sources**
Proteins (4 kcal/g)	Form important parts of muscles, bone, blood, enzymes, some hormones, and cell membranes; repair tissue; regulate water and acid-base balance; help in growth; supply energy	Meat, fish, poultry, eggs, milk products, legumes, nuts, soybeans
Carbohydrates (4 kcal/g)	Supply energy to cells in brain, nervous system, and blood; supply energy to muscles during exercise	Grains (breads and cereals), fruits, vegetables, milk
Fats (9 kcal/g)	Supply energy; insulate, support, and cushion organs; provide medium for absorption of fat-soluble vitamins	Saturated fats primarily from animal sources, palm and coconut oils, and hydrogenated vegetable fats; unsaturated fats from grains, nuts, seeds, fish
Vitamins	Promote (initiate or speed up) specific chemical reactions within cells	Abundant in fruits, vegetables, and grains; also found in meat and dairy products
Minerals	Help regulate body functions; aid in the growth and maintenance of body tissues; act as catalysts for the release of energy	Found in most food groups
Water	Makes up 50–70% of body weight; provides a medium for chemical reactions; transports chemicals; regulates temperature; removes waste products	Fruits, vegetables, and other liquids

REGULATE BODY PROCESSES   The second function of food is to regulate body processes. Although the raw fuel for biological and mechanical work comes from calories in the form of carbohydrates, fats, and proteins (or *macronutrients*), the systematic removal and utilization of energy from these nutrients requires an assortment of additional **micronutrients**. Vitamins, minerals, and water play crucial roles in regulating the body's processes related to activating energy release. The regulating of energy processes and tissue maintenance is referred to as human metabolism. *Human metabolism* is the sum total of all chemical and physical reactions that go on in living cells (see Chapter 8). Metabolic processes allow for the release and use of energy from food compounds, the making of new compounds, and the transporting of compounds from place to place. For example, certain vitamins are essential for facilitating the release of the energy found in food and for controlling growth of body tissues. Like vitamins, minerals also play a regulatory role in metabolism and are essential for the synthesis of nutrients.

MAINTENANCE, REPAIR, AND GROWTH   The third function of food is to supply the required nutrients for body tissue maintenance, repair, and growth. Nearly all body cells are constantly being replaced. For example, the red blood cells are useful for about a month and then must be replaced, and the cells that line the intestinal tract live less than a week. Various nutrients must be available to build the new cells for the body tissues: protein is a major material for red blood cells, muscle cells, and various enzymes; certain minerals like calcium and phosphorus make up the cells that form the skeletal system (see Chapter 10).

ESSENTIAL AND NONESSENTIAL NUTRIENTS   Six classes of nutrients are considered necessary in human nutrition: proteins, fats, carbohydrates, vitamins, minerals, and water (see Table 7.1). Some nutritional scientists further distinguish nutrients into **essential nutrients** and **nonessential nutrients**. The term *essential*

Micronutrients Nutrients required in small amounts; includes vitamins and minerals.

Essential nutrients Nutrients the body cannot make for itself; must be obtained from food.

Nonessential nutrients Nutrients made by the body from the foods we eat.

TABLE 7.2	The Essential Nutrients*			
Amino Acids	**Vitamins**	**Minerals**	**Fats**	**Water**
Isoleucine	Ascorbic acid	Calcium	Linoleic acid	
Leucine	(vitamin C)	Chlorine	Linolenic acid	
Lysine	Biotin	Chromium		
Methionine	Cobalamin	Cobalt		
Phenylalanine	(vitamin B_{12})	Copper		
Threonine	Folic acid	Iodine		
Tryptophan	Niacin (vitamin B_3)	Iron		
Valine	Pantothenic acid	Magnesium		
Arginine†	Pyridoxine	Manganese		
Histidine†	(vitamin B_6)	Molybdenum		
	Riboflavin	Phosphorous		
	(vitamin B_2)	Potassium		
	Thiamine	Selenium		
	(vitamin B_1)	Sodium		
	Vitamin A	Sulfur		
	Vitamin D	Zinc		
	Vitamin E			
	Vitamin K			

*Must be obtained from food

†Not essential for adults; needed for growth of children

SOURCE: Edlin, G., & Golanty, E. (2007). *Health and Wellness*, 9th ed. Sudbury, MA: Jones and Bartlett Publishers, 100.

nutrients describes nutrients the body cannot make for itself and that must be obtained from foods we eat. TABLE 7.2 lists the specific nutrients currently known to be essential. Essential nutrients are necessary for human life. Inadequate intake of essential nutrients can lead to certain disease states and, eventually, death.

Other nutrients either come from the foods we eat or can be made by the body. For example, the body can convert protein or fats into a carbohydrate, if needed. Since it is not crucial that we obtain them from food, we refer to these nutrients as *nonessential nutrients*. This is not to say that nonessential nutrients are unimportant, just that they can be made by the body.

Classes of Nutrients

Food can be divided into six classes and each class plays a different role.

As noted earlier, there are six classes of nutrients that your body needs for normal functioning and good health. These six classes—proteins, carbohydrates, fats, vitamins, minerals, and water—provide energy, regulate body processes, and contribute to the maintenance, repair, and growth of body structures. Each class can be further described by their composition, functions in the body, and dietary recommendations. The following sections examine these key differences.

Proteins

Protein is one of our most essential nutrients. The body uses it in more ways than any other nutrient. Protein was named after the Greek word *proteios*, meaning "of prime importance." The prime importance of protein is reflected by its uses in the body. The body uses proteins for new growth and to build such body proteins as hemoglobin, enzymes, hormones, and antibodies. Proteins constantly help to replace worn-out cells in the body. Protein has a number of physiological functions that are essential to optimal physical performance. People think of proteins as body-building nutrients, the material of strong muscles, and rightly so. Protein forms the structural basis for muscle tissue and is a major component of most enzymes in the muscle.

To appreciate the many vital functions of protein, we need to understand its structure. Protein is a complex chemical containing atoms of carbon, hydrogen, oxygen, and nitrogen that are combined in a structure called an **amino acid**. There are 20 different amino acids that are important to human nutrition. Humans can synthesize some amino acids in the body but cannot synthesize others. The 9 amino acids that the body cannot make are referred to as **essential amino acids** (see Table 7.2). Two of the essential amino acids, *lysine* and *tryptophan*, are poorly represented in most plant proteins. Thus, strict vegetarians should make special plans to ensure that their diet contains sufficient amounts of these two amino acids. It should be noted that all 20 amino acids are necessary for protein (synthesis) in the body and must be present simultaneously for optimal maintenance of body growth and function. Protein foods that contain all of the essential amino acids in adequate amount, and in the correct ratio to maintain nitrogen balance and allow for tissue growth and repair, are known as *complete proteins*. Excellent sources of complete protein are eggs, milk, meat, fish, poultry, and soybeans.

DIETARY RECOMMENDATION FOR PROTEIN The Food and Nutrition Board (FNB) recommends that healthy adults have a Recommended Dietary Allowance (RDA) of 0.8 grams of protein per kilogram (2.2 lb) of ideal body weight (Institute of Medicine [IOM], 2005). Ideal weight is used rather than actual weight, because protein is needed for lean body tissues, not for fat tissue. Thus, a 156-lb person needs approximately 56 grams of protein a day. Does the physically active individual or athlete need more protein in the diet? A joint position paper from the American Dietetic Association (ADA) and the Canada Dietetic Association states that all athletes, as well as those who train like athletes, need a little more protein than do sedentary people. They recommend 1.0 to 1.5 grams of protein per kilogram (0.5–0.8 g/lb) each day (ADA, 1993). Since many Americans and Canadians

Protein An essential nutrient that the body uses in more ways than any other.

Amino acid Complex chemical structure of protein, containing atoms of carbon, hydrogen, oxygen, and nitrogen.

Essential amino acids The nine amino acids that the body cannot make.

Protein sources consist of fish, meat, poultry, milk, and beans.

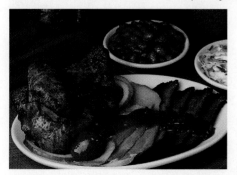
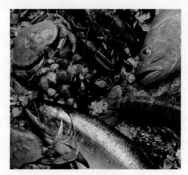
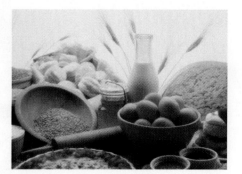

consume foods containing plenty of protein, they do not need protein supplements. It is important to realize that additional calories from protein are used for energy or stored as fat; protein is not an efficient source of energy.

Carbohydrates

Carbohydrates are the preferred energy source for most of the body's functions. Carbohydrates are found in all foods, but are especially plentiful in grains, fruits, and vegetables. Carbohydrates are organic compounds that contain carbon, hydrogen, and oxygen. A wide variety exist in nature and in the body. We will divide carbohydrates into two categories: simple and complex.

SIMPLE CARBOHYDRATES **Simple carbohydrates** are divided into one-sugar or two-sugar molecules. A one-sugar molecule is referred to as a **monosaccharide** (saccharide means "sugar" or "sweet"). More than 200 monosaccharides are found in nature, with the most common types being glucose, fructose, and galactose (FIGURE 7.3). Almost all of the body's cells use glucose as their chief energy source. Fructose is one of the sweetest sugars and is found in fruits and honey. Galactose is produced from milk sugar. Both must be converted to glucose to be used for energy by the cells.

The combination of two monosaccharides yields a **disaccharide**, of which sucrose, maltose, and lactose are formed. All three have glucose as one of their single sugars. Glucose occurs naturally in many fruits and vegetables. The most familiar source of sucrose is table sugar. Table sugar is a concentrated sweetener that is derived by refining the juice from sugar cane. Monosaccharides and disaccharides are known as simple carbohydrates, or simple sugars, because there is only one bond in each that must be broken down by the digestive enzymes before they can be absorbed by the blood.

COMPLEX CARBOHYDRATES **Complex carbohydrates** are known as polysaccharides. The term *polysaccharide* is used when three or more sugar molecules are linked. In fact, from 300 to 26,000 monosaccharides can be linked together to form a complex carbohydrate. The three most common forms of complex carbohydrates are starch, glycogen, and dietary fiber.

> **Carbohydrates** Organic compounds that contain carbon, hydrogen, and oxygen.
>
> **Simple carbohydrates** Either one-sugar or two-sugar molecules.
>
> **Monosaccharide** One-sugar molecule.
>
> **Disaccharide** Two-sugar molecule.
>
> **Complex carbohydrates** Called polysaccharides, these link three or more sugar molecules.

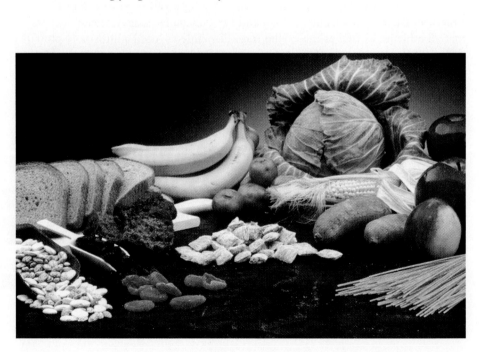

Carbohydrate sources consist of fruit, vegetables, and grains.

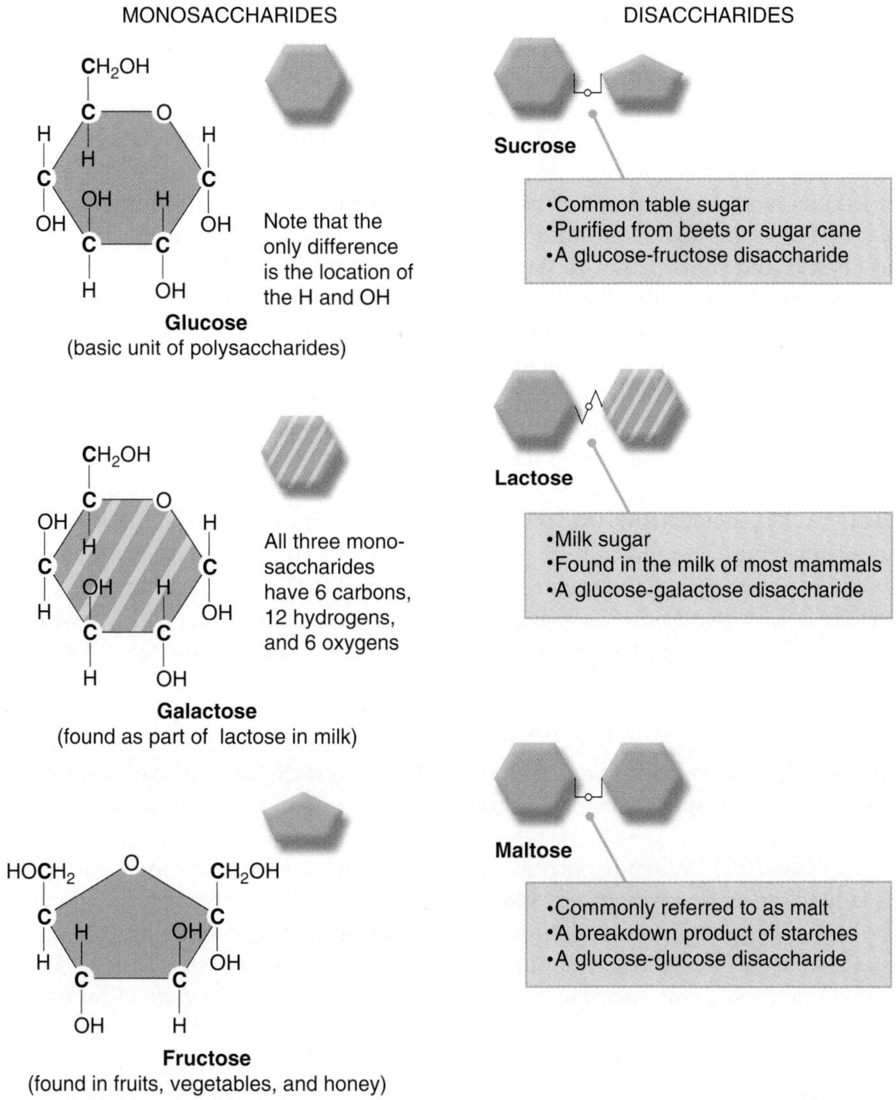

MONOSACCHARIDES

Glucose
(basic unit of polysaccharides)

Note that the only difference is the location of the H and OH

Galactose
(found as part of lactose in milk)

All three mono-saccharides have 6 carbons, 12 hydrogens, and 6 oxygens

Fructose
(found in fruits, vegetables, and honey)

DISACCHARIDES

Sucrose
- Common table sugar
- Purified from beets or sugar cane
- A glucose-fructose disaccharide

Lactose
- Milk sugar
- Found in the milk of most mammals
- A glucose-galactose disaccharide

Maltose
- Commonly referred to as malt
- A breakdown product of starches
- A glucose-glucose disaccharide

FIGURE 7.3 **Some Common Sugars.** Sucrose and fructose are the most common sugars in our diets.

Starches are the storage form of carbohydrates for plants. Grains such as wheat, rice, and corn are the richest food sources of starch. Other important sources include the foods from the legume family (peanuts, kidney beans, chickpeas, soybeans) and root vegetables (potatoes, yams).

As starch stores energy for plants, glycogen stores energy for humans and animals. If the blood delivers more glucose than the cells need, the liver and muscles take up a certain amount and build the polysaccharide **glycogen**. Glycogen plays an important role in the body as a readily available source of glucose, especially during physical activity (see Chapter 8). The well-nourished human body can store approximately 400 to 450 grams or 1500 to 2000 calories of energy (Wilmone & Costill, 2004). Excess glucose beyond what the body is able to use immediately, or deposit as glycogen, is stored as fat.

Starches Storage form of carbohydrates for plants.

Glycogen Storage form of sugar energy for humans and animals.

DIETARY RECOMMENDATION OF ENERGY-YIELDING CARBOHYDRATES Dietary recommendations state that carbohydrates should contribute 55 to 60 percent of the total daily energy intake. Simple refined sugars should account for 10 percent or less of total calories because they supply relatively few nutrients. The sugars in unrefined foods like fruits and vegetables are preferable because they are accompanied by many

Dietary fiber Diverse carbohydrate polysaccharides of plants that cannot be digested by the human stomach or small intestine.

Insoluble fibers Dietary fibers not soluble in water or metabolized by the intestines; make feces bulkier and softer, promoting decreased passage time.

Soluble fibers Dietary fibers soluble in water, metabolized in the large intestine; assist in removing cholesterol from the body.

Fats Members of a family of compounds called lipids.

Triglycerides Fatty acids that provide the body's largest energy store, act as insulation, transport fat-soluble vitamins, and contribute to satiety.

other nutrients. For active people, and for those involved in exercise training, the majority of carbohydrate calories should come from the complex variety.

Dietary fiber is a general term for diverse carbohydrate polysaccharides of plants that cannot be digested by the human stomach or small intestine. Technically, dietary fiber is not an essential nutrient, but it has demonstrated benefits of health maintenance and disease prevention making it a highly recommended functional food. Long praised as part of a healthy diet, fiber appears to reduce the risk of developing various conditions, including heart disease, diabetes, diverticular disease, and constipation (IOM, 2005; Pereira et al., 2004).

Dietary fiber exists in two basic forms: insoluble and soluble. **Insoluble fibers** are not dissolved in water or metabolized by the intestines; they make the feces bulkier and softer, thus decreasing passage time. They are made up mostly of cellulose, hemicelluloses, and lignins. **Soluble fibers** are dissolved in water and are metabolized in the large intestine; they assist in draining cholesterol from the body. They include pectins, gums, and mucilages.

DIETARY RECOMMENDATIONS FOR FIBER The Institute of Medicine's FNB recommends 20 to 35 grams of fiber per day, or 10 to 13 grams per 1000 calories (IOM, 2005). To achieve adequate dietary fiber intake, the FNB recommends you include at least two to three servings of whole grains as part of the daily servings of grains, five servings of fruits and vegetables, and legumes at least twice a week.

Fats

Fats (also known as lipids) are found in foods and in the body. Fats can be categorized into three main groups: triglycerides, cholesterol, and phospholipids.

TRIGLYCERIDES When people talk about body fat, or fat in their food, they are usually referring to triglycerides. **Triglycerides** provide many important functions in the body. These fatty acids constitute the body's largest energy store, provide insulation, transport fat-soluble vitamins, and contribute to satiety (satisfaction). More than 95 percent of our body fat is in the form of triglycerides. The chemical name

Fats sources include oil, ice cream, cheese, and margarine.

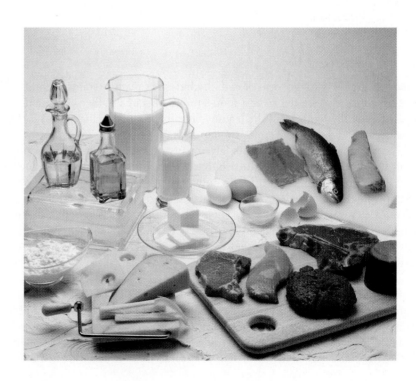

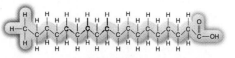

Stearic acid

Saturated fatty acid (no double bonds between carbon atoms)

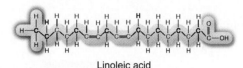

Oleic acid

Monounsaturated fatty acid (one double bond between carbon atoms)

Linoleic acid

Polyunsaturated fatty acid (two or more double bonds between carbon atoms)

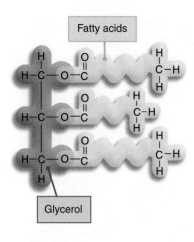

Fatty acids

Glycerol

Triglyceride

FIGURE 7.4 **Chemical Structure of Saturated and Unsaturated Fats.** Triglyceride consists of a molecule of glycerol with three fatty acids attached. Fatty acids can differ in the lengths of their carbon chains and degree of saturation.

helps explain itself. A triglyceride molecule consists of three fatty acid atoms attached to a glycerol molecule. Fatty acids are chains of carbon, oxygen, and hydrogen atoms (FIGURE 7.4). Fatty acids chains may differ from one another in two ways: chain length and saturation. The chain length affects the way fat is absorbed and its solubility in water (shorter chains are more soluble). Saturation refers to the chemical structure—specifically, to the number of hydrogens the fatty acid chain is holding. The basic structures of fatty acid molecules are *saturated* and *unsaturated*.

If every available bond from the carbons is holding a hydrogen atom, the fatty acid is saturated. In some fatty acids chains there is a place where hydrogens are missing; this is the point of unsaturation, and the fatty acid is unsaturated. If there is one point of unsaturation the chain is *monounsaturated* and if there is more than one point of unsaturation the chain is *polyunsaturated*.

Both plants and animals provide ready sources of fat. All dietary fats contain a mixture of saturated and unsaturated fatty acids (FIGURE 7.5). The type of fatty acid that predominates determines whether the fat is solid or liquid and whether it is characterized as saturated or unsaturated. Coconut and palm kernel oil, for example, contain high levels of saturated fatty acids and are relatively hard at room temperature. Oils such as soybean, canola, cottonseed, corn, and other vegetable oils contain higher levels of unsaturated fatty acids and are liquid at room temperature.

ESSENTIAL FATTY ACIDS The body can synthesize all the fatty acids it needs from carbohydrate, fat, or protein except for linoleic acid (omega-6) and alpha-linolenic acid (omega-3). Both are unsaturated fatty acids and, because they must be obtained from food, are referred to as **essential fatty acids** (see Table 7.2). These fatty acids are essential for the body because they participate in triggering immune

Essential fatty acids Support immune responses, form cell structures, regulate blood pressure, affect blood lipid concentration, and promote clot formation; must be obtained from food.

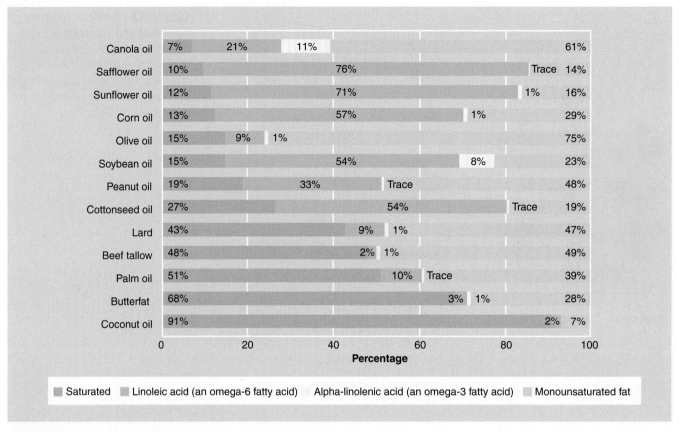

Canola oil — 7% | 21% | 11% | 61%
Safflower oil — 10% | 76% | Trace | 14%
Sunflower oil — 12% | 71% | 1% | 16%
Corn oil — 13% | 57% | 1% | 29%
Olive oil — 15% | 9% | 1% | 75%
Soybean oil — 15% | 54% | 8% | 23%
Peanut oil — 19% | 33% | Trace | 48%
Cottonseed oil — 27% | 54% | Trace | 19%
Lard — 43% | 9% | 1% | 47%
Beef tallow — 48% | 2% | 1% | 49%
Palm oil — 51% | 10% | Trace | 39%
Butterfat — 68% | 3% | 1% | 28%
Coconut oil — 91% | 2% | 7%

Percentage

■ Saturated   ■ Linoleic acid (an omega-6 fatty acid)   Alpha-linolenic acid (an omega-3 fatty acid)   ■ Monounsaturated fat

FIGURE 7.5 **Comparisons of Dietary Fats.**

responses, forming cell structures, regulating blood pressure, determining blood lipid concentration, and supporting clot formation. Linoleic acid is found in the seeds of plants and in the oils harvested from those seeds. Alpha-linolenic acid is found in fish such as salmon, tuna, trout, and sardines. Canola or soybean oil and nuts also supply these omega-3 fatty acids.

ENERGY SOURCE AND RESERVE   One gram of fat contains twice the energy (9 calories) of an equal gram of carbohydrate or protein. The utilization of fat provides energy at rest and during specific types of physical activity (see Chapter 8). We store most of our energy in the form of triglycerides, or body fat. Ideally, approximately 15 percent of body weight for males and 25 percent for females is fat (see Chapter 9). Each pound of body fat provides 3500 calories of energy; therefore, for an average male the energy stored in fat is about 100,000 calories. Compare this with the 2000 calories of stored energy from carbohydrate.

INSULATION AND PROTECTION   The layer of fat just beneath our skin is made up of triglycerides and insulates the body against extreme cold. Furthermore, approximately 4 percent of total body fat serves to protect vital organs such as the heart, liver, kidneys, brain, and spinal cord from injury as a result of trauma.

TRANSPORTING VITAMINS   Triglycerides and other fats in foods carry fat-soluble vitamins—vitamins A, D, E, and K—to the small intestine and aid their absorption. The ingestion of approximately 20 grams of fat per day serves this purpose. Without this fat, the fat-soluble vitamins are passed through the body and eliminated in the feces.

SATIETY   Triglycerides in foods help give us a full and contented feeling and off-set hunger feelings. The fat we eat takes much longer to be digested in the stomach than carbohydrate or protein. Fat also stimulates the release of hormones in the stomach that decrease hunger feelings. If you cut too much fat from your diet, you lose satiety value and may become hungry more quickly.

Trans Fats

Trans fats are unsaturated fatty acids that are formed when vegetable oils are processed to become more solid. This process is called *hydrogenation*. Foods are hydrogenated because the process increases the shelf life and flavor stability of these oils and the foods that contain them. Trans fat is found in vegetable shortenings and in some margarines, crackers, cookies, snack foods, and other foods. Although trans fats are unsaturated, they appear similar to saturated fats in terms of their effect on blood cholesterol levels. Many studies suggest that trans fats raise low-density lipoproteins (LDLs) and total blood cholesterol levels much like saturated fats, which increases the risk of coronary heart disease (Shapiro, 1997).

> **Trans fats** Unsaturated fatty acids formed when vegetable oils are processed (hydrogenation) and made more solid.
>
> **Phospholipids** Lipids made by the body and therefore not considered essential fatty acids.

Phospholipids and Cholesterol

Phospholipids and cholesterol make up the remaining 5 percent of lipids in the diet. **Phospholipids** are a component of all cells, and many types exist in the body; they are made by the body and therefore are not considered essential nutrients. Among these, the lecithins are of particular interest. *Lecithin* functions as a fat emulsifier in the small intestine, breaking fat into small globules that are suspended in water. This separation of fat in water helps create more fat surface area for the fat-digesting enzymes to work on. There is no need to supplement lecithin in your diet because the body makes its own lecithin and because it is so readily available in the diet through a variety of foods, including soybeans, nuts, egg yolks, beef, oatmeal, and wheat germ.

Cholesterol is vital to the body in a variety of ways. Cholesterol forms part of many important hormones and is an essential structural component of cells. However, like the lecithins, cholesterol can be manufactured by the body and therefore is not an essential nutrient. In addition to the cholesterol made by the body from fats, carbohydrates, or proteins, it can be obtained through eating foods of animal origin, such as eggs, red meat, and fish. Eating saturated fats raises your blood cholesterol level more than anything else in your diet. Elevated blood cholesterol levels have been shown to be related to an increased incidence of coronary heart disease (Expert Panel, 2001). The goal is to encourage people to eat less than 300 mg of cholesterol a day. In addition, less than 10 percent of their fat calories should come from saturated fat.

DIETARY RECOMMENDATIONS FOR FAT   Dietary fat is essential for the body because it provides us with a source of essential fatty acids and a means to transport fat-soluble vitamins. Although no specific RDA has been established for the total amount of fat, the FNB recommends a minimum daily amount of 3 to 6 grams, or 1 to 2 percent of your total calories from the essential fatty acids (IOM, 2005). Any diet that contains vegetable oils, seeds, nuts, soybeans, fish, and whole-grain foods provides enough linoleic acid (omega-6) and alpha-linolenic acid (omega-3) to meet the body's needs.

Although there is no established upper limit for fats, you should consume less than 10 percent of your calories from saturated and trans fats and less than 300 milligrams of cholesterol daily. These types are considered "bad" fats since they have a major effect on raising blood cholesterol levels that contribute to cardiovascular disease (Chapter 5). Fortunately, the unsaturated fats, or "good" fats, have been shown to protect against heart disease (Hu, Manson, & Willett, 2001). In fact, as will be discussed later in the chapter, it is recommended that between 20 to 35 percent of total calories come from fat, with the overwhelming majority being unsaturated fats (U.S. Department of Agriculture [USDA], 2005).

Vitamins

Vitamins are essential organic substances needed by the body to perform highly specific metabolic processes in the cells. They are indispensable nutrients because they can't be synthesized by the body and must be obtained from food. Additionally, for a substance to be classified as a vitamin, its absence from the diet over a period of time must lead to deficiency symptoms. For example, vitamin A deficiency over an extended period of time can cause blindness, and a lack of niacin can cause mental illness.

Vitamins contribute no energy to the body; instead they assist the enzymes that release energy from carbohydrate, fat, and protein. Thirteen different vitamins have been isolated, analyzed, and synthesized, and their recommended dietary intakes established (TABLE 7.3). They are needed in small amounts in the diet for normal function, growth, and maintenance of the body. In fact, the body requires only about 350 grams of vitamins from the nearly 1900 pounds of food consumed by the average adult during the year. Vitamins fall into two classes, fat-soluble and water-soluble. The solubility of a vitamin refers to how it is absorbed and transported, whether it can be stored, and how easily it is lost from the body.

The four **fat-soluble vitamins** (A, D, E, K) are absorbed into the body with fats. These vitamins travel with dietary fats through the bloodstream to reach the cells. They are not readily excreted by the body. Once absorbed, excessive amounts of fat-soluble vitamins are stored in the liver and fat cells until the body needs them. The ability to store fat-soluble vitamins makes daily ingestion of the fat-soluble vitamins unnecessary.

Nine vitamins are classified as water-soluble because they are transported throughout the watery medium of the body. **Water-soluble vitamins** are more readily excreted than fat-soluble vitamins and are not stored in tissues. Excess water-soluble vitamins are excreted through the urine.

Minerals

Minerals are inorganic substances that are vital to many body functions. Minerals help build strong bones and teeth, aid in accurate muscle function, help nervous systems transmit messages, help balance the amount of water in the body, and work closely with vitamins to perform our body's chemical and hormonal activities. Like vitamins, minerals do not provide any energy for the body. In the body, minerals are classified as **major minerals** if their requirement exceeds 100 milligrams per day and **trace minerals** if their requirement is less than 100 milligrams per day. TABLE 7.4 lists the minerals, their major functions, and their food sources.

Minerals can be found in most food items that we eat daily. For example, if you were to consume dark-green leafy vegetables, grain products, and meat and dairy products every day, you would get plenty of the minerals listed in Table 7.4.

In general, the human body maintains a proper balance of many minerals through a number of precise control mechanisms, but deficiencies and excesses of any mineral may disturb this balance. Some minerals interact and compete with each other, and consuming excesses of some minerals can affect the absorption of

---

Vitamins Essential organic substances needed by the body to perform highly specific metabolic processes in the cells.

Fat-soluble vitamins Vitamins A, D, E, K; must travel with dietary fats in the bloodstream to reach the cells.

Water-soluble vitamins Vitamins that can be transported throughout the body by a watery medium.

Minerals Inorganic substances vital to many body functions.

Major minerals Mineral requirements that exceed 100 mg per day.

Trace minerals Mineral requirements of less than 100 mg per day.

TABLE 7.3	Water-Soluble and Fat-Soluble Vitamins

Water-Soluble Vitamins	Why Needed?	Primary Sources	Deficiency Results in
Ascorbid acid (vitamin C)	Tooth and bone formation; production of connective tissue; promotion of wound healing; may enhance immunity	Citrus fruits, tomatoes, peppers, cabbage, potatoes, melons	Scurvy (degeneration of bones, teeth, and gums)
Biotin	Involved in fat and amino acid synthesis and breakdown	Yeast, liver, milk, most vegetables, bananas, grapefruit	Skin problems; fatigue; muscle pains; nausea
Cobalamin (vitamin B_{12})	Involved in single carbon atom transfers; essential for DNA synthesis	Muscle meats, eggs, milk, and dairy products (not in vegetables)	Pernicious anemia; nervous system malfunctions
Folacin (folic acid)	Essential for synthesis of DNA and other molecules	Green leafy vegetables, organ meats, whole-wheat products	Anemia; diarrhea and other gastrointestinal problems
Niacin	Involved in energy production and synthesis of cell molecules	Grains, meats, legumes	Pellagra (skin, gastrointestinal, and mental disorders)
Pantothenic acid	Involved in energy production and synthesis and breakdown of many biological molecules	Yeast, meats, and fish, nearly all vegetables and fruits	Vomiting; abdominal cramps; malaise; insomnia
Pyridoxine (vitamin B_6)	Essential fat synthesis, breakdown of amino acids, manufacture of unsaturated fats from saturated fats	Meats, whole grains, most vegetables	Weakness; irritability; trouble sleeping and walking; skin problems
Riboflavin (vitamin B_2)	Involved in energy production; important for health of the eyes	Milk and dairy foods, meats, eggs, vegetables, grains	Eye and skin problems
Thiamine (vitamin B_1)	Essential for breakdown of food molecules and production of energy	Meats, legumes, grains, some vegetables	Beri-beri (nerve damage, weakness, heart failure)

Fat-Soluble Vitamins	Why Needed?	Primary Sources	Deficiency or Excess Results in
Vitamin A (retinol)	Essential for maintenance of eyes and skin; influences bone and tooth formation	Liver, kidney, yellow and green leafy vegetables, apricots	Deficiency: night blindness; eye damage; skin dryness. Excess: loss of appetite; skin problems; swelling of ankles and feet
Vitamin D (calciferol)	Regulates calcium metabolism; important for growth of bones and teeth	Cod-liver oil, dairy products, eggs	Deficiency: rickets (bone deformities) in children; bone destruction in adults. Excess: thirst; nausea; weight loss; kidney damage
Vitamin E (tocopherol)	Prevents damage to cells from oxidation; prevents red blood cell destruction	Wheat germ, vegetable oils, vegetables, egg yolk, nuts	Deficiency: anemia; possibly nerve cell destruction
Vitamin K (phylloquinone)	Helps with blood clotting	Liver, vegetable oils, green leafy vegetables, tomatoes	Deficiency: severe bleeding

SOURCE: Edlin, G., & Golanty, E. (2007). *Health and Wellness*, 9th ed. Sudbury, MA: Jones and Bartlett Publishers, 109.

others; this is referred to as a mineral-mineral interaction. For example, iron and magnesium absorption will be hindered if too much calcium is taken in.

Another interaction that is important is the vitamin-mineral interaction. This refers to the importance of certain vitamins and minerals being available at the same time. Iron absorption is improved when it is consumed with vitamin C, and

TABLE 7.4	Essential Minerals		
Mineral	**Why Needed?**	**Primary Sources**	**Deficiency Results in**
Calcium	Bone and tooth formation; blood clotting; nerve transmission	Milk, cheese, dark-green vegetables, dried legumes	Stunted growth; rickets, osteoporosis; convulsions
Chlorine	Formation of gastric juice; acid-base balance	Common salt	Muscle cramps; mental apathy; reduced appetite
Chromium	Glucose and energy metabolism	Fats, vegetable oils, meats	Impaired ability to metabolize glucose
Cobalt	Constituent of vitamin B_{12}	Organ and muscle meats	Not reported in humans
Copper	Constituent of enzymes of iron metabolism	Meats, drinking water	Anemia (rare)
Iodine	Constituent of thyroid hormones	Marine fish and shellfish, dairy products, many vegetables	Goiter (enlarged thyroid)
Iron	Constituent of hemoglobin and enzymes of energy metabolism	Eggs, lean meals, legumes, whole grains, green leafy vegetables	Iron-deficiency anemia (weakness, reduced resistance to infection)
Magnesium	Activates enzymes; involved in protein synthesis	Whole grains, green leafy vegetables	Growth failure; behavioral disturbances; weakness, spasms
Manganese	Constituent of enzymes involved in fat synthesis	Widely distributed in foods	In animals; disturbances of nervous system, reproductive abnormalities
Molybdenum	Constituent of some enzymes	Legumes, cereals, organ meats	Not reported in humans
Phosphorus	Bone and tooth formation; acid-base balance	Milk, cheese, meat, poultry, grains	Weakness, demineralization of bone
Potassium	Acid-base balance; body water balance; nerve function	Meats, milk, many fruits	Muscular weakness; paralysis
Selenium	Functions in close association with vitamin E	Seafood, meat, grains	Anemia (rare)
Sodium	Acid-base balance; body water balance; nerve function	Common salt	Muscle cramps; mental apathy; reduced appetite
Sulfur	Constituent of active tissue compounds, cartilage, and tendon	Sulfur amino acids (methionine and cysteine) in dietary proteins	Related to intake and deficiency of sulfur amino acids
Zinc	Constituent of enzymes involved in digestion	Widely distributed in foods	Growth failure

SOURCE: Edlin, G., & Golanty, E. (2007). *Health and Wellness*, 9th ed. Sudbury, MA: Jones and Bartlett Publishers, 111.

the presence of vitamin D improves the absorption of calcium. Because of mineral-mineral and vitamin-mineral interactions, people should avoid taking individual supplements for minerals unless they have a specific condition that warrants it.

DIETARY RECOMMENDATIONS FOR VITAMINS AND MINERALS A well-balanced diet will satisfy all the vitamin and mineral requirements of most individuals, including those who are physically active. Select a wide variety of foods from all food groups. *For those receiving the RDA of vitamins and minerals, there is no research evidence that supplementation enhances exercise performance.* It is important to remember that excess vitamin and mineral intake does not improve health or exercise performance but it can be toxic. For example, excessive amounts of vitamin A can lead to weakness, headache, nausea, pain in the joints, and liver damage. Too much vitamin D may lead to vomiting, diarrhea, loss of weight, loss of muscle tone, and soft-tissue damage. Vitamin and mineral excesses generally occur as a result of supplementation.

SPECIAL NEEDS FOR IRON AND CALCIUM   Two minerals of special interest, especially for adolescents, adults over 50, and physically active individuals, are iron and calcium. Women need more of both nutrients than men. In all cases, individuals need to be particularly aware of obtaining good sources of nutrients in their diet.

The mineral *iron* has many diverse biological functions, but none more important than its role in the transport of oxygen in blood. Iron forms a major part of the hemogloblin in red blood cells. Red blood cells play a major role in aerobic capacity. Nearly 75 percent of the body's iron is found in hemogloblin. If neither diet nor body stores supply the iron needed, hemogloblin concentration levels eventually fall, leading to iron depletion and anemia. **Anemia** is a deficiency in red blood cells and is generally recognized to be the most common single nutritional deficiency, not just in developing countries but around the world.

Anemia Deficiency in red blood cells.

Several factors are responsible for iron deficiency, including inadequate dietary iron, absorption disturbances, illness, and exercise. Treatment of iron deficiency includes prudent use of MyPyramid (see **FIGURE 7.6**) and possibly iron supplements. High-iron foods come from the meat, poultry, fish, dry beans, eggs, and nuts group from MyPyramid and from fortified foods such as breakfast cereals. Women between the ages of 18 and 50 require 15 milligrams per day. Women over 50 and men over the age of 24 need 10 milligrams of iron daily. The higher RDA for young and middle-aged women is chiefly to counteract menstrual blood loss.

The body contains more *calcium* than any other mineral. Calcium's primary role in the body is that of forming and maintaining bones. Osteoporosis, a major health concern for women, is related to calcium deficiency (see Chapter 10). Calcium is also important for muscle contraction, nerve transmission, and cellular metabolism. Muscles cannot relax after contraction if blood calcium levels fall below a crucial point. Daily calcium intake allows good muscle contractions and relaxations during physical activity.

The milk, yogurt, and cheese group of MyPyramid and calcium-fortified foods (orange juice, breakfast cereals) provide the best sources of calcium. Adults need between 1000 and 1500 milligrams of calcium daily (see Chapter 10, Table 10.1). Surveys indicate that Americans consume only half of this requirement. If you are having difficulty maintaining a well-balanced diet, consider supplementing your diet with calcium.

Water

Water makes up about 60 percent of the body weight and is involved in virtually every body process. Water could be considered the most essential nutrient. Our bodies can survive deficiency of all the other nutrients for a few weeks or more, but can survive only a few days without water. Water serves as the body's transport solvent, distributing nutrients throughout the body and conducting waste products to be excreted through the water in urine and feces. Water serves as the body's reactive medium, participating in every chemical reaction in the body. Water plays a major role in regulating the maintenance of body temperature because it is able to absorb a significant amount of body heat with only a small change in its temperature. Because water is vital to these and other functions, it is essential to maintain a healthy level in the body.

Drink six to eight glasses of water a day.

Proper fluid replacement is important for both health and physical activity. The sedentary body loses about 2 to 3 liters of water each day through urination, perspiration, breathing, and defecation. To replace this water, the RDA recommendation is that, under normal dietary and environmental conditions, the average adult who expends 2000 calories a day should consume 2 to 3 liters, or about six to eight glasses, of water each day. In addition to the water people drink, nearly all foods provide water (IOM, 2004). Fruits and vegetables are generally high in water content, whereas many meats and fatty foods are low.

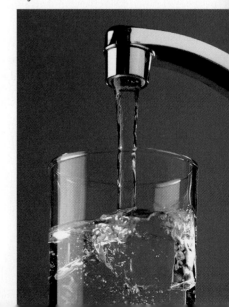

FIGURE 7.6 **MyPyramid.** The MyPyramid food guidance system allows individuals to personalize their diet plan based on gender, age, and level of physical activity. SOURCE: U.S. Department of Agriculture, Center for Nutrition Policy and Promotion. (n.d.). MyPyramid: Steps to a healthier you. Available: http://www.mypyramid.gov.

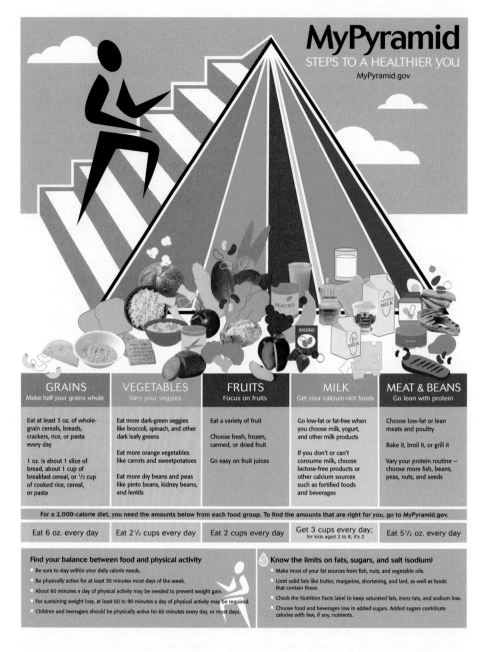

Water is a crucial nutrient for those engaged in physical activity, especially if the activity is strenuous and performed in extreme environmental temperatures and humidity. To find out how much water you need to replenish from losses occurring during exercise, weigh yourself before and after exercise; the difference is all water. One pound equals approximately two glasses of water. Plain cool water is the best choice for drinking because it leaves the digestive system rapidly, is quickly absorbed by tissues, and cools the body.

Functional Foods

We now know that the minimum diet for human growth, energy, and regulating body processes requires six classes of essential nutrients. Within the emerging area of food and nutrition science, however, is the expanding knowledge of the role of other physiologically active components in foods that provide health benefits beyond those supplied by the traditional nutrients. Examples include carotenoids, dietary fiber, flavonoids, and phenols, all of which can be found in fruits and vegetables (TABLE 7.5). The International Food Information Council (IFIC) defines

TABLE 7.5	Examples of Functional Components

Class/Components	Source(s)*	Potential Benefit(s)
Carotenoids		
Beta-carotene	Carrots, various fruits	Neutralizes free radicals that may damage cells; bolsters cellular antioxidant defenses
Lutein, zeaxanthin	Kale, collards, spinach, corn, eggs, citrus	May contribute to maintenance of healthy vision
Lycopene	Tomatoes and processed tomato products	May contribute to maintenance of prostrate health
Dietary (Functional and Total) Fiber		
Beta glucan†	Oat bran, rolled oats, oat flour	May reduce risk of coronary heart disease (CHD)
Insoluble fiber	Wheat bran	May contribute to maintenance of a healthy digestive tract
Soluble fiber†	Psyllium seed husk	May reduce risk of CHD
Whole grains†	Cereal grains	May reduce risk of CHD and cancer; may contribute to maintenance of healthy blood glucose levels
Fatty Acids		
Monounsaturated fatty acids (MUFAs)	Tree nuts	May reduce risk of CHD
Polyunsaturated fatty acids (PUFAs) and omega-3 fatty acids—ALA	Walnuts, flax	May contribute to maintenance of mental and visual function
PUFAs—omega-3 fatty acids, DHA/EPA	Salmon, tuna, marine and other fish oils	May reduce risk of CHD; may contribute to maintenance of mental and visual function
PUFAs—Conjugated linoleic acid (CLA)	Beef and lamb; some cheese	May contribute to maintenance of desirable body composition and healthy immune function
Flavonoids		
Anthocyanidins	Berries, cherries, red grapes	Bolster cellular antioxidant defenses; may contribute to maintenance of brain function
Flavanols—catechins, epicatechins, procyanidins	Tea, cocoa, chocolate, apples, grapes	May contribute to maintenance of heart health
Flavanones	Citrus foods	Neutralize free radicals that may damage cells; bolster cellular antioxidant defenses
Flavonols	Onions, apples, tea, broccoli	Neutralize free radicals that may damage cells; bolster cellular antioxidant defenses
Proanthocyanidins	Cranberries, cocoa, apples, strawberries, grapes, wine, peanuts, cinnamon	May contribute to maintenance of urinary tract health and heart health
Isothiocyanates		
Sulphoraphane	Cauliflower, broccoli, broccoli sprouts, cabbage, kale, horseradish	May enhance detoxification of undesirable compounds and bolster cellular antioxidant defenses
Phenols		
Caffeic acid, ferulic acid	Apples, pears, citrus fruits, some vegetables	May bolster cellular antioxidant defenses; may contribute to maintenance of healthy vision and heart health
Plant Stanols/Sterols		
Free stanols/sterols†	Corn, soy, wheat, wood oils, fortified foods and beverages	May reduce risk of CHD
Stanol/sterol esters†	Fortified table spreads, stanol ester dietary supplements	May reduce risk of CHD
Polyols		
Sugar alcohols—xylitol, sorbitol mannitol, lactitol	Some chewing gums and other food applications	May reduce risk of dental caries

(continued)

TABLE 7.5	Examples of Functional Components (continued)

Class/Components	Source(s)*	Potential Benefit(s)
Prebiotics/Probiotics		
Inulin, fructo-oligosaccharides (FOS), polydextrose	Whole grains, onions, some fruits, garlic, honey, leeks, fortified foods and beverages	May improve gastrointestinal health; may improve calcium absorption
Lactobacilli, bifidobacteria	Yogurt, other dairy and nondairy applications	May improve gastrointestinal health and systemic immunity
Phytoestrogens		
Isoflavones—daidzein, genistein	Soybeans and soy-based foods	May contribute to maintenance of bone health, healthy brain and immune function; for women, maintenance of menopausal health
Lignans	Flax, rye, some vegetables	May contribute to maintenance of heart health and healthy immune function
Soy Protein		
Soy protein†	Soybeans and soy based foods	May reduce risk of CHD
Sulfides/thiols		
Diallyl sulfide, allyl methyl trisulfide	Garlic, onions, leaks, scallions	May enhance detoxification of undesirable compounds; may contribute to maintenance of heart health and healthy immune system
Dithiolthiones	Cruciferous vegetables	Contribute to maintenance of healthy immune function

*Examples are not an all-inclusive list.

†FDA-approved health claim established for component.

SOURCE: International Food Information Council. (2004). Backgrounder—functional foods. Available: http://www.ific.org/nutrition/functional/index.cfm.

Functional foods Foods that contain significant levels of biologically active components that provide health benefits beyond basic nutrition.

functional foods as those that contain significant levels of biologically active components that provide health benefits beyond basic nutrition (IFIC, 2004). The increasing comprehension of the role of physiologically active food components, both from plant (*phytochemicals*) and animal (*zoochemicals*) sources, has notably changed the role of diet in health. Interest in functional foods continues to evolve as food and nutrition science has advanced beyond studying nutritional deficiencies to studying foods for biologically active components that impart health benefits or desirable physiological effects beyond basic nutrition. To obtain the many potentially beneficial components from functional foods, the best advice is to include foods from all of the food groups represented in MyPyramid.

Planning a Nutritious Diet

One of the most important features of a nutritious diet is to obtain all required nutrients through a reasonable calorie or energy intake approach. In other words, you should not only nourish your body with the proper amounts of nutrients but also understand that how much you eat contributes to your weight, which plays a major role in one's long-term health (see Chapter 9). Basically, you must meet your nutrient requirements within the constraints of your energy demands. Nutrient-calorie benefit ratio, or nutrient density, is a simple way to connect nutrients with calories.

Nutrient-Calorie Benefit Ratio and Why It Is Important

The American diet is said to be increasingly energy rich but nutrient poor. To help improve the nutrient-to-energy ratio, the 2005 *Dietary Guidelines for Americans* recommends that consumers replace some foods in their diets with more nutrient-dense options. **Nutrient-calorie benefit ratio (NCBR)** is defined as the amount of nutrient per energy unit, or the ratio of nutrients to calories. In essence, a food with high NCBR possesses a significant amount of a specific nutrient or nutrients per serving compared with its caloric content. We refer to these as "quality calories." For example, a candy bar contains much energy in the form of simple sugars but has few vitamins and minerals, so it has a low NCBR. Soybeans, on the other hand, have a moderate amount of calories but are rich in high-quality protein, healthy fats, complex carbohydrates, vitamins and minerals and sterols (a functional food component) and therefore have a high NCBR. Nutrient-dense foods give you the most nutrients for the fewest calories. In other words, nutrient-dense foods give you the biggest bang for the buck. You get lots of nutrients, and it doesn't cost you much in terms of calories.

Dietary Reference Intakes

Ever wonder how much of the nutrients listed in Table 7.2 you really need to eat every day to be healthy? The first set of recommendations, Recommended Dietary Allowances (RDAs), was published by the Institute of Medicine's Food and Nutrition Board of the National Academy of Sciences in 1941 and revised periodically over the years. The RDAs were originally designed to prevent nutritional deficiencies in large groups of people such as the armed forces and children in school lunch programs. From a statistical standpoint, this means that the RDAs were set to prevent nutritional deficiencies in 97 percent of the population. In other words, the RDAs are intentionally set somewhat higher than the body's actual physiological needs.

Times have changed. In 1993, the Food and Nutrition Board (FNB), working with Health Canada, began a major overhaul of the RDAs that continues today. With increased understanding of the relationship between nutrition and chronic diseases, the FNB is redefining nutrient requirements and developing new RDAs based on three overriding principles. The first two principles supporting the current revision are: (1) incorporating the concept of risk reduction for chronic diseases, not just prevention of nutrient deficiencies, and (2) recommending nutrient intakes that are thought to help people achieve good health by providing multiple reference points for nutrient intake instead of one number for each nutrient. The reference points are collectively referred to as the **Dietary Reference Intakes (DRIs)**. DRI serves as an umbrella term that includes the following values.

ESTIMATED AVERAGE REQUIREMENT (EAR) The Estimated Average Requirement (EAR) is estimated to meet the requirement of half the healthy individuals for a specific age-gender group. For example, the iron EAR for women of childbearing age will likely be different than for adult males. The EAR is used to assess nutritional adequacy of intakes of population groups. In addition, EARs are used to calculate RDAs.

RECOMMENDED DIETARY ALLOWANCE (RDA) The Recommended Dietary Allowance (RDA) is a goal for individuals and is based upon the EAR. Unlike earlier RDAs, these are designed to *reduce disease risk*, not just prevent deficiency. It is the daily dietary intake level that is sufficient to meet the requirements of 97 percent of all healthy individuals in a group and is meant for use by individuals. If

Nutrient-calorie benefit ratio (NCBR) Amount of nutrient per energy unit, or the ratio of nutrients to calories.

Dietary Reference Intakes (DRIs) Umbrella term that includes Estimated Average Requirement, Recommended Dietary Allowance, Adequate Intake, and Tolerable Upper Intake Level.

an EAR cannot be set, no RDA value can be proposed.

ADEQUATE INTAKE (AI)   Adequate Intake (AI) is used when an RDA cannot be determined. In other words, scientific data is not strong enough to come up with a final number, yet there is enough evidence to give a general guideline. Like the RDA, individuals can use this number to set their personal dietary goals.

TOLERABLE UPPER INTAKE LEVEL (UL)   The Tolerable Upper Intake Level (UL) is the highest level of daily nutrient intake that is likely to pose no risks of adverse health effects to almost all individuals in the general population. Anything above the UL might result in toxic reactions. The higher the intake, the higher the risk.

The third principle behind the nutrient revisions is that both essential nutrients and food components—deemed valuable even if not essential nutrients—will be considered. This principle allows the Food and Nutrition Board to consider components such as fiber and carotenoids.

Dietary Guidelines for Americans

The *Dietary Guidelines for Americans* provides general recommendations that focus attention on the association between diet and chronic diseases.

In recognition of the role that dietary factors play in promoting health and causing many major chronic diseases, the U.S. Departments of Agriculture (USDA) and Health and Human Services (USDHHS) periodically issue the *Dietary Guidelines for Americans*. The recommendations contained within the *Dietary Guidelines* provide authoritative advice for people 2 years and older about how proper dietary habits can promote health and reduce risk for major chronic diseases (USDHHS & USDA, 2005). The *Dietary Guidelines*, first published in 1980, are reviewed every 5 years by a committee of nutrition and health scientists who recommend changes based on current knowledge of the influence of diet on health and disease. The sixth edition of the *Dietary Guidelines*, published in 2005, conveys nine key messages. The major change from previous guidelines is that a stronger emphasis is placed on reducing calorie consumption and increasing physical activity.

The nine interrelated major messages and the key recommendations from the 2005 *Dietary Guidelines* are as follows (USDHHS & USDA, 2005).

Adequate Nutrients Within Calorie Needs

- Consume a variety of nutrient-dense foods and beverages within and among the basic food groups while choosing foods that limit the intake of saturated and trans fats, cholesterol, added sugars, salt, and alcohol.
- Meet recommended intakes within energy needs by adopting a balanced eating pattern, such as the USDA Food Guide or the Dietary Approaches to Stop Hypertension (DASH) Eating Plan.

Weight Management

- To maintain body weight in a healthy range, balance calories from foods and beverages with calories expended.
- To prevent gradual weight gain over time, make small decreases in food and beverage calories and increase physical activity.

Physical Activity

- Engage in regular physical activity and reduce sedentary activities to promote health, psychological well-being, and a healthy body weight.

- To reduce the risk of chronic disease in adulthood: Engage in at least 30 minutes of moderate-intensity physical activity, above usual activity, at work or home on most days of the week.
- For most people, greater health benefits can be obtained by engaging in physical activity of more vigorous intensity or longer duration.
- To help manage body weight and prevent gradual, unhealthy body weight gain in adulthood: Engage in approximately 60 minutes of moderate- to vigorous-intensity activity most days of the week while not exceeding caloric intake requirements.
- To sustain weight loss in adulthood: Participate in at least 60 to 90 minutes of daily moderate-intensity physical activity while not exceeding caloric intake requirements. Some people may need to consult with a health care provider before participating in this level of activity.
- Achieve physical fitness by including cardiovascular conditioning, stretching exercises for flexibility, and resistance exercises or calisthenics for muscle strength and endurance.

Food Groups to Encourage

- Consume a sufficient amount of fruits and vegetables while staying within energy needs. Two cups of fruit and 2.5 cups of vegetables per day are recommended for a reference 2000-calorie intake, with higher or lower amounts depending on the calorie level.
- Choose a variety of fruits and vegetables each day. In particular, select from all five vegetable subgroups (dark green, orange, legumes, starchy vegetables, and other vegetables) several times a week.
- Consume 3 or more ounce-equivalents of whole-grain products per day, with the rest of the recommended grains coming from enriched or whole-grain products. In general, at least half the grains should come from whole grains.
- Consume 3 cups per day of fat-free or low-fat milk or equivalent milk products.

Fats

- Consume less than 10 percent of calories from saturated fatty acids and less than 300 mg/day of cholesterol, and keep trans fatty acid consumption as low as possible.
- Keep total fat intake between 20 to 35 percent of calories, with most fats coming from sources of polyunsaturated and monounsaturated fatty acids, such as fish, nuts, and vegetable oils.
- When selecting and preparing meat, poultry, dry beans, and milk or milk products, make choices that are lean, low-fat, or fat-free.
- Limit intake of fats and oils high in saturated and/or trans fatty acids, and choose products low in such fats and oils.

Carbohydrates

- Choose fiber-rich fruits, vegetables, and whole grains often.
- Choose and prepare foods and beverages with little added sugars or caloric sweeteners, such as amounts suggested by the USDA Food Guide and the DASH Eating Plan.
- Reduce the incidence of dental caries by practicing good oral hygiene and consuming sugar- and starch-containing foods and beverages less frequently.

Sodium and Potassium

- Consume less than 2300 mg (approximately 1 teaspoon of salt) of sodium per day.
- Choose and prepare foods with little salt. At the same time, consume potassium-rich foods, such as fruits and vegetables.

Alcoholic Beverages

- Those who choose to drink alcoholic beverages should do so sensibly and in moderation—defined as the consumption of up to one drink per day for women and up to two drinks per day for men.
- Alcoholic beverages should not be consumed by some individuals, including those who cannot restrict their alcohol intake, women of childbearing age who may become pregnant, lactating women, children and adolescents, individuals taking medications that can interact with alcohol, and those with specific medical conditions.
- Alcoholic beverages should be avoided by individuals engaging in activities that require attention, skill, or coordination, such as driving or operating machinery.

Food Safety

- To avoid microbial foodborne illnesses:
  - Clean hands, food contact surfaces, and fruits and vegetables. Meat and poultry should not be washed or rinsed.
  - Separate raw, cooked, and ready-to-eat foods while shopping, preparing, or storing foods.
  - Cook foods to a safe temperature to kill microorganisms.
  - Chill (refrigerate) perishable food promptly and defrost foods properly.
  - Avoid raw (unpasteurized) milk or any products made from unpasteurized milk, raw or partially cooked eggs or foods containing raw eggs, raw or undercooked meat and poultry, unpasteurized juices, and raw sprouts.

In summary, the *Dietary Guidelines* are designed to help Americans choose diets that will meet nutrient requirements, promote health, support active lives, and reduce chronic disease risks. Research has shown that certain diets raise risks for chronic diseases. Such diets are high in fat, saturated fat, cholesterol, and salt and contain more calories than the body uses. They are also low in grain products, vegetables, fruit, and fiber.

The MyPyramid Food Guidance System

The MyPyramid food guidance system provides information to help implement the recommendations of the *Dietary Guidelines*. The MyPyramid symbol is a simple graphic design that is a visual reminder to make healthy food choices and be physically active each day (Figure 7.6) MyPyramid contains eight divisions. From left to right are the six color bands representing the five food groups of the pyramid (grains, vegetables, fruits, milk, and meat and beans) and oils. There are two other categories: physical activity, represented by a person climbing steps on the pyramid, and discretionary calories (candy, alcohol, or additional food from any other group) represented by the uncolored tip of the pyramid. MyPyramid is based on both the *Dietary Guidelines* and the Dietary Reference Intakes from the National Academy of Sciences, while taking into account current consumption patterns of Americans. The MyPyramid symbol illustrates six basic concepts (see Figure 7.6):

The MyPyramid food guidance system provides a wealth of information for you to apply in developing a nutritious diet and a physically active lifestyle.

- *Activity.* Activity is represented by the person climbing the steps of the pyramid.
- *Moderation.* Moderation is represented by the narrowing of each food group from bottom to top. The wider base stands for foods with little or no solid fats or added sugars. These should be selected more often. The narrower top area stands for foods containing added sugars and solid fats. The more active you are, the more these foods can fit into your diet. Wise selection of foods and beverages helps you control the amount of calories consumed and the total amount of fat, saturated fat, cholesterol, salt, sugars, and (if consumed) alcohol. Moderation allows you more flexibility to enjoy the variety of foods available to you.
- *Personalization.* Personalization is shown by the person on the steps, the slogan "Steps to a Healthier You," and the MyPyramid.gov URL. The MyPyramid website (http://www.MyPyramid.gov) helps individuals personalize their own MyPyramid by requesting their age, gender, and physical activity level.
- *Proportionality.* Proportionality is shown by the different widths of the food group bands. The widths suggest how much food a person should choose from each group.
- *Variety.* Variety is symbolized by the six color bands representing the five food groups of the pyramid and oils. This illustrates that foods from all groups are needed each day for good health. A varied diet includes many different foods from each of the MyPyramid five major food groups. It is generally agreed that people should not eat the same foods day after day, because no single food or foods supplies all the nutrients you need (TABLE 7.6).
- *Gradual improvement.* Gradual improvement is encouraged by the slogan "Steps to a Healthier You." It suggests that individuals can benefit from taking small steps to improve their diet and lifestyle each day.

TABLE 7.6	Variety from the Food Groups

Bread, Cereal, Rice, Pasta

Whole-Grain	Enriched	Grain Products with More Fat and Sugar
Brown rice	Bagels	Biscuit
Buckwheat groats	Cornmeal	Cake (unfrosted)
Bulgar	Crackers	Cookies
Corn tortillas	English muffins	Cornbread
Graham crackers	Farina	Croissant
Granola	Flour tortillas	Danish
Oatmeal	French bread	Doughnut
Popcorn	Grits	Muffin
Pumpernickel bread	Hamburger and hot dog rolls	Pie crust
Ready-to-eat cereals	Italian bread	Tortilla chips
Rye bread and crackers	Macaroni	
Whole-wheat bread, rolls, crackers	Noodles	
Whole-wheat pasta	Pancakes and waffles	
Whole-wheat cereals	Pretzels	
	Ready-to-eat cereals	
	Rice	
	Spaghetti	
	White bread and rolls	

(continued)

| TABLE 7.6 | Variety from the Food Groups (continued) |

Fruits

Citrus, Melons, Berries

Blueberries	Lemon
Cantaloupe	Orange
Citrus juices	Raspberries
Cranberries	Strawberries
Grapefruit	Tangerine
Honeydew melon	Watermelon
Kiwi	Ugli fruit

Other Fruits

Apple	Guava	Pineapple
Apricot	Grapes	Plantain
Asian pear	Mango	Plum
Banana	Nectarine	Prickly pear
Cherries	Papaya	Prunes
Dates	Passion fruit	Raisins
Figs	Peach	Rhubarb
Fruit juices	Pear	Star fruit

Vegetables

Dark-Green Leafy

Beet greens	
Broccoli	
Chard	
Chicory	
Collard greens	
Dandelion greens	
Endive	
Escarole	
Kale	
Mustard greens	
Romaine lettuce	
Spinach	
Turnip greens	
Watercress	

Deep Yellow

Carrots
Pumpkin
Sweet potato
Winter squash

Starchy

Breadfruit
Corn
Green peas
Hominy
Lima beans
Potato
Rutabaga
Taro

Dry Beans and Peas (Legumes)

Black beans
Black-eyed peas
Chickpeas (garbanzos)
Kidney beans
Lentils
Lima beans (mature)
Mung beans
Navy beans
Pinto beans
Split peas

Other Vegetables

Artichoke	Cauliflower	Lettuce	Summer squash
Asparagus	Celery	Mushrooms	Chinese cabbage
Bean and alfalfa sprouts	Cucumber	Okra	Tomato
Beets	Eggplant	Onions (mature and green)	Turnip
Brussels sprouts	Green beans	Radishes	Vegetable juices
Cabbage	Green pepper	Snow peas	Zucchini

Meat, Poultry, Fish, and Alternatives

Meat, Poultry, and Fish

Beef
Chicken
Fish
Ham
Lamb
Luncheon meats, sausage
Organ meats

Alternates

Pork
Shellfish
Turkey
Veal
Eggs
Dry beans and peas (legumes)
Nuts and seeds
Peanut butter
Tofu

(continued)

TABLE 7.6	**Variety from the Food Groups**

Milk, Yogurt, and Cheese

Lowfat Milk Products

Buttermilk

Lowfat cottage cheese

Lowfat milk (1%, 2% fat)

Lowfat or nonfat plain yogurt

Skim milk

Other Milk Products with More Fat or Sugar

Cheddar cheese

Chocolate milk

Flavored yogurt

Frozen yogurt

Fruit yogurt

Ice cream

Ice milk

Process cheeses and spreads

Puddings made with milk

Swiss cheese

Whole milk

Fats, Sweets, and Alcoholic Beverages

Fats

Bacon, salt port

Butter

Cream (dairy, nondairy)

Cream cheese

Lard

Margarine

Mayonnaise

Mayonnaise-type salad dressing

Salad dressing

Shortening

Sour cream

Vegetable oil

Sweets

Candy

Corn syrup

Frosting (icing)

Fruit drinks

Gelatin desserts

Honey

Jam

Jelly

Maple syrup

Marmalade

Molasses

Table syrup

Popsicles and ices

Sherbets

Soft drinks and colas

Sugar (white and brown)

Alcoholic Beverages

Beer

Liquor

Wine

SOURCE: A. Shaw, L. Fulton, C. Davis, and M. Hogbin. (1998). *Using the Food Guide Pyramid: A Resource for Nutrition Educators.* U.S. Department of Agriculture, Food, Nutrition, and Consumer Services, Center for Nutrition Policy and Promotion. Online: http://www.usda.gov:80/cnpp/using.htm.

The MyPyramid system is designed for individual differences and can be personalized for 12 levels of energy (caloric) needs, ranging from 1000 to 3200 calories per day depending on age, gender, and physical activity level (TABLE 7.7). It is flexible enough to help you make simple, small improvements in your food and lifestyle decisions and to match these steps with your own calorie needs, lifestyle, and food preferences. The suggested amounts of food from the basic food groups, subgroups, and oils to meet recommended nutrient intakes at 12 different calorie levels are shown in TABLE 7.8 . The table also shows the discretionary calorie allowance that can be accommodated within each calorie level, in addition to the suggested amounts of nutrient-dense forms of foods in each group (USDHHS & USDA, 2005).

To obtain more information about the MyPyramid food guidance system, access the USDA's interactive website (http://www.MyPyramid.gov). The messages regarding each of the food categories and the physical activity portion are further described in electronic print by clicking on the relevant category. The main messages in each category are described briefly in the following subsections.

GRAINS   The main message in the grain group of MyPyramid is to make at least half of the total grains eaten whole grains. The goal is to eat 3 or more ounce-equivalents of whole-grain products daily. Examples of whole grains are brown

TABLE 7.7 MyPyramid Food Intake Pattern Calorie Levels

	Males				Females		
Activity Level Age	Sedentary*	Mod. Active*	Active*	Activity Level Age	Sedentary*	Mod. Active*	Active*
2	1000	1000	1000	2	1000	1000	1000
3	1000	1400	1400	3	1000	1200	1400
4	1200	1400	1600	4	1200	1400	1400
5	1200	1400	1600	5	1200	1400	1600
6	1400	1600	1800	6	1200	1400	1600
7	1400	1600	1800	7	1200	1600	1800
8	1400	1600	2000	8	1400	1600	1800
9	1600	1800	2000	9	1400	1600	1800
10	1600	1800	2200	10	1400	1800	2000
11	1800	2000	2200	11	1600	1800	2000
12	1800	2200	2400	12	1600	2000	2200
13	2000	2200	2600	13	1600	2000	2200
14	2000	2400	2800	14	1800	2000	2400
15	2200	2600	3000	15	1800	2000	2400
16	2400	2800	3200	16	1800	2000	2400
17	2400	2800	3200	17	1800	2000	2400
18	2400	2800	3200	18	1800	2000	2400
19–20	2600	2800	3000	19–20	2000	2200	2400
21–25	2400	2800	3000	21–25	2000	2200	2400
26–30	2400	2600	3000	26–30	1800	2000	2400
31–35	2400	2600	3000	31–35	1800	2000	2200
36–40	2400	2600	2800	36–40	1800	2000	2200
41–45	2200	2600	2800	41–45	1800	2000	2200
46–50	2200	2400	2800	46–50	1800	2000	2200
51–55	2200	2400	2800	51–55	1600	1800	2200
56–60	2200	2400	2600	56–60	1600	1800	2200
61–65	2000	2400	2600	61–65	1600	1800	2000
66–70	2000	2200	2600	66–70	1600	1800	2000
71–75	2000	2200	2600	71–75	1600	1800	2000
76 and up	2000	2200	2400	76 and up	1600	1800	2000

*Calorie levels are based on the Estimated Energy Requirements (EER) and activity levels from the Institute of Medicine Dietary Reference Intakes Macronutrients Report, 2002.

Sedentary = less than 30 minutes a day of moderate physical activity in addition to daily activities.

Mod. active = at least 30 minutes up to 60 minutes a day of moderate physical activity in addition to daily activities.

Active = 60 or more minutes a day of moderate physical activity in addition to daily activities.

SOURCE: U.S. Department of Agriculture, Center for Nutrition Policy and Promotion. (2005, April). MyPyramid food intake pattern calorie levels. Available: http://www.mypyramid.gov/professionals/pdf_calorie_levels.html.

TABLE 7.8	MyPyramid Food Intake Patterns

Daily Amount of Food from Each Group

Calorie Level[1]	1000	1200	1400	1600	1800	2000	2200	2400	2600	2800	3000	3200
Fruits[2]	1 cup	1 cup	1.5 cups	1.5 cups	1.5 cups	2 cups	2 cups	2 cups	2 cups	2.5 cups	2.5 cups	2.5 cups
Vegetables[3]	1 cup	1.5 cups	1.5 cups	2 cups	2.5 cups	2.5 cups	3 cups	3 cups	3.5 cups	3.5 cups	4 cups	4 cups
Grains[4]	3 oz-eq	4 oz-eq	5 oz-eq	5 oz-eq	6 oz-eq	6 oz-eq	7 oz-eq	8 oz-eq	9 oz-eq	10 oz-eq	10 oz-eq	10 oz-eq
Meat and beans[5]	2 oz-eq	3 oz-eq	4 oz-eq	5 oz-eq	5 oz-eq	5.5 oz-eq	6 oz-eq	6.5 oz-eq	6.5 oz-eq	7 oz-eq	7 oz-eq	7 oz-eq
Milk[6]	2 cups	2 cups	2 cups	3 cups	3 cups	3 cups	3 cups	3 cups	3 cups	3 cups	3 cups	3 cups
Oils[7]	3 tsp	4 tsp	4 tsp	5 tsp	5 tsp	6 tsp	6 tsp	7 tsp	8 tsp	8 tsp	10 tsp	11 tsp
Discretionary calorie allowance[8]	165	171	171	132	195	267	290	362	410	426	512	648

Vegetable Subgroup Amounts (Cups per Week)

Calorie Level	1000	1200	1400	1600	1800	2000	2200	2400	2600	2800	3000	3200
Dark-green veg.	1	1.5	1.5	2	3	3	3	3	3	3	3	3
Orange veg.	0.5	1	1	1.5	2	2	2	2	2.5	2.5	2.5	2.5
Legumes	0.5	1	1	2.5	3	3	3	3	3.5	3.5	3.5	3.5
Starchy veg.	1.5	2.5	2.5	2.5	3	3	6	6	7	7	9	9
Other veg.	3.5	4.5	4.5	5.5	6.5	6.5	7	7	8.5	8.5	10	10

[1]**Calorie levels** are set across a wide range to accommodate the needs of different individuals. Table 7.7 can be used to help assign individuals to the food intake pattern at a particular calorie level.

[2]**Fruit group** includes all fresh, frozen, canned, and dried fruits and fruit juices. In general, 1 cup of fruit or 100 percent fruit juice, or ½ cup of dried fruit can be considered as 1 cup from the fruit group.

[3]**Vegetable group** includes all fresh, frozen, canned, and dried vegetables and vegetable juices. In general, 1 cup of raw or cooked vegetables or vegetable juice, or 2 cups of raw leafy greens, can be considered as 1 cup from the vegetable group.

[4]**Grains group** includes all foods made from wheat, rice, oats, cornmeal, or barley, such as bread, pasta, oatmeal, breakfast cereals, tortillas, and grits. In general, 1 slice of bread, 1 cup of ready-to-eat cereal, or ½ cup of cooked rice, pasta, or cooked cereal can be considered as 1 ounce-equivalent from the grains group. **At least half of all grains consumed should be whole grains.**

[5]**Meat and beans group:** In general, 1 ounce of lean meat, poultry, or fish, 1 egg, 1 Tbsp. peanut butter, ¼ cup cooked dry beans, or ½ ounce of nuts or seeds can be considered as 1 ounce-equivalent from the meat and beans group.

[6]**Milk group** includes all fluid milk products and foods made from milk that retain their calcium content, such as yogurt and cheese. Foods made from milk that have little to no calcium, such as cream cheese, cream, and butter, are not part of the group. Most milk group choices should be fat-free or low-fat. In general, 1 cup of milk or yogurt, 1.5 ounces of natural cheese, or 2 ounces of processed cheese can be considered as 1 cup from the milk group.

[7]**Oils** include fats from many different plants and from fish that are liquid at room temperature, such as canola, corn, olive, soybean, and sunflower oil. Some foods are naturally high in oils, like nuts, olives, some fish, and avocados. Foods that are mainly oil include mayonnaise, certain salad dressings, and soft margarine.

[8]**Discretionary calorie allowance** is the remaining amount of calories in a food intake pattern after accounting for the calories needed for all food groups—using forms of foods that are fat-free or low-fat and with no added sugars.

SOURCE: U.S. Department of Agriculture, Center for Nutrition Policy and Promotion. (2005, April). MyPyramid food intake patterns. Available: http://www.mypyramid.gov/professionals/pdf_food_intake.html.

rice, wild rice, oatmeal, buckwheat, bulgur, and whole-wheat bread, crackers, pasta, and tortillas.

VEGETABLES   The main message in the vegetable group of MyPyramid is twofold: (1) eat the recommended amounts of vegetables daily, and (2) choose a variety of vegetables throughout the week. The vegetables are listed in five subgroups based on nutrient content: dark-green, orange, starchy, dry beans and peas, and other vegetables. Any vegetable or 100 percent vegetable juice counts as a member of the vegetable group. Vegetables may be raw or cooked; fresh, frozen, canned, or dried/dehydrated; and may be whole, cut-up, or mashed. The recommended daily amount is listed in cups, rather than number of servings.

FRUITS   The main message in the fruit group of MyPyramid is to eat the recommended amounts of fruits and to choose a variety of fruits each day. Select whole or cut-up fruit as well as canned, frozen, and dried fruit rather than fruit juice for the most nutritional benefit. Fruit juices tend to be more calorie-dense and contain little fiber compared with whole fruits.

OILS   The main message in the fats and oils group of MyPyramid is to choose most fats from sources of monounsaturated and polyunsaturated fatty acids, such as fish, nuts, seeds, and vegetable oils. Saturated fats are also part of this section of MyPyramid. Keeping saturated fat below 10 percent of calories should be a primary focus, because this is the predominant fat that adversely affects blood lipid levels that increase the risk of cardiovascular disease.

MILK   The main message in the milk group of MyPyramid is to get your calcium-rich foods through low-fat or fat-free milk products such as liquid milk, yogurt, or cheese. If you can't or don't consume milk products, choose lactose-free products or other products such as hard cheeses and yogurt. Additionally, calcium-fortified foods and beverages such as soy beverages or orange juice may provide calcium.

MEAT AND BEANS   The main message in the meat and beans group of MyPyramid is to eat low-fat or lean meat when selecting meats and poultry. Lean meats, poultry, fish, eggs, dry beans and peas, nuts, and seeds all count toward meeting meat and bean group goals. The dry beans and peas, including soy products, are part of this group as well as the vegetable group.

PHYSICAL ACTIVITY   The main message of MyPyramid related to physical activity is to find your balance between food and physical activity. Encouraging physical activity at a level that can improve and be incorporated daily is given high importance in MyPyramid. The goal is to engage in regular physical activity and reduce sedentary activities. Making moderate physical activity part of your daily routine for at least 30 minutes per day promotes fitness and reduces the risk of many chronic diseases.

YOUR PERSONAL NUTRITION PLAN   To personalize a nutritional plan, you can go to www.MyPyramid.gov to obtain information that is specific to your energy needs and nutrient composition based on your physical activity level. You will be asked to enter your age, sex, and the amount of moderate or vigorous physical activity (such as brisk walking, jogging, biking, aerobics, or yard work) you do *in addition to your normal daily routine*, on most days of the week. For example, a 20-year-old female who jogs 30 minutes on most days of week would enter her age, gender, and the 30- to 60-minute level of daily physical activity into the online

MyPyramid program. The MyPyramid program will then calculate the recommended servings in each of the five major food groups and provide information on the amount of oils and discretionary calories per day based on these three characteristics. **FIGURE 7.7** shows the results of the calculations for this 20-year-old female jogger. Following the recommendations from this calculation will help this woman maintain a healthy weight and meet nutrient requirements. If this jogger decides to increase her physical activity level to 60-minutes or more daily, she would need to enter the new information using the 60-minute or more physical activity level. A new calorie amount and recommended servings would be calculated. This individualization is helpful because not all individuals of the same age and sex have the same physical activity level and energy needs.

The MyPyramid food guidance system provides a wealth of information for you to apply in developing your nutritious eating and physical activity lifestyle. The activities and assessments manual includes activities that enable you to use MyPyramid to evaluate the nutritional adequacy of your daily food choices. In

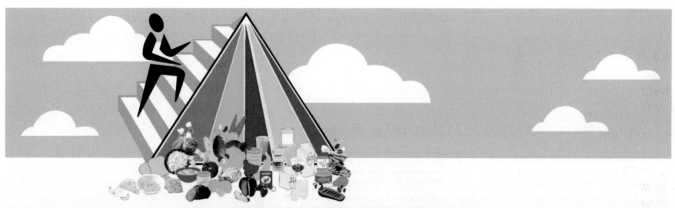

Based on the information you provided, this is your daily recommended amount from each food group.

GRAINS 7 ounces	VEGETABLES 3 cups	FRUITS 2 cups	MILK 3 cups	MEAT & BEANS 6 ounces
Make half your grains whole Aim for at least **3 1/2 ounces** of whole grains a day	**Vary your veggies** Aim for these amounts each week: **Dark green veggies** = 3 cups **Orange veggies** = 2 cups **Dry beans & peas** = 3 cups **Starchy veggies** = 6 cups **Other veggies** = 7 cups	**Focus on fruits** Eat a variety of fruit Go easy on fruit juices	**Get your calcium-rich foods** Go low-fat or fat-free when you choose milk, yougurt, or cheese	**Go lean with protein** Choose low-fat or lean meats and poultry Vary your protein routine-choose more fish, beans, peas, nuts, and seeds

Find your balance between food and physical activity	**Know your limits on fats, sugars, and sodium**
Be physically active for at least **30 minutes** most days of the week.	Your allowance for oils is **6 teaspoons a day**. Limit extras–solid fats and sugars–to **290 calories a day**.

Your results are based on a 2200 calorie pattern.   Name: _____

FIGURE 7.7 **Personalized MyPyramid Plan.** This plan is personalized for a 20-year-old woman who gets 30 to 60 minutes of daily physical activity.

summary, MyPyramid provides detailed guidelines for improving overall health through proper nutrition and physical activity.

Food Labeling

You know, as a health-conscious consumer, how important it is to choose foods that offer high nutritional value. But how can you be sure you are making the wisest selections of foods as you roll your grocery cart down the supermarket aisles? Considering that the average supermarket stocks over 40,000 different products and that many food manufacturers use health advertising claims to get you to purchase their products, you have to make many decisions in a short shopping trip.

Fortunately for you, the U.S. government requires that all manufactured foods must be labeled with the product name, name and address of the manufacturer, amount of product in package, ingredients listed in descending order by weight, and the **nutrition facts label**. An ingredients label that contains "wheat flour, malted barley flour, and salt" informs you that wheat flour is proportionally the largest ingredient and that the second largest is barley flour. The nutrition facts label (**FIGURE 7.8**) is a simple, graphical nutrition tool that can serve as a key to planning a healthful diet. The label provides comprehensive information on the nutri-

> **Nutrition facts label** Mandated food labeling designed to help consumers make appropriate choices.

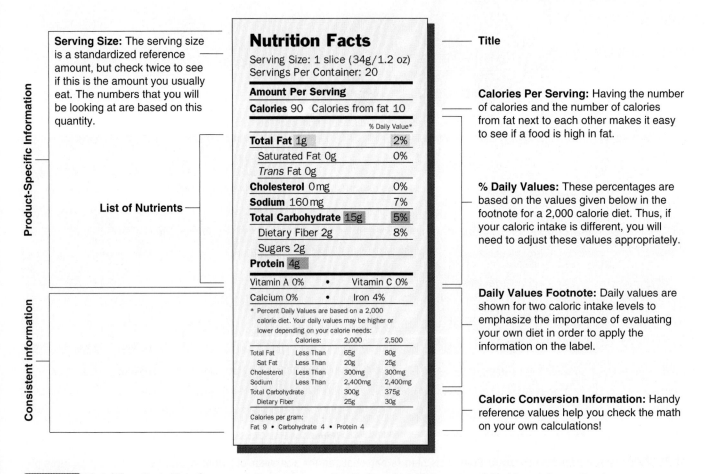

FIGURE 7.8 **Nutrition Facts Panel.** SOURCE: U.S. Department of Agriculture/U.S. Department of Health and Human Services.

tional composition of food products that facilitates comparison of food products and assists in the selection of foods for a diet that will meet the *Dietary Guidelines for Americans.*

Most of the information needed to adhere to the MyPyramid food guidance system is provided on the nutrition facts label. The following 15 nutrients must be listed: total calories, calories from fat, total fat, saturated fat, trans fat cholesterol, sodium, total carbohydrate, dietary fiber, sugars, protein, vitamin A, vitamin C, calcium, and iron. The 14 mandatory nutrients were selected because they are most relevant to our national health problems. If optional nutrients are listed by the manufacturer in order to make a health claim—for example, naming other essential vitamins and minerals, or whether the food is fortified or enriched with any of them—nutrition figures for these optional nutrients become mandatory as well. The types of descriptive words used to make health-related claims have specific meanings that are clearly defined by regulation (TABLE 7.9).

Another important way the nutrition facts label helps you meet the *Dietary Guidelines* is that % daily value is given for each nutrient. The *% daily value* is a measure of the contribution of one serving of the food product to the recommended daily intake of the nutrient-based on a daily intake of 2000 calories. This % daily value information permits comparison of food products without the need for calculations. Also, by scanning the % daily value column, you can see how a product's protein, carbohydrate, fiber, fat, and sodium fits within your total diet. Simple math calculations can help you keep track of how much of each of the various nutrients you have obtained for the day. All of this information can help you balance your food choices and develop improved eating habits.

HEALTH CLAIMS ON FOOD PRODUCTS The U.S. Food and Drug Administration (FDA) defines the health-related claims that manufacturers can use in labeling and advertising, in order to help consumers identify foods that are rich in nutrients and that may help to prevent chronic disease conditions. Manufacturers are allowed to make health claims about certain nutrients that are found naturally in foods. Claims must be balanced and based on current, reliable scientific studies and must be approved by the U.S. FDA.

To date, the following 14 health claims have been approved (FDA, 2005).

1. *Calcium and osteoporosis:* Adequate calcium may reduce the risk of osteoporosis. To carry this claim, a food must contain 20 percent or more of the daily value for calcium (200 mg) per serving, have a calcium content that equals or exceeds the food's content of phosphorus, and contain a form of calcium that can be readily absorbed and used by the body.

2. *Fat and cancer:* Low-fat diets decrease the risk for some types of cancers. To carry this claim, a food must meet the nutrient content claim requirements for "low-fat" or, if fish and game meats, for "extra lean."

3. *Fruits and vegetables and cancer:* Diets low in fat and rich in fruits and vegetables may reduce the risk of certain cancers. This claim may be made for fruits and vegetables that meet the nutrient content claim requirements for "low-fat" and that, without fortification, are a "good source" of at least one of the following: dietary fiber or vitamins A or C.

4. *Fiber-containing grain products, fruits, and vegetables and cancer:* Diets low in fat and rich in high-fiber foods may reduce the risk of certain cancers. To carry this claim, a food must be or must contain a grain product, fruit, or vegetable; meet the nutrient content claim requirements for "low-fat"; and, without fortification, be a "good source" of dietary fiber.

TABLE 7.9	Approved Nutrient Content Claims: What Words on Food Products Mean

Free: Food contains no amount (or trivial or "physiologically inconsequential" amounts). May be used with one or more of the following: fat, saturated fat, cholesterol, sodium, sugar, and calorie. Synonyms include *without*, *no*, and *zero*.

   Fat-free: Less than 0.5 mg of fat per serving.

   Saturated fat-free: Less than 0.5 of saturated fat per serving.

   Cholesterol-free: Less than 2 mg of cholesterol and 2 g or less of saturated fat and trans fat combined per serving.

   Sodium-free: Less than 5 mg of sodium per serving.

   Sugar-free: Less than 0.5 g of sugar per serving.

   Calorie-free: Fewer than 5 calories per serving.

Low: Food can be eaten frequently without exceeding dietary guidelines for one or more of these components: fat, saturated fat, cholesterol, sodium, and calories. Synonyms include *little*, *few*, and *low source of*.

   Low fat: 3 g or less per serving.

   Low saturated fat: 1 g or less of saturated fat; no more than 15% of calories from saturated fat and trans fat combined.

   Low cholesterol: 20 mg or less and 2 g or less of saturated fat per serving.

   Low sodium: 140 mg or less per serving.

   Low calorie: 40 calories or less per serving.

High: Food contains 20% or more of the daily value for a particular nutrient in a serving.

Good source: Food contains 10% to 19% of the daily value for a particular nutrient in one serving.

Lean and extra lean: The fat content of meal and main dish products, seafood, and game products.

Lean: Less than 10 g fat, 4.5 g or less saturated fat, and less than 95 mg of cholesterol per serving and per 100 g.

Extra lean: Less than 5 g fat, less than 2 g saturated fat, and less than 95 mg of cholesterol per serving and per 100 g.

Reduced: Nutritionally altered product containing at least 25% less of a nutrient or of calories than the regular or reference product. (*Note:* A "reduced" claim can't be used if the reference product already meets the requirement for "low.")

Less: Food, whether altered or not, contains 25% less of a nutrient or of calories than the reference food. *Fewer* is an acceptable synonym.

Light: This descriptor can have two meanings:

1. A nutritionally altered product contains one-third fewer calories or half the fat of the reference food. If the reference food derives 50% or more of its calories from fat, the reduction must be 50% of the fat.

2. The sodium content of a low-calorie, low-fat food has been reduced by 50%. Also, *light in sodium* may be used on a food in which the sodium content has been reduced by at least 50%.

   Note: The term *light* can still be used to describe such properties as texture and color as long as the label explains its meaning (e.g., "light brown sugar" or "light and fluffy").

More: A serving of food, whether altered or not, contains a nutrient that is at least 10% of the daily value more than the reference food. This also applies to fortified, enriched, and added claims, but in those cases, the food must be altered.

Healthy: A healthy food must be low in fat and saturated fat and contain limited amounts of cholesterol (less than 60 mg) and sodium (less than 360 mg for individual foods and less than 480 mg for meal-type products). In addition, a single-item food must provide at least 10% or more of one of the following: vitamins A or C, iron, calcium, protein, or fiber. A meal-type product, such as a frozen entrée or dinner, must provide 10% or two or more of these vitamins or minerals, or protein, or fiber, in addition to meeting the other criteria. Additional regulations allow the term *healthy* to be applied to raw, canned, or frozen fruits and vegetables and enriched grains even if the 10% nutrient content rule is not met. However, frozen or canned fruits or vegetables cannot contain ingredients that would change the nutrient profile.

Fresh: Food is raw, has never been frozen or heated, and contains no preservatives. *Fresh frozen*, *frozen fresh*, and *freshly frozen* can be used for foods that are quickly frozen while still fresh. Blanched foods also can be called fresh.

Percent fat free: Food must be a low-fat or a fat-free product. In addition, the claim must reflect accurately the amount of nonfat ingredients in 100 g of food.

Implied claims: These are prohibited when they wrongfully imply that a food contains or does not contain a meaningful level of a nutrient. For example, a product cannot claim to be made with an ingredient known to be a source of fiber (such as "made with oat bran") unless the product contains enough of that ingredient (in this case, oat bran) to meet the definition for "good source" of fiber. As another example, a claim that a product contains "no tropical oils" is allowed, but only on foods that are "low" in saturated fat, because consumers have come to equate tropical oils with high levels of saturated fat.

SOURCE: U.S. Food and Drug Administration. (1999, May). FDA backgrounder: The food label. http://www.cfsan.fda.gov/~dms/fdnewlab.html.

5. *Saturated fat and cholesterol and the risk of coronary heart disease:* Diets low in saturated fat and cholesterol decrease the risk for heart disease. A food must meet the definitions for low saturated fat, low cholesterol, and low-fat.

6. *Fruits, vegetables, and grain products that contain fiber, particularly soluble fiber, and the risk of coronary heart disease:* Diets low in fat and rich in soluble fiber sources may reduce the risk of heart disease. Fruits and vegetables must meet the definition for low saturated fat, low cholesterol, and low-fat, and contain, without fortification, at least 0.6 gram of soluble fiber.

7. *Whole grains and coronary heart disease:* Diets high in whole-grain food and other plant foods and low in total fat, saturated fat, and cholesterol may help reduce the risk of heart disease.

8. *Soy protein and risk of coronary heart disease:* Foods rich in soy protein as part of a low-fat diet may help reduce heart disease. The food must contain at least 6.25 grams of soy protein per serving.

9. *Sodium and high blood pressure:* Low-sodium diets may help lower blood pressure. A food must meet the description for low sodium.

10. *Potassium and high blood pressure and stroke:* Diets that contain good sources of potassium may reduce the risk of high blood pressure and stroke. The food must contain at least 350 milligrams of potassium and be low in sodium.

11. *Soluble fiber from certain foods, such as whole oats and psyllium seed husk, and heart disease:* Diets low in fat and rich in these types of fiber can help reduce the risk of heart disease. A food must be low in fat and contain at least 0.75 gram of soluble fiber.

12. *Plant sterol and stanol esters and reduced risk of heart disease:* Diets low in saturated fat and cholesterol that also contain several daily servings of plant sterols may reduce the risk of heart disease.

13. *Dietary sugar alcohols and dental caries (cavities):* Foods sweetened with sugar alcohols do not promote tooth decay. The gum needs to meet the definition of sugar free.

14. *Folate and neural tube defects:* Adequate folate status prior to and early in pregnancy may reduce the risk of neural tube defects. A food, including fortified foods, must be a good source or high source of folic acid.

Although these health claims have been approved by the FDA because of substantial supportive evidence, the FDA has recently approved "qualified health claims" for foods that scientific evidence suggests, but does not prove, may reduce disease risk (e.g., nuts and heart disease, tomatoes and cancer, calcium and heart disease). Additionally, other food products are being marketed with similar purposes in mind, but in many cases without substantial scientific support (FDA, 2005).

SERVING SIZES Knowing how much food is considered a serving is an important element of any nutrition plan. However, the serving size listed on the nutrition facts label may not be the same as the serving size for the food groups in MyPyramid. The serving sizes on the food label and MyPyramid serve different purposes. The serving size declared on the food label is to allow you to compare serving amounts from similar product categories. The serving sizes must be expressed in consumer-friendly units, such as ounces, cups, or gram weights. This means that all brands of tuna fish, for example, must use the same serving size (2 oz) on their labels. The serving sizes in the MyPyramid system are specified for each food group, using simple, easy-to-remember household units that allow people to *estimate visually* the amount of food they are eating (TABLE 7.10). In most cases the serving sizes are similar on food labels and in the MyPyramid system. It

TABLE 7.10 Playing with Pyramid Portions

GRAINS	1 cup dry cereal 4 golf balls	2 ounce bagel 1 hockey puck	1/2 cup cooked cereal, rice, or pasta tennis ball
VEGETABLES	1 cup of vegetables 1 baseball or 1 Rubik's cube		
FRUITS	1 large orange (equivalent of 1 cup of fruit) 1 softball		
OILS	1 teaspoon vegetable oil 1 die (11/16″ size)	1 Tablespoon salad dressing 1 jacks ball	
MILK	1 1/2 ounces of hard cheese 6 dice (11/16″ size)	1/3 cup shredded cheese 1 billiard ball or racquetball	
MEAT AND BEANS	3 ounces cooked meat 1 deck of playing cards	2 tablespoons hummus 1 ping pong ball	

SOURCE: Insel, P., Turner, R.E., & Ross, D. (2005). *Discovering Nutrition,* 2nd ed. Sudbury, MA: Jones and Bartlett Publishers.

is important to remember that the "serving size" is a unit of measure and may not be the *portion* an individual actually eats.

If you are not accustomed to judging the amount, or portion, of food you eat, you will find it helpful to weigh and measure foods for a brief time, using a food scale or measuring spoons or cups. This will help you become familiar with visually estimating a recommended serving size. Using the same size and type of bowl, plate, or glass will assist even further in learning to eyeball approximate serving sizes.

Dietary Supplements

The best way to get the nutrients you need to promote health is through the food you eat, not any supplements you might take. Nutrients are generally absorbed better from food than from tablets or capsules. Additionally, foods contain an array of nutrients that facilitate each other's absorption, whereas individual supplements must go it alone. If you stick to a healthy diet (MyPyramid and the *Dietary Guidelines*), you can obtain all the vitamins, minerals, fiber, calories, and other substances—presently known and yet to be discovered—that you need to maintain good health. However, if you do not consume a variety of foods as recommended by MyPyramid and the *Dietary Guidelines*, some supplements may help ensure that you get the adequate amounts of essential nutrients you need.

For example, multiple vitamin-mineral supplements, sometimes known as multivitamin-mineral (MVM) supplements, contain a variable number of essential and nonessential nutrients. Their primary purpose is to provide a convenient way to take a variety of supplemental nutrients from a single product in order to prevent vitamin or mineral deficiencies as well as to achieve higher intakes of nutrients believed to be of benefit above typical dietary levels. Many MVMs contain at least 100 percent of the daily value or RDA of all vitamins and minerals that have been assigned RDAs. Taking one MVM daily can provide you with dietary insurance against any diet deficiencies and may help to protect against future disease (Willet, 2001). However, one should always avoid megadoses (doses 10 times or more of the RDA) of vitamins and minerals.

Vegetarian Diets

Vegetarian diets depend largely or entirely on plant products and restrict intake of animal products. There are a variety of ways to be a vegetarian, ranging from being a strict vegetarian, eating no animal products of any kind, to being one who eats certain types of animal products.

Strict vegetarians are known as **vegans** because they eat no animal products. Most nutrients are obtained from breads, cereals, vegetables, fruits, legumes, seeds, and nuts. Less strict vegetarian diets include some foods derived from animals. **Ovovegetarians** include eggs (ovo) in their diet, and **lactovegetarians** include foods in the milk (lacto) group such as yogurt and cheese. An **ovolactovegetarian** eats both eggs and milk products. Finally, **semivegetarians** may eat fish and poultry, but do not eat red meat such as beef and pork.

The American Dietetic Association, in a position paper devoted to vegetarian diets, noted that such diets are healthful and nutritionally adequate, but deficiencies may occur if the diet is not planned appropriately (ADA, 1997). If foods are not selected carefully, the vegetarian may suffer nutritional deficiencies involving calories, vitamins, minerals, and protein. Vegetarians can modify their consumption of foods according to a modified food pyramid (**FIGURE 7.9**). The vegetarian pyramid presents a helpful plan for people wishing to avoid meats. The recommended number of servings of grains, vegetables, fruits, and milk products is iden-

Vegan A strict vegetarian who eats no animal products.

Ovovegetarian A vegetarian who includes eggs in the diet.

Lactovegetarian A vegetarian who includes milk in the diet.

Ovolactovegetarian A vegetarian who eats both eggs and milk products.

Semivegetarian A vegetarian who may eat fish and poultry, but not eat red meat.

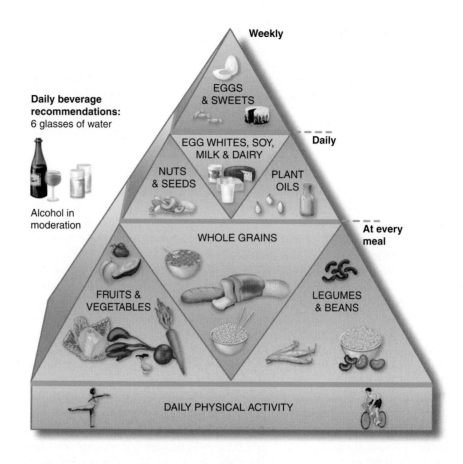

FIGURE 7.9 **The Vegetarian Food Guide Pyramid.** With careful planning, a diet that lacks animal products can be nutritionally complete. SOURCE: Copyright © 2000 Oldways Preservation and Exchange Trust. Reprinted with permission.

tical to the recommended amounts on MyPyramid. The major difference is the exclusion of meat in favor of legumes, nuts, seeds, and eggs.

Nutrition and Physical Activity

Good nutrition plays an important role in maximizing your capacity to maintain elevated levels of physical activity. In fact, most researchers feel that proper nutrition ranks right behind proper training principles and heredity in influencing exercise performance (Wilmore & Costill, 2004). This factor, however, may contribute to the widespread belief among those engaging in exercise that additional protein, vitamins, and minerals, sometimes in the form of energy bars or drinks, are necessary for optimal exercise performance. You will discover that the same diet principles that enhance health are advocated for exercise enthusiasts, along with a few commonsense guidelines for managing energy intake and fluid replacement. The following information will help you meet your nutrient needs when you participate in regular physical activity and is presented to dispel some myths related to exercise and food.

The ideal distribution of protein, carbohydrate, and fat for physically active individuals is comparable to the recommendations provided by the *Dietary Guidelines for Americans* and presented in MyPyramid (Figure 7.6). The main difference is in the quantity of calories consumed to produce the extra energy required by increased physical activity (see Chapter 8). As the amount of physical activity increases, so does the amount of energy required to maintain our energy

The diet recommended for the person who participates in physical exercise differs little in nutrient composition from the diet advised for any healthy individual.

reserves. Individuals who are highly active can expend high levels of daily energy, usually in a short period of time.

Similar to a healthy diet, a high-carbohydrate diet is probably the most important nutritional concern for regular exercisers. Carbohydrates are one of the main sources of energy for working muscles. Additionally, body carbohydrate stores (glycogen) are extremely important for maximizing the muscle glycogen stores that provide greater energy reserve for both aerobic and anaerobic activities. Therefore, heightened glycogen stores are important for increasing endurance and delay of fatigue. Because glycogen synthesis is directly related to dietary carbohydrate intake, it is recommended that 60 to 65 percent of the exerciser's total energy intake should come from carbohydrates.

Many exercisers, especially weight lifters and bodybuilders, feel that extra protein is needed to build muscle mass. Indeed, regular exercisers may require approximately 1.5 grams per kilogram of body weight compared to the Recommended Dietary Allowance of 0.8 gram per kilogram of body weight (Phillips, 2004). This increased requirement is minor. More important to remember is that the body's protein need is driven more by body-tissue maintenance, repair, and growth (see protein section) than energy needs. During exercise there is relatively little protein loss through energy metabolism. In fact, the limiting factor in the use of protein for tissue growth and repair is energy intake, not protein intake (Brooks, Fahey, & Baldwin, 2005). This means that you must first meet your energy requirements with an adequate intake of carbohydrates and then determine your protein requirements via the biologically driven protein-grams-per-kilogram ratio method. This has been referred to as the *protein-sparing* effect of protein.

Following the serving recommendations of the MyPyramid system for diary products and meat or meat substitutes will provide the necessary daily RDA protein requirements. Americans already eat more protein than they need and do not require protein supplements. Excess protein is used as energy and can be stored as body fat. Furthermore, too much protein can increase calcium loss (contributing to osteoporosis) and put an added burden on the kidneys and liver, which are required to filter out the nitrogen by-product (ketones) of the protein.

Probably the second most important dietary principle for regular exercisers is to consume the right amount of fluids before, during, and after exercise. Losing as little as 2 to 3 percent of body weight by dehydration can adversely affect exercise performance. Moreover, if exercisers are not careful about avoiding dehydration, they run the risk of heat exhaustion and even heat stroke. Water and fluids are essential to maintaining good hydration and body temperature.

Increased muscular activity from exercise leads to an increase in heat production in the body. The body's chief way to lose heat is evaporation from the skin. To keep the body cool, sweat losses can exceed a liter in a 1-hour period under normal conditions, and be even higher in extremely hot and humid conditions. Any lost body weight during exercise should be replaced with equal amounts of fluids immediately following the exercise. If exercise is longer than an hour or in extremely warm and humid conditions, or if body weight drops more than 3 percent, regular intervals of fluid replacements during exercise is imperative. Cool water (refrigerator cold) is the best choice. The addition of electrolytes (through "sport" drinks like All Sport, Gatorade, and Powerade) is generally not justified. Sweat is about 99 percent water and only 1 percent electrolytes and other substances.

As you learned earlier, vitamins and minerals play an important role in the metabolism of carbohydrates, protein, and fats. Physical activity slightly increases the need for some vitamins and minerals (iron, calcium, and ascorbic acid, to name a few) because of the increased metabolism. However, these demands for vitamins and minerals can be easily met through the increased calories consumed from carbohydrate-rich foods. Remember, people who exercise are at an advantage because they need to eat more than sedentary people to account for their increased caloric expenditure, thereby providing their bodies with more vitamins and minerals. Vitamin and mineral supplements are generally not needed if you follow the MyPyramid food guidance system.

Physical Activity and Health Connection

Sound nutritional advice for good health is also sound nutritional advice for physical activity. Although proper exercise and sound nutrition habits may confer health benefits separately, a reduction in risk factors can be maximized when both are part of a healthy lifestyle. A healthy diet may prevent disease in a variety of ways, but the health benefits multiply when healthful nutrition and proper exercise are combined. For example, dieting and aerobic exercise may combat obesity independently (see Chapter 9), but together sound eating practices and participation in a physical activity program are more effective.

Proper nutritional practices may complement physical activity as a means to enhance health status. Nutrition forms the foundation for physical activity; it provides both the fuel for mechanical work and the elements for extracting and using the potential energy contained within the fuel. Food also provides the essential elements for the synthesis of new tissue and the repair of existing cells. A nutrient-dense diet provides the minerals for strong bones and muscles. Adequate consumption of water helps keep you hydrated when you are active in warm climates. Expending energy through physical activity helps maintain healthy body composition. As you increase your level of physical activity, you will find that you are much more successful if you are also following sound nutritional practices.

concept connections

1. **Nutrition plays a major role in our overall health.** Today, scientific studies indicate that diet and nutrition often play a crucial role in the development and progression of chronic diseases that are the major killers of adults: cardiovascular disease, stroke, high blood pressure, diabetes, and some types of cancer. Obesity and osteoporosis also have been associated with faulty nutrition. Consequently, sensible lifelong eating habits play an important role in maintaining good health and preventing chronic disease.

2. **Nutrients provide energy, regulate body processes, and nourish tissues.** These major functions are essential for life.

3. **Food can be divided into six classes and each class plays a different role.** Proteins, carbohydrates, and fats are macronutrients that provide the raw fuel for both biological and mechanical energy requirements. Vitamins, minerals, and water play crucial roles in regulating the body's processes related to activating energy release.

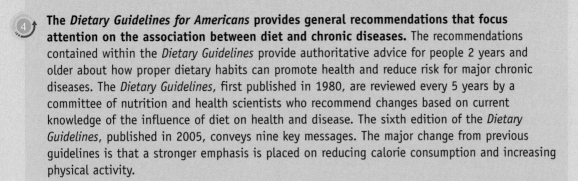

4 The *Dietary Guidelines for Americans* provides general recommendations that focus attention on the association between diet and chronic diseases. The recommendations contained within the *Dietary Guidelines* provide authoritative advice for people 2 years and older about how proper dietary habits can promote health and reduce risk for major chronic diseases. The *Dietary Guidelines*, first published in 1980, are reviewed every 5 years by a committee of nutrition and health scientists who recommend changes based on current knowledge of the influence of diet on health and disease. The sixth edition of the *Dietary Guidelines*, published in 2005, conveys nine key messages. The major change from previous guidelines is that a stronger emphasis is placed on reducing calorie consumption and increasing physical activity.

5 The MyPyramid food guidance system provides a wealth of information for you to apply in developing a nutritious diet and a physically active lifestyle. The MyPyramid symbol is a simple graphic design that is a visual reminder to make healthy food choices and be physically active each day. MyPyramid was based on both the *Dietary Guidelines* and the Dietary Reference Intakes from the National Academy of Sciences, while taking into account current consumption patterns of Americans. The MyPyramid system is designed for individual differences and can be personalized for 12 levels of energy (caloric) needs, ranging from 1000 to 3200 calories per day depending on age, gender, and physical activity level. It is flexible enough to help you make simple, small improvements in your food and lifestyle decisions and to match these steps with your own calorie needs, lifestyle, and food preferences.

6 The diet recommended for the person who participates in physical exercise differs little in nutrient composition from the diet advised for any healthy individual. The most important dietary concerns for regular exercisers are meeting their increased caloric requirements with complex carbohydrates and drinking enough fluids before, during, and after exercise to ensure proper hydration.

Terms

Nutrients, 109
Digestion, 109
Macronutrients, 109
Calorie, 110
Micronutrients, 111
Essential nutrients, 111
Nonessential nutrients, 111
Protein, 113
Amino acid, 113
Essential amino acids, 113
Carbohydrates, 114
Simple carbohydrates, 114
Monosaccharide, 114
Disaccharide, 114
Complex carbohydrates, 114

Starches, 115
Glycogen, 115
Dietary fiber, 116
Insoluble fibers, 116
Soluble fibers, 116
Fats, 116
Triglycerides, 116
Essential fatty acids, 117
Trans fats, 119
Phospholipids, 119
Vitamins, 120
Fat-soluble vitamins, 120
Water-soluble vitamins, 120
Minerals, 120
Major minerals, 120

Trace minerals, 120
Anemia, 123
Functional foods, 126
Nutrient-calorie benefit ratio (NCBR), 127
Dietary Reference Intakes (DRIs), 127
Nutrition facts label, 138
Vegan, 143
Ovovegetarian, 143
Lactovegetarian, 143
Ovolactovegetarian, 143
Semivegetarian, 143

making the connection

Meeting with the nutritionist at the university health center, Mary learns that she is meeting all of her daily nutrient requirements for vitamins and minerals, including iron and calcium. Mary is relieved to discover that, by following the MyPyramid food guidance system and its basic principles of variety, balance, and moderation, she is obtaining all the needed nutrient requirements to maintain her physically active lifestyle.

Critical Thinking

1. Like Mary, we sometimes rely on dietary supplements. What supplements are you currently taking or have you taken? For each supplement, list natural foods that you could have eaten that would have provided you the same nutritional value as the supplement.
2. Identify three barriers you face in trying to follow the *Dietary Guidelines for Americans*. For each barrier, identify a strategy and timeline to overcome each barrier.
3. You are one of 12 students at your university who are asked to assist the dietetics staff in developing healthy, nutritious, and appealing meals for college students. Using your nutrition knowledge, develop a well-balanced menu for breakfast, lunch, and dinner.
4. Go to a local health food store (these are often found in a shopping mall). Walk through the store, looking at the products and their health claims. Find two products, identify the claims made, and note any scientific research that support the claim. Would you, based on the information provided, use this product? Why or why not?

References

American Dietetic Association. (1993). Position of the American Dietetic Association and the Canadian Dietetic Association: Nutrition for physical fitness and athletic performance for adults. *Journal of the American Dietetic Association* 93:691–696.

American Dietetic Association. (1997). Position of the American Dietetic Association: Vegetarian diets. *Journal of the American Dietetic Association* 97(11):1317–1321.

American Medical Association. (1999). Nutritional basics: Nutrition information that will make a difference in your health. Online: http://www.ama-assn.org/insight/gen_hlth/nutrinfo/nutrinfo.htm.

Brooks, G.A., Fahey, T.D., & Baldwin, K.M. (2005). *Exercise Physiology: Human Bioenergetics and Its Applications*, 4th ed. Boston: McGraw Hill.

Bush, M. (2005). Understanding the forces that influence our eating habits. *Canadian Journal of Public Health* 96(Suppl. 3):4.

Expert Panel on Detection, Evaluation, and Treatment of High Blood Cholesterol in Adults. (2001). Executive summary of the third report of the National Cholesterol Education Program (NCEP) Expert Panel on Detection, Evaluation, and Treatment of High Blood Cholesterol in Adults. *Journal of the American Medical Association* 285:2486–2497.

Food and Drug Administration, Center for Food Safety and Applied Nutrition. (2005). Qualified health claims subject to enforcement discretion. Online: http://www.cfsan.fda.gov/~dms/qhc-sum.html.

Hu, F.B., Manson, J.E., & Willett, W.C. (2001). Types of dietary fat and risk of coronary heart disease: A critical review. *Journal of the American College of Nutrition* 20:5–19.

Institute of Medicine, Food and Nutrition Board. (2004). *Dietary Reference Intakes for Water, Potassium, Chloride, and Sulfate*. Washington, DC: National Academy Press.

Institute of Medicine, Food and Nutrition Board. (2005). *Dietary Reference Intakes for Energy, Carbohydrate, Fiber, Fat, Fatty Acids, Cholesterol, Protein, and Amino Acids (Macronutrients)*. Washington, DC: National Academy Press.

International Food Information Council Foundation. (2004, May). Functional foods. Online: http://www.ific.org/nutrition/functional/index.cfm.

Pereira, M.A., O'Reilly, E., Augustsson, K., Fraser, G.E., et al. (2004). Dietary fiber and risk of coronary heart disease: A pooled analysis of cohort studies. *Archives of Internal Medicine* 164:370–376.

Phillips, S.M. (2004). Protein requirements and supplementation in strength sports. *Nutrition* 20:689–695.

Shapiro, S. (1997). Do *trans* fatty acids increase the risk of coronary heart disease? A critique of the epidemiologic evidence. *American Journal of Clinical Nutrition* 66(Suppl.):1011S–1017S.

United States Department of Agriculture. (2005). MyPyramid. Online: http://MyPyramid.gov.

United States Department of Health and Human Services & U.S. Department of Agriculture. (2005). Dietary Guidelines for Americans 2005: Executive summary. Online: http://www.health.gov/dietaryguidelines/dga2005/document/html/executivesummary.htm.

Willett, W.C. (2001). *Eat, Drink and Be Healthy*. New York: Simon & Schuster.

Wilmore, J., & Costill, D. (2004). *Physiology of Sport and Exercise*, 3rd ed. Champaign, IL: Human Kinetics.

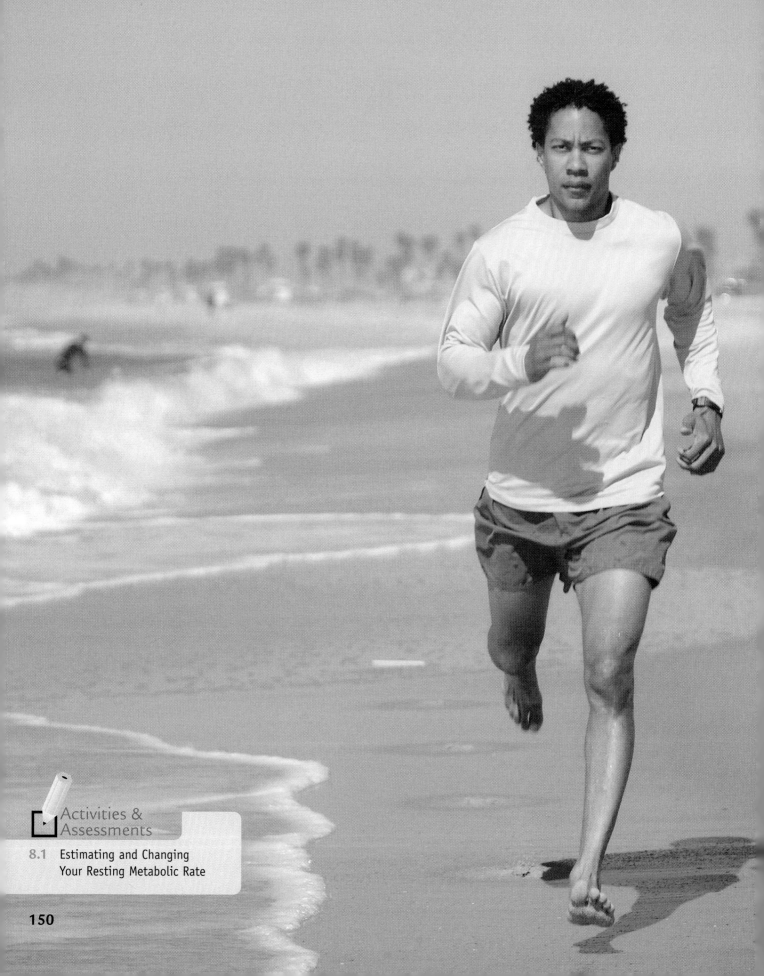

Metabolic Health

8

what's the connection?

Fred noticed that some people could eat just about anything and never put on weight, while some who became overfat didn't appear to eat any more than their slim friends. Fred knew the answer had something to do with how energy is used and stored in the body, but he wasn't sure what factors make people use and store energy differently. As part of a class project, Fred decided to research the process by which energy is utilized in the human body. He thought this might help him to understand why some people store excess fat and others don't.

concepts

1. Metabolism is the transfer, storage, and utilization of energy in the human body.

2. Your metabolism at rest is called the resting metabolic rate, or RMR.

3. Physical activity has a profound effect on your metabolism.

4. Metabolic disorders may lead to obesity, eating disorders, and other conditions that can negatively affect your health.

5. We are in the midst of an obesity epidemic in the United States.

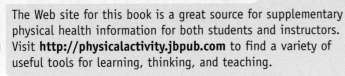

http://physicalactivity.jbpub.com

The Web site for this book is a great source for supplementary physical health information for both students and instructors. Visit **http://physicalactivity.jbpub.com** to find a variety of useful tools for learning, thinking, and teaching.

Metabolism is the transfer, storage, and utilization of energy in the human body.

Introduction

This chapter will establish the link between your metabolism and your health. In order to function, all living beings must take in energy, transfer it into a useable form, store what is needed, and eliminate what is not. This process is referred to as **metabolism**. There are many factors that influence your metabolism, including genetics, gender, body size, eating habits, and physical activity. Physical activity has a profound effect on energy intake, storage, and utilization (metabolism). This chapter also touches on several metabolic disorders and explains how they may affect your metabolic health.

Energy Balance, Transfer, and Storage

Our ability to balance, transfer, and store energy determines, to a large extent, our fitness, our health, and our body composition. The intensity of our activities is limited by how rapidly we can transfer energy. Our energy intake and our energy expenditure regulate whether we gain or lose weight. The importance of our metabolic health cannot be overlooked (Kaplan & Dietz, 1999).

First Law of Thermodynamics

Metabolism Process whereby the body takes in energy, converts it to a useable form, stores what is needed, and eliminates what is not.

First law of thermodynamics Energy can neither be created nor destroyed.

Substrates Sources of energy that can be used by our bodies.

Thermic effect A warming effect; occurs when physically active, digesting food, or increasing energy expenditure in any other way.

The **first law of thermodynamics** states that energy can neither be created nor destroyed. The energy used by the human body for movement and to power biological work comes from the food we eat. The three sources of food energy used by humans are carbohydrates, fats, and proteins (Chapter 7). When our body uses energy, we don't destroy it. Rather, we transfer the energy into a useable form (adenosine triphosphate, or ATP), send it to our surrounding environment (heat energy), or store it in our bodies (most commonly as adipose tissue). Your ability to balance the transfer, utilization, and storage of energy determines your metabolic health.

When we consume carbohydrates, fats, or proteins, we must first break them down to **substrates** that can be used by the body. Carbohydrates are reduced to glucose, fats to triglycerides, and proteins to amino acids. Of these three fuel sources, fats supply the most energy per unit of weight. For example, 1 gram of either carbohydrate or protein will contain approximately 4 kilocalories (kcal) of energy. For each gram of fat we consume, we receive 9 kcal of energy. Therefore, more energy is available in foods higher in fat than in foods higher in either protein or carbohydrate.

Heat is one of the by-products when food is broken down and used for energy. The heat production can actually be measured, and this **thermic effect** of breaking down food, transferring it, using it to power biological work, storing excess amounts in the body, and exchanging energy with our environment determines your metabolic rate. Sweating during physical activity releases the body's heat produced during the transfer of energy.

Your metabolic rate is composed of three factors: (1) the thermic effect of feeding, (2) your resting metabolic rate, and (3) the thermic effect of physical activity (Wilmore, 1994). Of these three, the greatest contributor to daily energy expenditure is your resting metabolic rate (**FIGURE 8.1**).

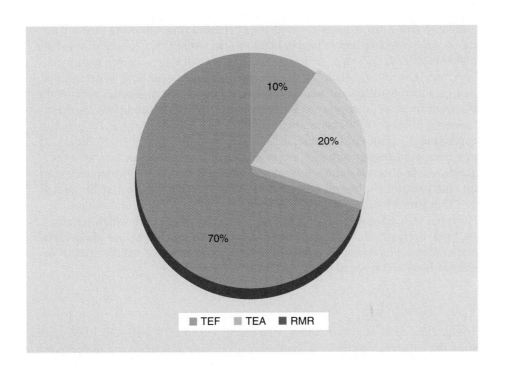

FIGURE 8.1 **Components of Energy Expenditure.** Three major factors contribute to our daily energy expenditure: the thermic effect of feeding (TEF), the thermic effect of physical activity (TEA), and the resting metabolic rate (RMR). SOURCE: Data from J.H. Wilmore. (1994). Exercise, obesity, and weight control. *President's Council on Physical Fitness and Sports Research Digest* 1(6).

The Thermic Effect of Feeding

The process of digesting food requires energy. The warming sensation that we feel after eating is due to the release of heat produced through the digestive process. This warming sensation also explains why we feel a bit drowsy after eating. Warmth relaxes the body. Roughly 10 percent of your daily energy expenditure is due to the thermic effect of feeding (TEF) (Wilmore, 1994).

Resting Metabolic Rate and Basal Metabolism

Two terms are commonly used to describe a person's metabolic rate. The first term, **resting metabolic rate (RMR)**, reflects energy expenditure in a normal rested state. The second term, **basal metabolic rate (BMR)**, represents energy expenditure under carefully controlled conditions, in which a person spends the night in a clinical facility, fasts for 12 hours, has no activity preceding measurement, and minimizes emotional excitement. BMR reflects the basic energy requirements of the body necessary to sustain life. Measurement of BMR is difficult and must be performed in a strictly controlled environment.

Most research on metabolism focuses on the resting metabolic rate. Your RMR accounts for 60 to 75 percent of the total energy you expend each day (Wilmore, 1994). It reflects the normal energy requirement of your body while it is in a state of rest. The RMR is usually low per unit of time when compared with energy expenditure while we are active, but because we spend a greater proportion of our time in a rested state, our RMR contributes significantly to total daily energy expenditure.

Several factors influence the RMR. Large people tend to have higher metabolic rates because they have more mass that requires energy. People with a great concentration of lean muscle mass also have higher metabolic rates because muscle is more active tissue than fat and it expends more energy, even in a resting state. We

Your metabolism at rest is called the resting metabolic rate, or RMR.

Resting metabolic rate (RMR) A person's rate of energy use at rest.
Basal metabolic rate (BMR) Basic energy requirement necessary to sustain life.

also know that RMR remains elevated for a period of time following physical activity. Men tend to have higher metabolic rates than women, and young people have higher metabolic rates than seniors. Your genetics will also influence your metabolic rate. The rate at which cellular processes occur in your body is determined by a combination of genetic and environmental factors. Your genetics provide the blueprint for all cellular processes and set up the necessary conditions for these processes to occur. Your environment supplies the necessary triggers for genetic expression to occur. For example, if you have the genetics to be tall, cellular processes will cause growth to occur at a rate greater than in a person with the genetics to be short. However, if we don't provide the proper environmental stimuli (good nutrition, physical activity, lack of disease), the growth may be stunted.

Your natural resting metabolic rate will be influenced by your genetics. However, your RMR may be altered by environmental factors to which you are exposed. Being physically active will raise your RMR. The advantage of having a higher metabolic rate is that more of the energy you consume will be used to sustain the body and less will end up stored as adipose tissue.

The Thermic Effect of Activity

The thermic effect of activity (TEA), the energy expended above your RMR, represents the energy necessary to accomplish a given task or activity and includes anything from a small turn of the head while seated to an all-out physical workout. Your TEA accounts for the remainder (15–30 percent) of your daily energy expenditure (Wilmore, 1994). You may also experience a carryover effect from physical activity on your metabolic rate. Some evidence suggests that physical activity causes a higher metabolic rate that remains elevated for a period of time after the activity has been completed.

Diet and Metabolic Rate

The body will adjust each of these three components of total energy expenditure when there are major increases or decreases in the energy intake. With very low calorie diets, your RMR, TEF, and TEA decrease. Your body attempts to conserve its energy stores to balance the lowered energy consumption associated with dieting. Resting metabolic rate may decrease by 20 to 30 percent or more within weeks after someone begins a very low calorie diet (Wilmore, 1994). With overeating, RMR and TEF increase to prevent the unnecessary storage of a large number of calories, although the adjustment may not be large enough to prevent an increase in body fat. It is speculated that these adaptations are under the control of the **sympathetic nervous system** (controls involuntary bodily functions) and play a major role in controlling weight around a given **set point** (the concept that your body prefers to maintain a certain body weight) (Wilmore, 1994).

Energy Balance

To maintain a healthy metabolic profile, you must balance your energy intake with your energy expenditure. If you expend more than you consume, you decrease energy stores in your body. If you consume more than you expend, you increase energy stores in your body.

The typical human consumes an average of 2500 kcal per day, or nearly 1 million kcal per year. We also know that the average adult gains 1.5 pounds of fat each year. This gain represents an imbalance between energy intake and expenditure of only 5250 kcal per year, or less than 15 kcal per day (Wilmore, 1994). It has been proposed that body weight is regulated within a narrow range similar to the way in which body temperature is regulated. When people go to extremes of

Physical activity has a profound effect on your metabolism.

Sympathetic nervous system Part of the autonomic nervous system; helps prepare the body for physical activity.

Set point Level of resting metabolism that your body naturally prefers. Some research suggests that our metabolic rate will return to its set point even if we try to change our metabolism through modifying our diet.

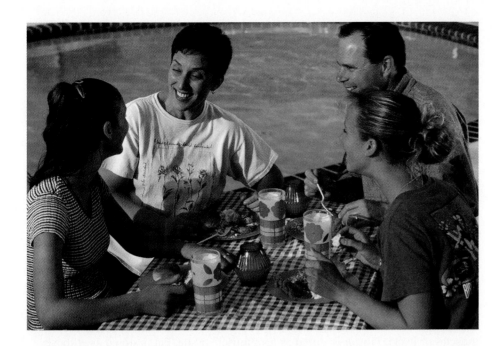

A sound eating approach is an important aspect of maintaining a healthy metabolic profile.

food consumption by eating too much or going on a starvation diet, they usually return to their original weight when allowed to go back to their normal eating patterns (Wilmore, 1994).

Energy Transfer

Energy transfer in the human body involves the breakdown of carbohydrates, fats, and proteins for the eventual formation of ATP. The breakdown of ATP causes the release of energy that powers all biologic work. Our metabolic systems function to ensure that we have an adequate amount of ATP available when the body needs it. When we initially require energy for movement, we draw upon stores of ATP in the muscle (intramuscular ATP). We only have limited amounts of intramuscular ATP, so we must quickly replenish these stores by breaking down **creatine phosphate**, glucose, triglyceride, and amino acids. Small amounts of creatine phosphate in our muscles require that we rely primarily upon glucose, triglyceride, and amino acids. Carbohydrate is the preferred fuel source because it can be used with or without oxygen present. We rely on carbohydrate when intensity of physical activity is high. However, the amount of carbohydrate we have stored in the body is limited, so we eventually turn to triglyceride to power long-term physical activity (**FIGURE 8.2**).

Most people have almost unlimited energy stored in their body in the form of adipose tissue. Adipose tissue is the stored form of triglyceride. Each pound of adipose tissue contains 3500 kcal of energy. To expend this amount of energy, you would have to run 35 miles! In fact, when we tire during physical activity, it is not because we do not have adequate amounts of energy in our body. It is usually because we have run low on carbohydrates or are experiencing orthopedic stress (pounding on our joints).

To utilize body fat as a fuel source, low-level metabolism of carbohydrate must be occurring. This is because a by-product of the breakdown of carbohydrates is required to break down fat (triglycerides); thus, we must maintain a baseline level of carbohydrate metabolism if we wish to utilize our stored fat. The statement "Fats burn in a carbohydrate flame" expresses this relationship.

Creatine phosphate Fuel source used in the body to replenish ATP; stored in small amount, it depletes rapidly.

FIGURE 8.2 **Energy Systems.**
We rely on a blend of various energy pathways to power physical activity. SOURCE: Insel, P., Turner, R.E., and Ross, D. (2006). *Discovering Nutrition,* 2nd ed. Sudbury, MA: Jones and Bartlett Publishers.

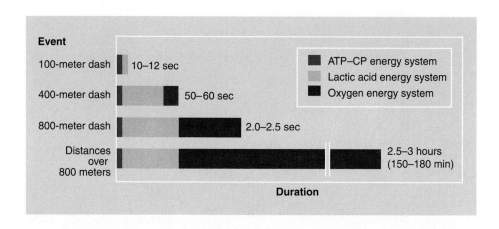

Energy Storage

Energy from the food we eat is stored in our bodies in three ways. *Carbohydrates* are usually stored as either glucose (in the muscles and blood) or glycogen (in the muscles or liver). *Protein* is stored as lean muscle tissue. *Fat* is stored as adipose tissue. Remember that excess energy from any food source can be converted and stored as adipose tissue. Thus, it is important not only to avoid consuming excessive amounts of fat but also to avoid excessive carbohydrates and proteins.

The energy needed to power physical activity is drawn first from the energy stores in muscle, second from energy circulating in the blood, and third from energy stores throughout the body. Because carbohydrate is the only fuel source that can be used without oxygen present, it plays a crucial role in energy utilization. If we eat a low-carbohydrate diet, or exercise to extreme levels, we start to burn muscle tissue as fuel in an attempt to make up for low levels of carbohydrate.

Anaerobic Metabolism

Anaerobic metabolism refers to the transfer of energy when there is a limited amount of oxygen available. This occurs when we are first starting to move and also when we are active at high intensity. At these times, the need for energy is greater than the speed at which the blood can deliver oxygen. The only fuel source that can be used anaerobically is carbohydrate. Physical activity of high intensity (sprinting, weight lifting) is referred to as *anaerobic exercise.* When we use carbohydrate anaerobically, one of the by-products is an accumulation of **lactic acid**. The hydrogen ions released during the formation of lactic acid upset the acid-base balance in the body, leading to muscle fatigue. This explains why we can only be active at high intensities for short periods of time. As the intensity of the activity diminishes, adequate amounts of oxygen are delivered and the lactic acid is reconverted to **pyruvic acid**, which can then be used as a fuel source.

Aerobic Metabolism

Aerobic metabolism refers to the process whereby energy is transferred in the presence of oxygen. In aerobic metabolism, energy demand does not outpace oxygen delivery. Your heart and circulatory system are able to deliver oxygen in sufficient quantities to meet the body's needs for energy transfer. In this circumstance, you initially use

Lactic acid By-product of the anaerobic breakdown of carbohydrate; it upsets the acid-base balance in tissues and disrupts muscle function.

Pyruvic acid By-product of the breakdown of glucose metabolism. If oxygen is not present, pyruvic acid is converted into lactic acid. If oxygen is present, pyruvic acid is further broken down to provide energy for movement.

carbohydrate as a fuel source and then shift to fat as the primary source. If the intensity remains relatively low, this type of activity can go on indefinitely. The only limiting factors will be orthopedic stress and low levels of carbohydrate.

Physical Activity and Metabolism

When we are physically active, our metabolic rate increases to meet the energy demands of the activity. If we are engaged in high-intensity physical activity, our metabolic rate is higher per unit of time. If we engage in lower-intensity, longer-duration activity, our metabolic rate is elevated for a longer period of time. In both cases, our energy expenditure is significantly higher than at rest. Understanding this concept is important to understanding energy balance in the body. From an energy storage and energy reduction standpoint, the total caloric output at the end of the day is the primary determinant of whether you gain or lose body fat. Although higher-intensity activity may result in greater energy expenditure per unit of time, the short duration during which we can maintain high-intensity activity may result in lower total energy expenditure at the end of the day compared with performing lower-intensity activity for longer periods of time. For this reason, and because it is safer for most people, it is usually recommended that people interested in reducing adipose tissue stores participate in low- to moderate-intensity activity for longer periods of time. For those interested in optimal fitness, or for those with time restrictions that do not allow longer activity sessions, higher-intensity activities are an option. Remember that you can break your activity session into multiple segments and still receive the same benefits as if all the activity were performed during one extended session.

Physical activity has an impact on your RMR and the thermic effect of food. However, the contribution of physical activity to total daily energy expenditure is primarily a result of increased energy expenditure during the activity (Melby & Hill, 1999). In other words, although being active may affect your metabolic rate during recovery, and in some cases even during rest, physical activity has its greatest impact on energy expenditure during the time in which you are active. The energy expended in physical activity will vary both with the characteristics of the activity (frequency, intensity, duration) and the individual (body weight, aerobic capacity, skill level) (Melby & Hill, 1999). More activity results in greater energy expenditure.

Energy expenditure does not return to baseline levels immediately following physical activity. How much physical activity contributes to the magnitude and duration of postactivity energy expenditure is controversial and appears to be related to the frequency, intensity, duration, and type of activity performed (Melby & Hill, 1999). Some research suggests that physical activity will raise your resting metabolic rate for an hour or longer after you finish working out, whereas other research suggests that your metabolic rate returns to normal levels much more rapidly.

The intensity of your physical activity affects the magnitude of the postactivity elevation of metabolic rate more than the duration of the activity. The intensity and duration of the types of activity sessions engaged in by most nonathletes typically results in a return of metabolic rate to baseline values within 5 to 40 minutes following the activity (Melby & Hill, 1999). In individuals capable of performing high-intensity, long-duration activities, the postactivity energy expenditure may be higher and could be a significant contributor to total energy requirements (Melby & Hill, 1999).

An active lifestyle helps to maintain a healthy metabolism.

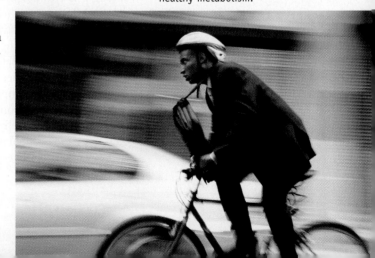

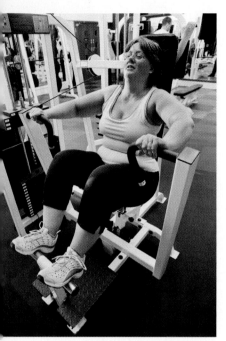

Resistance training is an important component of fat-loss programs.

Hormones Substances secreted by the glands of the endocrine system that regulate cellular function.

Less is known about the effects on postactivity energy expenditure following resistance training, but recent data suggest that high-intensity weight lifting may elevate energy expenditure above baseline values for several hours. However, novice weight lifters may not be capable of training at the intensities required to bring about a prolonged elevation of postactivity energy expenditure (Melby & Hill, 1999). For those individuals who experience increases in muscle mass as a result of resistance training, increases in resting metabolic rate usually result. Because muscle tissue is metabolically more active than adipose tissue, if you increase the percentage of muscle mass in your body, you increase your metabolic rate. Therefore, resistance training should be incorporated as one component of fat and body composition management programs.

Building Muscle Mass

The ability to gain lean body mass is dependent on four major factors: (1) proper nutrition, (2) overload resistance training, (3) genetic predisposition, and (4) secretion of the **hormones** associated with tissue growth. A variety of other factors, including body mass, gender, and motivation, will also have an impact on how much muscle you can gain.

In some people, it is possible to observe body mass increases of approximately 20 percent during the first year of regular heavy resistance training (Butterfield, Kleiner, Lemon, & Stone, 1995). These initial gains usually occur at a faster rate and to a greater magnitude than subsequent gains. The reduction in the degree of further benefit occurs because once you have started a resistance training program, you have less room for improvement. In other words, you tend to approach your genetic potential. After a few years of systematic training, gains may be only 1 to 3 percent per year (Butterfield et al., 1995).

Affecting resting metabolic rate through weight training is not a short-term endeavor. Skeletal muscle burns about 13 kcal per kg of body weight when a person is at rest. A typical man (154 lb) has about 28 kg of skeletal muscle. His muscles at rest burn about 22 percent of the calories his body uses. The brain and the liver use about the same number of calories as do his skeletal muscles. If the man lifts weights and gains 2 kg (4.4 lb) of muscle, his metabolic rate would increase by 24 kcal per day—not a very large amount. The average amount of muscle that men gain after lifting weights for 12 weeks is 2 kg. Women will gain less. So, in the short term, adding muscle mass through weight training is not easy, and its effect on resting metabolic rate is limited. However, if muscle mass is added gradually over a number of years, a greater percentage of the body's weight becomes muscle, which then can have a substantial impact on resting metabolic rate.

Impact of Physical Activity on TEF and RMR

Changes in chronic physical activity may influence the other components of energy expenditure, specifically the TEF and RMR. It is likely that the effect of physical activity on TEF is fairly small, with the benefits on weight control of being active resulting more from the increased energy expenditure during the activity than from its impact on TEF (Melby & Hill, 1999).

There is some uncertainty as to whether changes in physical activity alter RMR independently of changes in fat-free mass (Melby & Hill, 1999). Some data suggest that RMR may be chronically elevated in individuals who engage in daily, high-intensity, prolonged physical activity. It is unclear whether the increase in RMR is caused by the residual effects of acute activity or by an actual long-term change in metabolism. It has been speculated that the amount of activity performed by nonathletes for the purpose of weight control is typically of much lower intensity and duration than would be needed to increase RMR permanently (Melby & Hill, 1999).

Inactivity and Metabolism

In direct opposition to the relationship of physical activity and metabolism, we see that being inactive lowers the metabolic rate and increases the likelihood of storing excess adipose tissue. Inactivity results in a lower lean-mass percentage of body composition. Muscle responds to physical activity by becoming stronger and **hypertrophying**. Muscle also responds to inactivity by becoming weaker and *atrophying*. As your percentage of muscle tissue decreases, your metabolic rate also decreases.

We also know that as your activity level declines, a greater percentage of your day is spent in an inactive state. Since physical activity itself has a thermic effect, this component of daily energy expenditure is also decreased. The end result is that your total caloric expenditure is lower when you are inactive than when you are active. Based on the relationship of total caloric expenditure and total caloric consumption, we can see that if we lower caloric expenditure by being inactive, we must either decrease caloric consumption by eating less or see an increase in adipose tissue storage (increased percentage of body fat). As we increase our percentage of body fat, our metabolism is decreased further, a vicious circle that leads to obesity.

Metabolic Abnormalities

A healthy metabolic rate is necessary for good health. If your metabolic rate wanders from its natural state, your health may suffer. A metabolic rate that is either too high or too low can bring on several conditions that may be detrimental to your health.

Metabolic disorders may lead to obesity, eating disorders, and other conditions that can negatively affect your health.

Hypertrophy Increase in cell size. Adipose tissue (fat cells) hypertrophies when there is too much food; muscle cells hypertrophy when stressed through resistance training.

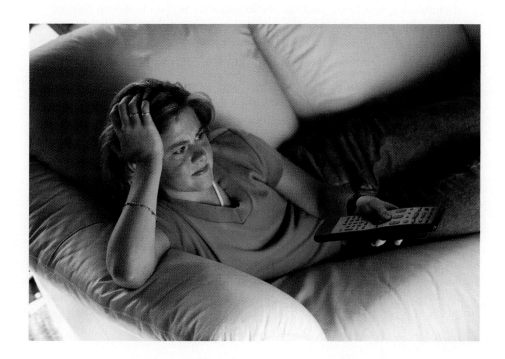

Inactivity may result in many metabolic disorders.

Body Composition

Body composition refers to the components that make up the human body. (For more information on body composition management, see Chapter 9.) Generally speaking, these components are divided into a two-component model (fat and fat-free mass) or a four-component model (fat, mineral, muscle, and water). Body composition is more important than body weight when determining the health of an individual. Weight only informs someone of how much they weigh; it does not inform them of the composition (how much is fat, bone, and muscle) of the weight.

To understand the importance of knowing your body composition, you need to understand the concepts of **overweight** and **underweight** versus **overfat** and **underfat**. Traditionally, people have compared their weight to a height-weight chart. These charts were originally developed by life insurance companies to establish premiums. They categorize people as being underweight, overweight, or of acceptable weight. The concern with these charts is that a person's weight does not always accurately represent the composition of that weight. Individuals who are very muscular, have dense bones, or are in optimal physical condition may be labeled as being overweight and therefore unhealthy. On the other hand, someone who has poor muscular development, porous bones, and is not in optimal physical condition might be categorized as being of acceptable weight and considered to be healthy. In terms of metabolic health, being overfat or underfat is a health problem, whereas being overweight or underweight may not be a problem, depending on the composition of the weight.

Body fat is normally categorized as either essential or nonessential. *Essential fat* is the fat necessary for normal physiologic functioning. Body fat plays an important role in thermal insulation, vitamin transfer and storage, nervous system function, reproductive function, hormone synthesis, cell structure, and energy storage and utilization (Chapter 7). Having too little essential fat in your body can lead to physiological dysfunction.

Excess energy stored in your body in the form of adipose tissue is not necessary for normal physiological function. This additional storage fat is referred to as *nonessential fat*. Too much nonessential fat leads to overfatness and obesity.

Determining how much body fat we should have is open to debate. Several standards, ranging from traditional normative data to criterion-referenced standards, have been proposed. Normative data are based on comparing your body fat score to data gathered on a representative population. In others words, a researcher might collect body composition data on a large group of adults. Your body composition score would then be compared to this data set. The potential problem with using normative data is that it only tells you how you compared to the data set. Normative data provide little information about your health status. You may find out that your score is equal to the average score of the data set; however, you don't know if the average score of the data set is overfat, underfat, or falls into a healthy fatness zone.

Due to the limitations of normative data in body composition analysis, experts who study this area of health and fitness have begun relying more on criterion-referenced standards. *Criterion-referenced standards* are standards that have been developed through an analysis of **epidemiological studies**, expert opinion, and normative data. The experts have determined levels of body fatness that are related to health and disease and not so closely associated with averages. Criterion-referenced standards define healthy zones of body fatness and zones where one would be considered at increased risk for disease. These standards also help to demonstrate that it is just as dangerous to be underfat as it is to be overfat (TABLE 8.1).

Overweight Having a body weight above levels recommended for a certain height.

Underweight Having a body weight below levels recommended for a certain height.

Overfat Having body fat levels above recommended levels for good health.

Underfat Having body fat levels below what is recommended for good health.

Epidemiological studies Studies of diseases, their causes, and their spread.

TABLE 8.1	Criterion-Referenced Standards for Healthy Fat Zones		
	Essential Fat*	Healthy Fat Zone	Overfat
Men	3%	3–25%	25%
Women	12%	12–30%	30%

*If your body fat percentage drops below this level, you are considered underfat and are putting yourself at increased health risk.

Regional Fat Distribution and Disease

Body fat is stored in various locations throughout the human body. The majority is stored directly under the skin (*subcutaneously*). This layer of fat provides for cushioning, makes a body feel soft, and provides thermal insulation. We also store fat around our internal organs (*viscerally*). Several factors determine where we store our fat and how much fat we store, including genetics, activity levels, food consumption, and hormones.

ANDROID AND GYNOID PATTERNS   Men and women tend to store fat in different locations. Men typically store extra fat around the abdominal region. Women tend to store additional fat in the hips, thighs, and buttocks. The male pattern of fat storage is referred to as the *android* (derived from a Greek word meaning "male") pattern. The female pattern of body fat storage is termed the *gynoid* pattern. You will also hear these patterns referred to as the apple-shaped pattern (male) and pear-shaped pattern (female). These patterns are determined by secretion of the hormones responsible for the development of secondary sexual characteristics. In fact, as men and women age and hormone secretion levels diminish, their body fat storage patterns start to resemble each other more closely.

Research has indicated that the android pattern is associated with a higher risk for the development of cardiovascular disease. This is thought to be related to the fact that the android pattern represents visceral fat storage around the internal organs, whereas the gynoid pattern is more peripheral and away from internal organs.

Metabolic Abnormalities and Disease

Several factors can lead to metabolic abnormality and disease. These include genetic predisposition, lifestyle patterns (eating and activity patterns), and environment (access to nutritious foods). Genetic factors may *predispose* us, or put us at higher risk, for the development of metabolic abnormalities. If we have the genetic predisposition for metabolic disease, it does not mean that we are doomed to develop the disease. It does mean that we must be extremely vigilant and avoid exposing ourselves to environmental factors that could trigger the disease. For instance, if we come from a long line of obese individuals, we are not necessarily doomed to be obese. However, for people with the genetic predisposition for obesity, it can be more difficult to maintain a healthy body composition. These individuals must be more careful to eat moderately and nutritiously while making regular physical activity an important part of their lives. If people with a genetic predisposition for obesity carefully watch how much and what they eat and maintain an active lifestyle, they limit their risk for the development of this metabolic disorder.

A modest amount of physical activity provides a lot of protection against degenerative diseases.

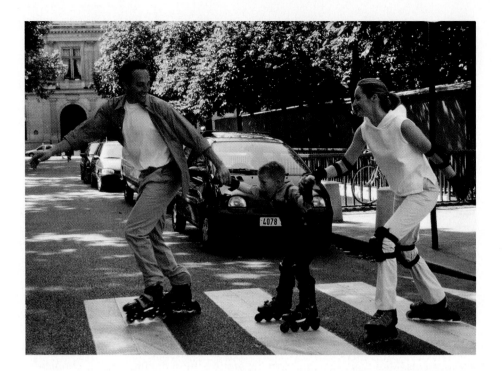

We must also realize that if most of our relatives are large people, the chances of our becoming very thin are not good. Many people put themselves through much anxiety, and even choose unwise weight loss and diet techniques, in an attempt to change their body type. This may be nothing short of impossible and thus potentially very harmful. We must think of weight (body fat) in much the same way we think of height. If all of our relatives are short, the odds are against our being tall.

Some common forms of metabolic disorder and disease include hyperinsulinemia, elevated levels of cholesterol and blood lipids, increased blood pressure, and obesity. *Hyperinsulinem*ia is a condition in which there is an excessive amount of insulin in the blood. This can result in low blood sugar levels and possibly lead to insulin shock. Elevated levels of blood cholesterol and blood lipids are dangerous because they may increase the likelihood of plaque forming within the arteries, potentially leading to a heart attack or stroke. Obesity (severe overfatness), is related to all of the metabolic disorders just mentioned. Being obese places you at a greater risk for numerous diseases.

A disease that has garnered increased interest lately related to overweight and being sedentary is metabolic syndrome (also called syndrome X). Metabolic syndrome (National Institutes of Health [NIH], 2005; Grundy et al., 2005) is diagnosed when a patient exhibits three of the following:

- Visceral adiposity: a waist girth of 102 cm (40 in.) or greater for men, and 88 cm (35 in.) or greater for women
- Elevated blood pressure: 130/85 or higher or the use of blood pressure medications
- Insulin resistance: a fasting glucose level of 110 mg/dL or greater
- Low HDL/high triglycerides: HDL less than 40 mg/dL for men and less than 50 mg/dL for women
- Triglycerides above 150 mg/dL

Metabolic syndrome is a recognized disease that received an ICD-9 code (allowing physicians to bill insurance companies for this disease) in 2001 (NIH, 2005). This condition is important because more than 87 percent of patients who experienced a fatal coronary event had exposure to at least one of these risk factors. It has been estimated that 86 million Americans will have metabolic syndrome by 2025 (NIH, 2005).

Obesity

Obesity is associated with 5 of the 10 leading causes of death and disability in the United States: heart disease, some forms of cancer, type 2 diabetes, stroke, and high blood pressure (Centers for Disease Control and Prevention [CDC], 2005; Daniels et al., 2005)). The laws of thermodynamics dictate that an energy surplus is the cause of all obesity; if we take in more energy from eating than we expend through physical activity, then we will store energy (Melby & Hill, 1999). An energy surplus occurs when food consumption increases, energy expenditure decreases, or both. The best research available suggests that a low level of physical activity is a major factor contributing to the high prevalence of obesity in the United States. A sedentary lifestyle resulting in fewer kcal expended than consumed leads to the excess kcal being stored in the body as adipose tissue or fat. It must be understood that physical activity contributes to weight loss only if it creates a negative energy balance. A negative energy balance will not occur if we start eating more to meet the energy demands brought on by physical activity or if physical activity levels decline, or both (Melby & Hill, 1999). Chapter 9 presents the challenge of achieving and maintaining a healthy body composition in more detail.

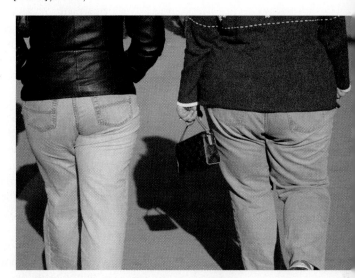

America is in the midst of an obesity epidemic.

Eating Disorders

In our society, metabolic health disorders are not only associated with excessive consumption of food but also with the underconsumption of food (FIGURE 8.3). Certain segments of our society are under constant pressure to be thin. This pressure may come from society, from families and peers, or it may be self-imposed. Individuals may practice nutritional behaviors that are unhealthy in an attempt to

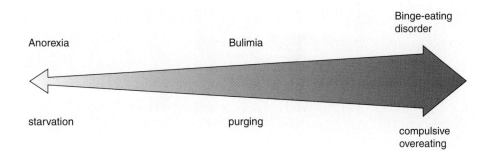

Anorexia

Bulimia

Binge-eating disorder

starvation

purging

compulsive overeating

FIGURE 8.3 **The Eating Disorder Continuum.** Anorexia and bulimia are part of a continuum of disordered eating that also includes binge eating. SOURCE: Insel, P., Turner, R.E., and Ross, D. (2006). *Discovering Nutrition*, 2nd ed. Sudbury, MA: Jones and Bartlett Publishers.

Anorexia nervosa Eating disorder in which individuals incorrectly believe they are overfat; resultant excessive dieting leads to health problems.

Bulimia nervosa Eating disorder in which individuals binge-eat and then force themselves to vomit.

We are in the midst of an obesity epidemic in the United States.

achieve thinness. Two eating disorders are associated with the drive to be thin. The first, **anorexia nervosa**, is a condition that occurs when individuals develop a severe misconception of their body image and believe that they are too fat even if their body fat levels are dangerously low. Anorexic individuals starve themselves in an attempt to reduce their weight. This leads to malnutrition, and the person's health will suffer correspondingly. Anorexia nervosa may be fatal.

Bulimia nervosa is another condition related to metabolic health. Bulimic individuals binge-eat and then force themselves to vomit so the energy in the food will not be absorbed. Bulimia is an attempt to lose weight while continuing to eat more than the body requires. In addition to the likelihood of being malnourished, a bulimic individual may also sustain throat and mouth injury due to the vomiting of stomach acids, and eye injury from ruptured blood vessels.

Anorexia and bulimia are conditions that require professional counseling and treatment. If someone you know practices these behaviors, they should be referred to qualified practitioners for treatment. For more information on anorexia and bulimia, see Chapter 9 and this book's web site, http://physicalactivity.jbpub.com.

An Obesity Epidemic

The citizens of the United States are the fattest population on earth. Over the last 30 years, Americans have gotten progressively fatter (FIGURE 8.4): current figures indicate that approximately 65 percent of the adult population is overfat, and close to one-third are obese (CDC, 2005). Perhaps even more alarming are the statistics that indicate that over one-quarter of adolescents are overfat. If these trends continue, we will see increasing health care costs, higher insurance rates, and a greater percentage of our population dying from obesity-related diseases. Some people are quick to blame genetics for this increased rate of obesity. However, the increased rate of obesity has far outdistanced the rate at which genetics can change.

FIGURE 8.4 **Rise in Overweight in the United States.** The incidence of overweight has increased over the last three decades.

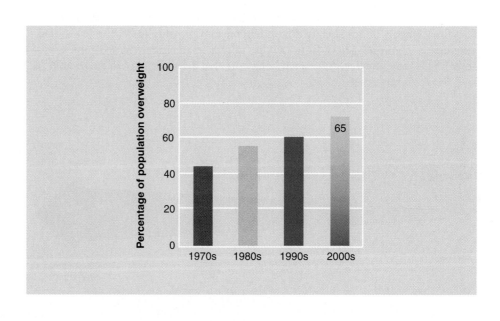

Physical Activity and Health Connection

Your metabolism is directly connected to your health. If your metabolic system is functioning properly, your body will be able to transfer, store, and utilize energy efficiently. However, if you have a metabolic disorder, you may develop several conditions that can lead to life-threatening situations. Physical activity is an important component of metabolic health. To prevent metabolic disorders such as obesity, you must make sure that your energy expenditure balances your energy consumption. Physical activity plays a major role in increasing your metabolic rate and total energy expenditure. Being active makes it easier to ensure that your energy expenditure keeps pace with your energy consumption.

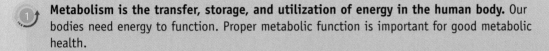

concept connections

1. **Metabolism is the transfer, storage, and utilization of energy in the human body.** Our bodies need energy to function. Proper metabolic function is important for good metabolic health.

2. **Your metabolism at rest is called the *resting metabolic rate*, or RMR.** In all living bodies, there is a baseline rate of cellular activity required to keep the body functioning. All cellular activity requires the exchange of energy. The rate of energy exchange when the body is in a relaxed state is the resting metabolic rate.

3. **Physical activity has a profound effect on your metabolism.** Any increase in cellular function increases your metabolism. Physical activity increases your rate of cellular function while active and results in an elevated metabolic rate during the recovery period following physical activity. Performing physical activity that builds muscle mass will even affect your resting metabolic rate. Muscle is more active tissue than fat, even at rest. By increasing your muscle mass, you increase the percentage of metabolically active tissue in your body.

4. **Metabolic disorders may lead to obesity, eating disorders, and other conditions that can negatively affect your health.** Your body typically does an amazing task in balancing energy expenditure against energy consumption. However, in certain individuals, factors including lifestyle, genetics, and societal pressures may lead to the development of metabolic disorders. Metabolic disorders such as obesity, anorexia, and bulimia can have severe consequences. It is important to identify symptoms of metabolic disorders and seek treatment as soon as possible.

5. **We are in the midst of an obesity epidemic in the United States.** Figures indicate that close to two-thirds of the adult population are overfat and approximately one-third may be clinically obese. This alarming information demonstrates the need for action to reduce the negative consequences associated with obesity. Obesity is related to several serious medical conditions and results in increasing health care costs for all Americans. The best recommendation for reducing the incidence of obesity is to encourage physical activity and good nutritional habits.

Terms

Metabolism, 152

First law of thermodynamics, 152

Substrates, 152

Thermic effect, 152

Resting metabolic rate (RMR), 153

Basal metabolic rate (BMR), 153

Sympathetic nervous system, 154

Set point, 154

Creatine phosphate, 155

Lactic acid, 156

Pyruvic acid, 156

Hormones, 158

Hypertrophy, 159

Overweight, 160

Underweight, 160

Overfat, 160

Underfat, 160

Epidemiological studies, 160

Anorexia nervosa, 164

Bulimia nervosa, 164

making the connection

Fred now understands why people develop different body builds. He plans to use the information he has learned about energy transfer, storage, and utilization to his advantage. Fred has decided to begin a program designed to lower his body fat and increase his muscle mass through healthy eating and increased physical activity. He thinks he will be able to stick with his new program because his goals are realistic and based on what he has learned about energy metabolism and health.

Critical Thinking

1. Like Fred, we can find information a powerful tool in understanding ourselves. Identify three factors that affect metabolism. For each, describe how this factor may or may not affect your metabolism.

2. There are many different body builds. Looking at your parents, siblings, and friends, what are some possible explanations for the different body build each has?

References

Butterfield, G., Kleiner, S., Lemon, P., & Stone, M. (1995). Roundtable: Methods of weight gain in athletes. *Sports Science Exchange* 6(3).

Centers for Disease Control and Prevention. (2005). Physical activity and good nutrition: Essential elements to prevent chronic diseases and obesity. Online: http://www.cdc.gov/nccdphp/publications/aag/dnpa.htm.

Daniels, S.R., Arnett, D.K., Eckel, R.H., Gidding, S.S., Hayman, L.L., Kumanyika, S., Robinson, T.N., Scott, B.J., St. Jeor, S., & Williams, C.L. (2005). AHA scientific statement. Overweight in children and adolescents: Pathophysiology, consequences, prevention, and treatment. *Circulation* 111:1999–2012.

Grundy, S.M., Cleeman, J.I., Daniels, S.R., Donato, K.A., Eckel, R.H., Franklin, B.A., Gordon, D.J., Krauss, R.M., Savage, P.J., Smith, S.C., Spertus, J.A., & Costa, F. (2005). Diagnosis and management of the metabolic syndrome: An American Heart Association/National Heart, Lung, and Blood Institute scientific statement. *Circulation*. 112:e285–e290.

Kaplan, J.P., & Dietz, W.H. (1999). Caloric imbalance and public health policy. *Journal of the American Medical Association* 282(16):1579–1581.

Melby, C.L., & Hill, J.O. (1999). Exercise, macronutrient balance, and body weight regulation. *Sports Science Exchange* 12(1).

National Institutes of Health. (2005). National Cholesterol Education Program. Online: http://www.nhlbi.nih.gov/about/ncep.

Wilmore, J.H. (1994, May). Exercise, obesity, and weight control. *President's Council on Physical Fitness and Sports Research Digest* 1(6).

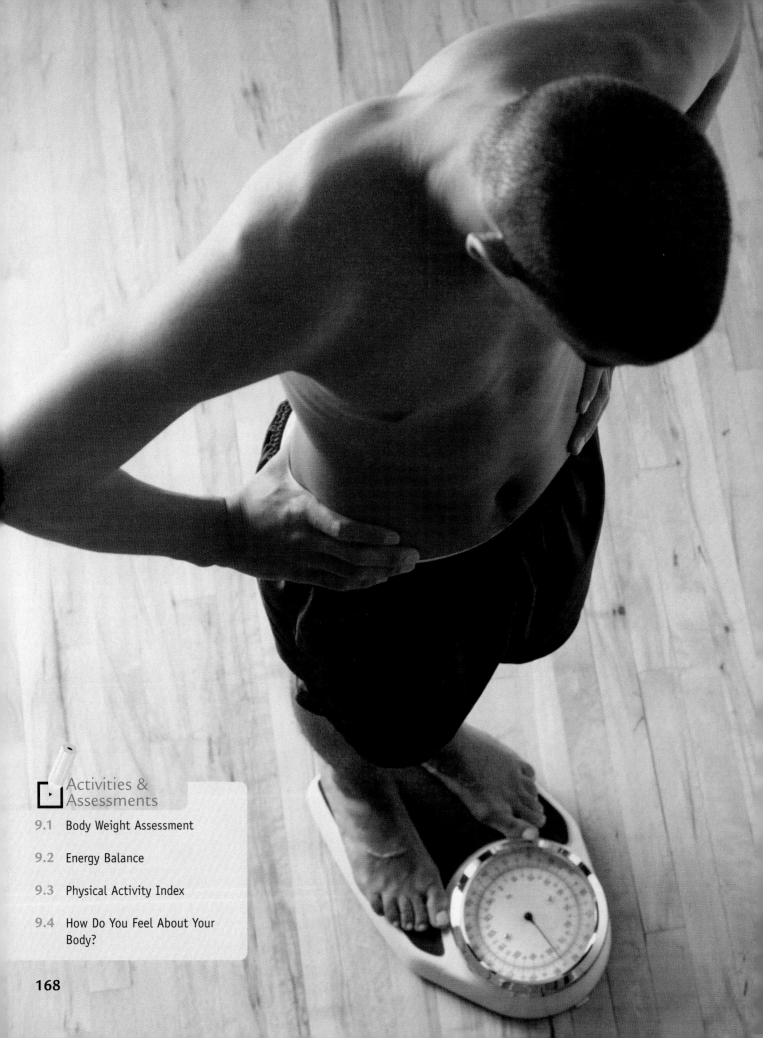

Activities &
Assessments

9.1   Body Weight Assessment

9.2   Energy Balance

9.3   Physical Activity Index

9.4   How Do You Feel About Your
      Body?

Achieving and Maintaining a Healthy Weight

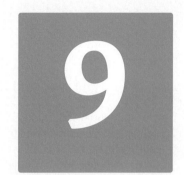

9

what's the connection?

Melinda is a freshman in college; she is 5'6" tall and weighs about 130 pounds. Previously, when Melinda was happy, she looked in the mirror and thought "Hey, I am not that bad!" However, if Melinda was in a bad mood, she would think "I am so fat!" and get mad at herself. Recently, things are not going well in Melinda's life and, when she looks in the mirror, she often sees herself as fat. It seems to her that the weight is piling on and she cannot stop it. To Melinda, every part of her body looks bigger—her legs, her arms, her face—and she hates it. Melinda thinks "I just want to be thin. I never really noticed how fat I was until yesterday when I looked in the mirror." Melinda is not sure what to do. "I don't eat that much. Really I eat only a little, and I'm not sure why I even eat that." Melinda is thinking about stopping eating altogether so she can lose all this weight.

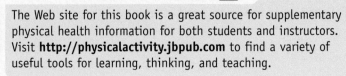

http://physicalactivity.jbpub.com

The Web site for this book is a great source for supplementary physical health information for both students and instructors. Visit **http://physicalactivity.jbpub.com** to find a variety of useful tools for learning, thinking, and teaching.

concepts

1. Achieving and maintaining a healthy body weight has been identified as a major public health challenge in the United States.

2. The body mass index (BMI) uses weight and height to produce a number that enables health professionals to gauge risk of weight-related illnesses.

3. Individuals with more upper body fat than lower body fat tend to have a more adverse metabolic profile and an increased risk for diabetes and cardiovascular disease, whereas lower body fat is less harmful in this respect.

4. A body composition analysis allows for the assessment of the percentage of fat versus the percentage of fat-free tissue.

5. Obesity is a complex disorder with multiple contributing factors.

6. A lifestyle approach that includes regular physical activity and a nutritious diet is essential in achieving and maintaining a healthy weight.

7. A negative sign of dissatisfaction with body weight, when basing it on the "ideal" weight portrayed by the mass media, is the development of eating disorders.

Achieving and maintaining a healthy body weight has been identified as a major public health challenge in the United States.

Introduction

Achieving and maintaining a healthy body weight has been identified as a major public health challenge in the United States (U.S. Department of Health and Human Services [USDHHS], 2001). Data show that based on the weight-for-height standards developed by the National Institutes of Health (NIH), two-thirds of adult Americans are now overweight, and that number continues to rise (Hedley et al., 2004). Furthermore, nearly one-third of young people aged 6–19 years are considered to be either at risk for overweight or overweight, double the rate from 20 years ago (Hedley et al., 2004). These prevalence rates raise fear because of their implications for Americans' health. According to the NIH and the Centers for Disease Control and Prevention (CDC), being overweight or obese increases an individual's risk for developing over 35 major diseases (National Institute of Diabetes and Digestive and Kidney Diseases [NIDDK], 2005; CDC, 2005a). **FIGURE 9.1** outlines the health risks related to overweight and obesity.

Considerable health care dollars are spent each year on the treatment and management of obesity-related diseases, including high blood pressure; diabetes mellitus; dyslipidemia (abnormalities in blood lipid and lipoprotein concentrations); coronary artery disease and stroke; respiratory problems, including obstructive sleep apnea (interrupted breathing during sleep) and asthma; osteoarthritis (wearing away of the joints); gallstones; and certain cancers, including endometri-

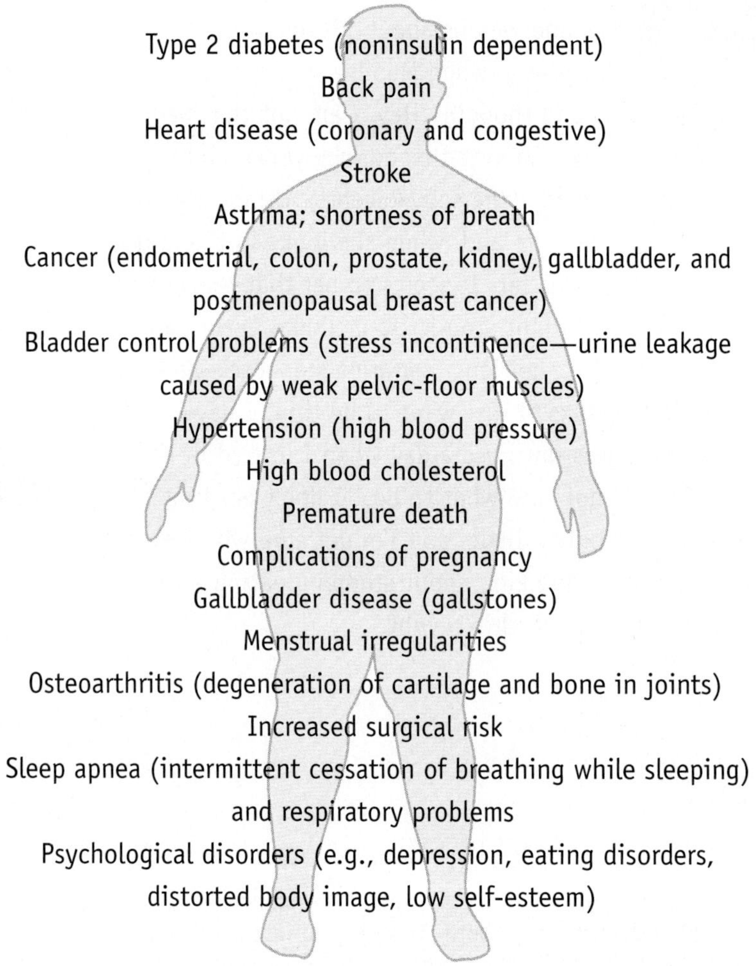

FIGURE 9.1 **Health Risks for Overweight and Obese People.** Overweight people have a greater likelihood of developing certain health problems.

Type 2 diabetes (noninsulin dependent)
Back pain
Heart disease (coronary and congestive)
Stroke
Asthma; shortness of breath
Cancer (endometrial, colon, prostate, kidney, gallbladder, and postmenopausal breast cancer)
Bladder control problems (stress incontinence—urine leakage caused by weak pelvic-floor muscles)
Hypertension (high blood pressure)
High blood cholesterol
Premature death
Complications of pregnancy
Gallbladder disease (gallstones)
Menstrual irregularities
Osteoarthritis (degeneration of cartilage and bone in joints)
Increased surgical risk
Sleep apnea (intermittent cessation of breathing while sleeping) and respiratory problems
Psychological disorders (e.g., depression, eating disorders, distorted body image, low self-esteem)

al, breast, prostate, and colon cancer. Federal officials have estimated that treating obesity-related illnesses costs about $93 billion annually (NIDDK, 2004), or nearly 10 percent of total health care expenditures (Finkelstein, Fiebelkorn, & Wang, 2004). The lifetime health care costs are comparable to those attributable to cigarette smoking (Thompson et al., 1999).

Higher levels of weight are associated with increased mortality and reduced life expectancy (Fontaine et al., 2003). Individuals with excess body weight experience decreased physical function, vitality, and quality of life (Lean, Han, & Seidell, 1999; Fine et al., 1999). Being overweight or obese may result in *psychosocial morbidity*, where an individual suffers from psychological and social consequences due to depression, social stigma, and discrimination (Douketis & Feldman, 1994). Our modern culture idealizes thinness and disparages obesity (Latner, Stunkard, & Wilson, 2005). Because weight is an important aspect of appearance in our society, especially for women, it seems likely that basing one's self-esteem on appearance would be a particular risk factor for mental health (FIGURE 9.2). Indeed, those who are overweight and base their self-esteem on their appearance have lower self-esteem, more symptoms of depression, and more symptoms of eating disorders (Jambekar, Quinn, & Crocker, 2001). Furthermore, overweight or obese individuals have suffered from weight bias and discrimination in various areas of society, including employment practices, salary and promotion decisions, education and housing opportunities, and the portrayal of obese persons in popular media as physically unattractive, lazy, and lacking in willpower (Puhl & Brownell, 2001; Greenberg et al., 2003). Not surprisingly, many overweight or obese individuals are dissatisfied and preoccupied with their weight and body image (Friedman, Reichmann, Costanzo, & Musante, 2002).

Health experts use the terms *overweight* and *obesity* as nouns to reflect conditions characterized by excessive and unhealthy amounts of body fat that lead to an increase in disease risks. Therefore, the characterization of people as overweight and obese has to be evaluated within the context of their overall health. The current prevailing scientific consensus is that the increased health risks blamed on being

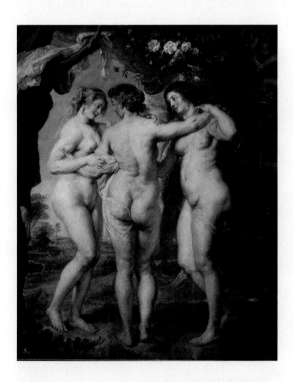 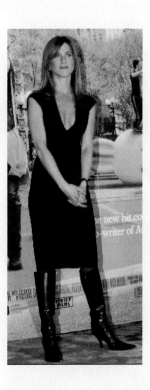

FIGURE 9.2 **Changing Standards.** Voluptuous women were once considered the female ideal (A); in today's society, Jennifer Aniston embodies a popular standard (B).

FIGURE 9.3 **Get Out and Move.** Regular physical activity is important at all weight levels.

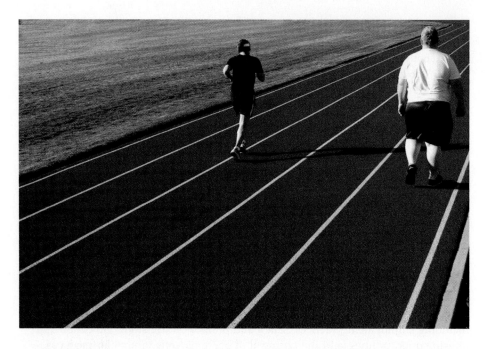

overweight and obese are really the result of many overweight people being out of shape and having detrimental diets and other unhealthful habits. Therefore, one's weight is not just about the numbers on the scale and body image, but also about the lack of regular physical activity and poor eating habits. Engaging in regular physical activity and following proper eating habits have a positive impact on one's health no matter what one's current weight may be (FIGURE 9.3 and FIGURE 9.4).

This chapter is divided into three basic sections. The first section provides an overview of the current medical literature on the relationship between weight and health. This section provides a better understanding of how America's public health authorities determine if you are medically at risk based on your current

FIGURE 9.4 **Be an Informed Consumer.** Reading food labels to compare calorie content is important to understanding your overall caloric intake.

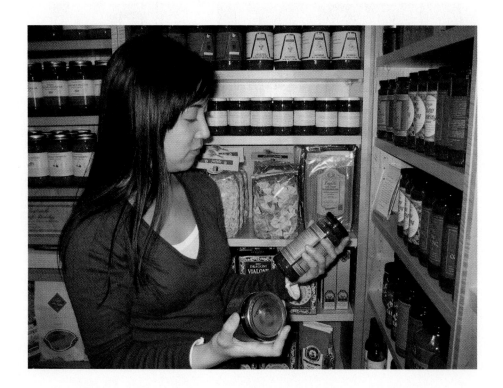

weight and related conditions. The second section provides an overview of your body's intricate mechanism for maintaining a healthy weight and how this mechanism can be altered. The third section provides information related to a lifestyle approach to maintaining a healthy weight that focuses on developing a lifelong commitment to regular physical activity and suitable eating practices that are sustainable and enjoyable.

Overweight and Obesity and Health Risk

To understand both the statistics and the significance of health risk related to overweight and obesity, it is important to know how they are defined and measured. **Overweight** is generally defined as weight that exceeds the threshold of a health criterion standard. The health criterion standard is based on the relationship of weight to morbidity (disease) or mortality (death) outcomes. In quantifiable terms, it refers to a body weight that is at least 10 percent over an ideal weight for a specified height (National Heart, Lung, and Blood Institute [NHLBI], 2000). Many people who are classified as overweight are also overfat, and the health risks they face are due to the latter condition. **Obesity**, like overweight, is a weight that exceeds the threshold of a health criterion standard, but to a greater degree. The health criterion standard for obesity refers to a body weight that is at least 30 percent over an ideal weight for a specified height (NHLBI, 2000).

The excessive weight mentioned in these definitions generally refers to an excessive amount of body fat in relation to lean body mass. The proportion of lean tissue—bone, muscle, and water—to fat tissue and the distribution of fat tissue are important to health and is the basis of body composition. If a person's weight is disproportionally fat, he or she will have greater health risks than someone whose ratio of fat to lean tissue mass is better proportioned. Clinical or laboratory measures to determine fat weight and fat-free weight (body composition) are discussed following an explanation of the two most common measures to screen for whether a person is overweight: the body mass index (BMI) and waist circumference. BMI and waist circumference are simple, inexpensive, and reliable measurements known as *anthropometrics*—measures of body size and proportions that provide an initial screening for overfatness and potential health risk.

Overweight A weight that exceeds the threshold of a health criterion standard.

Obesity A weight that exceeds the threshold of a health criterion standard to a greater degree than overweight.

Body Mass Index

The BMI uses weight and height to produce a number that enables health professionals to gauge risk of weight-related illnesses. The BMI criterion standards recommended by the National Heart, Lung, and Blood Institute (NHLBI) Expert Panel on the Identification, Evaluation, and Treatment of Overweight and Obesity in Adults are as follows: underweight, BMI less than 18.5; normal or healthy weight, BMI of 18.5 to 24.99; overweight or preobesity, BMI of 25.0 to 29.9; and class 1, 2, and 3 obesity, BMI of 30 to 34.99, 35 to 39.99, and 40.0 or greater, respectively (NHLBI, 2000) (TABLE 9.1). Therefore, an adult BMI under 18.5 or greater than 25.0 indicates a potential health risk. The link between being screened with a BMI classified as underweight or overweight/obese and the chance of becoming ill is not definite. The research is ongoing; however, when data from large groups of people from the general population are analyzed, a J-shaped association is found between BMI and mortality rate (FIGURE 9.5). For example, BMIs lower than 18.5 are associated with a slight increase in mortality; as weights increase past BMIs of 25 or greater, a successively larger association with mortality is represented. This successively larger association between increasing weight and risk of death is visually represented by the slight increase (20 to 30 percent) as BMI rises from 25 to 27 and the steeper increase (60 percent) as BMI rises above 27.

The body mass index (BMI) uses weight and height to produce a number that enables health professionals to gauge risk of weight-related illnesses.

TABLE 9.1	Body Mass Index Classifications
BMI (kg/m^2)	**Classification**
<18.5	Underweight
18.5–24.9	Normal weight
25.0–29.9	Overweight
30.0–34.9	Obesity class 1
35.0–39.9	Obesity class 2
>40	Obesity class 3 (extreme obesity)

Although the greatest number of deaths is associated with the overweight categories, there is an increased risk of death for underweight as well. This primarily results from *unhealthy* underweight people, not *healthy* underweight people. Most deaths associated with a low BMI are usually among elderly people who have suffered from underlying chronic diseases that cause low body weight. Cancer, heart failure, chronic lung disease, alcoholism, depression, a digestive disease, malnourishment, eating disorders, and osteoporosis (low bone density) are associated with low body weight as well as ill health. The key to knowing whether there is a link between underweight and disease is in determining whether low body weight is voluntary or involuntary, explained or unexplained. An underweight person in poor health should be medically evaluated to rule out an underlying disease or medical condition. For example, many college students are socialized to believe their worth and power comes from rigid cultural definitions of beauty, including thinness. The emphasis on extreme thinness, to which women are quite susceptible, may lead to the development of eating disorders—a severe medical condition that involves serious disturbances in eating behavior, such as the extreme and unhealthy reduction of food intake. Eating disorders are discussed at the end of this chapter.

Adult BMIs are calculated using a mathematical formula that takes into account both a person's height and weight. BMI equals a person's weight in kilograms divided by height in meters squared (BMI = kg/m^2). The metric and English formulas to calculate your BMI, as well as addresses to online calculators, are available in the activities and assessment manual. (TABLE 9.2) has already calculated the

FIGURE 9.5 **BMI and Mortality.** People with a very low or high BMI have a higher relative mortality rate.

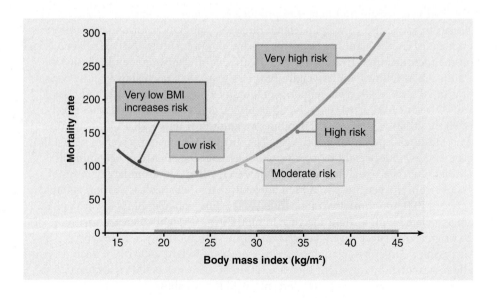

TABLE 9.2   Body Mass Index Table

	Normal						Overweight					Obese											Extreme Obesity														
BMI	19	20	21	22	23	24	25	26	27	28	29	30	31	32	33	34	35	36	37	38	39	40	41	42	43	44	45	46	47	48	49	50	51	52	53	54
Height (inches)																		Body Weight (pounds)																		
58	91	96	100	105	110	115	119	124	129	134	138	143	148	153	158	162	167	172	177	181	186	191	196	201	205	210	215	220	224	229	234	239	244	248	253	258
59	94	99	104	109	114	119	124	128	133	138	143	148	153	158	163	168	173	178	183	188	193	198	203	208	212	217	222	227	232	237	242	247	252	257	262	267
60	97	102	107	112	118	123	128	133	138	143	148	153	158	163	168	174	179	184	189	194	199	204	209	215	220	225	230	235	240	245	250	255	261	266	271	276
61	100	106	111	116	122	127	132	137	143	148	153	158	164	169	174	180	185	190	195	201	206	211	217	222	227	232	238	243	248	254	259	264	269	275	280	285
62	104	109	115	120	126	131	136	142	147	153	158	164	169	175	180	186	191	196	202	207	213	218	224	229	235	240	246	251	256	262	267	273	278	284	289	295
63	107	113	118	124	130	135	141	146	152	158	163	169	175	180	186	191	197	203	208	214	220	225	231	237	242	248	254	259	265	270	278	282	287	293	299	304
64	110	116	122	128	134	140	145	151	157	163	169	174	180	186	192	197	204	209	215	221	227	232	238	244	250	256	262	267	273	279	285	291	296	302	308	314
65	114	120	126	132	138	144	150	156	162	168	174	180	186	192	198	204	210	216	222	228	234	240	246	252	258	264	270	276	282	288	294	300	306	312	318	324
66	118	124	130	136	142	148	155	161	167	173	179	186	192	198	204	210	216	223	229	235	241	247	253	260	266	272	278	284	291	297	303	309	315	322	328	334
67	121	127	134	140	146	153	159	166	172	178	185	191	198	204	211	217	223	230	236	242	249	255	261	268	274	280	287	293	299	306	312	319	325	331	338	344
68	125	131	138	144	151	158	164	171	177	184	190	197	203	210	216	223	230	236	243	249	256	262	269	276	282	289	295	302	308	315	322	328	335	341	348	354
69	128	135	142	149	155	162	169	176	182	189	196	203	209	216	223	230	236	243	250	257	263	270	277	284	291	297	304	311	318	324	331	338	345	351	358	365
70	132	139	146	153	160	167	174	181	188	195	202	209	216	222	229	236	243	250	257	264	271	278	285	292	299	306	313	320	327	334	341	348	355	362	369	376
71	136	143	150	157	165	172	179	186	193	200	208	215	222	229	236	243	250	257	265	272	279	286	293	301	308	315	322	329	338	343	351	358	365	372	379	386
72	140	147	154	162	169	177	184	191	199	206	213	221	228	235	242	250	258	265	272	279	287	294	302	309	316	324	331	338	346	353	361	368	375	383	390	397
73	144	151	159	166	174	182	189	197	204	212	219	227	235	242	250	257	265	272	280	288	295	302	310	318	325	333	340	348	355	363	371	378	386	393	401	408
74	148	155	163	171	179	186	194	202	210	218	225	233	241	249	256	264	272	280	287	295	303	311	319	326	334	342	350	358	365	373	381	389	396	404	412	420
75	152	160	168	176	184	192	200	208	216	224	232	240	248	256	264	272	279	287	295	303	311	319	327	335	343	351	359	367	375	383	391	399	407	415	423	431
76	156	164	172	180	189	197	205	213	221	230	238	246	254	263	271	279	287	295	304	312	320	328	336	344	353	361	369	377	385	394	402	410	418	426	435	443

SOURCE: Adapted from National Heart, Lung, and Blood Institute. (1998). *Clinical Guidelines on the Identification, Evaluation, and Treatment of Overweight and Obesity in Adults: The Evidence Report.* Bethesda, MD: National Institutes of Health.

math and metric conversions. To determine your BMI, find your height on the left side of the chart and go straight across from that point until you come to your weight in pounds. The number at the top of the column is your BMI for your height and weight. Compare your BMI with the recommended classifications in Table 9.1.

If you were classified as overweight or obese, you should try not to gain any additional weight. You may even begin thinking about a small decrease of 10 percent of your total body mass. But before you take action, it is important to look at other factors—namely, your waist circumference and conditions associated with being overweight or obese—when it comes to assessing your overall risk for developing a chronic health condition. Before discussing waist circumference and associated conditions, the advantages and limitations of BMI will be addressed.

The BMI is an easy and quick noninvasive method to assess weight-related health status. You only need to measure your height in inches (without shoes) and weight in pounds (obtained with minimal clothing—only undergarments). The BMI is not gender specific, and therefore is appropriate for all men and nonpregnant women over 20 years of age. For children and teenagers, weight status is defined differently than it is for adults. Because children and teenagers are still growing, and boys and girls develop at different rates, BMIs for children 2 to 20 years old are determined by comparing their weight and height against growth charts that take their age and gender into account (see the Activities and Assessment Manual).

There is much evidence to support the predictive power of BMI in risk assessment since it provides a more accurate measure of total body fat compared with the assessment of body weight alone (NHLBI, 2000). Given that BMI correlates well with health risk, it is one of the many tools available to identify individuals who would benefit from weight loss, thus lowering their risk of developing a chronic disease condition.

Although a BMI measurement may be good in predicting health risks associated with excess weight due to fat, including high blood pressure, diabetes mellitus, and coronary heart disease, as the name suggests, it measures body mass, not body fat. Any measure of obesity that relies primarily on weight, an indirect estimate of body fat, has limitations. A high BMI may indicate obesity, but a high value may also occur in people who are not overfat. The BMI may overestimate fatness in lean, muscular athletes or people with high bone densities. Conversely, older individuals who have gained fat, lost muscle and bone mass due to a sedentary lifestyle, or lost weight to an underlying chronic illness may have a BMI in the normal healthy range, but actually be at greater risk for disease due to a higher percentage of body fat. Determining whether an individual is obese from simply being overweight or because of increased muscle mass, or is underweight because of a lack of muscle tissue, requires body composition techniques for quantifying fat mass and fat-free mass. Finally, the BMI provides no information about fat distribution (site of fat), which may be as important a risk factor as how much fat you have—and perhaps more important.

Body Fat Distribution

Fat is not uniformly distributed in the body. The major fat depot is subcutaneous (under the skin) and makes up about 80 percent of all body fat. In the obese and nonobese states, there are characteristic gender differences in the distribution of subcutaneous fat. Nonobese women have relatively more subcutaneous fat in the gluteofemoral (thigh/hip/butt) area than in other subcutaneous regions, whereas in nonobese men the subcutaneous fat is distributed in a uniform fashion. The gen-

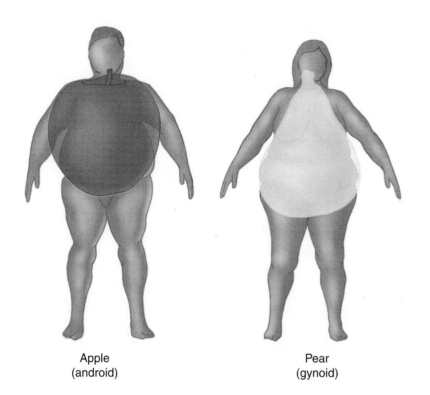

Apple
(android)

Pear
(gynoid)

FIGURE 9.6 **Body Fat Distribution.**
Men and women who have large body fat deposits centrally located in their waists tend to have a higher risk of diabetes and cardio-vascular disease than individuals with the same amount of fat locat-ed below the waist. (A) Overweight males typically have central fat deposits (apple-shaped bodies). (B) Overweight females often have excess body fat below the waist (pear-shaped bodies).

der differences are more pronounced in obesity (**FIGURE 9.6**). Obese men usually accumulate fat in the subcutaneous abdominal area. This male obesity is called upper body, central, android, or apple-shaped obesity. Obese women usually accu-mulate subcutaneous fat in the lower part of the abdominal area and the glute-ofemoral region. This female type of obesity is called lower body, peripheral, gynoid, or pear-shaped obesity. The link between gender and regional obesity is not absolute. There are many women (especially after menopause) who have upper body fat distribution, and many men who have lower body fat distribution.

The relationship of body fat distribution to metabolic abnormalities and dis-ease is now well recognized. Individuals with more upper body fat than lower body fat tend to have a more adverse metabolic profile and an increased risk for diabetes and cardiovascular disease, whereas lower body fat is less harmful in this respect. More specifically, the fat inside the abdomen cavity surrounding the organs (visceral fat) contributes to these metabolic abnormalities by producing chemicals and hormones that make a person more vulnerable to a number of obe-sity-related complications (**FIGURE 9.7**). The mechanisms linking to the metabolic disturbances are not fully understood. The portal system is the most common the-ory. In a nutshell, the portal theory suggests that visceral fat—fat within the trunk and middle of the body—secretes free fatty acids that flow into the liver through the portal vein, the vein that carries blood from the abdominal organs to the liver. Too much fat may mean too many free fatty acids. Too many free fatty acids com-ing through the portal vein seem to make the liver produce too much glucose. With so much glucose, the body pumps out more insulin to try to control the sugar's high levels. Over time, this vicious cycle might contribute to a dreaded con-dition known as metabolic syndrome (see Chapter 8).

Individuals with more upper body fat than lower body fat tend to have a more adverse metabolic profile and an increased risk for diabetes and cardiovascular disease, whereas lower body fat is less harmful in this respect.

FIGURE 9.7 **Visceral Fat.** The fat lying deep within the body's abdominal cavity (shown here in cross section) may pose an especially high risk for metabolic disturbances.

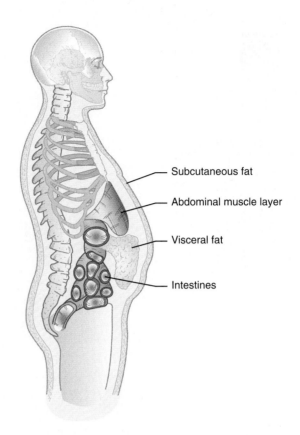

Subcutaneous fat

Abdominal muscle layer

Visceral fat

Intestines

Waist Circumference

Subcutaneous abdominal fat correlates well with intraabdominal fat (visceral fat), so for many people, the modest measuring tape provides an easy and reliable way of telling if additional inches around the waist constitute health risk. To assess waist circumference, locate the upper hip and place a measuring tape in a horizontal plane around the waist while standing (**FIGURE 9.8**). The measurement should be taken at the narrowest point on the torso and made with the abdominal muscles relaxed (not pulled in). Men who have a waist circumference greater than 40 inches (>102 cm) and women who have a waist circumference greater than 35 inches (>88 cm) are at higher risk for developing type 2 diabetes, hypertension, and cardiovascular disease.

Many health experts believe that because fat around the waist is so hazardous to heart health, measuring waist circumference may actually provide a more accurate method of assessing overweight and obesity risks than BMI. TABLE 9.3 integrates both the BMI and waist circumference to estimate risk status. For BMI classifications of normal, overweight, and class I obesity (18.5–24.9, 25.0–29.9, and 30.0–34.9, respectively), the inclusion of a high waist circumference increases the overall disease risk for type 2 diabetes, hypertension, and cardiovascular disease to a greater degree than BMI by itself. Furthermore, it has been shown that increases or decreases in waist circumference measures, even in the absence of BMI changes, are important predictors of cardiovascular risk factors (Lemieux et al., 2000).

If you were classified as overweight based on your waist circumference measurement, your focus should be on "waist loss," or losing inches, not necessarily pounds. You can reduce your chances of getting many metabolic diseases by 50 percent or more just by losing a couple of inches. The most promising way to go about losing those inches and significantly reducing the amount of visceral fat you

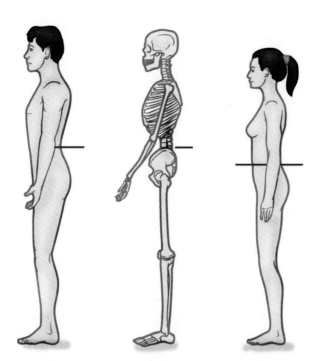

FIGURE 9.8 **Measuring-Tape Position for Waist Circumference in Adults.**

carry around is through regular physical activity (College of Family Physicians of Canada, 2004). According to researchers from Duke University Medical Center, the more exercise you do, the more of this type of dangerous fat you will lose (Slentz et al., 2005). Researchers found that elevated amounts of exercise (jogging 15 to 20 miles a week) can reverse the amount you have, and some moderate exercise (brisk 30-minute walks six times per week) can stop your visceral fat from increasing. These effects occurred over a fairly short time period. If, on the other hand, you remain inactive, more likely than not you risk building up large amounts of visceral fat in your body.

TABLE 9.3   Classification of Overweight and Obesity by BMI and Waist Circumference, and Associated Disease Risk*

BMI (kg/m²)	Obesity Class	Men ≤ 102 cm (≤ 40 in.) Women ≤ 88 cm (≤ 35 in.)		> 102 cm (> 40 in.) > 88 cm (> 35 in.)
Underweight	< 18.5	—	—	—
Normal†	18.5–24.9	—	—	May increase risk
Overweight	25.0–29.9	—	Increased	High
Obesity	30.0–34.9	I	High	Very high
	35.0–39.9	II	Very high	Very high
Extreme obesity	≥ 40	III	Extremely high	Extremely high

*Disease risk for type 2 diabetes, hypertension, and cardiovascular disease.

†Increased waist circumference can also be a marker for increased risk, even in persons of normal weight.

SOURCE: National Heart, Lung, and Blood Institute. (2000). *The Practical Guide: Identification, Evaluation, and Treatment of Overweight and Obesity in Adults* (NIH Publication No. 00-4084). Washington, DC: U.S. Department of Health and Human Services.

Risk Factors for Diseases and Conditions Associated with Overweight and Obesity

Besides being classified as overweight or obese based on BMI and waist circumference measures, there are risk factors for diseases and conditions associated with overweight and obesity that need to be assessed (TABLE 9.4) (NHLBI, 2000). The treatment algorithm shown in **FIGURE 9.9** graphically identifies the timing of this risk assessment in step 6. According to this treatment guideline, for people who are considered obese (BMI ≥ 30) or overweight (BMI of 25 to 29.9) or who have a high waist circumference (> 40 inches for men and > 35 inches for women) and two or more risk factors (step 7), weight loss is recommended (step 8). It is important to know that even a small weight loss (10 percent of current body mass) or losing a couple of inches around the waist will help lower one's risk of developing diseases associated with overweight and obesity. Prevention of weight gain with physical activity and diet is indicated for any individual with a BMI of 25 to 29.9 and two or more comorbidities (TABLE 9.5).

Age and the duration of overweight and obesity can have a powerful harmful impact on developing a chronic disease, particularly in young adults. Approximately 25 to 30 percent of adult obesity cases begin with being overweight during childhood or adolescence (Dietz, 2004). A history of being overweight in childhood that persists into adulthood is associated with more severe complications of obesity later in life. The steadily increasing incidence of overweight children and teenagers raises concern about the health of these youth as they approach adulthood. As with obese adults, overweight children have an increased risk of developing a number of health conditions and diseases, such as diabetes mellitus, high blood pressure, high blood lipids, fatty liver, orthopedic problems, sleep apnea, eating disorders, and symptoms of depression (**FIGURE 9.10**).

TABLE 9.4	**Risk Factors and Conditions to Consider If Overweight or Obese**

Risk Factors

High blood pressure (hypertension)

High LDL cholesterol ("bad" cholesterol)

Low HDL cholesterol ("good" cholesterol)

High triglycerides

High blood glucose (sugar)

Family history of premature heart disease

Physical inactivity

Cigarette smoking

Diagnosed Conditions

Established coronary heart disease

Presence of other atherosclerotic diseases (e.g., peripheral artery disease or symptomatic carotid artery disease)

Type 2 diabetes

Sleep apnea

Osteoarthritis

SOURCE: National Heart, Lung, and Blood Institute. (2000). *The Practical Guide: Identification, Evaluation, and Treatment of Overweight and Obesity in Adults* (NIH Publication No. 00-4084). Washington, DC: U.S. Department of Health and Human Services.

Treatment Algorithm*

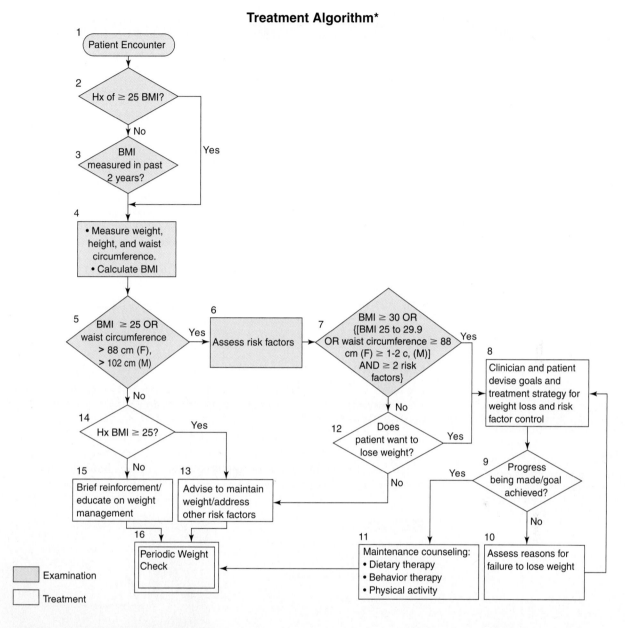

* This algorithm applies only to the assessment for overweight and obesity and subsequent decisions based on that assessment. It does not include any initial overall assessment for cardiovascular risk factors or diseases that are indicated.

FIGURE 9.9 **Treatment Algorithm.** This algorithm is used to assess overweight and obesity and to guide health practitioners in the assessment and subsequent treatment planning process. SOURCE: National Heart, Lung, and Blood Institute. (2000). *The Practical Guide: Identification, Evaluation, and Treatment of Overweight and Obesity in Adults* (NIH Publication No. 00-4084). Washington, DC: U.S. Department of Health and Human Services.

The process of assessment utilizing BMI, waist circumference, and risk factors for diseases and conditions associated with overweight and obesity can help people realize that change is needed to support their health. These assessment results may suggest treatment approaches related to lifestyle change strategies (see Figure 9.9). In addition to these assessments, knowing one's body composition brings additional information to the screening profile.

TABLE 9.5	A Guide to Selecting Treatment				
			BMI category		
Treatment	25–26.9	27–29.9	30–34.9	35–39.9	≥40
Diet, physical activity, and behavior therapy	With comobidities	With comorbidities	+	+	+
Pharmacotherapy		With comorbidities	+	+	+
Surgery			With comorbidities	With comorbidities	With comorbidities

Prevention of weight gain with lifestyle therapy is indicated in any patient with a BMI = 25 kg/m², even without comorbidities, while weight loss is not necessarily recommended for those with a BMI of 25–29.9 kg/m² or a high waist circumference, unless they have two or more comorbidities.

Combined therapy with a low-calorie diet, increased physical activity, and behavior therapy provides the most successful intervention for weight loss and weight maintenance.

Consider pharmacotherapy only if a patient has not lost 1 pound per week after 6 months of combined lifestyle therapy.

The + represents the use of indicated treatment regardless of comorbidities.

SOURCE: National Heart, Lung, and Blood Institute. (2000). *The Practical Guide: Identification, Evaluation, and Treatment of Overweight and Obesity in Adults* (NIH Publication No. 00-4084). Washington, DC: U.S. Department of Health and Human Services.

A body composition analysis allows for the assessment of the percentage of fat versus the percentage of fat-free tissue.

Body Composition

The major problem is not weight itself; it is excessive body fat. Weight is a measure of the entire body, including fat tissue and fat-free tissue. A body composition analysis allows for the assessment of percentage of fat versus percentage of fat-free tissue. Body fat percentage is simply the percentage of fat your body contains. If you are 150 pounds and 10 percent fat, it means that your body consists of 15 pounds of fat and 135 pounds of lean body mass (muscle, bone, organ tissue, blood, and everything else). One's percentage of fat can range between 2 and 70

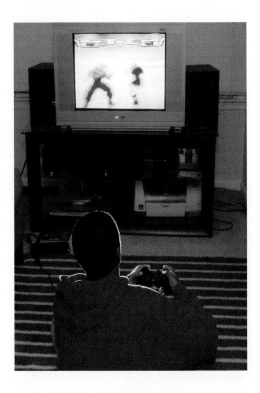

FIGURE 9.10 Today's Youth. Many young Americans are following sedentary lifestyles that place them at greater health risks.

percent of body weight. Determining cutoff points for acceptable body fat percentages requires first considering essential body fat and storage fat allowances. **Essential body fat** is required for normal physiologic functioning and is stored in bone marrow, the heart, lungs, liver, kidneys, intestines, muscles, central nervous system, and other major tissues and organs. Due to hormones and the ability to bear children, women typically have up to four times more essential fat than men—12 to 15 percent versus 3 to 5 percent.

Storage fat is body fat above essential body fat levels that accumulates in adipose tissue (fat cells). Some storage fat is advised for both males and females. Storage fat is needed to protect internal organs from trauma, serve as insulation, and provide an important energy reserve. As an energy storage repository, it provides 3500 calories in every pound of adipose tissue, which is nearly double the calories stored as glycogen (Chapter 7). Storage fat accumulates when energy intake (calories consumed) exceeds energy expenditure (calories burned). Desirable storage levels for both men and women are estimated to be between 8 and 20 percent.

Many health experts use the percentage of body fat in assessing health risk. When body fat percentage is used in conjunction with BMI, it can help differentiate people who are overweight because of lean body mass from those who are overweight because of fat. An ideal body fat percentage is one that meets your body's fundamental need for normal physiological functioning and energy needs but does not create health risks (**FIGURE 9.11**). Although there are no perfect criterion standards for ideal body fat percentage, most health experts agree that fat percentages that range from 10 percent to 25 percent and 20 percent to 30 percent for men and women, respectively, are considered to be below average or average risk (American Dietetic Association [ADA], 1993; Lohman, 1992). *Obesity* is the term used to define excessive accumulation of body fat that places individuals at greatest risk. This is usually designated by a body fat percentage that exceeds 25 per-

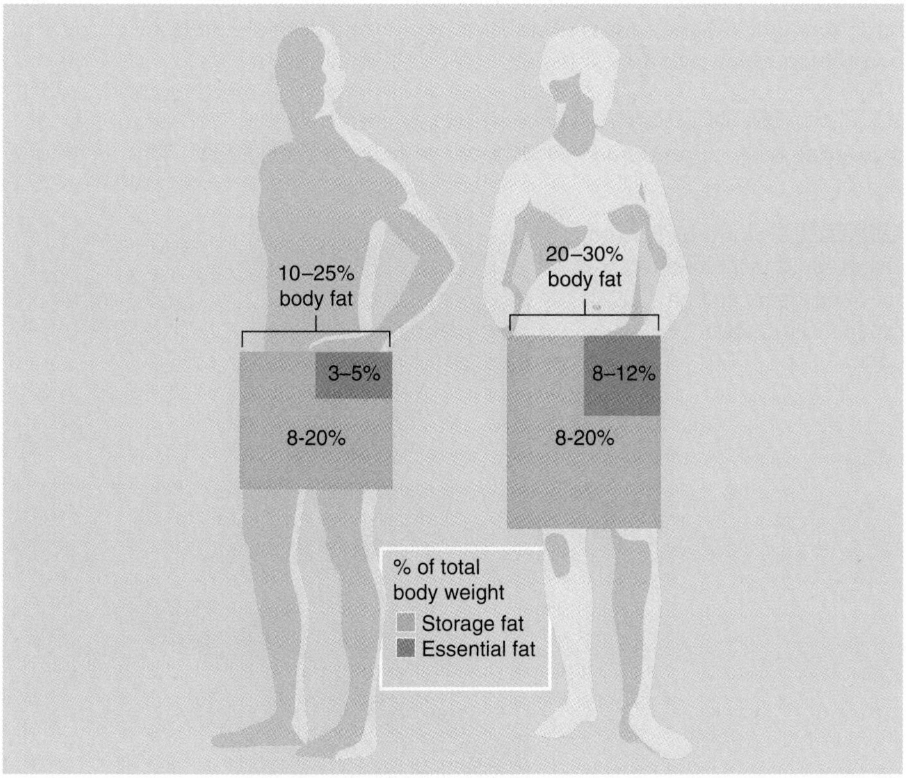

Essential body fat Fat that is required for normal healthy functioning.

Storage fat Body fat, above essential levels, that accumulates in adipose tissue.

FIGURE 9.11 **Body Fatness of a Typical Man and Woman.** SOURCE: Data compiled from American Dietetic Association (1993), Nutrition for physical fitness and athletic performance for adults—Position of ADA and the Canadian Dietetic Association. *Journal of the American Dietetic Association* 93:691–697.

cent in males and 30 percent for females. Fortunately, even minor fat reduction reduces and improves the conditions associated with obesity.

ASSESSING BODY COMPOSITION Direct measurement of body composition in living human beings is not feasible, so various models for indirect estimation of the constituents of the body have been developed. Indirect measurement techniques give estimates of the percentage of body fat, fat-free mass, muscle, bone density, hydration, or other body components. Each method uses one or more measurable body components (such as skinfold thickness, resistance, etc.) to make educated predictions about the other components. All of these methods are subject to measurement error and have basic assumptions that do not always hold true. In fact, even the most accurate techniques have measurement errors in the 2 to 4 percent range. According to the National Institutes of Health, no trial data exist to indicate that one method of measuring body fat is better than any other for following overweight and obese individuals to assess the effects of both dietary and physical activity programs. The following sections address three commonly used body composition measurement tools.

SKINFOLD TESTING The **skinfold technique** is an anthropometric technique that measures subcutaneous fat, the fat located just under your skin throughout your body. This technique requires special calipers and an experienced tester to ensure accuracy and repeatability on future testing. The tester lifts a fold of skin and fat between the thumb and forefinger, pulls it away from the underlying muscle, and then measures the fold (**FIGURE 9.12**). The five most commonly measured sites are the triceps (back of upper arm), subscapular (upper back), suprailiac (just above the hip bone), abdomen (either side of the umbilicus), and the frontal thigh. The values obtained are inserted into an appropriate skinfold formula to calculate body fat percentage. Skinfolds can have a standard error of 3 to 4 percent. Thus, a person with a skinfold estimate of 12 percent body fat may, in actuality, fall between 8 and 16 percent. Skinfold testing is easy to perform, however, and can be administered very quickly, and thus is useful as a monitoring device to indicate changes in body composition over time.

UNDERWATER WEIGHING The most widely used laboratory procedure for measuring body composition is **underwater weighing** (**FIGURE 9.13**). This technique

> **Skinfold technique** Measure of subcutaneous fat at various body sites using special calipers.
>
> **Underwater weighing** Technique to measure body fat percentage that requires weighing a person underwater as well as on land.

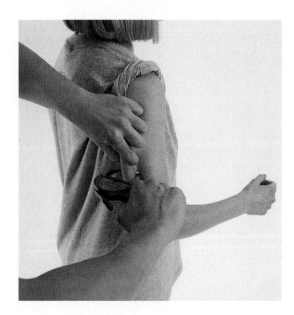

FIGURE 9.12 **Skinfold Testing.** The skinfold technique requires special calipers and an experienced tester.

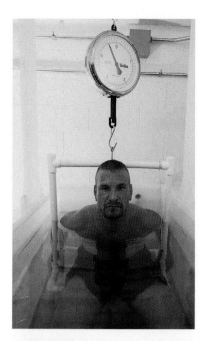
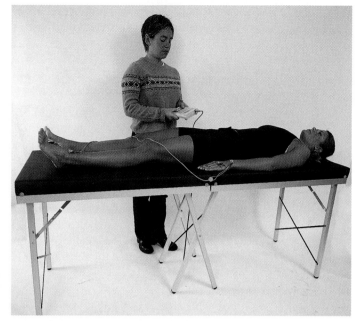

FIGURE 9.13 **Measuring Methods.** (Left) Body fat is measured using the underwater weighing method. (Right) Bioelectrical impedance is another method used to measure body fat.

is considered a more precise assessment of body fatness than skinfolds but requires special equipment and highly trained personnel and is time-consuming. This method uses the *Archimedes principle*, which states that when a body is submerged in water, there is a buoyant counterforce equal to the weight of the water that is displaced. Because bone and muscle are denser than water, a person with a larger percentage of fat-free mass will weigh more in the water and have a lower percent body fat value. Conversely, fat floats; therefore, a large amount of fat mass will make the body lighter in the water, and have a higher percent body fat value. This technique provides a density measurement from which the percentage of body fat can be calculated. If each test is performed correctly according to the recommended protocol, the standard error is 1.5 percent.

BIOELECTRICAL IMPEDANCE   In **bioelectrical impedance**, a harmless, low-level, signal-frequency electrical current is passed through the person's body by electrodes placed on the wrist and an ankle (see Figure 9.13). The amount of resistance and the body size are used to calculate body fat percentage. Since body fat contains less water and fewer electrolytes than lean body mass, it exhibits a greater resistance (impedance) to the flow of an electrical current. If done correctly using properly calibrated equipment, the standard error is 3 percent. Testing is quick and painless.

In summary, further assessment utilizing body composition analysis may significantly add to the criteria used in assessing your health risk related to obesity-related conditions. The next section provides an explanation of your body's intricate mechanism of weight control. Weight control has become an obsession with many in contemporary America. Whether you count the number of people unhappy with their shape, the percentage on a diet, or the billions of dollars spent on diet programs, books, foods, and supplements, the figures all show that our society has become more obsessed with weight in the past decade or two than ever before. Although many still attempt to obtain an ideal body weight to enhance

> **Bioelectrical impedance**
> Technique to measure body fat percentage that passes a harmless, low-level, single-frequency electrical current through the body using electrodes placed on the wrist and ankle.

their appearance, a growing number are trying to control their weight because they see it as a serious health problem that needs to be solved.

Maintaining a Healthy Body Weight

Maintaining a healthy body weight should be a simple matter. It demands that one maintain a balance between energy intake and energy output—in other words, balancing calories consumed with calories expended (FIGURE 9.14). Since both can be calculated fairly accurately and without elaborate equipment, the conscientious individual should have no problem maintaining a healthy weight. In reality, however, maintaining healthy weight over a lifetime is a constant battle for a majority of Americans. Many factors affect how much or how little food a person eats and how that food is processed, or metabolized, by the body, and therefore maintaining a healthy body weight can be a challenge. To understand the intricate mechanism of weight control, we examine the relationship between calorie intake and expenditure.

Energy Intake: Hunger, Appetite, and Satiety

Supplying enough energy to support the many functions of the body at work and play is one of the chief functions of food. Energy intake is simply calories consumed in the form of macronutrients (protein, carbohydrates, and fats) and alcohol (see Figure 9.14). As discussed in Chapter 7, protein and carbohydrates contain 4

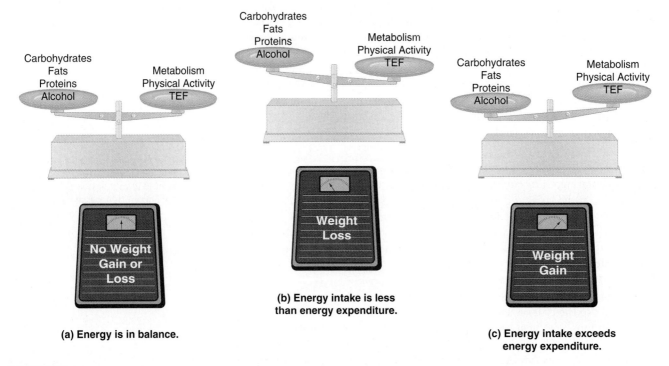

(a) Energy is in balance.

(b) Energy intake is less than energy expenditure.

(c) Energy intake exceeds energy expenditure.

FIGURE 9.14 **Energy Balance Equation.** (a) When energy expenditure equals energy intake, the body maintains its weight. (b) When energy expenditure is greater than energy intake, the body loses weight. (c) When energy expenditure is less than energy intake, the body gains weight.

calories per gram and fats 9 calories per gram. Alcohol contains 7 calories per gram, but does not provide any substantial nutrients. To be able to control your food intake (energy intake) and maintain a healthy weight, you need to understand why you feel the need to eat.

Our eating behaviors involve both physiological and psychological factors. Hunger is the physiological need for food. Numerous physiological signals tell us we are hungry, such as an empty or growling stomach, a decrease in blood glucose levels, and alterations in circulating hormones (e.g., increased glucagons and ghrelin and decreased insulin) (FIGURE 9.15). Appetite is the psychological desire to eat, and is associated with sensory experiences or aspects of food such as the sight and smell of food, emotional cues, social situations, and cultural conventions. Stressful situations often stimulate or repress appetite. Appetite is learned and relates to the desire for specific types of food and eating experiences, instead of food in general. Appetite helps select the quality and balance of food as learned by an individual in his or her environment. Whereas hunger acts as the more basic drive, appetite is more of a reflection of eating experiences. At times we are not hungry but have an appetite (such as seeing a tempting dessert after eating a full meal) or may be hungry but have no appetite (such as when we are sick).

You can use appetite to control hunger when it comes to maintaining a healthy weight. If you wait to eat until you are physiologically hungry, you may eat four or five times the amount you need to fill the necessary nutritional stores. Many people skip meals to try to lose weight and then end up pigging out. It is relatively easy to fight off your appetite but nearly impossible to fight off your hunger. To prevent this situation from occurring, eat nutrient-dense balanced meals every day and avoid allowing yourself to become physiologically hungry by using your appetite to control your hunger.

Satiety is the physiological and psychological feeling of fullness that stops hunger and appetite signals. As was true for hunger and appetite, a number of factors influence the experience of fullness, including stomach distention, elevations in blood glucose and glycogen stores, and alternations in circulating hormones.

HUNGER, SATIATION, AND SATIETY

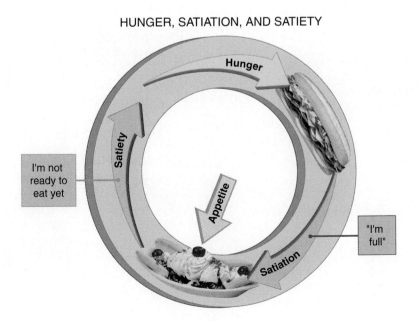

FIGURE 9.15 Hunger, Satiation, and Satiety. Hunger, satiation, and satiety are internal cues that influence eating behavior.

Fostering a full feeling can be helpful in managing your weight. Here are a few ideas for choosing foods that will help fill your stomach up without filling you out.

* Foods high in water content are known to promote a feeling of fullness. Foods with a high water content and low energy density include fruits, vegetables, low-fat milk, cooked grains, lean meats, fish, poultry, and beans. Dishes such as soups, stews, and some pasta dishes are high in water content and may have low energy density depending on preparation.

* Fiber, like water, has no calories but does add weight to the food; thus, it promotes a feeling of fullness. Fiber is not digested and gives structure or bulk to natural foods such as fruits and vegetables; food high in fiber tends to be very filling.

* Slow down when you eat to allow your stomach time to give a proper "gut check" report to the brain so it can register that you are full.

* Seek out unprocessed foods, which tend to have a low energy density or few calories per weight.

Energy Expenditure: How We Use Calories

Our metabolism is the rate at which the body uses energy (calories) to support all basic functions essential to sustain life, plus all energy requirements for additional activity and digestive processes. There are three components to human metabolism, hence determining our energy needs. These components are the resting metabolic rate, the thermic effect of food, and the thermic effect of activity (**FIGURE 9.16**).

Resting metabolic rate (RMR) is the largest part of total metabolism and accounts for 60 to 75 percent of calories burned in a day (Wildman & Miller, 2004). This is the amount of calories needed to run all essential functions and chemical reactions while in a rested and quiet state. The functions included are the respiratory process, the pumping of blood around the body, nerve transmission, producing and transporting substances, cell growth and maintenance, tissue repair, and temperature regulation. RMR is relatively stable for a given individual, but sig-

FIGURE 9.16 **Major Components of Energy Expenditure.** The majority of daily energy expenditure is used to maintain physiological functions. Energy expended by athletes during physical activity and exercise is significant and could equal or exceed the energy needed for maintaining resting energy expenditure. The thermic effect of food is the energy required to digest, absorb, transport, metabolize, and store food.

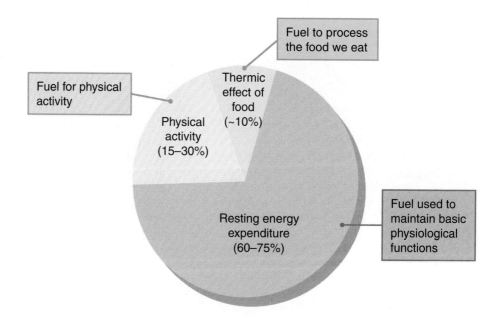

nificant differences in RMR can be found when comparing different individuals. Many factors can influence RMR, including the following:

- *Age.* RMR slows with age, due to a loss in muscle tissue but also due to hormonal and neurological changes. After 20 years of age, RMR decline about 2 percent per decade.
- *Gender.* Generally, men have faster metabolisms than women because they tend to be larger and have less body fat.
- *Glands.* Thyroxin (produced by the thyroid gland) is a key RMR regulator. The more thyroxin produced, the higher the RMR. If too much thyroxin is produced, RMR can actually double. If too little thyroxin is produced, RMR may shrink to 30 to 40 percent of normal. In some people, the thyroid gland does not function properly, and as a result the organ produces too much or too little thyroid hormone.
- *Muscle-to-fat ratio.* Muscle cells are about eight times more metabolically demanding than fat cells. So the greater our proportion of muscle to fat, the faster our metabolic rate.
- *Crash dieting, starving, or fasting.* Starvation or serious abrupt calorie reduction can dramatically reduce RMR by up to 30 percent. Restrictive low-calorie weight loss diets may cause your RMR to drop as much as 20 percent.
- *Infection or illness.* RMR increases because the body has to work harder to build new tissues and create an immune response.
- *Environmental temperature.* If temperature is very low or very high, the body has to work harder to maintain its normal temperature; this increases RMR.
- *Drugs.* Some drugs, such as caffeine and nicotine, increase the RMR.

The **thermic effect of food (TEF)** is used to describe the energy expended by our bodies in order to eat and process (digest, transport, metabolize, and store) food. We expend energy by burning calories. The calories needed to eat and process food are fairly constant, usually about 10 percent of the total calories taken in. For example, a person who consumes 2500 calories per day will expend approximately 250 calories a day to metabolize food. The more calories eaten, the more energy is used to digest them, but it's in proportion to total calories. Variance in the type of macronutrients eaten affects TEF. Processing protein requires the greatest amount of energy, with estimates ranging as high as 30 percent. Dietary fat, on the other hand, is so easily processed and stored as body fat that there is little thermic effect, perhaps only 2 or 3 percent. The amount of energy required to process carbohydrates falls between that of protein and fat.

The **thermic effect of activity (TEA)** is the energy costs for skeletal muscle contraction and relaxation. As noted previously, RMR is measured with the person at rest; any physical activity will raise the metabolic activity above the RMR and thus increase energy expenditure. The energy we expend in voluntary physical activity is the most variable component of our calorie requirements. Muscles need energy to contract. The more muscles we contract and the more frequently we contract them, the more calories we burn. In addition, metabolic rate increases during physical activity and remains elevated for some time after physical activity. The more active one is, the more calories one requires. Physical activity has a profound effect on human energy expenditure and contributes 20 to 30 percent to the body's total energy output; however, some endurance athletes can actually meet or exceed estimated RMR rates.

Although energy intake is easily measured and can be regulated by consulting caloric intake charts, regulating and determining energy output are slightly more

Thermic effect of food (TEF) The energy expended by our bodies in order to eat and process (digest, transport, metabolize, and store) food.

Thermic effect of activity (TEA) The energy expended in skeletal muscle contraction and relaxation.

complex. The Activities and Assessment Manual provides worksheets to calculate daily energy requirements, and Appendix B lists the energy costs of various activities.

In summary, maintaining a healthy weight is a general matter of energy balance, as illustrated in Figure 9.14. To maintain body weight, energy intake (calories) and energy expenditure must be equal. When calories consumed are greater than energy expended, individuals gain weight. When energy expenditure exceeds caloric intake, weight loss occurs. It is important to remember that all of us from time to time have short-term weight fluctuations. This is normal because it is easy to become dehydrated, leading to losing a couple pounds of water weight within a few days, or because we don't eat exactly the same amount of calories every day or don't do the same level of physical activity every day. However, when weight consistently increases or decreases, we have an energy imbalance, and we need to look into that. In the United States, the energy imbalance is tilted to weight gain for a majority of children and adults.

Causes of Overweight and Obesity

What is becoming increasingly difficult for researchers to explain is why this imbalance in the energy balance equation occurs. Until recently, the major causes of obesity were thought to be behavioral in nature—that is, due to excessive energy intake and deficient energy expenditure (people eating too much and exercising too little). This idea led many health professionals, and thus, the public, to believe that excess weight reflects a lack of will power on the part of the overweight and obese. However, recent research provides evidence that obesity is a complex disorder with multiple contributing factors. There is no one cause of obesity. A combination of behavioral, psychological, genetic, physiological, metabolic, hormonal, sociocultural, and environmental factors acting together over time can contribute to weight gain and obesity (**FIGURE 9.17**). Separating one cause from another is not an easy diagnostic task when looking at individuals. For example, obesity tends to run in families, suggesting a genetic link, yet families also share common dietary, physical exercise, and lifestyle habits that may also contribute to obesity.

Genetics determines the "body-weight ballpark" each person is born into. So there is no denying the fact that biology is at work when it comes to understanding body weight. Genes affect a number of weight-related processes in the body, including influences on fat metabolism and the regulation of certain hormones, which may affect appetite and contribute to obesity. Several genes have been iden-

Obesity is a complex disorder with multiple contributing factors.

FIGURE 9.17 **Multiple Factors Contribute to Obesity.** There is no one cause of obesity.

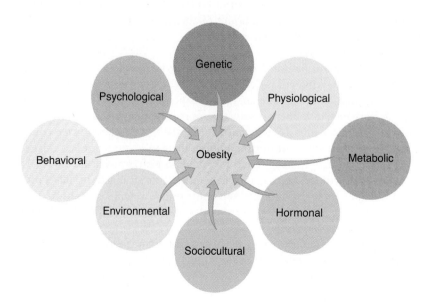

tified as contributors to obesity, and researchers at the CDC are constructing a human obesity gene map in hope of finding genetic targets in humans that may lead to the development of new treatments (CDC, 2005b). These genetic discoveries related to obesity are particularly promising for a better understanding of obesity in some individuals who have a genetic tendency to gain weight and store fat.

Although some people may have genes that permit them to become obese, it still is their environment that determines if they actually do become obese. In other words, while recognizing that genetic differences may predispose an individual toward obesity, it is important to understand that these differences can be overcome by changes in one's environment, such as being physically active and eating right. So despite obesity having strong genetic determinants, the genetic composition of the population cannot change rapidly; therefore, the large increase in obesity in our current population must reflect changes in other factors.

Interest in the physiological factors related to obesity focuses on the **set point theory**, which proposes that a regulatory system exists in the human body that is designed to maintain body weight at some fixed level. Similar to other regulated physiological variables in the body (e.g., blood glucose, body temperature) that are maintained within certain limits, the body seeks to protect against pressures to be too heavy or too thin. The level of the body's fat stores is thought to be determined by a mechanism in the brain called the **adipostat**. The adipostat establishes a set point for a fixed amount of body fat just as a thermostat regulates heat according to a preset temperature. The brain maintains this set point by regulating the expenditure or storage of energy until fat stores meet the level determined by the adipostat. A set point above the ideal healthy weight presents a difficult struggle for the obese individual. Unknown to the person who has been diligently dieting, the brain is busily undermining the efforts by working to restore weight to the set point. The adipostat may do this by activating the sensation for hunger, so that more calories are consumed, or by slowing the metabolism.

Just because our body aggressively maintains a stable amount of body fat at a target level doesn't mean the target level can't be changed. Many health scientists believe that the set point can be changed. If we go back to the analogy of the thermostat, they are saying that the "body fat thermostat" has a dial, and we can turn the dial to a new setting by fine-tuning our lifestyle. The dial of the thermostat is turned by a combination of the type and amount of physical activity we do, the levels of nutrients we eat, and the amount of stress we have in our lives. The lifestyle factor that can lower the set point more than any other is regular physical activity. So if we want to turn the dial to a new setting permanently, we have to make permanent changes in our lifestyle. This means that the strategy we adopt should be suitable for the long term, not just a strategy for losing weight in the short term.

Two hormones of great interest in the study of obesity are leptin and cortisol. A gene in fat cells called the *ob* gene makes leptin. As discussed previously, our eating patterns are regulated by feeding and satiety centers located in the hypothalamus and pituitary glands in the brain that respond to signals indicating high fat stores and hunger (see Figure 9.15). Substances critical to this process include glucose (sugar), insulin, and leptin. Rising levels of leptin appear to signal the hypothalamus to suppress appetite, and falling levels to stimulate appetite. Interestingly, overweight people tend to have higher levels of leptin, and leptin levels fall as weight is lost. This system works as a self-balancing biological mechanism, particularly to prevent starvation by stimulating appetite as weight is lost, and to reduce appetite as weight is gained. This raises the question of why obesity occurs at all, given that obese people have high levels of leptin. It has been theorized that obese people may have insensitivity to leptin that stops the signal reaching the brain, and that the body is overproducing leptin in an attempt to compensate for the insensitivity.

Set point theory A theory that proposes that a regulatory system exists in the human body that is designed to maintain body weight at some fixed level.

Adipostat Brain mechanism that establishes a set point for a fixed amount of body fat.

Cortisol is a hormone produced by the adrenal gland when the body is under stress. Your hypothalamus, via the pituitary gland, directs the adrenal glands to secrete cortisol. Cortisol is released as part of one's daily hormonal cycle, but can also be released in greater amounts in reaction to acute and chronic stressors—both physical and emotional—as part of the body's fight-or-flight response that is essential for survival (Chapter 13). One of the functions of cortisol is to trigger a glucocorticoid effect—helping the body produce blood sugar from proteins. Excess glucose is then used for lipogenesis (fat production). There have been a number of studies that have examined the release of cortisol during acute and chronic stress, and the physiologic effects that this hormone has on the body, especially how it contributes to the deposition of visceral fat particularly in the abdominal region (Bjorntorp & Rosmond, 2000). Many health experts have linked oversecretion of cortisol with obesity and increased fat storage in the body.

Cortisol is thought to affect weight gain and metabolism in a number of ways. Being an inbuilt defense mechanism (fight-or-flight response), it temporarily shuts down certain bodily functions and activates others to deal with the emergency situation. It also increases appetite. Most overweight people can attest to an understanding of "comfort eating" and resultant weight gain during times of stress. It is an evolutionary response to make a person eat, particularly something sweet, to urgently boost blood glucose levels for the energy to either fight or fly from a stressful situation. Similarly, it shuts down or significantly slows down your metabolic rate as your body seeks to preserve its energy supplies. The effect on weight gain from those two factors is obvious. Although it may be possible for a person to have malfunctioning adrenal glands that simply overproduce cortisol, in most cases the real solution is to practice various relaxation and stress-releasing activities or eliminate sources of ongoing stress (Chapter 13).

Most cases of obesity occur now in people with normal physiology who live in a sociocultural environment characterized by a sedentary lifestyle and ready access to abundant food. Eating foods high in calories and low in nutrients is common in our daily diets (Chapter 7). Food manufacturers know how taste, smell, and texture increase the human appetite, and engineer food accordingly (Sclafani, 1996). The increased availability of convenience foods, changes in food preparation, and eating out more often are additional factors that contribute to overeating among Americans (Harnack, 2000) and are major contributing factors to Americans consuming 12 percent more calories than they were only a few decades ago (CDC, 2005a).

In conjunction with an increase in energy consumption is a concurrent decrease in energy expenditure. Everyone who leads a sedentary lifestyle is at risk for obesity. Systematic survey trend data collected over the last couple of decades regularly indicate that the majority of adults are not engaging in the recommended amount of physical activity. Thus, this provides evidence that reduced physical activity, and subsequent decrease in energy expenditure, is a potentially important contributor to obesity.

A sedentary lifestyle and obesity play against each other in a no-win game; that is, lack of physical activity contributes to fat gain, and fat gain makes it more difficult to be physically active. The tendency in America is toward an unhealthy weight gain with age. As you age, bone and muscle mass tend to decrease. A sedentary lifestyle accelerates the problem of bone and muscle loss. All physical activity involves muscular movement that requires the expenditure of calories and contributes to lean-tissue maintenance (**FIGURE 9.18**). In other words, body fatness is not only responsible for general weight gain in sedentary individuals but also for making up more of the lean weight they may have once had.

To summarize, the increased prevalence of overweight and obesity in America has been largely attributed to an increased consumption of energy-dense and low-nutrient food, which is simultaneously flavorful, pleasurable, and accessible, and a decreased level of caloric expenditure due to a sedentary lifestyle. This increase in

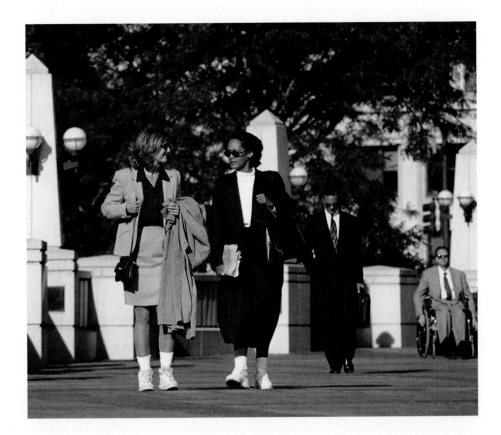

FIGURE 9.18 Get into the Habit. Regular movement is a good way to burn calories.

energy intake and decrease in energy expenditure leads to an unbalancing of the energy equation (see Figure 9.14).

A Lifestyle Approach to Achieving and Maintaining a Healthy Weight

A lifestyle approach to weight maintenance focuses on developing a lifelong commitment to a way of life that achieves and maintains a healthy body composition relative to physical and psychological functioning. The most important components in this approach are regular physical activity and eating a healthy nutritious diet. By focusing on these two major components, you will be able to avoid the effects of creeping obesity or the negative consequences of repeated weight gains and losses. Based on the self-assessments provided in the activities and assessment manual, you may be currently at a healthy weight. If you are at a healthy weight and have a low risk of obesity-related diseases, you ought to read the following as a way to prevent weight gain in the future. If the self-assessments indicate that you may be overweight or at risk for an obesity-related condition, and you are ready to make a change, the following will provide essential information to assist you with initial fat loss and maintenance of this loss in the long term. Remember that small victories in weight loss—often as little as 10 percent of total body mass—can result in positive effects on health and well-being, even if an ideal weight remains elusive.

Using the Energy Balance Equation
DETERMINING YOUR ENERGY BALANCE EQUATION   An objective assessment of your average daily energy intake and energy expenditure provides the basis for *unbalancing* the energy equation. To determine your average daily calorie intake,

A lifestyle approach that includes regular physical activity and a nutritious diet is essential in achieving and maintaining a healthy weight.

keep a careful daily food intake record using the worksheets found in the activities and assessment manual. When it comes to healthy eating, it's what you take in over a number of days that counts, not just one day. Withhold judgment regarding your diet until a week's worth of recording food intake has been completed. By avoiding early analysis, you can learn much about your individuality related to your food habits, which is an important aspect of the evaluation process. In addition, your food intake record will provide a more accurate picture of your average daily caloric and nutrient intake. At the same time you are recording your caloric intake you should be recording your daily caloric expenditure. Again, avoid analysis of your daily caloric energy expenditure activities until a week has passed. After determining this important baseline information, you will be able to proceed to develop an effective strategy to achieve a negative energy balance.

UNBALANCING THE ENERGY EQUATION   The best way to create a negative energy balance is through a combination of reduced caloric intake and increased caloric expenditure. The recommended amount of fat loss in a week is 1 pound. This is best accomplished by creating a 3500 weekly calorie deficit or 500 daily calorie deficit (remember, 1 pound of fat equals 3500 calories). Generally, you do not want to attempt to shed more than 1 pound of body fat per week. Increasing the weekly energy deficit above 3500 calories could cause a significant loss of muscle tissue and be counterproductive to your body composition goal of losing body fat. As discussed earlier, although either lowering your caloric intake (dietary modification) or increasing energy expenditure (exercise modification) can be effective independently in obtaining the recommended 3500 weekly calorie deficit, a combination of the two produces the best results. In other words, reducing daily caloric intake by 250 calories and increasing daily physical activity by 250 calories will generally produce the best results. As you will discover in the next sections, the advantages of one technique counterbalance the disadvantages of the other. For example, caloric restriction produces a rapid reduction of resting metabolic rate, substantially decreasing energy expenditure, whereas exercise increases resting metabolic rate, thereby negating the dietary effects.

It is important to note that you will not necessarily get bigger using an exercise program when trying to lose fat. For example, if you are losing fat weight through a healthful combination of exercising and eating nutritiously, your actual overall weight may stay constant even as you get leaner and smaller. Why? Because fat loss and muscle gain may occur together. Muscle is much more compact and dense than fat. It actually takes up less space than fat does because of that. That makes sense, right? Fat, on the other hand, is very soft and jelly-like and is a lot bigger than muscle. By that we mean it takes up more space than muscle does. So although your dress size or pant size may drop, your weight may not.

This lifestyle intervention strategy for fat loss is built on the sound premise that individuals can modify their own behaviors related to managing and maintaining a focus on healthy eating and increased physical activity. However, it is often difficult to motivate people with this sound physiological approach to losing 1 pound of fat per week when they read or hear about such quick fixes as "lose 10 pounds in 1 week" or "lose 30 pounds in 1 month." These ads may lead people to abandon basic fat-loss principles. Rather than defining success solely in terms of general weight loss, a more fitting focus would be on shedding excess body fatness that increases your overall health risk. Any plan to shed excess body fat should include strategies for maintaining or enhancing the level of lean body tissues to provide a more healthy weight. This approach requires a thorough understanding of body fatness and health. This pattern of thinking is consistent with our emphasis on a lifestyle approach that is sustainable and enjoyable.

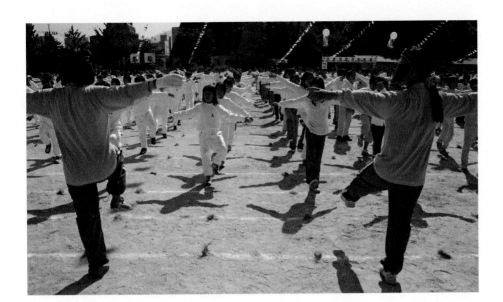

FIGURE 9.19 **The Opportunities Are Endless.** Physical activity of any kind is generally considered an important component in a fat-loss program.

Physical Activity and Fat Loss

Physical activity is one of the most important components of any fat-loss program (**FIGURE 9.19**). In addition, accumulated evidence has shown that physical activity is the best predictor for maintaining weight loss (Mcinnis, Franklin, & Rippe, 2003). Therefore, describing the benefits of physical activity related to fat loss and maintenance will provide you with added incentives to become, or stay, physically active.

PHYSICAL ACTIVITY BURNS CALORIES The immediate function of physical activity in a fat-loss program is simply to increase the level of energy expenditure—helping to unbalance the caloric equation so that there is a greater amount of energy output. Physical activity is the most important way to increase the calories you burn. The calorie-expending effects of physical activity are cumulative and substantial. This means that even mild to moderate increases in physical activity can be beneficial. For example, 40 to 60 minutes of walking expends approximately 350 calories. Performing this activity five times a week would contribute to 1750 calories expended or shedding half a pound of fat. Increasing the intensity or duration of physical activity (or participating in a formal exercise program) can further increase the number of calories burned.

PHYSICAL ACTIVITY AMELIORATES OBESITY-ASSOCIATED DISEASES
Physical activity benefits your health even if you don't lose weight. Physical activity has positive effects on blood pressure, blood fat levels, and insulin insensitivity (type 2 diabetes), independent of those produced by weight loss alone.

PHYSICAL ACTIVITY LEADS TO "WAIST LOSS" Physical activity is the best modifier of visceral fat. Research has demonstrated that physical inactivity leads to a significant increase in this potentially dangerous fat, while regular amounts of physical activity can lead to significant decreases in such fat over a fairly short time period (Slentz et al., 2005). Maintaining a normal waistline by adopting a regular physical activity program and a moderate eating plan will help you avoid midriff weight gain (the apple shape), which puts you at greater risk for diabetes and heart disease.

PHYSICAL ACTIVITY COMPENSATES FOR RMR DECLINE   A well-documented change that occurs during dietary restriction of calories is a considerable reduction in resting metabolic rate. This decline can reach up to 40 percent of RMR after a brief time, significantly reducing overall calorie expenditure by the body. Physical activity increases the metabolic rate both during activity and afterward.

PHYSICAL ACTIVITY MINIMIZES LOSS OF LEAN BODY MASS   Muscle is metabolically active—it requires calories. The more muscle you have, the more calories you need to sustain it, and the more calories you can eat and still lose weight. The use of physical activity in a weight loss program provides protection against a loss of lean tissue routinely seen with diet-only weight loss programs. Aerobic and weight-resistance activities contribute to the conservation of lean tissue in different ways. Aerobic physical activities utilize the oxygen energy system that requires the mobilization and metabolism of the body's fat storage (Chapter 8). Weight-resistance activities (weight training) burn calories as well. In addition, weight-resistance activities help stimulate muscular development (Chapter 11), preventing significant losses of lean body tissue that generally occur during calorie-restricting diets.

PHYSICAL ACTIVITY SUPPRESSES APPETITE   To some degree, regular physical activity appears to contribute to the normal functioning of the brain's feeding control mechanisms. A sensitive balance between energy expenditure and food intake is apparently not maintained very well in physically inactive people. This lack of precision in regulating food intake may account for some of the increasing obesity observed in America (Weinsier et al., 1998). Individuals who are regularly physical active are better able to match daily energy intake with daily expenditure.

PHYSICAL ACTIVITY CAN LOWER SET POINT   The set point theory proposes that a regulatory system exists in the human body that maintains body weight at some fixed level. Instead of a simply genetic determination, set point is now believed to be under control of environmental factors. The environmental factor that can lower set point more than any other is regular, sustained physical activity (Bennett, 1995). A lower set point can make maintaining a lower percentage of body fat much easier.

PHYSICAL ACTIVITY IMPROVES PSYCHOLOGICAL WELL-BEING   A weight problem or poor body image may contribute to lower self-esteem, guilt, depression, anxiety, and distress. Physical activity can enhance self-esteem and reduce depression, anxiety, and stress through both physiological and psychological mechanisms (Chapter 13). Increased psychological well-being can enhance compliance with a weight loss program as well as helping the individual to cope with societal pressure.

   As you can see, physical activity plays an integral role in a healthy weight loss program. Another key component is healthy eating.

Healthy Eating and Fat Loss

The foundation for any healthy eating plan for fat loss should be built from the *Dietary Guidelines for Americans* and the MyPyramid food guidance system (Chapter 7). To incorporate their guidelines into a fat-loss program, particular attention must be given to serving size and to choosing mainly nutrient-dense foods.

FOOD INTAKE MODIFICATION   Using your estimated daily caloric intake, develop a daily caloric plan that reduces your calories by 250 each day. (Avoid daily caloric restriction plans of 1200 calories or less.) As for the diet itself, the corner-stone of any meal plan should be MyPyramid, which builds upon and comple-ments the *Dietary Guidelines* (Chapter 7). MyPyramid recommends a variety of foods, with a notable emphasis on grains, fruits, and vegetables. Moreover, it helps you establish a tolerable, enjoyable, and stable eating pattern that is consistent with a healthy lifestyle approach to fat loss. Finally, the *Dietary Guidelines* advo-cates the moderation of fat, sugar, and alcohol consumption, all of which are important in weight loss.

Although not designed to be calorie-specific management tools, both MyPyramid and the *Dietary Guidelines* are relevant and valuable tools for healthy menu planning related to body fat loss. You just need to pay special attention to the serving size and select nutrient-dense foods.

Choosing foods with a high nutrient-calorie benefit ratio can easily be accom-plished by choosing natural and unrefined foods from the food groups. Avoid refined and processed foods (refined sugar) as much as possible. Since you will be encouraged to participate in a regular physical activity program, it is important to maintain a good macronutrient ratio composed of 55 to 65 percent of your total calories from carbohydrates (preferably complex carbohydrates), 20 to 25 percent from protein, and 10 to 20 percent from fat (Kleiner, 1998). Dietary fat is not a ter-rible thing, but when you are limiting your calories, as on a fat-loss program, the calories are better spent on carbohydrates (to fuel your activity) and protein (to maintain your muscle tissue). Research has shown that, during negative energy balance, slightly more protein (1.2 grams per 2.0 pounds of body weight) is required to maintain muscle mass. Finally, sources of complex carbohydrates, such as grain products and vegetables, not only allow you to feel energetic for longer periods of time but also are generally higher in other important nutrients.

EATING STYLE MODIFICATION   Obesity is as much a result of how we eat as it is of what we eat. Although what we eat contributes to our fat-loss efforts, so do our eating styles. Eating styles can be hard to change. Correcting problem areas will make a big difference in your success with fat loss. Therefore, it is important to evaluate your eating styles.

EMOTIONAL EATING   One of the primary reasons for keeping a food diary is to have a written record of your moods and the events occurring just prior to eating. How you feel and what's going on around you before you eat are significant; our emotions strongly influence our eating behavior. By keeping an accurate food diary that includes this information, your eating style will become more visible to you. This may include eating when you are stressed or depressed. Once you become aware of the precursors causing unnecessary eating behaviors, a conscious effort can be made to avoid them.

FOCUS ON BODY FAT, NOT WEIGHT   Do not build everything around "losing weight." Too many people focus their dietary restriction program on weight loss and not fat loss. They get up every day and check their weight on the scale. They are depressed if they did not lose anything and elated if they lost weight. You want to focus on losing body fat. You could lose weight and get fatter if you are dieting incorrectly! What matters is your level of body fatness, not your weight.

EAT SMALLER, MORE FREQUENT MEALS   Do not skip meals or go more than 3 to 4 hours without eating. Skipping a meal often leads to bingeing at the next

FIGURE 9.20 **Rethink Snacks.** Fruits and vegetables make excellent snacks for either maintaining or losing weight.

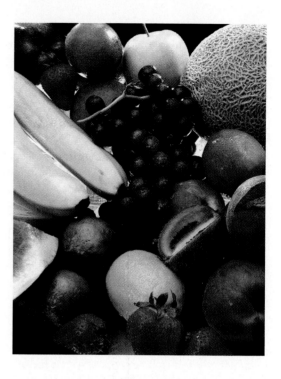

meal, which initiates an up-and-down energy and nutrient pattern. When meals are more than 6 hours apart, plan strategic healthy snacks. You can obtain many nutrients, and energy, by choosing your snacks wisely and eating them in moderation. Include fresh fruits and vegetables and avoid cookies, candies, ice cream, and potato chips (**FIGURE 9.20**).

EAT SLOWLY You will probably overeat if you eat too quickly. It takes about 20 to 30 minutes for your stomach to signal the brain that you are full. Put your eating utensil down between bites and chew your food thoroughly.

Body Image and Weight

Most of us are well aware of how much we weigh, and we typically equate our weight with our body image or appearance. **Body image** is the picture one has of one's body, what it looks like to one's self, and how one thinks it looks to others. This image can be accurate or inaccurate and is often subject to change. The relationship between body image and weight is complicated.

Although you may have a perception of an ideal body weight for appearance, this ideal body weight may or may not be in accord with optimal health. Most research effort has attempted to find an ideal body weight for reducing the risk of disease. An increasing number of Americans, however, attempt to achieve an unrealistic weight and shape based on the fashion industry's ideal body. This "ideal" standard is one of extreme thinness for females and exaggerated muscularity for males. These so-called ideals have been created by the fashion and advertising industry to sell products. For people who try to live up to this standard of "perfection," the defining characteristic for ideal weight and size is perceived body image.

People should not attempt to base their weight or shape on our society's glamour approach. Choosing unrealistic weight loss goals in response to societal ideals can set you up for failure and perpetuate unhealthy choices (**FIGURE 9.21**). To improve body image, as well as self-esteem, it is important to learn to like our-

Body image The picture one has of one's body, what it looks like to one's self, and how one think it looks to others.

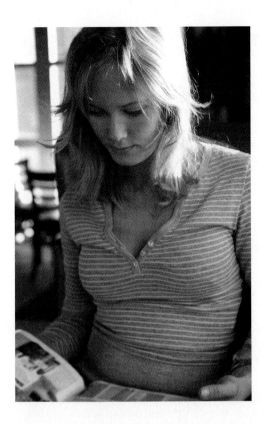

FIGURE 9.21 **Media Messages.** The "ideal" body promoted by the fashion industry may influence distorted images in individuals, particularly women.

selves and to take care of ourselves through healthy lifestyle choices that do not emphasize weight loss at the expense of psychological and physical health.

Unfortunately, some people become so focused on their image and body weight that they feel pressured to match the "ideal" portrayed in magazines and on television. This can lead to major discontent with body weight. A negative sign of dissatisfaction with body weight, when basing it on the "ideal" weight portrayed by the mass media, is the development of eating disorders. The term **eating disorders** refers to a wide range of harmful eating behaviors used in an attempt to lose weight or achieve a thin appearance. These dangerous behaviors range from severe restriction of food intake to binge eating and purging.

Eating disorder patterns are far-reaching, affecting more than 5 million women and approximately 1 million men in the United States (National Institute of Mental Health [NIMH], 2001). Nearly 90 percent of these destructive eating patterns begin before the age of 20, with the majority lasting anywhere from 1 to 15 years. Eating disorders are not due to a failure of will or behavior; rather, they are real, treatable medical illnesses in which certain maladaptive patterns of eating take on a life of their own (NIMH, 2001). Without treatment, up to 20 percent of people with serious eating disorders die. With treatment, that number falls drastically to 2 to 3 percent. With proper treatment, about 60 percent of people with eating disorders recover. They maintain a healthy weight and feel stronger and more positive about life in general. Anorexia nervosa and bulimia nervosa are the two most severe forms of eating disorders (TABLE 9.6).

Anorexia Nervosa

Anorexia nervosa literally means "loss of appetite." This definition is misleading, in that a person with anorexia nervosa becomes hungry, but repudiates the hunger because of an irrational fear of eating and becoming fat. Anorexia nervosa is characterized by a distorted body image, self-starvation, and extreme weight loss.

A negative sign of dissatisfaction with body weight, when basing it on the "ideal" weight portrayed by the mass media, is the development of eating disorders.

Eating disorder Refers to a wide range of harmful eating behaviors used in the attempt to lose weight or achieve a lean appearance.

TABLE 9.6	Anorexia Nervosa and Bulimia Nervosa Symptoms

Anorexia Nervosa Symptoms

- Resistance to maintaining body weight at or above a minimally normal weight for age and height
- Intense fear of gaining weight or becoming fat, even though underweight
- Disturbance in the way in which one's body weight or shape is experienced, undue influence of body weight or shape on self-evaluation, or denial of the seriousness of the current low body weight
- Infrequent or absent menstrual periods (in females who have reached puberty)

Bulimia Nervosa Symptoms

- Recurrent episodes of binge eating, characterized by eating an excessive amount of food within a discrete period of time and by a sense of lack of control over eating during the episode
- Recurrent inappropriate compensatory behavior in order to prevent weight gain, such as self-induced vomiting or misuse of laxatives, diuretics, enemas, or other medications (purging); fasting; or excessive exercise
- The binge eating and inappropriate compensatory behaviors both occur, on average, at least twice a week for 3 months
- Self-evaluation is unduly influenced by body shape and weight

SOURCE: Melissa Spearing, Public Information and Communications Branch, National Institute of Mental Health (NIMH). (2001). *Eating Disorders: Facts About Eating Disorders and the Search for Solutions.* Expert assistance provided by NIMH Director Steven E. Hyman, MD, and NIMH staff members Bruce N. Cuthbert, PhD, Regina Dolan-Sewell, PhD, Benedetto Vitiello, PhD, Clarissa K. Wittenberg, and Constance Burr. Editorial assistance provided by Margaret Strock and Lisa D. Alberts. NIH Publication No. 01-4901.

Because of extreme weight loss, females with anorexia nervosa often suffer from a lack of menstrual periods (amenorrhea) due to too little body fat. Furthermore, excessive weight loss increases rates of bone loss (osteoporosis), muscle loss, and dehydration. When body fat is severely limited and muscle tissue is lost, the body turns to its organs in a critical search for energy, and the vicious cycle of wasting away continues. Victims lose the ability to function effectively and put themselves in a life-threatening physical condition.

Bulimia Nervosa

Bulimia means to "eat like an ox." Bulimia nervosa is characterized by uncontrollable cycles of binge eating followed by purging through forced vomiting or the abuse of laxatives and diuretics. During a binge, individuals lose control over their eating and may quickly consume large amounts of food—up to 20,000 calories in a single binge. Bulimic individuals are afraid of being fat and follow the binge with efforts to redress uncontrolled eating by purging the food from their bodies or by fasting (**FIGURE 9.22**).

The person suffering from bulimia nervosa is usually in a normal weight range, but may suffer from weight fluctuations of 10 or more pounds over short periods of time due to alternating binges and purging/fasting. This binge–purge cycle puts a tremendous strain on the body. In repeated vomiting, the stomach acid can erode tooth enamel and even the esophagus. Additionally, nutrient deficiencies may occur from vomiting and the use of laxatives.

Compulsive Overeating

Compulsive eaters are similar to those with bulimia nervosa in that they may eat large amounts of food in a short period of time and exhibit a lack of control

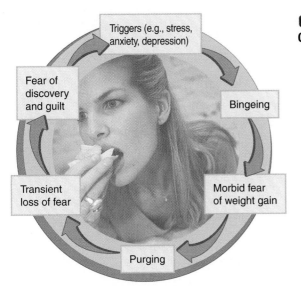

FIGURE 9.22 The Binge–Purge Cycle of Bulimia.

Triggers (e.g., stress, anxiety, depression)

Bingeing

Morbid fear of weight gain

Purging

Transient loss of fear

Fear of discovery and guilt

regarding their eating. However, compulsive eaters do not purge, and thus they usually become obese, thereby encountering all the health risks of obesity. They may eat continually throughout the day as a means to cope with stress and other emotionally issues.

Compulsive Exercising

With an eating disorder, too much exercise, or compulsive exercising, is just another outlet of behavior. Those who have symptoms of compulsive exercise usually have episodes of repeated exercising beyond the requirements of what is considered safe. They will find time at any cost to exercise (including cutting classes and taking off from work) and will work out for hours. The main goal of exercise usually is to burn calories and relieve the guilt from just having eaten or binged, or to give themselves permission to eat ("I can't eat unless I have exercised or know I will exercise"). Compulsive exercise is another way to purge, and afflicted individuals use exercise as another way to cope with their emotions and anxiety about their weight.

Female Athlete Triad

The female athlete triad, or simply the triad, is a combination of three coexistent conditions: disordered eating, amenorrhea, and osteoporosis. The depiction of the triad as a triangle was developed to demonstrate the interrelationship among the three disorders normally considered independent medical conditions (**FIGURE 9.23**). Alone or in combination, triad disorders can reduce physical performance and have serious medical and psychological consequences.

The triad is most associated with physically active girls and women as well as elite athletes. Females who are most susceptible are those who reach and maintain unrealistically low levels of body weight or body fat or both. The same inner and societal pressures that contribute to the development of eating disorders help initiate the triad. Additional factors that are specific to athletes include sport-related emphasis on body weight and body fat, perfectionism, lack of nutrition knowledge, the drive to excel at any cost, and pressure to lose weight from coaches, judges, and significant others.

Treatment for Eating Disorders

The treatments for disordered eating patterns are complex and most often require professional help. Anorexia nervosa treatment, depending on the duration of the

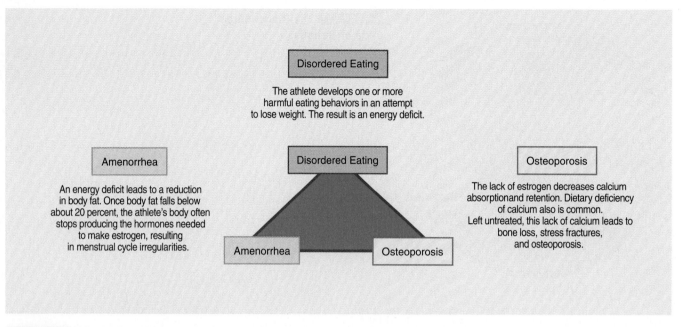

FIGURE 9.23 **The Female Triad.** The depiction of the triad as a triangle demonstrates the interrelationship among the three disorders normally considered independent medical conditions.

illness, generally begins with medical treatment to address the physical destruction and to restore the body to a sufficient weight. This generally requires hospitalization. Once health is stabilized, the psychological factors underlying the anorexia nervosa need to be addressed through psychotherapy.

Initial treatment for bulimia nervosa or compulsive eating disorders involves the elimination of the eating pattern. Unlike anorexia nervosa, most bulimia nervosa and compulsive eating disorders do not require hospitalization. They do, however, require professional assistance to uncover the system of thinking that led to the disordered eating. Changing the thinking pattern is necessary for successful treatment.

Self-help and supports groups are extremely beneficial adjuncts to treatment by professionals. Family, friends, and support groups all play an important role in helping the person with disordered eating to start and maintain a treatment program.

Physical Activity and Health Connection

Healthy weight management includes a lifelong commitment to a healthy lifestyle. Two elements involved in attaining and maintaining a healthy body weight are eating a nutritious diet and performing regular physical activity. Adequate nutrition and decreased calorie intake are important goals of diet modification for decreasing body fatness. Sufficient physical activity is equally important because it expends excessive fat storage and enhances lean body mass. Moreover, physical activity offsets the harmful effects of a number of morbid conditions that are attributed to excessive body fat storage. The goals of physical activity related to achieving and maintaining a healthy body weight should be based on activities that are enjoyable and can be performed consistently.

concept connections

1. **Achieving and maintaining a healthy body weight has been identified as a major public health challenge in the United States.** Data show that based on the weight-for-height standards developed by the National Institutes of Health (NIH), two-thirds of adult Americans are now overweight, and that number continues to rise. These prevalence rates raise fear because of their implications for Americans' health. According to the NIH and the Centers for Disease Control and Prevention, being overweight or obese increases an individual's risk for developing over 35 major diseases.

2. **The body mass index (BMI) uses weight and height to produce a number that enables health professionals to gauge risk of weight-related illnesses.** The BMI criterion standards recommended by the National Heart, Lung, and Blood Institute Expert Panel on the Identification, Evaluation, and Treatment of Overweight and Obesity in Adults are as follows: underweight, BMI greater than 18.5; normal or healthy weight, BMI of 18.5 to 24.99; overweight or preobesity, BMI of 25.0 to 29.9; and class 1, 2, and 3 obesity, BMI of 30 to 34.99, 35 to 39.99, and 40.0 or greater, respectively. An adult BMI under 18.5 or 25.0 or greater may indicate health risk.

3. **Individuals with more upper body fat than lower body fat tend to have a more adverse metabolic profile and an increased risk for diabetes and cardiovascular disease, whereas lower body fat is less harmful in this respect.** More specifically, the fat inside the abdomen cavity surrounding the organs (visceral fat) contributes to metabolic abnormalities by producing chemicals and hormones that make a person more vulnerable to a number of obesity-related complications.

4. **A body composition analysis allows for the assessment of the percentage of fat versus the percentage of fat-free tissue.** Knowing one's body composition brings additional information to the screening profile. When body fat percentage is used in conjunction with BMI, it can help differentiate people who are overweight because of lean body mass from those who are overweight because of fat. Most important, the percentage of fat assists in predicting health risk. An ideal body fat percentage is one that meets your body's fundamental need for normal physiological functioning and energy needs but does not create health risks.

5. **Obesity is a complex disorder with multiple contributing factors.** There is no one cause of obesity. However, most cases of obesity occur now in people with normal physiology who live in a sociocultural environment characterized by a sedentary lifestyle and ready access to abundant food.

6. **A lifestyle approach that includes regular physical activity and a nutritious diet is essential in achieving and maintaining a healthy weight.** A lifestyle approach to weight maintenance focuses on developing a lifelong commitment to a way of life that achieves and maintains a healthy body composition relative to physical and psychological functioning. This approach requires a lifelong commitment to healthful behaviors that emphasize eating practices and regular physical activities that are sustainable and enjoyable. The goal of maintaining weight through lifestyle efforts is desirable for good physical and psychological health and to avoid the effects of creeping obesity or the negative consequences of repeated weight gains and losses.

7. **A negative sign of dissatisfaction with body weight, when basing it on the "ideal" weight portrayed by the mass media, is the development of eating disorders.** The term *eating disorders* refers to a wide range of harmful eating behaviors used in an attempt to lose weight or achieve a thin appearance. These dangerous behaviors range from severe restriction of food intake to binge eating and purging.

Terms

Overweight, 173
Obesity, 173
Essential body fat, 183
Storage fat, 183
Skinfold technique, 184
Underwater weighing, 184

Bioelectrical impedance, 185
Thermic effect of food (TEF),
  189
Thermic effect of activity (TEA),
  189
Set point theory, 191

Adipostat, 191
Body image, 198
Eating disorder, 199

making the connection

Melinda realizes that what is important is not a weight based on her self-image, but a weight based on healthy physical and psychological functioning. In recognizing these important differences she decides to have a body composition assessment completed. She schedules an appointment with the university wellness center, choosing the skinfold technique. Furthermore, she decides to make an appointment to discuss her self-image with the university's counseling center.

Critical Thinking

1. From the vignette, how would you assess Melinda's preoccupation with her weight? What factors influence her concerns about her weight? Do you believe she has an unhealthy obsession with her weight?

2. On your campus, identify and briefly describe the resources available for students regarding healthy weight management and eating disorders.

3. Your housemate, Joan, goes on a new fad diet that was recently reported by a respected national morning TV show. Joan reports that this new diet will allow her to lose 10 pounds by Saturday (6 days from now). Explain to Joan why this fad diet will not work, and if she were to lose the 10 pounds in 6 days, what would likely happen.

4. As a residence hall assistant (RA) you have been asked by your floor to talk about obesity and how as college freshmen they can manage their weight sensibly. In your talk discuss healthy weight, overweight and obesity, body mass index, and the importance of good nutrition and physical activity.

References

American Dietetic Association. (1993). Nutrition for physical fitness and athletic performance for adults: Position of ADA and the Canadian Dietetic Association, *Journal of the American Dietetic Association* 93:691–697.

American Psychiatric Association. (1994). *Diagnostic Criteria from DSM-IV*. Washington, DC: American Psychiatric Association.

Bennett, W.I. (1995). Beyond overeating [Editorial]. *New England Journal of Medicine* 332:621.

Bjorntorp, P., & Rosmond, R. (2000). Activity of the hypothalamic-pituitary-adrenal axis in different phenotypes. *International Journal of Obesity Related Metabolic Disorders* 24(Suppl. 2):S80–S85.

College of Family Physicians of Canada. (2004). Primary care-based physical activity and dietary counseling in the prevention and control of type 2 diabetes. Literature review. Online: http://www.cfpc.ca/English/cfpc/programs/patie nt%20care/type%202%20diabetes%20education/ literary%20review/default.asp?s=1.

Centers for Disease Control and Prevention. (2005a). Overweight and obesity: Health consequences. Online: http://www.cdc.gov/nccdphp/dnpa/ obesity/consequences.htm.

Centers for Disease Control and Prevention. (2005b). Obesity and genetics: A public health perspective. Online: http://www.cdc.gov/genomics/info/ perspectives/obesity.htm.

Dietz, W.H. (2004). Overweight in childhood and adolescence. *New England Journal of Medicine* 350:855–857.

Douketis, J., & Feldman, W. (1994). Prevention of obesity in adults. In *Canadian Guide to Clinical*

Preventive Health Care. Ottawa, Canada: Health Canada, 574–584.

Fine, J.T., Colditz, G.A., Coakley, E.H., et al. (1999). A prospective study of weight change and health-related quality of life in women. *Journal of the American Medical Association* 282:2136–2142.

Finkelstein, E., Fiebelkorn, I.C., & Wang, G. (2004). State-level estimates of annual medical expenditures attributable to obesity. *Obesity Research* 12:1824.

Fontaine, K., Redden, D., Wang, C., Westfall, A., & Allison, D. (2003). Years of life lost due to obesity. *Journal of the American Medical Association* 289:187–193.

Friedman, K.E., Reichmann, S.K., Costanzo, P.R., & Musante, G.J. (2002). Body image partially mediates the relationship between obesity and psychological distress. *Obesity Research* 10(1):33–41.

Greenberg, B.S., Eastin, M., Hofschire, L., Lachlan, K., & Brownell, K.D. (2003). Portrayals of overweight and obese individuals on commercial television. *American Journal of Public Health* 93:1342–1348.

Harnack, L.J. (2000). Temporal trends in energy intake in the United States: An ecologic perspective. *American Journal of Clinical Nutrition* 71:1478–1484.

Hedley, A.A., Ogden, C.L., Johnson, C.L., Carroll, M.D., Curtin, L.R., & Flegal, K.M. (2004). Prevalence of overweight and obesity among U.S. children, adolescents and adults, 1999–2002. *Journal of the American Medical Association* 29:2847–2850.

Jambekar, S., Quinn, D.M., & Crocker, J. (2001). Effects of weight and achievement primes on the self-esteem of college women. *Psychology of Women Quarterly* 25:48–56.

Kleiner, S.M. (1998). *Power Eating*. Champaign, IL: Human Kinetics.

Latner, J.D., Stunkard, A.J., & Wilson, G.T. (2005). Stigmatized students: Age, sex, and ethnicity effects in the stigmatization of obesity. *Obesity Research* 13(7):1226–1231.

Lean, M.E., Han, T.S., & Seidell, J.C. (1999). Impairment of health and quality of life using new U.S. federal guidelines for the identification of obesity. *Archives of Internal Medicine* 159:837–843.

Lemieux, I., Pascot, A., Couillard, C., Lamarche, B., Tchernof, A., Almeras, N., et al. (2000). Hypertriglyceridemic waist: A marker of the atherogenic metabolic triad (hyperinsulinemia; hyperapolipoprotein B; small, dense LDL) in men. *Circulation* 102(2):179–184.

Lohman, T.G. (1992). *Advances in Body Composition Assessment*. Champaign, IL: Human Kinetics.

Mcinnis, K.J., Franklin, B.A., & Rippe, J.M. (2003). Counseling for physical activity in overweight and obese patients. *American Family Physician* 67:1249–1256.

National Institute of Diabetes and Digestive and Kidney Diseases. (2004). Statistics related to overweight and obesity: The economic costs. Online: http://www.win.niddk.nih.gov/statistics/index.htm.

National Institute of Diabetes and Digestive and Kidney Diseases. (2005). Do you know the health risks of being overweight? Online: http://win.niddk.nih.gov/publications/health_risks.htm.

National Heart, Lung, and Blood Institute. (2000). *The Practical Guide, Identification, Evaluation, and Treatment of Overweight and Obesity in Adults* (NIH Publication No. 00-4084). Washington, DC: U.S. Department of Health and Human Services.

National Institute of Mental Health. (2001). *Eating Disorders: Facts About Eating Disorders and the Search for Solutions* (NIH Publication No. 01-4901). Bethesda, MD: National Institutes of Health.

Puhl, R., & Brownell, K.D. (2001). Bias, discrimination and obesity. *Obesity Research* 9:788–805.

Sclafani, A. (1996). Dietary obesity. In Stunkard, A. J., Wadden, T.A., eds. *Obesity Theory and Therapy*, 2nd ed. New York: Raven Press.

Seccareccia, F., Lanti, M., Menotti, A., et al. (1998). Role of body mass index in the prediction of all cause mortality in over 62,000 men and women. The Italian RIFLE pooling project. *Journal of Epidemiology and Community Health* 52:20–26.

Slentz, C.A., Aiken, L.B., Hounmard, J.A., Bales, C.W., Johnson, J.L., Tanner, C.J., Duscha, B.D., & Kraus, W.E. (2005). Inactivity, exercise, and visceral fat. STRRIDE: A randomized, controlled study of exercise intensity and amount. *Journal of Applied Physiology* 99:1613–1618.

Thompson, D., Eldelsberg, J., Graham, A.C., et al. (1999). Lifetime health and economic consequences of obesity. *Archives of Internal Medicine* 159:2177–2183.

United States Department of Health and Human Services. (2001). *The Surgeon General's Call to Action to Prevent and Decrease Overweight and Obesity*. Washington, DC: U.S. Government Printing Office.

Weinsier, R.L., Hunter, G.R., Heini, A.F., Goran, M.I., & Sell, S.M. (1998). The etiology of obesity: Relative contribution of metabolic factors, diet, and physical activity. *American Journal of Medicine* 105:145–150.

Wildman, R.C., & Miller, B.S. (2004). *Sports and Fitness Nutrition*. Belmont, CA: Thompson and Wadsworth.

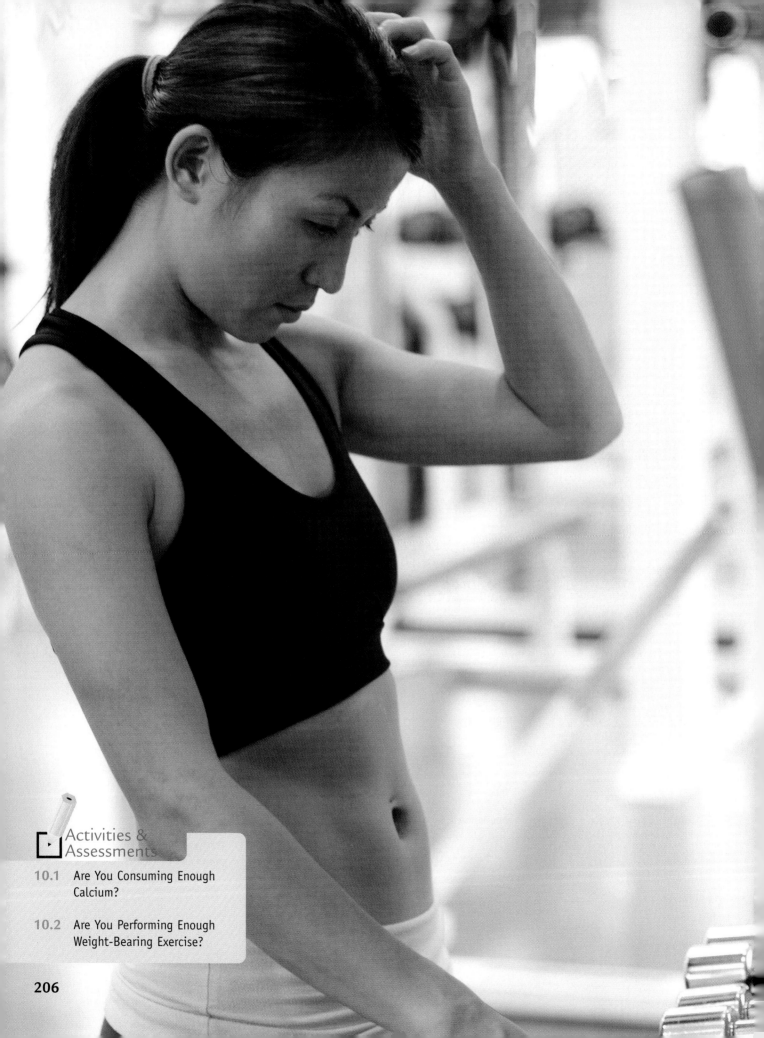

Activities &
Assessments

10.1   Are You Consuming Enough
       Calcium?

10.2   Are You Performing Enough
       Weight-Bearing Exercise?

206

Achieving Optimal Bone Health

what's the connection?

Julie is a sophomore in college and is concerned about her skeletal health. Her biggest concern is developing osteoporosis, a chronic metabolic disease that causes excessive skeletal weakness and increases her chance for developing bone fractures later in life. Julie watched her grandmother suffer from a broken hip as a result of osteoporosis and therefore is quite aware of its crippling effects. Julie pays close attention to her diet, making sure to fulfill her daily requirements of calcium and vitamin D. Moreover, she has recently been reading about the importance of physical activity and its role in preventing osteoporosis. Julie is interested in "making the connection" by beginning a safe and effective physical activity program to build and maintain a strong skeletal system.

concepts

1. Bones do more than provide structural support; they protect vital organs and support essential metabolic processes.

2. Three types of cells are involved in bone formation and resorption: osteoblasts, osteocytes, and osteoclasts.

3. To maintain bone mass, bone formation must occur at the same rate as bone resorption.

4. Physical activity enhances bone density through both weight-bearing and resistance-training exercises.

5. Osteoporosis is a chronic disease process characterized by progressive bone loss for both males and females.

6. Osteoporosis can be affected by genetic, hormonal, nutritional, and lifestyle factors.

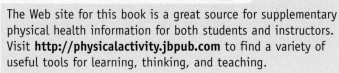

http://physicalactivity.jbpub.com

The Web site for this book is a great source for supplementary physical health information for both students and instructors. Visit **http://physicalactivity.jbpub.com** to find a variety of useful tools for learning, thinking, and teaching.

Paget's disease A disease whose precise cause is unknown but that is a consequence of both genetic and environmental factors, such as a viral infection that triggers the osteoblasts to try to repair the damage (infection) by forming new bone. However, the new formation is disrupted, leading to weakness and deformities in the bone.

Osteogenesis imperfecta A disease caused by abnormalities in the collagen matrix within the bone, resulting in a weak structure and the potential for multiple fractures.

Rickets A deficiency of vitamin D (usually seen in children), causing weak bones and deformation due to overgrowth of cartilage at the ends of the bones. In adults, this condition leads to softening of the bone, leading to fracture and deformity.

Bones do more than provide structural support; they protect vital organs and support essential metabolic processes.

Cartilage Semi-rigid tissue that provides support.

Collagen The principle substance in connecting fibers and tissues, and in bones.

Resorption The loss of substance (bone, in this case) through physiological or pathological means.

Osteoblasts Bone-forming cells.

Osteocytes A bone cell responsible for the maintenance and turnover of the mineral content of surrounding bone.

Osteoclasts A cell in developing bone concerned especially with the breaking down of unnecessary bone parts.

Introduction

Structural strength and energy are necessary contributors to a healthy and active lifestyle from childhood into old age. To live well, one must not only practice positive cardiovascular fitness and nutrition habits but must also strive to maintain optimal bone health. Like many of our body's systems, the bones can be affected by disease. A common bone disease affecting many Americans is osteoporosis, which will be discussed in detail later in the chapter. Although many therapeutic advances are now available to prevent and treat some bone disorders, there are others that are more difficult to avoid, such as **Paget's disease**, **osteogenesis imperfecta**, and **rickets**, which can lead to a downward spiral in physical health and quality of life, including losing the ability to walk, stand up, or even dress yourself (U.S. Department of Health and Human Services [USDHHS], 2004b). Fortunately, there is a great deal that we can do to contribute to our own bone health. Practicing the behaviors of healthy nutrition, daily physical activity, and regular medical screenings, Americans of all ages can maintain strong bones and healthier lives. This chapter reviews the structure and formation of bone, the nutritional and physical activity recommendations for preserving healthy bones, and the effects of aging and metabolic changes on bone health.

Understanding Bone Physiology

Beyond the structural support provided by the skeleton, some of the bones (ribs, skull) protect our vital internal organs (heart, lungs, brain). Bone also plays a major role in daily metabolic processes: bones produce cells that contribute to the formation of red and white blood cells and platelets, store fat needed for cellular energy production, and both release and absorb calcium to regulate blood levels.

Bone Structure

Bone and cartilage are forms of connective tissue in the human body. **Cartilage** is a semi-rigid connective tissue that provides firm, flexible support. Bone is a more specialized and harder form of connective tissue (Rhoades & Pflanzer, 1996). Healthy bone is light, rigid, of high tensile strength, and not brittle (Ng, Romas, Donnan, & Findlay, 1997). As fetal development begins, the skeleton is made entirely of cartilage. This cartilaginous framework serves as the template for the bone to come later. Mature bone (**FIGURE 10.1**) consists of inorganic bone minerals, calcium, and phosphate precipitates that are incorporated into the organic support material known as osteoid. **Collagen** makes up 95 percent of the osteoid substance (Rhoades & Pflanzer, 1996).

BONE CELLS   Three types of cells are involved both in bone formation and in **resorption** of mature bone: osteoblasts, osteocytes, and osteoclasts.

   Osteoblasts are immature bone cells that deposit new bone around the outside of the bone. When they are surrounded by mineralized bone, they become mature bone cells and are then called **osteocytes**. **Osteoclasts** digest, or absorb, bony tissue. They remove old bone tissue so that its components can be absorbed into the circulation. This process is known as resorption.

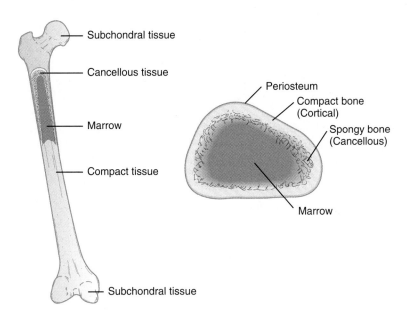

FIGURE 10.1 **Bone and Its Parts.**

Bone Formation

Although the diameter of bones can change throughout our lifetimes, bones grow in length only while the skeleton develops; this growth usually ends in adolescence. Longitudinal bone growth occurs at the ends of long bones at the epiphyseal plate (Ackermann, 1992). The epiphyseal plate is where cartilage synthesis and bone replacement form an area of active growth. Chrondrocytes, or chondroblasts (cells like osteoblasts), synthesize the cartilage. Bone replacement, by osteoblasts, begins in the center of the cartilage and proceeds outward (Rhoades & Pflanzer, 1996). This process of bone formation occurs in layers. As chondrocytes are surrounded and trapped by the cartilage, new chondrocytes replace them on top of the cartilage for continued synthesis of the collagen matrix. The cartilage calcifies, the chondrocytes begin to die off, and the calcified material begins to erode. Osteoblasts move into the area and begin bone replacement. This continuous activity of cartilage synthesis, calcification, erosion, and osteoblast invasion forms the zone of active bone formation (Rhoades & Pflanzer, 1996).

Chondrocyte activity is greatly influenced by hormones. Growth hormone is considered the major stimulus to bone growth and is an important regulator in the growth of young children. Around puberty, the epiphyseal plates of long bones begin to stop responding to hormonal stimulus (Rhoades & Pflanzer, 1996). When adult height is reached, the epiphyseal plate is sealed from the marrow by a thin plate of bone (Ackermann, 1992). Bone formation is now complete, and the process of bone remodeling begins.

Bone Remodeling

Bone, like the kidneys and heart, is a live tissue that continually remodels itself to maintain **bone mineral density (BMD)** and to repair small damage (microtrauma) and large damage (fractures) that may occur over time. Most individuals reach peak bone mass around the age of 28, at which time BMD is then maintained by a process called **remodeling** (Endocrine Web, 2006).

Remodeling involves the breaking down or removing of old bone (resorption) by osteoclasts, which are large, active cells that live in the central portion of the bone. This is followed up by the activity of cells called osteoblasts, which assist

Three types of cells are involved in bone formation and resorption: osteoblasts, osteocytes, and osteoclasts.

Bone mineral density (BMD) Usually expressed as the amount of mineralized tissue in the scanned area, it is a risk factor for fractures.

Remodeling The ongoing dual processes of bone formation and bone resorption after cessation of growth.

To maintain bone mass, bone formation must occur at the same rate as bone resorption.

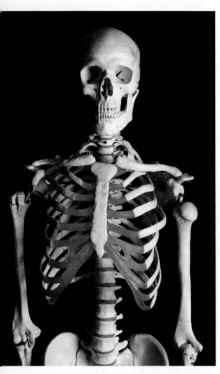

The human skeleton consists of 206 bones. These bones support your body and allow you to move.

Physical activity at all ages is essential to improve and maintain bone health.

with new bone formation. Basically, as long as everything does its job, the rate of breakdown and buildup maintains itself, and BMD remains optimal. However, any factor that causes greater bone removal than bone building leads to a loss of bone mass, simply because new bone formation can't keep up. This is what accounts for the gradual loss of bone density as a person ages and results in more fragile bones (Endocrine Web, 2006).

This lifelong remodeling process preserves the mechanical integrity of the skeleton. The adult skeleton undergoes bone remodeling 24 hours a day, 7 days a week. Remodeling is under the control of a number of hormones, including estrogens, androgens, vitamin D, and the parathyroid hormone, which regulates calcium levels in the blood (Cosman, 2005).

The same factors that encourage bone formation as a young adult affect the maintenance of bone mass during adult years. The most important influences are calcium intake, reproductive hormone status, normal parathyroid gland function, and physical activity. We will take a look in this chapter at how these influences affect the health of your skeleton.

Nutrition and Physical Activity for Bone Health

To achieve optimal bone health, and to continue to build new bone as you get older, good nutrition and consistent physical activity are necessary.

Nutritional Recommendations

Good nutrition is not only critical for strong bones but also for proper functioning of the heart, muscles, and nerves. It is important to eat a well-balanced diet containing a variety of foods. Nutrients that are key for bone health are calcium and vitamins D and C.

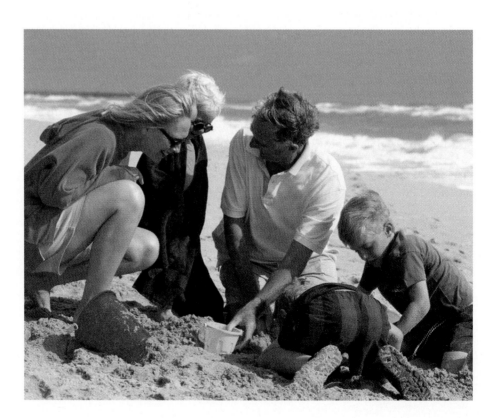

TABLE 10.1	Daily Calcium Requirements by Age and Sex

Age and Gender	Adequate Daily Intake of Calcium (mg)
Infants, male or female, 0–6 months	210
Infants, male or female, 7–12 months	270
Children, male or female, 1–3 years	500
Children, male or female, 4–8 years	800
Males and females, 9–18 years	1300
Males and females,* 19–50	1000
Males and females,† 51 years and older	1200
Pregnant or lactating female, 14–18 years	1300
Pregnant or lactating female, 19–50 years	1000

*If you are female and in menopause, you should increase your calcium intake to 1200 mg.

†Some clinicians recommend 1500 mg of calcium per day for postmenopausal women.

SOURCE: I.M. Alexander. (2006). *100 Questions and Answers About Osteoporosis and Osteopenia*. Sudbury, MA: Jones and Bartlett, 95.

CALCIUM INTAKE   Calcium balance is important for achieving peak bone mass and maintaining bone mass throughout your life. Although calcium alone will not prevent osteoporosis, it is considered an essential ingredient in the diet regardless of gender or age, and may be particularly beneficial for children, adolescents, and young adults to ensure maximal bone density at maturity (National Osteoporosis Foundation [NOF], 2005a). Yet, many Americans do not consume enough calcium. Let's take a closer look at just how much calcium an individual needs in his or her diet.

The Food and Nutrition Board of the Institute of Medicine (IOM) updated its recommended amounts for calcium in 1997. (TABLE 10.1) lists adequate intakes of important bone nutrients. These recommendations differ by age group and are intended for healthy individuals. The highest amount of calcium (1300 mg per day) is recommended for children and adolescents because this is a period of rapid bone growth and maturational development. Also shown in Table 10.1 are age-appropriate calcium intakes for pregnant and lactating women. It is important to realize that too much of a good thing can also be detrimental. The IOM defines the safe upper limit of calcium as 2500 mg per day without increasing the risk of adverse side effects (USDHHS, 2004a).

CALCIUM SOURCES   How do you obtain calcium in your daily diet? Many Americans obtain a majority of their calcium by consuming common dairy products such as milk, cheese, and yogurt. Most adults can meet the recommended requirements by drinking three 8-ounce glasses of milk each day in combination with the calcium obtained in their normal daily diet. Low-fat and nonfat dairy products are good choices because of their reduced fat content. Other favorable selections are foods that are fortified with calcium, such as cereal, nonfat milk, and orange juice (USDHHS, 2004a). Fruits, vegetables, and grains also provide calcium, but the amount of calcium absorbed varies by the food type. For example, it would take almost 8 cups of spinach to yield the same amount of calcium found in 1 cup of milk (USDHHS, 2004a).

For individuals who find it difficult to achieve optimal calcium intake from their daily dietary habits, calcium supplements may be necessary to meet the needed requirements. Two commonly available supplements are calcium carbonate and calcium citrate. Those who take supplements should note that:

- All major forms of calcium are best taken with meals.
- Calcium from supplements is best taken in small doses (500–600 mg at one time).
- Supplements may differ in their absorbability due to manufacturing practices (IOM, 1997).
- All calcium sources—food or supplement—reduce the absorption of iron, so calcium and iron supplements should be taken at different times (USDHHS, 2004a).

To assist in planning a diet containing adequate levels of calcium, TABLE 10.2 provides a list of sources and the percent daily value of calcium they contain.

LACTOSE INTOLERANCE   In some cases, an individual's digestive system may lack the enzyme, lactose, needed to break down milk sugar when consumed, making them lactose intolerant and incapable of ingesting dairy products without intestinal distress. TABLE 10.3 suggests alternative methods for acquiring adequate levels of calcium.

VITAMIN D   Vitamin D is essential to the absorption of calcium and bone health. The link between calcium absorption and vitamin D is comparable to that of a locked door and a key. Vitamin D is the key that unlocks the door and allows calcium to leave the intestine and enter the bloodstream. Vitamin D also helps the kidneys resorb calcium that would otherwise be excreted in the urine. Adults should consume approximately 200 IU per day of vitamin D and may safely take in up to about 1000 IU per day if needed.

There are two sources of vitamin D: sunlight and dietary intake. Most individuals can obtain adequate levels of vitamin D through exposure to sunlight in the warmer months or exposure of the hands, arms, and face to sunlight for 10 to 15 minutes, two to three times a week. This method is not practical for others, who will therefore need to increase their levels of vitamin D through their diet. Primary food sources include fortified milk and cereals, egg yolk, and fish oils (USDHHS, 2004a). To help you make the right choices and obtain the correct amounts, see TABLE 10.4.

BONE ROBBERS   You need not only be aware of nutrients that build strong bones but must also be aware of substances that deplete nutrients from your body, referred to as "bone robbers" (McIlwain & Bruce, 1998). Common bone robbers are sodium, protein, and caffeine. A diet high in sodium and protein may cause increased urinary loss and a negative calcium balance. Coffees and colas containing caffeine may be bone robbers of concern today. A diet with a high caffeine intake also causes loss of bone calcium. Recent studies suggest that excessive caffeine intake may contribute to osteoporosis.

Physical Activity Recommendations

Physical activity should be engaged in throughout a lifetime to promote overall health as well as bone integrity. The foundation of a physical activity regimen for overall health involves following the Surgeon General's report on Physical Activity and Health, which recommends a "minimum of 30 minutes of physical activity of moderate intensity (such as brisk walking) on most, if not all days of the week" (USDHHS 1996).

Many studies have investigated the role of physical activity and bone health and reported that physical activity is necessary for bone acquisition and mainte-

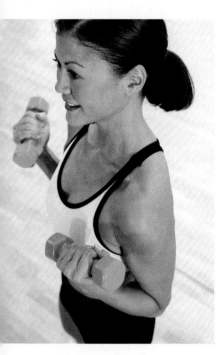

Weight-bearing activity is key for maintaining bone density.

Physical activity enhances bone density through both weight-bearing and resistance-training exercises.

TABLE 10.2	Selected Food Sources of Calcium	
Food	Calcium (mg)	% Daily Value
Sardines, canned in oil, with bones, 3 oz	324	32
Cheddar cheese, 1½ oz shredded	306	31
Milk, nonfat, 8 fl oz	302	30
Yogurt, plain, low fat, 8 oz	300	30
Milk, reduced fat (2% milk fat), no solids, 8 fl oz	297	30
Milk, whole (3.25% milk fat), 8 fl oz	291	29
Milk, buttermilk, 8 fl oz	285	29
Milk, lactose reduced, 8 fl oz	285–302	20–30
(content varies slightly according to fat content, average = 300 mg)		
Cottage cheese, 1% milk fat, 2 cups unpacked	276	28
Mozzarella, part skim, 1½ oz	275	28
Tofu, firm, with calcium, ½ cup	204	20
Orange juice, calcium fortified, 6 fl oz	200–260	20–26
Salmon, pink, canned, solids with bone, 3 oz	181	18
Pudding, chocolate, instant, made with 2% milk, ½ cup	153	15
Tofu, soft, with calcium, ½ cup	138	14
Breakfast drink, orange flavor, powder prepared with water, 8 fl oz	133	13
Frozen yogurt, vanilla, soft serve, ½ cup	103	10
Ready-to-eat cereal, calcium fortified, 1 cup	100–1000	10–100
Turnip greens, boiled, ½ cup	99	10
Kale, raw, 1 cup	90	9
Kale, cooked, 1 cup	94	9
Ice cream, vanilla, ½ cup	85	8.5
Soy beverage, calcium fortified, 8 fl oz	80–500	8–50
Chinese cabbage, raw, 1 cup	74	7
Tortilla, corn, ready to bake/fry, 1 medium	42	4
Tortilla, flour, ready to bake/fry, one 6" diameter	37	4
Sour cream, reduced fat, cultured, 2 Tbsp	32	3
Bread, white, 1 oz	31	3
Broccoli, raw, ½ cup	21	2
Bread, whole wheat, 1 slice	20	2
Cheese, cream, regular, 1 Tbsp	12	1

SOURCES: U.S. Department of Agriculture, Agricultural Research Service. (2002). *USDA Nutrient Database for Standard Reference, Release 15*. Online: http://www.nal.usda.gov/fnic/foodcomp; and R.P. Heaney, M.S. Dowell, K. Rafferty, and J. Bierman. (2000). Bioavailability of the calcium in fortified soy imitation milk, with some observations on method. *American Journal of Clinical Nutrition* 71(5):1166–1169.

nance throughout adulthood. Physical activity plays an important role in benefiting bone health specifically because bone mass is responsive to mechanical loads (stress) placed on the skeleton. In other words, bone becomes stronger and denser when you place demands on it, such as when you play a game of tennis or jump rope. Two types of exercise are important for increasing and maintaining bone density: weight-bearing and resistance-training exercises (NOF, 2005b). Weight-bearing exercises include activities in which your muscles and bones work against gravity or in which your lower body bears your body weight. Jogging, walking, and stair climbing are good examples of common weight-bearing activities. Safe and effective resistance-training exercises can be found in Chapter 11. Your muscles must be challenged by using weight resistance to improve muscle and bone

TABLE 10.3	Tips for Those with Lactose Intolerance

- Seek out and choose dairy and other calcium-rich foods with lower amounts of lactose. Alternative choices might include yogurt with live cultures (which provide bacterial lactase that digests the lactose); hard cheeses like cheddar, Colby, Swiss, and parmesan (the production process for these cheeses breaks down the lactose); and lactose-free or lactose-reduced products (including milk without lactose).
- Gradually increase the amount of lactose-containing foods consumed over a period of weeks to develop the capability to digest lactose.
- Consume nondairy products that contain high levels of calcium, such as fortified soy products or fortified cereal or orange juice.

SOURCE: U.S. Department of Health and Human Services. (2004). *Bone Health and Osteoporosis: A Report of the Surgeon General*, Chapter 7, p. 7. Rockville, MD: U.S. Department of Health and Human Services, Office of the Surgeon General.

strength. Evidence suggests that the skeleton responds proactively to resistance training and short bouts of high-load impact, such as jumping for the lower body and weight lifting for the upper body. These types of activities can promote the building of muscle mass as well as the promotion of balance and coordination.

Unfortunately, research has yet to establish a specific set of exercises for improving bone health, but instead offers a set of principles to follow:

- Physical activity will only affect bone at the skeletal sites that are stressed (or loaded) by the activity.
- For bone gain to occur, the stimulus must be greater than that which the bone usually experiences. Static loads applied to muscle (such as standing) do not promote increased bone mass.

Good nutrition is essential for optimal bone health.

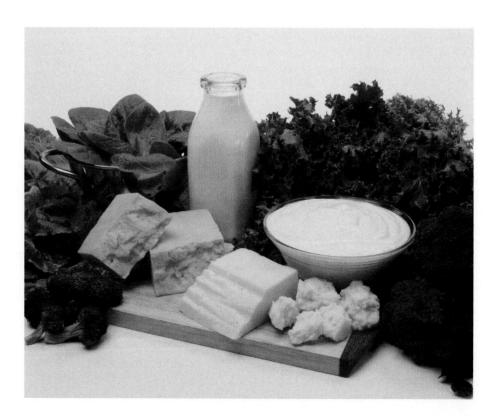

TABLE 10.4	Dietary Sources of Vitamin D	
Food	Serving Size	Vitamin D (IU)
Milk	1 cup	98
Baked herring	3 oz	1775
Baked salmon	3 oz	238
Canned tuna	3 oz	136
Sardines	1 oz	77
Raisin bran cereal	¾ cup	42
Pork sausage	1 oz	31
Egg yolk	1	25

SOURCE: U.S. Department of Agriculture, Agricultural Research Service. (2002). *USDA Nutrient Database for Standard Reference, Release 15*. Online: http://www.nal.usda.gov/fnic/foodcomp.

- Complete lack of activity (immobility, paralysis, bed rest) causes bone loss.
- General physical activity most days of the week, coupled with weight-bearing, strength-building, and balance-enhancing activities two or more times a week, is effective for promoting bone health in most people.
- Any activity that causes impact (e.g., jumping or skipping) may increase bone mass more than low- to moderate-intensity endurance-type activities.
- Load-bearing physical activities (e.g., jumping) need not be engaged in for long periods of time to provide benefits to skeletal health. Five to ten minutes of physical activity that incorporates 50 three-inch jumps per day should suffice for most adults.
- Physical activities should include a variety of loading patterns to promote increased bone mass. Be creative in finding ways to add other weight-bearing activities to your daily life. See TABLE 10.5 for a list of weight-bearing exercises for adults.
- Consult a physician or physical therapist if orthopedic conditions or other medical conditions make these physical activity guidelines difficult or unsafe to follow.

Osteoporosis

Osteoporosis, literally meaning "porous bones," is a metabolic disease characterized by excessive skeletal fragility, as noted earlier. Bone loss is so common that most people consider it a normal process of aging. However, osteoporosis is a preventable and unnecessary occurrence in most individuals (USDHHS, 2004a).

The onset of osteoporosis occurs most often in women after menopause. As the U.S. population ages, the incidence of osteoporosis will increase, with a subsequent increase in cost to the health care industry. Since osteoporosis is a painful and debilitating disease that can impact a person's quality of life, prevention and early treatment are important issues for all ages. Some changes in bone health are considered permanent; therefore, prevention becomes the primary "cure" for osteoporosis (FIGURE 10.2).

Postmenopausal osteoporotic individuals undergo a high rate of bone turnover. Osteoblastic activity cannot meet the rate of osteoclastic bone resorption. Bones are thin and brittle due to the loss of mineralization. The decreased bone

Osteoporosis is a chronic disease process characterized by progressive bone loss for both males and females.

Osteoporosis Literally means "porous bones"; a metabolic disease resulting in bone loss and bones that fracture easily.

TABLE 10.5	Weight-Bearing Exercise for Adults

Weight-Bearing, High-Impact, and/or Resistance Activities
Stair climbing
Hiking
Dancing
Jogging
Downhill and cross-country skiing
Aerobic dancing
Volleyball
Basketball
Gymnastics
Weight lifting or resistance training
Soccer
Jumping rope

Weight-Bearing, Low-Impact Activities
Walking
Treadmill walking
Cross-country ski machines
Stair-step machines
Rowing machines
Water aerobics
Deep-water walking
Low-impact aerobics

Minimal Weight-Bearing, Nonimpact Activities
Lap swimming
Indoor cycling
Stretching or flexibility exercises (avoid forward-bending exercises)
Yoga
Pilates

SOURCE: National Osteoporosis Foundation. (2003). *Boning Up on Osteoporosis: A Guide to Prevention and Treatment*. Washington, DC: Author.

FIGURE 10.2 **Osteoporosis.** Microscopically, normal bone (top) is much stronger than osteoporotic bone (bottom).

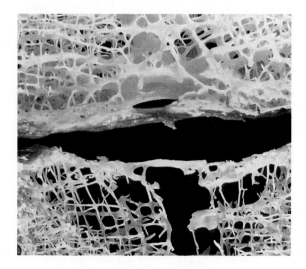

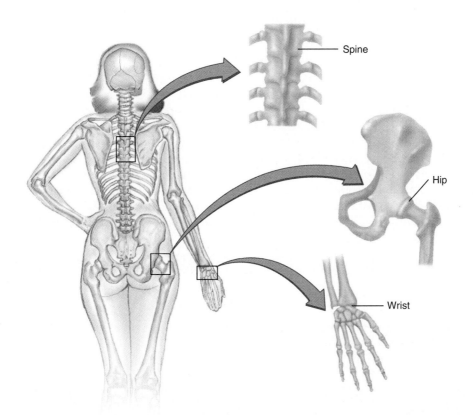

FIGURE 10.3 **Postmenopausal Risk for Fracture.** The wrist, spine, and hip are easily fractured in someone with osteoporosis.

Spine

Hip

Wrist

mass puts the individual at an increased risk for fracture, most often fractures of the hip, spine, and wrist (FIGURE 10.3).

The annual cost of osteoporosis in the United States is estimated to be $18 billion. Currently, 10 million Americans are affected, and 34 million more have low bone mass, placing them at risk for osteoporosis. This cost of osteoporosis is expected to increase over the next decade due to the overall aging of the population. Part of the cost of osteoporosis is related to the morbidity of the disease. Only 50 percent of individuals who suffer a hip fracture are able to return home or live independently after injury, and the estimated cost of hip fractures could reach $240 billion by the year 2040 (USDHHS, 2004a).

Osteoporosis affects both men and women; however, 80 percent of those affected are women. While postmenopausal women may exhibit bone loss due to estrogen deficiency, men entering their older years may develop osteoporosis due to testosterone deficiency. Men may be treated with testosterone therapy; however, this treatment puts them at risk for enlargement of the prostate (Francis, 1999).

Since osteoporosis is often not diagnosed until fractures occur, prevention is considered the most cost-effective approach. Prevention focuses on two main objectives: (1) achieving optimal bone density in the first two to three decades of life, and (2) maintaining bone density and decreasing rate of bone loss in later years. Physical activity and good nutrition are key elements in meeting these preventive strategies.

Osteoporosis can be affected by genetic, hormonal, nutritional, and lifestyle factors.

Risk Factors

The many risk factors that influence osteoporosis (TABLE 10.6) can be grouped into four categories: genetic, hormonal, nutritional, and lifestyle factors.

GENETIC FACTORS Race, heredity, and gender influence bone fragility. Typically, white and Asian women are at greater risk for developing osteoporosis and related fractures; Hispanic and black women have greater bone mineral density (BMD) and are at less risk for developing osteoporosis (however, they are still at some risk). In addition, women with a family history of osteoporosis are considered to be at increased risk. Daughters of women with spinal fractures generally have lower BMD in the spine. Although most research has focused on the mother's history of osteoporosis, research shows that the father's history is also important. Furthermore, women with relatives who have a dowager's hump (FIGURE 10.4) or

TABLE 10.6	Risk Factors for Fracture

Older age (>65 years)

Fracture after age 45

First-degree female relative with a fracture in adulthood

Self-report health as "fair" or "poor"

Current tobacco use

Weight less than 127 lbs.

Menopause prior to age 45 years

Amenorrhea

Lifelong low calcium intake

Excess alcohol consumption

Poor vision despite correction

Falls

Minimal weight-bearing exercise

Medical conditions

   Hyperthyroidism

   Chronic lung disease

   Endometriosis

   Malignancy

   Chronic hepatic or renal disease

   Hyperparathryoidism

   Vitamin D deficiency

   Cushing's disease

   Multiple sclerosis

   Sarcoidosis

   Hemochromatosis

Medications

   Oral glucocorticoids

   Excess thyroxine replacement

   Antiepileptic medications

   Gonadal hormone suppression

   Immunosuppressive agents

SOURCE: U.S. Department of Health and Human Services. (2004). *Bone Health and Osteoporosis: A Report of the Surgeon General,* Chapter 10. Rockville, MD: U.S. Department of Health and Human Services, Office of the Surgeon General.

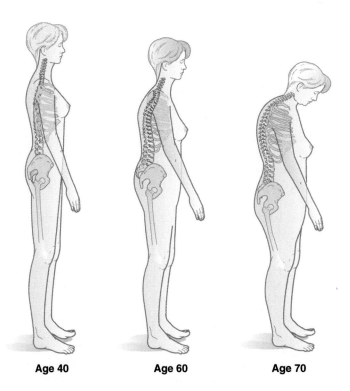

Age 40   **Age 60**   **Age 70**

FIGURE 10.4 **Progression of Dowager's Hump.** Women with postmenopausal osteoporosis tend to experience numerous fractures in the bones of their spine (vertebrae) as they age. Eventually these vertebrae can collapse, causing the spine to curve. Such curvature causes loss of height, a tilted rib cage, a dowager's hump, and a protruding abdomen.

have incurred low-trauma fractures have a positive family history of osteoporosis (USDHHS, 2004a).

Gender also plays a major role in bone fragility. The prevalence of osteoporosis and related fractures is substantially greater in women than in men. This is a result of lower bone mass and bone density among women. Why? Men have larger skeletons, their bone loss starts later in life and progresses more slowly, and they do not experience menopause.

HORMONAL FACTORS Hormonal status greatly influences bone fragility, and menstrual history is a key component. Risk of bone fragility also increases for women after menopause because bone loss accelerates with reduction in estrogen production (Cosman, 2005). Hormonal changes of menopause cause the loss of about 11 percent of bone during the first 5 years after menopause and an additional 5 percent during the next 20 years (Nordin et al., 1990). Men with hypogonadism are at special risk for bone loss. (Hypogonadism is a failure of the testes to function normally. It is treated with replacement testosterone therapy.)

Amenorrhea is a condition associated with BMD that may result from excessive exercise or eating disorders. Achieving high bone mineral density is critical during adolescence, but amenorrhea lowers estrogen levels, which can cause a loss of bone mass and increase the risk of osteoporosis later in life. Amenorrhea in young women is of concern because achieving peak bone mass in the second and third decades seems to be an important indicator for lifetime fracture risk. Although physical activity may affect estrogen hormone levels and indirectly affect bone density, low body fat is more likely the culprit.

Estrogen and other sex hormones have been reported to stimulate osteoblastic activity weakly. Estrogens are female sex hormones that are responsible for the development and maintenance of a woman's secondary sex characteristics (development of breasts, for example), and following menstruation, estrogens stimulate the rebuilding of the uterine lining. Ovaries are the primary source of estrogen. Estrogens are probably the most important hormone controlling bone mass loss.

Amenorrhea Absence of menstrual periods.

Estrogens inhibit bone resorption by modifying osteoclast function. Estrogen replacement therapy is one treatment used to prevent the onset of osteoporosis; however, its many side effects make it an unpopular treatment for many women (USDHHS, 2004a).

A condition referred to as *female athlete triad* is chronic overexercising accompanied by disordered eating, amenorrhea, and osteoporosis (Beck & Shoemaker, 2000). Chronic overexercising has been associated with reduced bone mass in premenopausal women. The overexercising and unbalanced diet disrupts the body's hormones enough to impair the influence of estrogens on the skeletal system. Despite the weight-bearing exercise, the lack of estrogen accelerates bone resorption and bone loss.

NUTRITIONAL FACTORS   As noted earlier, a general well-balanced diet is recommended, with special attention to adequate calcium, vitamin C, and vitamin D.

LIFESTYLE FACTORS   Another risk factor for osteoporosis is physical inactivity. Prolonged inactivity decreases bone mass. Regular exercise has been shown to stimulate bone formation and retard bone mass reduction. Studies also support the principle that weight-bearing exercise can promote and preserve bone strength (USDHHS, 2004a).

Use of cigarettes, alcohol, and certain medications (for example, long-term use of glucocorticoids in treating arthritis, asthma, lupus, and other diseases of the lungs, kidneys, and liver) also affects bone mass negatively. Women who smoke cigarettes experience an earlier menopause, a higher incidence of vertebral compression fractures, a decreased bone mineral density, and a lower urinary estrogen level. Alcohol abuse, a lifestyle factor, has devastating effects on bone mass. On average, alcoholics exhibit low BMD and a subsequent increased risk of fracture (Wardlaw, 1993). First, alcohol is thought to depress bone formation by directly reducing osteoblastic activity. Second, dietary intakes of heavy drinkers are often lacking in essential nutrients. Finally, alcohol intoxication gives rise to social situations that favor accidents and falls (USDHHS, 2004a).

Prevention and Detection of Osteoporosis

Osteoporosis diagnosis often begins with a thorough physical examination, which includes an oral history, recording of complaints of height loss, a review of overall nutrition and medication intake, and observations of stature, carriage, and spine curvature (Woodhead & Moss, 1998) (**FIGURE 10.5**). Spinal osteoporosis is often characterized by loss of stature.

BONE MINERAL DENSITY TESTS   BMD tests measure bone density in various body sites: the hip, spine, wrist, finger, kneecap, shinbone, and heel (**FIGURE 10.6**). A bone density test can detect osteoporosis before a fracture occurs, predict your risk of fracturing in the future, determine your rate of bone loss and monitor the effect of treatment. The test is conducted at intervals of 1 year.

The BMD tests vary in the type of bone measured (trabecular, cortical, or both), precision (deviation based on multiple measurements, generally represented on a percentage basis as a coefficient of variation), accuracy (variation in quality of bone measured versus real content of bone), and radiation dose (Black et al., 1992) (TABLE 10.7).

What do your BMD test results mean? A normal bone density is called a "T-score." This means you have the bone density of a normal young adult and have no risk for fractures. The World Health Organization (1994) has established the following mineral density diagnostic criteria for women who have experienced no fragility fractures. These criteria provide a basic diagnostic framework:

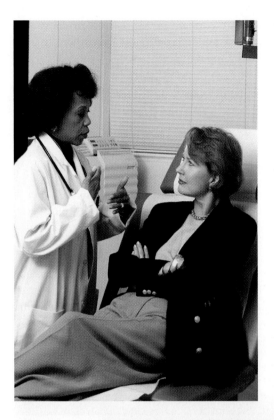

FIGURE 10.5 **An Examination to Diagnose Osteoporosis Can Involve Several Tests.** Before performing these tests, your health care professional will record information about your medical history and lifestyle in an initial physical exam.

TABLE 10.7	Types of BMD Tests	

Acronym	Name	Measures
DXA	Dual-energy X-ray absorptiometry	Spine, hip, or total body
SXA	Single-energy X-ray absorptiometry	Wrist or heel
RA	Radiographic absorptiometry	Uses an X-ray of the hand and a small metal wedge to calculate BMD
DPA	Dual-photon absorptiometry	Spine, hip, or total body
SPA	Single-photon absorptiometry	Wrist
QCT	Quantitative computed tomography	Wrist

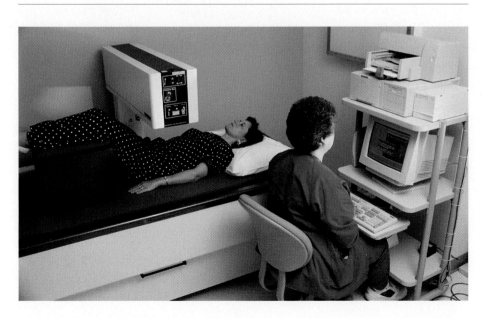

FIGURE 10.6 **Bone Mineral Density Test.** Bone mineral density tests are painless, noninvasive, and safe. Bone density may be measured in the spine, hip, wrist, finger, kneecap, shin bone, or heel, depending on the machine.

- Normal bone mineral density is within 1 standard deviation (SD) of the young adult mean. (*Standard deviation* is a measure of variation in a distribution.)
- **Osteopenia**, or low bone mass, is a bone mineral density between 1 and 2.5 SD of the young adult mean.
- Osteoporosis is defined as a value greater than 2.5 SD below the young adult mean.

Osteopenia Low bone mass.

Physical Activity and Health Connection

Maintaining optimal bone health requires a lifestyle that includes a balanced diet and a healthy physical activity program. A diet that pays close attention to calcium intake through dairy and other foods is important. If the diet does not contain enough calcium naturally, calcium supplements may be needed.

Bone is a living tissue that responds to exercise by becoming more dense and stronger. Weight-bearing and resistance exercises increase bone mass and density. Therefore, weight-bearing physical activities (e.g., dancing, walking) and resistance activities (e.g., weight lifting, swimming) are essential for improving and maintaining optimal bone health.

TABLE 10.8 gives a summary of recommendations for bone health.

TABLE 10.8   Summary Recommendations for Bone Health

	Calcium (mg/Day)	Vitamin D (IU/Day)	Physical Activity	Bone Density Testing	Patients at Increased Risk
Infants					
0–6 months	210	200	Interactive play.	As clinically indicated in high-risk patients.	
6–12 months	270				
Children and adolescents					Frequent fractures; anorexia; amenorrhea; chronic hepatic, renal, gastrointestinal, or autoimmune disease.
1–3 years	500	200	Moderate to vigorous activity at least 60 minutes per day. Emphasize weight-bearing activity.	As clinically indicated in high-risk patients.	
4–8 years	800				
9–18 years	1300				
Adults					Individuals with risk factors in Table 10.6.
18–50 years	1000	200	Moderate activity at least 30 minutes per day on most, preferably all, days of the week. Emphasize weight-bearing activity. Fall prevention programs, modified for the frail elderly and spine fracture patients.	As clinically indicated in high-risk patients.	
51–70 years	1200	400		Bone density testing by DXA in all women over age 65; consider in women under age 65 with risk factors. No consensus on men.	
>70 years	1200	600			

SOURCE: U.S. Department of Health and Human Services. (2004). *Bone Health and Osteoporosis: A Report of the Surgeon General,* Chapter 10. Rockville, MD: U.S. Department of Health and Human Services, Office of the Surgeon General.

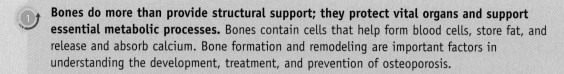

concept connections

1. **Bones do more than provide structural support; they protect vital organs and support essential metabolic processes.** Bones contain cells that help form blood cells, store fat, and release and absorb calcium. Bone formation and remodeling are important factors in understanding the development, treatment, and prevention of osteoporosis.

2. **Three types of cells are involved in bone formation and resorption: osteoblasts, osteocytes, and osteoclasts.** *Osteoblasts* are immature cells that when surrounded by mature bone cells become osteocyctes. *Osteoclasts* absorb bony tissue.

3. **To maintain bone mass, bone formation must occur at the same rate as bone resorption.** Bone remodeling is the lifelong renewal process of the skeletal system. This process allows for bone to be removed and new bone generated. This process of new bone forming at the same rate as resorption is critical, because without this balance osteoporosis can take place.

4. **Physical activity enhances bone density through both weight-bearing and resistance-training exercises.** Bone becomes stronger and denser when one places demands on it, such as jogging or playing tennis. Physical activity is necessary for bone acquisition and maintenance throughout adulthood.

5. **Osteoporosis is a chronic disease process characterized by progressive bone loss for both males and females.** Millions of Americans suffer from osteoporosis and the bone fractures that result from it. Optimal physical activity and nutrition habits when young are key elements to an osteoporosis prevention program.

6. **Osteoporosis can be affected by genetic, hormonal, nutritional, and lifestyle factors.** Recognizing common osteoporosis risk facts will help in understanding effective prevention strategies and will be useful in decreasing the incidence and prevalence of osteoporosis.

Terms

Paget's disease, 208

Osteogenesis imperfecta, 208

Rickets, 208

Cartilage, 208

Collagen, 208

Resorption, 208

Osteoblasts, 208

Osteocytes, 208

Osteoclasts, 208

Bone mineral density (BMD), 209

Remodeling, 209

Osteoporosis, 215

Amenorrhea, 219

Osteopenia, 222

making the connection

Julie now knows that, while her bones may seem to be rigid and unchanging, they are actually more like muscles, capable of strengthening with use or weakening without use. Each time a bone is moved, it bends ever so slightly, just enough to stimulate electrical and biochemical changes that stimulate bone formation. The more force, the greater the bending, the greater the stimulus for new bone formation (up to a point). In addition to maintaining the Recommended Daily Intake (RDI) for calcium, Julie knows that a regular physical activity program keeps the density of bone constant or contributes to increased bone mass. Julie now understands that the threat of osteoporosis doesn't just come from a low calcium intake, but from a sedentary lifestyle. She is encouraged to know that by monitoring her dietary habits and participating in a regular weight-bearing physical activity program, she now has the right tools to live strong and live well.

Critical Thinking

1. Like Julie, many people do not understand that both physical inactivity and low calcium intake are key factors in the development of osteoporosis. You have been asked by a local ninth-grade health teacher to explain to her students the importance of physical activity and nutrition in preventing osteoporosis (a condition that is the last thing on most ninth-graders' minds). In 250 words or less, explain their importance.

2. Review the factors that affect osteoporosis (genetic, hormonal, nutritional, and lifestyle). Review your family history to determine if you are at risk of osteoporosis. Then select two other factors and, based on your current behaviors, decide what behaviors you could change that would assist in preventing osteoporosis. List them.

3. "Physical activity and nutrition are key elements in achieving optimal bone density during the first 20 to 30 years of life and maintaining bone density throughout life." Provide information that supports that statement.

References

Ackermann, U. (1992). *Essentials of Human Physiology*. St. Louis, MO: Mosby-Year Book.

Beck, B.R., & Shoemaker, M.R. (2000). Osteoporosis: Understanding key risk factors and therapeutic options. *The Physician and Sportsmedicine* 28(2):69ff.

Black, D.M., et al. (1992). Axial and appendicular bone density predict fractures in older women. *Journal of Bone Mineral Research* 14(3):633–638.

Cosman, F. (2005). The prevention and treatment of osteoporosis: A review. *General Medicine* 7(2):73.

Endocrine Web. (n.d.) Osteoporosis: Maintenance of strong bones as an adult . . . How do we avoid osteoporosis? Online: http://www.endocrineweb.com/osteoporosis/adult.html.

Francis, R.M. (1999). The effects of testosterone on osteoporosis in men. *Clinical Endocrinology* 50(4):411–414.

Institute of Medicine. (1997). *Dietary Reference Intakes for Calcium, Phosphorus, Magnesium, Vitamin D, and Fluoride*. Washington, DC: National Academy Press.

McIlwain, H.H., & Bruce, D.F. (1998). *The Osteoporosis Cure*. New York: Avon.

National Osteoporosis Foundation. (2005a). Prevention: Calcium and vitamin D. Online: http://www.nof.org/prevention/calcium.htm.

National Osteoporosis Foundation. (2005b). Prevention: Exercise for healthy bones. Online: http://www.nof.org/prevention/exercise.htm.

Ng, K.W., Romas, E., Donnan, L., & Findlay, D.M. (1997). Bone biology. *Balliere's Clinical Endocrinology and Metabolism* 11(1):1–22.

Nordin, B.E.C., Need, A.H., Chatterton, B.E., Horowitz, M., & Morris, H.A. (1990). The relative contributions of age and years since menopause to postmenopausal bone loss. *Journal of Clinical Endocrinology* 70(1):83–88.

Rhoades, R., & Pflanzer, R. (1996). *Human Physiology*. Philadelphia: WB Saunders.

United States Department of Health and Human Services. (1996). *Physical Activity and Health: A Report of the Surgeon General*. Atlanta, GA: U.S. Department of Health and Human Services, Centers for Disease Control and Prevention.

United States Department of Health and Human Services. (2004a). *Bone Health and Osteoporosis: A Report of the Surgeon General*. Rockville, MD: U.S. Department of Health and Human Services, Office of the Surgeon General.

United States Department of Health and Human Services. (2004b). By 2020, one in two million Americans over age 50 will be at risk for fractures from osteoporosis or low bone mass [News release]. Online: http://www.hhs.gov/news.

Wardlaw, G.M. (1993). Putting osteoporosis in perspective. *Journal of the American Dietetic Association* 93(9):1000–1006.

Woodhead, G.A., & Moss, M.M. (1998). Osteoporosis: Diagnosis and prevention. *The Nurse Practitioner* 23(11):18–35.

World Health Organization. (1994). *Assessment of Fracture Risk and Its Application to Screening for Postmenopausal Osteoporosis* (Technical Report Series 843). Geneva, Switzerland: Author.

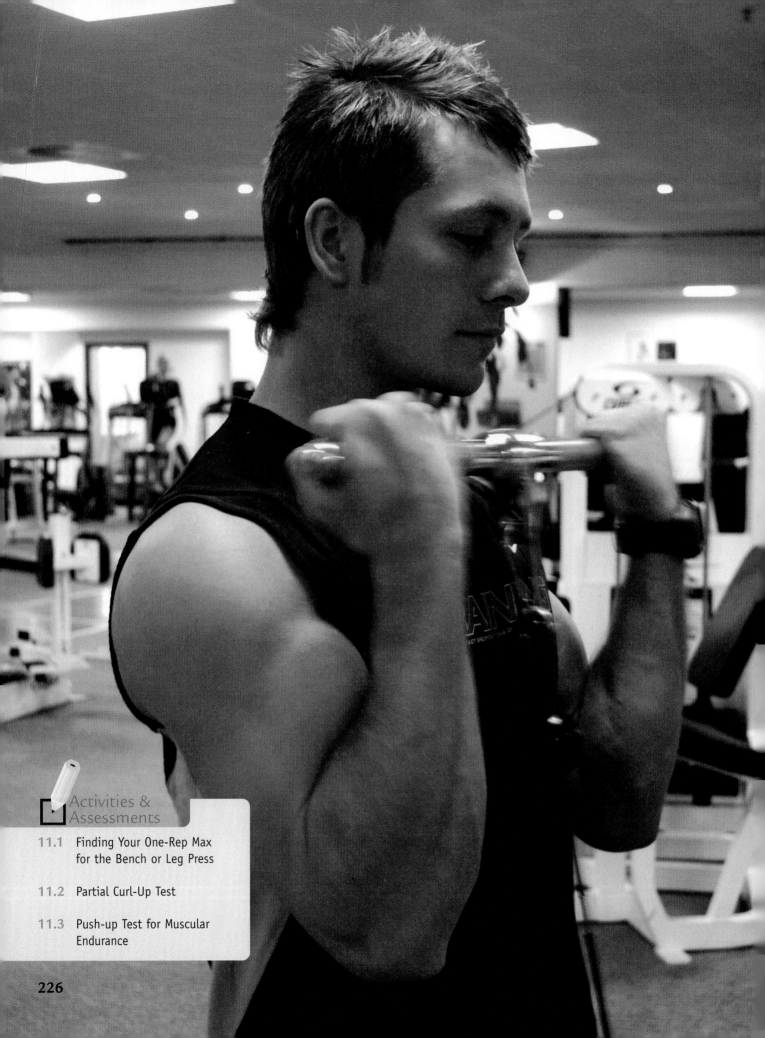

Activities &
Assessments

11.1   Finding Your One-Rep Max
        for the Bench or Leg Press

11.2   Partial Curl-Up Test

11.3   Push-up Test for Muscular
        Endurance

Muscular Strength and Endurance

what's the connection?

Beth wants to improve her muscular strength to lessen the possibility of developing osteoporosis as she ages. She's interested in including resistance training in her activity program. Beth has toyed with weights at the health club on occasion, but has never really been serious about performing resistance training with goals and outcomes in mind. She decides to search the Internet for information on how to get the most out of a resistance training program. Beth knows she has to be careful to screen suggestions from the Internet, but hopes she can get the information she needs.

concepts

1. *Strength* refers to a muscle's ability to generate maximal force.

2. Significant health benefits are associated with resistance training.

3. Muscles that are stressed by resistance training get stronger and increase in size (hypertrophy), while muscles that are neglected get weaker and shrink in size (atrophy).

4. You can develop muscular strength and endurance through a variety of resistance training programs.

5. Individuals of any age can benefit from resistance training.

http://physicalactivity.jbpub.com

The Web site for this book is a great source for supplementary physical health information for both students and instructors. Visit **http://physicalactivity.jbpub.com** to find a variety of useful tools for learning, thinking, and teaching.

Strength refers to a muscle's ability to generate maximal force.

Significant health benefits are associated with resistance training.

Circuit weight training Method of training that involves moving from station to station, performing different exercises at each station.

Protein filaments Strands of protein (actin and myosin) that give muscle its structure and functional ability.

Actin Thin protein filament found in muscle; plays an important role in muscle movement.

Sarcomere The functional unit of a muscle. The site where muscle movement takes place.

Myosin Thick protein filament found in muscle; plays an important role in muscle movement.

Introduction

This chapter focuses on the importance of good muscular strength and endurance and their relationship to good health. It provides information on how to assess your muscular strength and endurance and how to formulate a program to optimize the development of these important assets.

Muscles provide the force that allows our bodies to move. As muscles contract they pull on the bones to which they are connected. The many complex physical movements of which the human body is capable are the result of this simple action. *Muscular strength* refers to a muscle's ability to generate maximal force. The stronger a muscle, the more force it can generate. *Muscular endurance* refers to a muscle's ability to sustain a given force over an extended period of time or to repeat a muscle action for several repetitions.

Muscle fitness is important in many ways. Fit muscles allow us to perform the tasks of daily living with less stress; help to protect our joints from injury; aid in sport and activity performance; assist in developing and maintaining strong bones, thereby reducing the risk for osteoporosis (Chapter 10); and have a positive effect on our metabolism (Brill et al., 2000; Stone et al., 2000).

Building muscles that are strong and have good endurance can improve your health. In addition to increasing bone mineral density, regular resistance training lowers your percentage of body fat, increases your lean body mass, decreases your insulin response to changing levels of glucose, lowers your baseline insulin levels, and increases your insulin sensitivity (American College of Sports Medicine [ACSM], 2006; Pollock & Vincent, 1996). The last three factors are related to your body's ability to use sugars as fuel and aid in the prevention of diabetes. Resistance training maintains or improves your HDL levels, maintains or decreases your LDL levels, regulates your diastolic blood pressure at rest, increases your VO$_2$max (**circuit weight training**), improves your endurance, improves your physiologic function, and increases your basal metabolism (ACSM, 2006; Mayo & Kravitz, 1999; Pollock & Vincent, 1996). All of these factors help to insure a healthy cardiovascular system and guard against cardiovascular disease.

Seniors who perform regular resistance training have discovered that it helps to improve their ability to resist falls, improves their balance, and helps to prevent (or rehabilitate) low-back pain (Pollock & Vincent, 1996). These improvements are vital in maintaining independent living.

Muscular Anatomy and Physiology

To understand how muscles get stronger and more enduring, we must look at some basic muscular anatomy and physiology. Muscles are composed of water, **protein filaments**, and several key minerals. Tendons are connective tissues that function to connect muscle to bones (**FIGURE 11.1**). The membranes that form the tendons both surround, and are a part of, the muscles. When the muscles contract, the tendons exert forces on the bones, causing the bones to move.

Sliding Filament Theory

It is the protein filaments, located within the muscles, that cause muscle movement to occur. The filaments responsible for movement are called *actin* and *myosin*. **Actin** filaments are made of thin protein and located within the functional unit of a muscle cell, or **sarcomere**. **Myosin** filaments are thicker protein strands that must connect with the actin for movement to happen. Oar-like projections

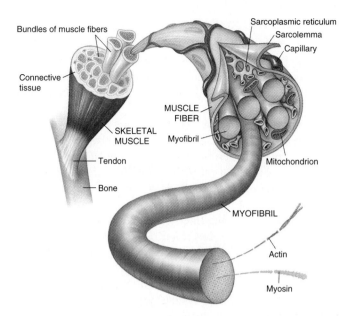

FIGURE 11.1 **The Structure of Skeletal Muscle.** A tendon connects your muscles to bone.

(myosin cross bridges) extend from the myosin and connect to active sites on the actin when the muscle is stimulated by an electrical impulse. As the muscle is stimulated, energy is released, and the connected cross bridges swivel and rotate (**FIGURE 11.2**). This pulls the actin filaments over the myosin filaments, and the muscle shortens. As long as the muscle remains stimulated and energy is released, the muscle will remain in this shortened state. When the stimulus is removed, the cross bridges detach and the filaments slide back over each other until they regain their elongated, resting state. The process of protein filaments moving over the top of each other is referred to as the *sliding filament theory of muscle contraction*.

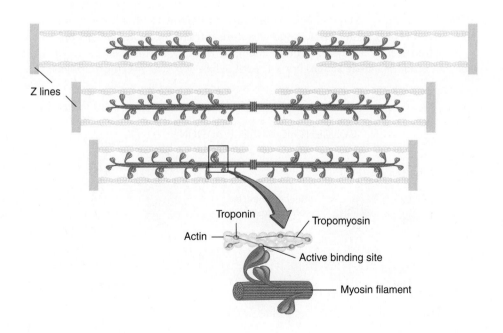

FIGURE 11.2 **Contraction of Muscle Fibers.** Your muscle filaments connect and slide to make your muscles move.

Muscle Fibers and Motor Units

The protein filaments found within our muscles join together to form muscle fibers. There are two types of muscle fibers: slow-twitch and fast-twitch. Most muscles in our body have a composition that contains both slow- and fast-twitch fibers. The function of the muscle and our genetics determine which one is available in the greater quantity.

Slow-twitch fibers are endurance fibers. They have a better blood supply than fast-twitch fibers, more mitochondria (sites of energy transfer), and greater aerobic capacity. Muscles that perform aerobic activities and muscular endurance training improve the functional abilities of the slow-twitch fibers. Slow-twitch fibers allow us to perform activities for extended periods of time or to repeat an activity again and again.

Fast-twitch fibers are the power fibers. They allow us to generate a great deal of force in a short period of time. Since their blood supply is not as rich as slow-twitch fibers, fast-twitch fibers fatigue more rapidly. Sprint training and heavy resistance training develop the functional capacity of our fast-twitch fibers.

A motor unit is composed of a nerve and all of the fibers in a muscle that are *innervated* (connected to the nervous system) by that single nerve. Some motor units contain relatively few muscle fibers. These tend to be slow-twitch motor units. Motor units that contain large numbers of muscle fibers tend to be fast-twitch motor units. The more muscle fibers in a motor unit, the greater the force-generating capacity of that motor unit. One reason fast-twitch motor units are capable of generating a great deal of power is because each motor unit contains many muscle fibers. Fast-twitch motor units also have larger nerves than do slow-twitch motor units. This allows for greater speed of conduction of the nervous impulse that controls the muscle.

Eccentric and Concentric Muscle Action

A muscle can be in one of four states of motion. The first is the normal relaxed state in which muscle activity is at a minimum. The second is when the muscle develops tension, but does not move. This is referred to as a **static contraction**. The third is when the muscle shortens under tension. This state is called a **concentric muscle action**. For example, when you bend your arm at the elbow to lift an object from a table, your biceps brachii muscle undergoes concentric movement (**FIGURE 11.3**).

The fourth state is when the muscle lengthens under tension. This state is called an **eccentric muscle action**. For example, when you are lowering an object

Static contraction A state in which the muscle develops tension but does not move.

Concentric muscle action Muscle movement in which the muscle shortens while under tension.

Eccentric muscle action Muscle movement in which the muscle lengthens while under tension.

FIGURE 11.3 **Concentric Muscle Action.** Your muscles shorten during concentric action.

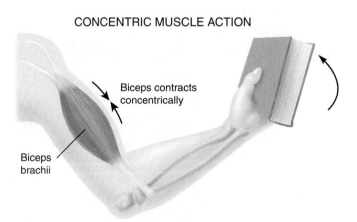

CONCENTRIC MUSCLE ACTION

Biceps contracts concentrically

Biceps brachii

ECCENTRIC MUSCLE ACTION

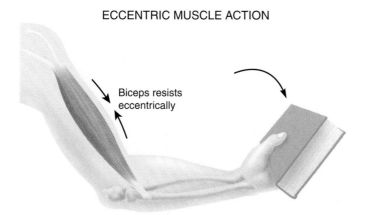

Biceps resists
eccentrically

FIGURE 11.4 **Eccentric Muscle Action.** Your muscles lengthen during eccentric action.

back to a table and controlling how fast the object is moving by regulating how slowly you allow your arm to straighten out, your biceps muscle is undergoing eccentric muscle action (**FIGURE 11.4**). Eccentric muscle action is more stressful to the muscle than concentric muscle action because the myosin cross bridges are being stretched while they are under tension (Dolezal, Potteiger, Jacobsen, & Benedict, 2000). Many people believe that eccentric muscle activity may be responsible for the soreness you sometimes feel when you do too much resistance training too soon (Dolezal et al., 2000).

Focusing the early stages of a resistance training program on proper form, using light resistance, and emphasizing the concentric portion of a lift can minimize this pain. Once the body has adapted to the stress of regular resistance training, greater emphasis may be placed on eccentric muscle action with less likelihood of pain. It has been demonstrated that eccentric resistance training is important is achieving maximal benefit from a strength training program. Eccentric muscle action adds to the total work of resistance training, and the use of typical concentric-eccentric repetitions contributes to enhanced muscle strength and muscle fiber size (Kraemer, 1992).

Agonists, Antagonists, Synergists, Neutralizers

Muscles can perform many different functions, depending on the demands placed upon them (**FIGURE 11.5**). If a muscle is called upon to be responsible for the primary action of a desired movement, it is called the **agonist**, or prime mover. A muscle that resists the prime mover and helps to maintain joint integrity is called an **antagonist**. If we look at the example of raising a glass from a table, the biceps muscle of the upper arm that causes the arm to bend at the elbow would be considered the agonist. The triceps muscle in the back of the upper arm resists the biceps and helps keep the elbow from dislocating. In this scenario, the triceps would be acting as an antagonist.

Muscles can also act as **synergists** if they assist the agonist, but are not primarily responsible for carrying out the movement. In the above example, the brachial radialis (a muscle that crosses the elbow and connects to the forearm) would act as a synergist. A **neutralizer**, or fixator, is a muscle whose action prevents unwanted activities of muscles not directly involved in the movement you wish to carry out. For example, the abdominal muscles frequently act as neutralizers to support the spinal column when the arm is bent at the elbow.

Agonist Muscle that acts as the prime mover; the muscle most responsible for a movement.

Antagonist Muscle that resists the agonist; helps to maintain joint stability.

Synergists Muscles that assist the agonist.

Neutralizer Muscle that prevents unwanted activity in muscles not directly involved in performing a movement.

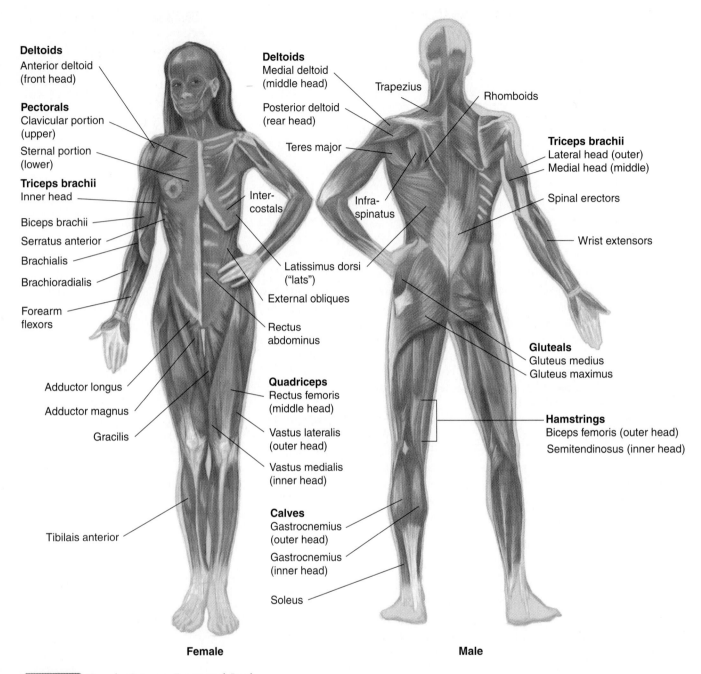

Deltoids
Anterior deltoid (front head)

Pectorals
Clavicular portion (upper)
Sternal portion (lower)

Triceps brachii
Inner head

Biceps brachii

Serratus anterior

Brachialis

Brachioradialis

Forearm flexors

Adductor longus

Adductor magnus

Gracilis

Tibilais anterior

Deltoids
Medial deltoid (middle head)

Posterior deltoid (rear head)

Teres major

Inter-costals

Latissimus dorsi ("lats")

External obliques

Rectus abdominus

Quadriceps
Rectus femoris (middle head)

Vastus lateralis (outer head)

Vastus medialis (inner head)

Calves
Gastrocnemius (outer head)

Gastrocnemius (inner head)

Soleus

Female

Trapezius

Rhomboids

Triceps brachii
Lateral head (outer)
Medial head (middle)

Spinal erectors

Wrist extensors

Infra-spinatus

Gluteals
Gluteus medius
Gluteus maximus

Hamstrings
Biceps femoris (outer head)
Semitendinosus (inner head)

Male

FIGURE 11.5 **Muscle Groups, Front and Back.**

Getting Stronger, Building Size, Toning Up

Muscles that are stressed by resistance training get stronger and increase in size (hypertrophy), while muscles that are neglected get weaker and shrink in size (atrophy).

In order for muscles to become stronger, they must regularly be exposed to more stress than they are exposed to under normal resting conditions. A stronger muscle is one that can produce more force. Muscles that are stressed will grow in size (hypertrophy) and become stronger. Hypertrophy occurs when a muscle is regularly challenged to produce near-optimal levels of force. The structure of the muscle then changes by increasing the size of its protein filaments. Once this happens, the muscle is capable of producing greater force.

The degree to which hypertrophy occurs is dependent on four factors. The first is the amount and type of resistance training you perform. The second is making sure that you are eating a nutritious diet containing adequate amounts of carbohydrate, fat, and protein. Although you must consume adequate amounts of the essential amino acids to build muscle daily, the role of protein consumption in muscle mass development is overstated. Total dietary energy, specifically carbohydrate energy, is the most important nutritional factor affecting muscle gain (Butterfield, Kleiner, Lemon, & Stone, 1995). Carbohydrate provides the main source of fuel for a muscle used to generate force. Excessive intake of protein will not speed up the development of muscle mass or cause greater muscle mass to occur.

The third factor is the genetics for large-muscle growth, and the fourth is secretion of adequate amounts of the hormones responsible for causing muscle to grow (testosterone, androgens, human growth hormone). This last factor explains one reason why some people gain more muscle mass than others. If you produce large volumes of testosterone, androgens, and human growth hormone, and combine this production with proper training, good genetics, and proper nutrition, you will have greater muscle mass development. Men produce more of these hormones, so men tend to have the capacity for more muscle mass development than women. Most women can practice regular heavy resistance training, increase their strength tremendously, and not develop large bulky muscles.

It takes approximately 8 to 12 weeks to experience signs of muscular hypertrophy. People will show improvements in strength before this time (usually 2 weeks after starting a program); however, this improvement is mainly due to improvements in lifting technique, better coordination, and **neuromuscular adaptations**. The neuromuscular adaptations include the ability to selectively recruit the muscle fibers necessary to perform a given activity, the ability to synchronize the firing of these muscle fibers, and the ability to call more muscle fibers into action. Changes in muscular endurance will begin almost immediately. In as few as 2 weeks you should see some improvement in your muscular endurance.

Some people achieve body mass increases of about 20 percent during the first year of regular heavy resistance training; however, later gains slow down substantially because we tend to approach our genetic potential relatively early in a training program. After a few years of resistance training, gains will level off at only 1 to 3 percent per year (Butterfield et al., 1995). Muscles must be regularly exposed to the stress that resistance activity supplies or the muscle fibers will become weaker and actually shrink in size. This process is called muscle atrophy.

Toning muscles involves training the muscle to maintain a tonic state (a state in which the muscle maintains a degree of tension). A toned muscle feels more firm than an untoned muscle. It is important to remember that *you cannot change fat to muscle* because they are different cells; however, you *can* increase the size of one while reducing the size of the other.

Isotonic, Isokinetic, and Isometric Training

There are a variety of ways in which you can train a muscle to become stronger and more enduring. The three different types of training are **isometric**, **isotonic**, and **isokinetic** training. Isometric training occurs when the muscle is put under tension but the length of the muscle does not change. An example of an isometric exercise would be pushing against an immovable object such as a wall. The prefix *iso* means "the same" and *metric* refers to length, so *isometric* means the muscle maintains the same length when under tension.

Isotonic training involves muscular movement, but the resistance stays the same. An example would be lifting a barbell with 100 pounds on it. The weight stays the same throughout the lift. *Tonic* refers to tension, so *isotonic* means "the

Neuromuscular adaptations Changes in the function of the nervous and muscular systems brought on by exposure to regular resistance training. These changes include the ability to selectively recruit motor units, to synchronize the recruitment of these units, and to maintain a state of equilibrium throughout the movement.

Isometric Form of resistance training in which the muscle is stationary while under tension.

Isotonic Form of resistance training in which there is movement.

Isokinetic Form of resistance training in which the speed of movement is controlled.

You can develop muscular strength and endurance through a variety of resistance training programs.

same tension." There are two types of isotonic training methods. The first involves set resistance training, in which the resistance remains the same throughout the muscular action. The best example of this type of resistance training is free weights. The second type of isotonic training involves machines that provide variable resistance as you move through the range of motion associated with a muscular activity. An example would be performing exercises on a Nautilus machine. The Nautilus camshaft causes the chain that provides resistance to move over varying lengths, thereby altering the resistance that is provided. This allows for variations in the resistance that the muscle must work against as it moves through its range of motion.

The third type of training is isokinetic training. *Kinetic* refers to the energy of movement, so *isokinetic* means "the same energy." Isokinetic training is similar to variable-resistance isotonic training, with the key differences that with isokinetic training the speed of movement is controlled and the resistance is accommodating. By controlling the speed, the energy involved in the movement is regulated. *Accommodating resistance* refers to resistance that varies based on the force generated by the person performing the activity. The harder you work, the more resistance you receive. Isokinetic devices, such as the Cybex Orthotron, control the speed of motion and provide accommodating resistance through the use of hydraulics. These machines may use gas, water, or oil-based hydraulics to control speed and resistance. An example of how hydraulics can do this would be to consider a door with an automatic closer. If you allow the door to close at its preset rate, it takes little effort to move the door. However, if you try to speed the door up, the amount of resistance increases.

Isometric exercises provide you with the opportunity to train anywhere. Since there is no equipment required, you are not dependent on a workout facility to perform isometric exercises. There is also no cost associated with isometric exercise. Disadvantages of isometric training include the need to perform the exercise at multiple angles to get the full range of motion involved. It's also difficult to gauge the intensity of your workout because you don't see any resistance being lifted. Isometric training may be dangerous for those with high blood pressure or cardiovascular disease. Since you are holding a position and creating tension, *isometric training raises blood pressure.*

Isotonic training is the preferred method of training for people who perform regular resistance exercise and will probably be your form of choice. The advantages of isotonic training are that you can easily train through the full range of motion, you can isolate individual muscles to make sure they are properly stressed, and you can more easily gauge the intensity of your exercise by watching how much resistance you are lifting. The disadvantages of isotonic resistance training include being somewhat dependent on equipment, the cost associated with access to that equipment (either by purchasing it or by paying for membership at a health club), and the potential for injury through improper use of the equipment.

The major advantage to isokinetic training is that the resistance adjusts to the force you generate. This is important if you are rehabilitating injured or weak

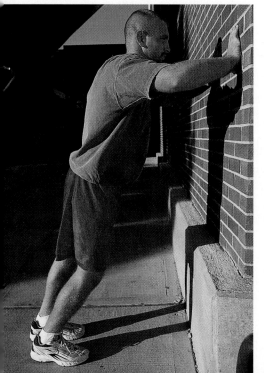
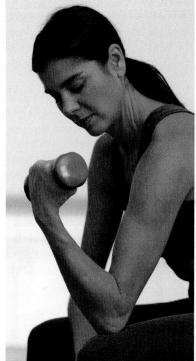

(Left) Pushing against an immovable object is a form of isometric resistance training. (Right) Lifting dumbbells is a form of isotonic resistance training.

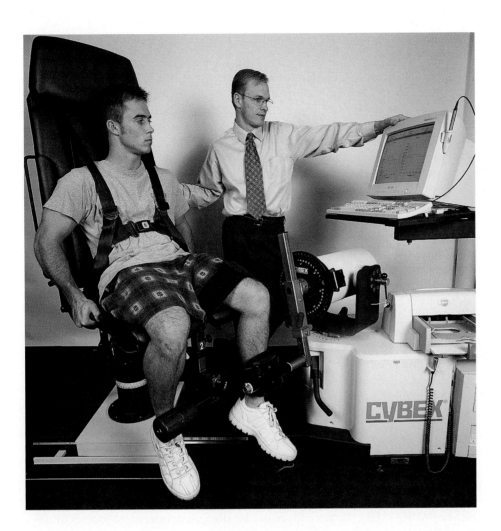

Exercise using a Cybex machine is a form of isokinetic resistance training.

muscles. The disadvantages of isokinetic training include the high cost of the equipment, lack of access to this type of equipment (it is found mostly in rehabilitation clinics), and the inability to isolate individual muscle groups easily.

Resistance Training Guidelines

As with the guidelines for cardiovascular physical activity (Chapter 4), there are two sets of guidelines for resistance training. The first guideline is for those people seeking basic health benefits. Basic health benefits are associated with good health, but not optimal health. Some individuals only wish to perform the amount of physical activity that will bring about some protection against degenerative disease, are not overly concerned about their level of fitness, and are not willing to perform the amount of exercise required to bring about optimal health and fitness.

Others may wish to bring about optimal protection against degenerative disease and higher levels of fitness. The second set of guidelines is for those seeking optimal health and fitness benefits. The basic health benefit guidelines require less time and effort. The optimal health and fitness guidelines build upon the basic health benefit guidelines and require more time and effort. In either case, resistance training should be an integral part of everyone's physical activity program.

ACSM Guidelines

According to the American College of Sports Medicine, resistance training should be progressive in nature, rhythmic, individualized, performed at a moderate to slow speed, involve full range of motion, provide a stimulus to all the major muscle groups, and not interfere with normal breathing (ACSM, 2006). For those seeking basic health benefits, a single set of 8 to 12 exercises that condition the major muscle groups 2 to 3 days per week is recommended (ACSM, 2006) (TABLE 11.1). Most people should be able to complete 8 to12 repetitions of each exercise; however, for those unaccustomed to resistance training, and for more frail people, 10 to 15 repetitions with lighter loads may be more appropriate (ACSM, 2006; Pollock & Vincent, 1996). The major muscle groups include the arms, shoulders, chest, abdomen, back, hips, and legs (ACSM, 2006).

There is some debate as to how many **reps** (repetitions) and **sets** you should do. A *rep* is the number of times you perform a movement. For example, if you are performing a bicep curl (grasping a dumbbell and lifting it to your shoulder by bending your elbow), each time you take the dumbbell to your shoulder and then back to its original starting position, you have completed one rep. A *set* is a series of reps.

Eighty to 90 percent of strength gains can be achieved using single-set regimens when compared to multiple-set types of programs (Pollock & Vincent, 1996). Multiple-set types of programs may provide for optimal fitness and muscle growth, and are recommended if time allows (ACSM, 2006). However, since time is an important factor for program compliance, the single-set guidelines seem appropriate for the majority of the population (Pollock & Vincent, 1996). Multiple-set regimens may not be appropriate for older, nonathletic individuals (Pollock & Vincent, 1996).

> **Reps** Repetitions; a rep occurs each time a muscle action is performed.
>
> **Sets** Groups of repetitions.

Muscular Strength Training

BASIC PRINCIPLES Training for muscular strength development focuses on the physical conditioning concepts of overload, progression, specificity, and recovery. In order for a muscle to hypertrophy, or increase in size, the muscle must work

TABLE 11.1	A Sample Resistance Training Workout
1. Legs	Quad extensions
	Hamstring curls
2. Back	Lat pull-downs
	Bent-over rows
3. Chest	Bench press
	Bent-arm flys
4. Shoulders	Seated press
	Shoulder shrugs
5. Arms	Bicep curls
	Tricep extensions
6. Abdomen	Sit-ups/curl-ups/crunches
7. Groin	Lunges

against resistance greater than that to which it is normally exposed (overload). The best way of accomplishing this task is to have the muscle work at a level exceeding 85 percent of its maximal capacity. Exactly how much weight 85 percent of maximal capacity is will be based on the fitness level of the individual. Someone who has not previously performed resistance exercise will be working against a much lighter load than someone who has been training for years.

The principle of progression is important in training for muscular strength development. *Progression* refers to the logical and systematic application of the overload principle. Frequently, misinformed or overeager people will attempt to do too much too soon when they begin a physical activity program that includes resistance training. The result is pain, and potentially an injury, which will have severely negative effects on adherence. Resistance training programs must be entered into wisely and gradually. You must allow your body time to adjust to the rigors of training for muscular strength. You should undergo assessment to determine exactly how much resistance you need.

If you wish to develop strength in specific muscle groups, you must perform activities that stress those muscles. This concept (specific activities for specific outcomes) is referred to as the *principle of specificity*. Ideally, you will be able to select activities that isolate the muscles you wish to develop. By isolating muscles, you can ensure that they are being overloaded properly. For instance, if you wish to stress the chest muscles (pectorals) optimally, you should perform activities in which the chest muscles are the prime movers. Bench pressing and bent-arm flies are two activities that do this (FIGURE 11.6 and FIGURE 11.7).

It is also important to remember to apply the principle of recovery to your muscular strength program. Occasionally, people fall into the trap of thinking that the more frequently you perform an exercise, the more rapidly you will see improvement in fitness. This supposition does not always hold true. In fact, if you do not allow adequate recovery time, your body will not have the chance to rebuild itself and make the structural changes necessary for muscular growth to occur. It is best to allow 48 to 72 hours of recovery time between training sessions in which a muscle or group of muscles is maximally stressed. This does not mean that we must remain inactive during this time. We can perform activities that stress other parts of our bodies or other aspects of our fitness while we allow those segments that were maximally stressed time to recover.

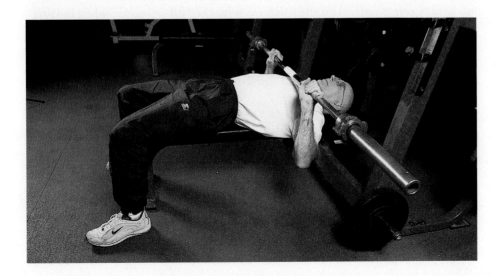

FIGURE 11.6 **Principle of Specificity.** The bench press specifically stresses the chest muscles.

FIGURE 11.7 **Principle of Specificity.** Bent-arm flies can also be used to strengthen the chest muscles.

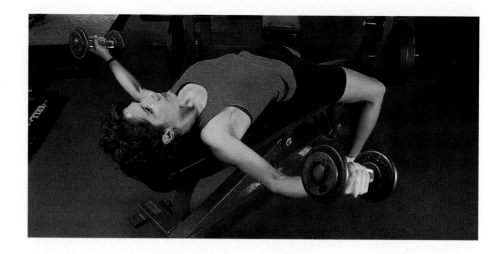

PROPER FORM AND TECHNIQUE   Any resistance training program should focus initially on proper form and technique. By doing so, you will not only improve the safety of the activities you perform but also increase the gains you receive. As stated earlier, you must stress the muscle you wish to develop in order for it to get larger and stronger. If you improperly perform a resistance training activity, you may in fact be stressing things (joints, muscles, tendons) that were not the intended target areas for improvement. At any resistance training facility you will see that many people incorrectly perform activities, putting themselves at risk for injury and reducing the possibility for achieving their desired outcomes.

BREATHING   It is important to remember to breathe properly when performing resistance training exercises. Improper breathing can put you at risk for injury. It is recommended that you breathe out while exerting force and breathe in when returning (not exerting force). For example, when performing the bench press exercise, you would breathe in when lowering the bar to your chest and breathe out when pressing the bar upward.

You should *never hold your breath when lifting*, particularly when you are exerting force. This may bring about a condition called the **Valsalva maneuver**. The valsalva maneuver occurs when the windpipe is blocked off (as occurs when holding your breath). Pressure in your lungs begins to build up, which in turn causes an increase in blood pressure. Higher blood pressures put you at risk for a stroke, heart attack, or hemorrhage. By breathing out when exerting force, you greatly reduce this risk.

Valsalva maneuver Condition that occurs when you hold your breath and exert force (grunting action); causes elevated blood pressure that increases the risk for stroke, heart attack, or hemorrhage.

Muscular Endurance Training

Many of the same principles that govern training for muscular strength govern training for muscular endurance. The principles of overload, progression, specificity, and recovery all apply to muscular endurance training. The major differences between strength and endurance training are the amount of resistance applied and the number of repetitions performed. For optimal gains in muscular endurance, it is recommended that you train at an intensity that ranges between 50 and 65 percent of your maximal capacity. As with strength training, the amount of resistance applied will be dependent on the fitness level of the person. To gain muscular endurance benefits, you apply less stress than you would if you were seeking strength gains, but you perform more repetitions of the activity for longer periods of time.

Training for Power

Training for power is very similar to training for strength, with the major difference that power training requires greater speed. By definition, *power* means that work is accomplished at a high rate of speed. Power is best developed through explosive training. Because of the dynamic nature of power training, there is a high risk of injury. Power training is usually reserved for those individuals who have already developed a good degree of muscular fitness. When performing power training, you must try to move the resistance rapidly without forsaking proper form.

TABLE 11.2 contains sample regimens that may be used to train for muscular strength, endurance, or power.

Developing a Personalized Program

There are many variations of training routines that you can follow. The basic guidelines have been spelled out in this chapter. More information can be obtained by visiting websites that cater to those interested in strength and muscular endurance training.

ASSESSMENT   As with the performance of cardiovascular physical activity (Chapter 4), you should begin any resistance training program with proper assessment. Assessment is important to establish beginning workloads, to monitor progress, and to enhance safety. Two sample assessments are included in the activities and assessment manual. One shows how to measure your one-repetition maximum (1-RM) for the bench press, and the other shows how to measure your abdominal endurance. You can follow the same procedures to determine the 1-RM for any other muscle or to find the muscular endurance capacity of other muscle groups. Several other self-assessments are available on the Web, or you may elect to have a qualified professional help with your assessment.

FINDING QUALIFIED PROFESSIONAL HELP   When instructed by a qualified professional in the strength training field, you can learn to lift safely and effectively. A "strength coach" can teach you how to lift with proper form, demonstrate

TABLE 11.2	Sample Training Regimens for Strength, Endurance, or Power			
Training	Strength	Endurance	Power	Power (Core)
Exercises	8–12	8–12	8–12	3–5
Repetitions	8–12	10–15	8–12	3–5
Sets	1–3	3–5	3–5	3–5
Intensity	> 85% 1-RM	50–65% 1-RM	50–65% 1-RM	75–85% 1-RM
Days per week	2–3	2–3	2–3	2–3
Training speed	Slow to moderate	Slow to moderate	Fast, with little or no rest between sets	Fast, with little or no rest between sets

These are basic guidelines. Additional sets or combinations of sets and repetitions may elicit greater gains.

SOURCE: Core power recommendations are modified from National Strength and Conditioning Association (2000), *Essentials of Strength Training and Conditioning*, 2nd ed. Colorado Springs, CO: Author.

proper spotting techniques, and help you develop a sound resistance training program. You must be careful when seeking a strength coach. Don't rely on the assumption that everyone who lifts regularly knows what they are doing. We suggest that you ask at your health club to locate a person certified through one of the major professional organizations. The National Strength and Conditioning Association offers a certification for a strength and conditioning specialist (CSCS). The American College of Sports Medicine offers a certified health-fitness instructor and a Personal Trainer certification. More information on these certifications can be found at the websites of these organizations.

SELECTING EQUIPMENT AND EXERCISES When selecting exercise equipment for resistance training, there are three overriding factors that must be considered. The first is safety. The equipment should fit your body comfortably and be sturdy enough to withstand the stress applied during a resistance training program. When using machines, the axis of rotation for any piece of equipment should be aligned with the center of the joint on your body that will be performing the activity. Safety straps should be worn to help you maintain proper body alignment. Seek out professional instruction on how to use the equipment safely and effectively.

The second factor is effectiveness. In order to develop muscular strength and endurance, your physical activity program must be designed in such a way as to optimize the time spent in training. With resistance training equipment, a great deal of time may be lost in adjusting the resistance or the equipment. The best advice we can give is to try out any piece of equipment before deciding to purchase it or incorporate it into your program.

The third factor is expense. Resistance training does not need to be expensive. Obviously, if you are interested in using gold-plated barbells or participating in the swankiest fitness facility, resistance training can be expensive. However, your muscles do not know or care what form of resistance is being applied. You can overload your muscle by pushing against an immovable object, by lifting buckets with varying amounts of sand or water, or by performing calisthenics in water. The key to developing muscular fitness is the regular application of resistance. With a little imagination, you can find a variety of ways of applying this resistance.

SAMPLE EXERCISES As stated previously, there are a variety of activities in which you can participate to enhance your muscular strength, endurance, and power. We have subdivided some of these activities into what we refer to as *basic lifts* and *advanced lifts*. The basic lifts require little time to learn proper technique, work the major muscle groups as recommended by the ACSM (2006), and are safe if performed properly (FIGURE 11.8 through FIGURE 11.25).

The advanced lifts are designed for those seeking optimal health and fitness goals, or those competing in sports. They require more time to learn proper technique (professional instruction is required), place a great deal of stress on specific areas of the body, and are associated with a higher risk for injury (FIGURE 11.26 through FIGURE 11.35).

ORDER OF EXERCISES For most beginners, it is better to alternate between agonists and antagonists when setting the order of exercises. It is also better to start with the large muscle groups and then move to the smaller muscle groups. For example, you might want to perform leg extensions followed by leg curls (flexion), and then move on to calf raises. Another example would be to perform bench presses followed by lat (latissimus dorsi) pull-downs, and then move on to tricep extensions.

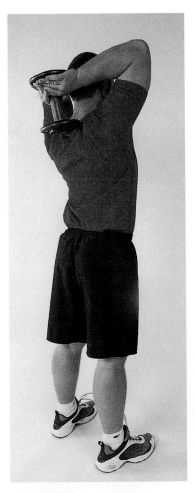

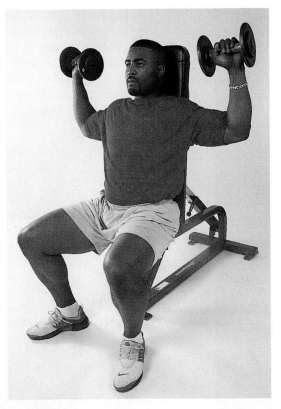

FIGURE 11.9 **Shoulder Exercises.** Seated press.

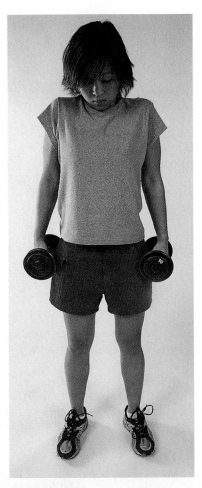

FIGURE 11.8 **Arm Exercises.**
Tricep extension.

FIGURE 11.10 **Neck Exercises.**
Shoulder shrugs.

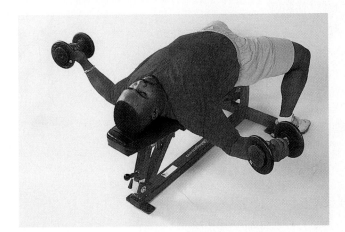

FIGURE 11.11 **Chest Exercises.** Bent-arm flies.

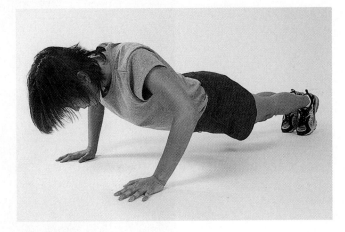

FIGURE 11.12 **Chest Exercises.** Push-ups.

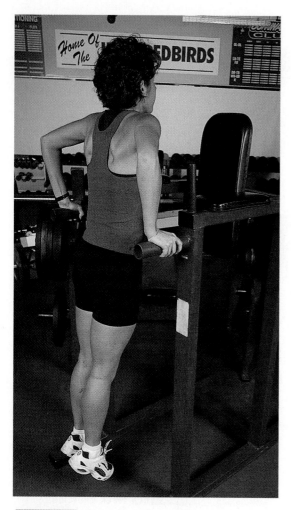

FIGURE 11.13 **Chest Exercises.** Dips.

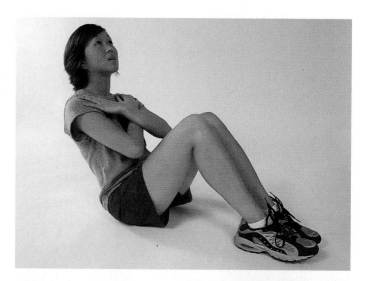

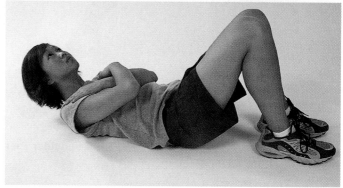

FIGURE 11.14 **Abdomen Exercises.** Sit-up (upper), curl-up (lower).

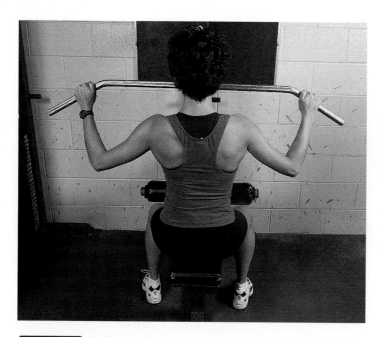

FIGURE 11.15 **Back Exercises.** Lat pull-down.

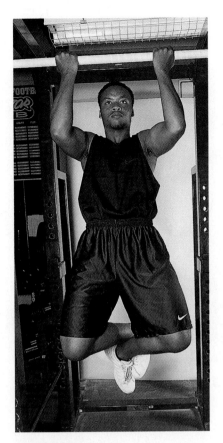 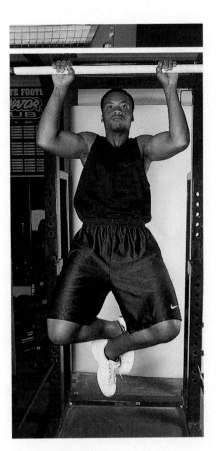

FIGURE 11.16 **Back Exercises.** Curl-up (left); pull-up (right).

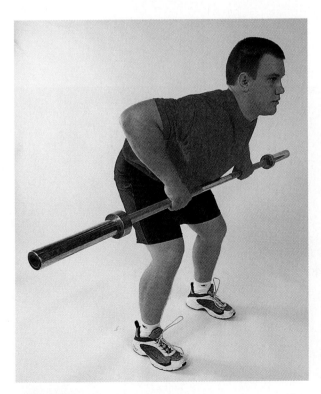

FIGURE 11.17 **Back Exercises.** Bent-over rows.

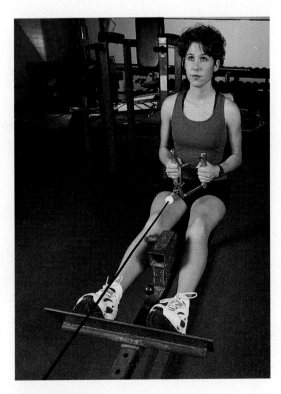

FIGURE 11.18 **Back Exercises.** Seated rows.

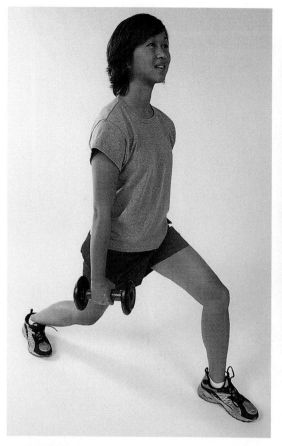

FIGURE 11.19 **Groin Exercises.** Lunges.

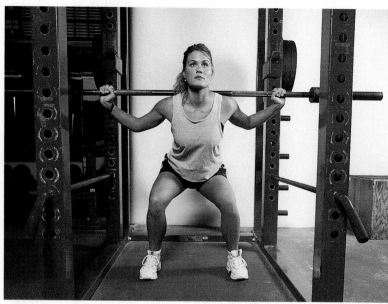

FIGURE 11.20 **Leg Exercises.** Squats.

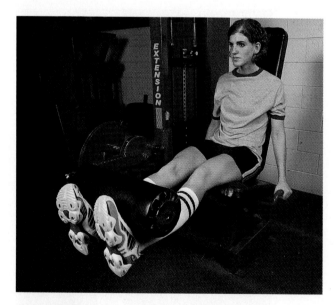

FIGURE 11.21 **Leg Exercises.** Quad extension.

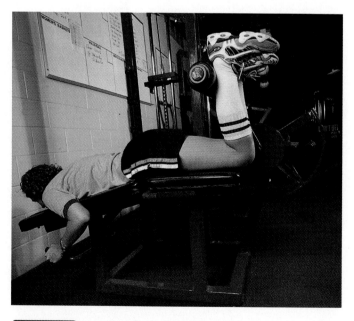

FIGURE 11.22 **Leg Exercises.** Hamstring curl.

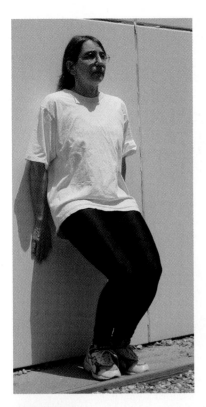

FIGURE 11.23 **Leg Exercises.** Wall sit.

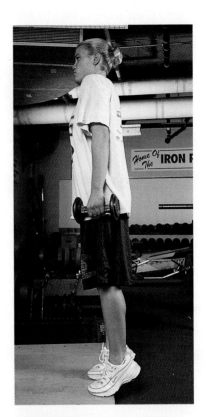

FIGURE 11.24 **Leg Exercises.** Calf raise.

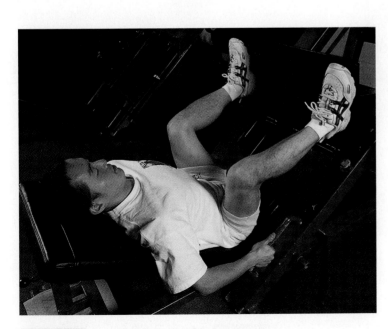

FIGURE 11.25 **Leg Exercises.** Double-leg press.

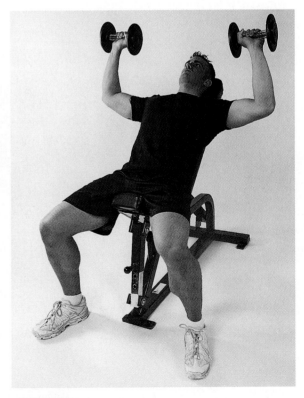

FIGURE 11.26 **Advanced Lifts.** Incline bench press (chest and shoulders).

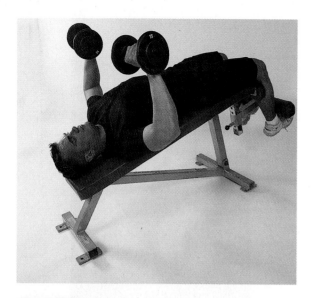

FIGURE 11.27 **Advanced Lifts.** Decline bench press (chest and shoulders).

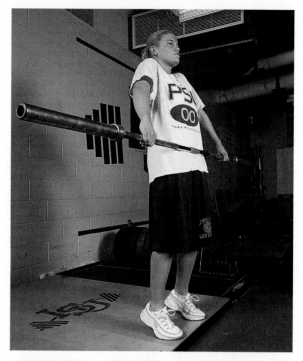

FIGURE 11.28 **Advanced Lifts.** Snatch pull (legs, buttocks, and back).

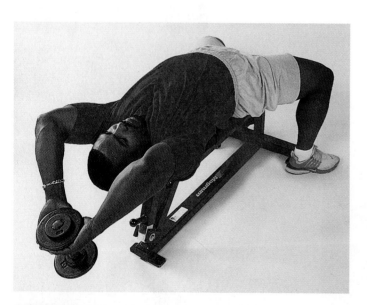

FIGURE 11.29 **Advanced Lifts.** Bent-arm pullover (lats).

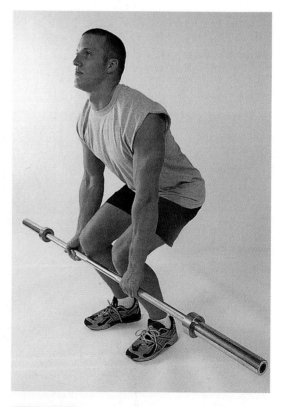

FIGURE 11.30 **Advanced Lifts.** Dead lift (legs, buttocks, and back).

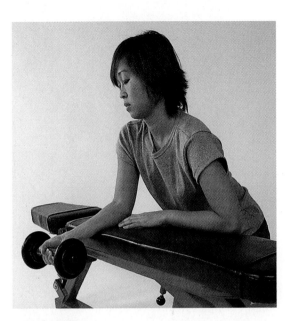

FIGURE 11.31 **Advanced Lifts.** Wrist curl (wrist flexors).

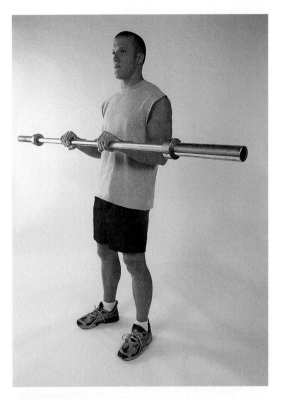

FIGURE 11.32 **Advanced Lifts.** Reverse bicep curl (biceps and forearms).

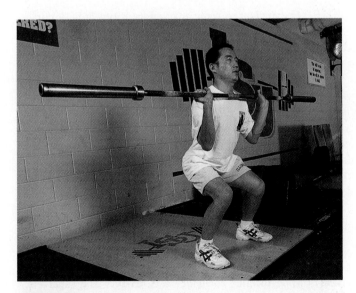

FIGURE 11.33 **Advanced Lifts.** (Upper) Power clean, starting position. (Lower) Extending the bar overhead. (Most major muscle groups.)

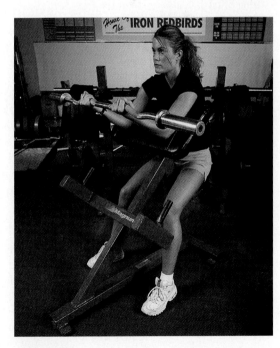

FIGURE 11.34 **Advanced Lifts.** Preacher curl (biceps).

FIGURE 11.35 **Advanced Lifts.**
Concentration curl (biceps).

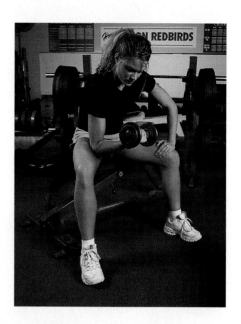

Periodization Form of resistance training in which a training program is subdivided into sections, or periods; the focus of training in each period varies, allowing for a greater overall adjustment to occur.

Pyramiding A gradual increase in the weight being lifted with a corresponding reduction in the number of repetitions until the one-repetition maximum is reached; this is followed by a gradual decrease in the resistance being lifted and an increase in the number of repetitions, until the exerciser returns to the initial load.

Plyometrics Form of resistance training that uses bounding-type exercises to overload muscles; recoil from bounding activity utilizes stored elastic energy in the connective tissue that runs through the muscle to improve performance.

Compound sets Consecutive performance of two sets of exercises that stress the same muscle group.

Tri-sets Consecutive performance of three sets of exercises that stress the same muscle group.

Supersets Consecutive performance of two sets of exercises that stress one muscle group and its antagonist without a rest period separating the sets.

FREE WEIGHTS VERSUS MACHINES Most people who perform resistance training use either free weights or machines. Machines tend to be used more by beginners, those who may have difficulty with balance, and those who have limited space to perform resistance training. Machines allow for an application of resistance in a guided or restricted manner (Stone et al., 2000).

Free weights tend to be used by those who want to isolate individual muscles, are interested in developing control and balance when lifting, and want to engage in a wide variety of activities. It has been suggested that free weights allow for more mechanical specificity (more lifelike movements) than machines and therefore provide a superior method for training (Stone et al., 2000). Most "serious" lifters use free weights.

WEIGHT ROOM ETIQUETTE If you elect to train in a weight room, it is important to follow the rules for safety and to maintain harmony with others who may be using the facility. Always remember to return any equipment to its proper storage place after you use it. Don't hog equipment or stations. If someone is waiting and it won't take major equipment adjustment, ask if he or she wishes to alternate sets with you. Use a spotter to assist you with lifts. Good spotters not only make your workout safer but also allow you to work until complete fatigue. Be aware of your environment. Pay attention to what is going on around you and keep your eyes open for equipment that may place you in danger. Always use collars on dumbbells and barbells. Don't use equipment unless you have been instructed about its use, and don't use defective equipment. In sum, have a healthy respect for the equipment and for those around you.

Specialized Training Routines

There are several variations of resistance training programs that have seen increased interest over the years. These include circuit weight training, **periodization**, **pyramiding**, **plyometrics**, and performing **compound sets**, **tri-sets**, and **supersets**.

CIRCUIT WEIGHT TRAINING Circuit weight training involves setting up a series of stations at which you perform different weight training (and/or aerobic) exercises. You can use any combination of exercises included in the basic lifts outlined earlier. By limiting time between stations, you can develop muscular strength, muscular endurance, and aerobic capacity. Improvements in VO₂max of 5 percent have been associated with circuit weight training (ACSM, 2006).

PERIODIZATION *Periodization* refers to varying the resistance training program at regular time intervals to bring about optimal gains in strength, power, motor performance, and/or muscle hypertrophy (Fleck, 1999). For example, you can subdivide the year into four cycles. During the first cycle, you may focus on the development of muscular strength. During the second cycle, you may focus on the development of muscular power. During the third cycle, you may focus on the development of muscular endurance. And, during the fourth cycle, you may focus on cross training to allow adequate recovery from the three resistance training cycles. In the case of a competitive athlete, a goal may be to bring about peak physical performance for a major competition (Fleck, 1999). The utilization of the training cycles allows the muscles to be stressed throughout the year without being stressed in the same way at all times. This will decrease the risk of injury while reducing the potential for boredom.

Advantages of programs that include periodization are greater strength gains, greater gains in lean body mass and total body weight, greater decreases in percentage of body fat, and greater overall fitness gains than nonperiodized multiple-set and single-set programs (Fleck, 1999).

PYRAMIDING *Pyramiding* refers to a progression of sets during a resistance workout. The individual may start with a set consisting of a relatively light load and multiple repetitions (reps). For the next set, the load is increased and the number of reps decreased. This continues until the individual is lifting maximally with a minimal number of reps. The person then continues by performing more sets during which the resistance is reduced and the number of reps increased (FIGURE 11.36).

PLYOMETRICS *Plyometrics* involves the use of bounding-type exercises to overload muscle groups. For example, depth jumping involves jumping off an elevated platform, landing on a surface, and then immediately performing a maximal verti-

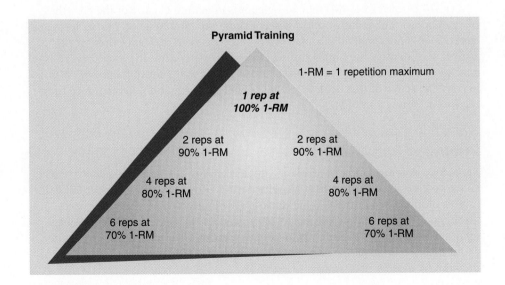

Pyramid Training

1-RM = 1 repetition maximum

1 rep at
100% 1-RM

2 reps at
90% 1-RM

2 reps at
90% 1-RM

4 reps at
80% 1-RM

4 reps at
80% 1-RM

6 reps at
70% 1-RM

6 reps at
70% 1-RM

FIGURE 11.36 **Pyramid Training.** The illustration is an example of using a pyramid training protocol.

cal leap. Plyometric training is favored by some athletes because it allows them to train at a normal speed of movement and overloads the muscles in a way not possible with other training techniques. The disadvantage associated with plyometric training lies in the high potential for injury, due to the ballistic nature of the activity. You must have well-conditioned muscles to perform plyometrics safely.

COMPOUND AND TRI-SETS   Compound sets and tri-sets involve performing two (compound) or three (tri) exercises in a row that stress the same muscle groups. This ensures that the muscle group is optimally fatigued and increases the likelihood that it will get stronger faster. The disadvantage of using compound and tri-sets is that you increase the likelihood of injuring a muscle or joint and increase the discomfort and pain sometimes associated with resistance training.

SUPERSETS   *Supersetting* involves performing a set of exercises for one muscle group and, with no rest period between sets, immediately performing a set of exercises for the antagonist of that group. Supersetting is designed to ensure that both muscle groups are actively fatigued. If done correctly, supersetting has the potential to speed up the development of muscular strength. The major disadvantage is the discomfort associated with this technique and its high rate of injury.

For more information on these specialized training formats, it is recommend that you check with a certified strength training professional or consult references that focus on these topics.

Resistance Training Across the Life Span

Individuals of any age can benefit from resistance training.

Resistance training can and should be performed across the life span (Brill et al., 2000). You are never too old or too young to benefit from resistance training. Infants grasping their parents' fingers are performing a type of resistance training. We must remember not to fall into the trap of associating resistance training solely with weight rooms. Any type of resistance (water, body weight, free weights) can be used to bring about improvement in function.

Resistance training can be performed safely at any age if some commonsense guidelines are followed. In particular, preadolescent children should avoid maximal resistance training. In this age group, maximal resistance training (lifting at or beyond 70 percent of 1-RM) may bring about premature closure of the growth plate in bones. The focus of preadolescent programs should be on proper form and supervision. Older individuals may wish to decrease the resistance they work against and increase the number of repetitions they perform. In either case, resistance training can help to build and maintain strong and enduring muscles. It is beyond the scope of this book to provide detailed information on resistance training for the young and old.

Self-Image and Training

Resistance training can have a positive impact on how we look—and how we feel about how we look. Strong, firm muscles permit better posture and a certain gracefulness of movement. Muscles that don't fatigue easily make us feel energized throughout the day. Numerous books have detailed the impact of body language upon our own moods and on how others receive us. Generally, people feel better about themselves when they are fit. Muscular fitness plays an important role in providing a healthy body image.

Resistance Training's Impact on Metabolism

Resistance training increases our lean muscle mass. Lean muscle mass is metabolically more active than any other tissue found in the body. By increasing lean body mass we can actually increase our metabolic rate. This means that we are capable of expending energy at a greater rate even when sleeping. The advantages of this state are that we can consume more food and store fewer calories. See Chapter 8 for more information.

Physical Activity and Health Connection

Resistance training is an integral component in the comprehensive health program promoted by the major health organizations, including the American College of Sports Medicine, the American Heart Association, the American Association of Cardiovascular and Cardiopulmonary Rehabilitation, and the Surgeon General's Office (Feigenbaum & Pollock, 1999). Resistance training will make your muscles stronger and supply them with more endurance. Resistance training will guard against injury, prevent or rehabilitate low-back disorders, and increase metabolism, thereby having a positive impact on the body composition profile. Increased bone density and lower risk of osteoporosis are other reasons why everyone should regularly incorporate resistance training into their physical activity programs.

concept connections

1. **Strength refers to a muscle's ability to generate force.** Muscles generate force by contracting. Muscular strength refers to the amount of force a muscle can generate. Stronger muscles are capable of generating more force than weaker muscles.

2. **Significant health benefits are associated with resistance training.** Resistance training makes muscles stronger and more enduring. It helps guard against injury and prevents and rehabilitates low-back disorders. It will also help to increase your bone density, thereby decreasing the probability of your developing osteoporosis. It has positive effects on metabolic rate, allowing you to attain a healthy body composition profile.

3. **Muscles that are stressed by resistance training get stronger and increase in size (hypertrophy), while muscles that are neglected get weaker and shrink in size (atrophy).** A muscle will get stronger if it is physically stressed. The best way to stress a muscle physically is by incorporating resistance training into your physical activity program. A muscle that is not regularly exposed to stress atrophies and becomes weaker.

4. **You can develop muscular strength and endurance through a variety of resistance training programs.** The form of resistance you use to stress your muscles is not as important as the way in which you use the resistance. For this reason, you can perform a variety of activities using a variety of items to perform resistance training.

5. **Individuals of any age can benefit from resistance training.** Since muscles need to be stressed to function well, resistance training should be performed from the cradle to the grave. Infants who grasp their parent's finger are performing resistance training. To maintain functional independence as we age, resistance training should be performed throughout the life span.

Terms

Circuit weight training, 228
Protein filaments, 228
Actin, 228
Sarcomere, 228
Myosin, 228
Static contraction, 228
Concentric muscle action, 230
Eccentric muscle action, 230
Agonist, 231

Antagonist, 231
Synergists, 231
Neutralizer, 231
Neuromuscular adaptations, 233
Isometric, 233
Isotonic, 233
Isokinetic, 233
Reps, 236
Sets, 236

Valsalva maneuver, 238
Periodization, 248
Pyramiding, 248
Plyometrics, 248
Compound sets, 248
Tri-sets, 248
Supersets, 248

making the connection

Beth feels confident about her resistance training program. She has started to develop a program focused on muscular endurance. Beth understands that she must start gradually and work on proper form and safety. She has already noticed an increased feeling of self-confidence since she started resistance training.

Critical Thinking

1. What are the major differences between training to improve muscular strength and training to improve muscular endurance?
2. What factors determine how large and strong a person can become?
3. What principles of training are important when developing a resistance training program?
4. In addition to using free weights, how else might one perform resistance training?
5. In what ways does resistance training improve your health?

References

American College of Sports Medicine. (2006). *ACSM's Guidelines for Exercise Testing and Prescription,* 7th ed. Philadelphia: Lippincott, Williams & Wilkins.

Brill, P.A., Macera, C.A., Davis, D.R., Blair, S.N., & Gordon, N. (2000). Muscular strength and physical function. *Medicine and Science in Sports and Exercise* 32(2):412–416.

Butterfield, G., Kleiner, S., Lemon, P., & Stone, M. (1995). Roundtable: Methods of weight gain in athletes. *Gatorade Sports Science Exchange* 6(3).

Dolezal, B.A., Potteiger, J.A., Jacobsen, D.J., & Benedict, S.H. (2000). Muscle damage and resting metabolic rate after acute resistance exercise with an eccentric overload. *Medicine and Science in Sports and Exercise* 32(7):1202–1207.

Feigenbaum, M.S., & Pollock, M.L. (1999). Prescription of resistance training for health and disease. *Medicine and Science in Sports and Exercise* 31(1):38–45.

Fleck, S.J. (1999). Periodized strength training: A critical review. *Journal of Strength and Conditioning Research* 13(1):82–89.

Kraemer, W.J. (1992). Involvement of eccentric muscle action may optimize adaptations to resistance training. *Gatorade Sports Science Exchange* 4(41).

Mayo, J.J., & Kravitz, L. (1999). A review of the acute cardiovascular responses to resistance exercise of healthy young and older adults. *Journal of Strength and Conditioning Research* 13(1):90–96.

Pollock, M.L., & Vincent, K.R. (1996, December). Resistance training for health. *President's Council on Physical Fitness and Research Digest* 2(8):1–5.

Stone, M.H., Collins, D.C., Plisk, S.P., Haff, G., & Stone, M.E. (2000). Training principles: Evaluation of modes and methods of resistance training. *Strength and Conditioning Journal* 22(3):65–76.

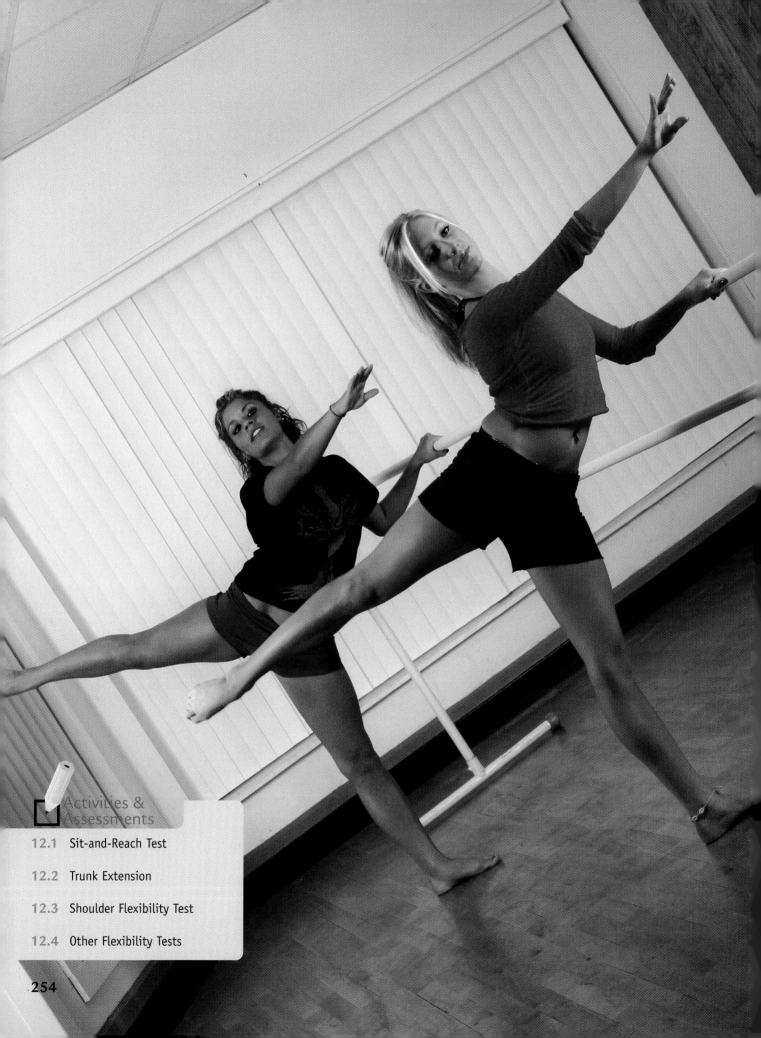

Activities &
Assessments

12.1   Sit-and-Reach Test

12.2   Trunk Extension

12.3   Shoulder Flexibility Test

12.4   Other Flexibility Tests

Stretching and Flexibility

what's the connection?

Bob works out regularly, but he has not paid much attention to incorporating flexibility exercises into his physical activity routine. Recently, Bob has noticed that his lower back gets sore in the morning following a highly active day. Bob can't remember any sudden trauma to his back, and the pain subsides as he gets up and starts moving around. He remembers hearing something about low-back pain being related to poor muscular fitness and in particular, poor flexibility. Bob decides to do some investigating to see what he can find out about the relationship between low-back pain and flexibility.

concepts

1. Many factors influence the amount of flexibility you have at a joint.

2. Sense receptors located in your muscles and tendons play an important role in developing good flexibility.

3. Three common categories of flexibility exercises are static, ballistic, and PNF.

4. Guidelines for improving flexibility suggest stretching a muscle and holding the position for 10 to 30 seconds.

5. Good flexibility protects against injury, enhances your ability to be physically active, and helps maintain an independent lifestyle.

6. Most low-back pain is caused by poor muscular fitness.

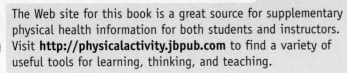

http://physicalactivity.jbpub.com

The Web site for this book is a great source for supplementary physical health information for both students and instructors. Visit **http://physicalactivity.jbpub.com** to find a variety of useful tools for learning, thinking, and teaching.

Introduction

This chapter focuses on the importance of maintaining good flexibility. It provides instruction on developing a flexibility program and examples of stretching exercises. The chapter explores the relationship between good flexibility and good health.

Flexibility refers to the range of motion available at a joint. Many factors can influence range of motion, including anatomical structure of the joint (how the bones are aligned), muscle temperature, disease status, muscle and tendon **elasticity** and **compliance**, age, sex, activity status, and **tissue interference**. Anatomical structure varies from joint to joint in our own bodies, and there is a great deal of variation among individuals. Since range of motion is in part determined by our joint structure, this anatomical variation can have profound effects on flexibility.

Length of bone also affects range of motion. A common test of hamstring flexibility, the sit-and-reach test, demonstrates this point. When performing the sit-and-reach, you sit down with your legs straight out in front of you (FIGURE 12.1). Placing your hands on top of each other, you lean as far forward as possible. Your flexibility is assessed based on how far you can reach. If the test is not modified, limb length discrepancies may have a major impact on the results. For example, someone with short legs and long arms will score better than someone with long legs and short arms.

Muscle temperature has a direct impact on flexibility because it affects muscle elasticity and compliance. *Elasticity* and *compliance* refer to the muscle's ability to stretch beyond its normal resting length and then return to its initial length once the forces causing the stretch are removed. When a muscle is cold, its elastic and compliant properties are diminished; when it is warm, the muscle is more pliable (stretchy). If you warm a muscle, or perform stretching activities, on warm days, you will have better flexibility than if you stretch cold muscles on cold days.

Many factors influence the amount of flexibility you have at a joint.

Elasticity Degree to which a material resists deformation and quickly returns to its normal shape.

Compliance Ease with which a material is elongated or stretched; the opposite of stiffness.

Tissue interference Occurs when either muscle or fat tissue physically blocks a movement, restricting a joint's full range of motion.

Flexibility is important throughout the life span.

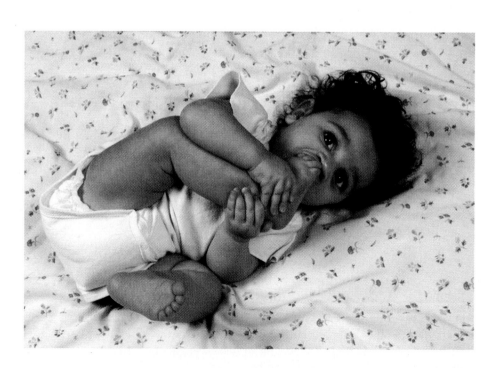

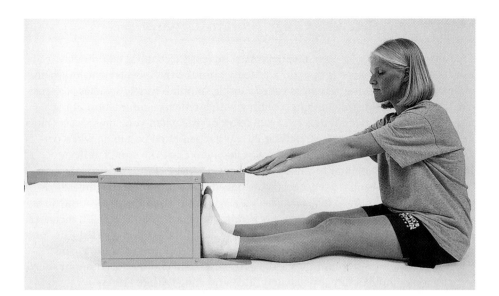

FIGURE 12.1 **Sit-and-Reach Test.** A sit-and-reach test can be used to assess your hamstring flexibility.

Certain diseases can diminish flexibility. They can limit compliance of a muscle, of a muscle's tendon, or of the ligaments that connect the bones. We lose flexibility if we lose muscle and tendon compliance. Loss of muscle and tendon elasticity and compliance may be caused by disuse. Stretching exercises can improve muscle and tendon compliance by regularly making the muscle move through its full range of motion. Over a period of time, muscles and tendons that are stretched and then relaxed become more pliable.

As we age, the elastic and compliant properties of our muscles and tendons naturally diminish. This can lead to a loss of flexibility. However, we now know that the rate and degree at which this natural aging process occurs can be limited by performing stretching activities regularly (American College of Sports Medicine [ACSM], 2006; Knudson, Magnusson, & McHugh, 2000). We can delay the onset of age-related flexibility loss, and we can also minimize the impact of age on our functional ability.

In most cases, women are more flexible than men. This is due in part to anatomic differences (for example, differences in hip joint structure), but hormonal influences on muscle compliance also contribute to male/female flexibility differences.

Tissue interference refers to the possibility that either muscle or fat tissue may physically block a movement and restrict a joint's ability to provide full range of motion. For instance, an obese individual, or a person with highly developed muscle mass, may find that the fat mass or muscle mass physically blocks some movement. This can become a problem if the muscle is prevented from moving through its full range of motion. The affected muscle and tendon may shorten, thereby decreasing flexibility.

Several of these factors are beyond our control (anatomic structure, age, sex). We do, however, have the ability to manipulate other factors, such as activity status, muscle temperature, disease status, muscle and tendon elasticity and compliance, and tissue interference. We can enhance our flexibility by performing stretching exercises daily and by maintaining an active lifestyle.

Improving your flexibility helps to maintain an independent, active lifestyle.

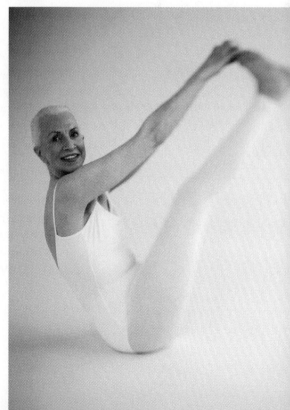

Muscle Spindles and Golgi Tendon Organs

Throughout the body we have **proprioceptors**, or sense receptors, that provide feedback to the central nervous system. Located within the thick center portion (belly) of our muscles are sense receptors called muscle spindles. **Muscle spindles** are sensitive to rapid forceful stretching, responding with a reflexive contraction of the muscle called the stretch reflex. A **stretch reflex** occurs when your muscle contracts in response to rapid forceful stretching. If you happen to be bouncing when performing a stretching exercise, you are more likely to elicit the stretch reflex. Bouncing has the potential to cause muscle injury.

Our tendons also have sense receptors imbedded within them that are called Golgi tendon organs. **Golgi tendon organs** are sensitive to rapid forceful contractions and cause a reflexive relaxation to occur within the muscle. As the tension increases in the muscle and tendon, these sense receptors detect the tension and regulate further muscle action. Muscle action might be inhibited to induce relaxation. This reflex inhibition can prevent injury from excessive strain and may account for short-term increases in flexibility immediately after stretching (ACSM, 1998).

Muscle Elasticity and Compliance

Our muscles are held together by a series of elastic connective tissues that both surround each muscle and are found throughout each muscle. These connective tissues come together at the ends of the muscles into tendons. It is the tendons that connect muscle to bone. When we move a muscle, we stretch these connective tissues. When the muscle relaxes, the connective tissue recoil helps the muscle return to its original resting length.

Stretching exercises have their greatest impact on the connective tissues of the muscle and tendon. By regularly stretching these connective tissues, the elastic and compliant properties of the tissues are enhanced. Stretching results in a short-term increase in muscle and tendon length, and a lasting increase through alteration in the surrounding connective tissue matrix (ACSM, 1998).

Types of Stretching Exercises

To perform stretching exercises, you can select several different methods. All have advantages and disadvantages, so choose the one that best fits your individual needs and the type of physical activity you are about to perform.

Static Stretching

Static stretching moves a muscle into a position where the muscle is stretched slightly beyond its normal range of motion. A slight discomfort, but no pain, should be felt. The muscle is then held in this position for 10 to 30 seconds. The nonmoving state of the muscle gives static stretching its name. This type of stretching activity is recommended prior to starting physical activity. It is one of the safest methods of stretching.

A potential disadvantage of static stretching is that it may take a good deal of time to stretch out all of your muscles. For this reason, multiple-joint stretching is recommended. By performing static multiple-joint stretching activities, you can stretch more than one muscle group at a time.

Sense receptors located in your muscles and tendons play an important role in developing good flexibility.

Proprioceptors Sense receptors that provide feedback to our central nervous system.

Muscle spindles Sense receptors sensitive to rapid forceful stretching that cause a reflexive contraction of the muscle.

Stretch reflex Reflexive response to forceful rapid stretching that causes a muscle to contract.

Golgi tendon organs Sense receptors sensitive to rapid forceful contractions that cause a reflexive relaxation to occur within the muscle.

Static stretching Elongating a muscle and holding that position.

Three common categories of flexibility exercises are static, ballistic, and PNF.

Ballistic Stretching

Ballistic stretching, an exaggerated form of dynamic stretching, utilizes a bouncing motion to move a muscle beyond its normal range of motion. This type of stretching activity has the potential to cause injury if the muscle is not properly warmed up, or if the bouncing is too forceful and rapid. However, since most physical activity is dynamic in nature, the body can handle dynamic stretching if it is performed properly. This type of stretching is recommended only when the muscle is adequately warmed up, after static stretching has been performed, and when the dynamic stretches are performed slowly. An advantage to this type of stretching is that you can stretch rather rapidly. The major disadvantage is that you are at greater risk of injury.

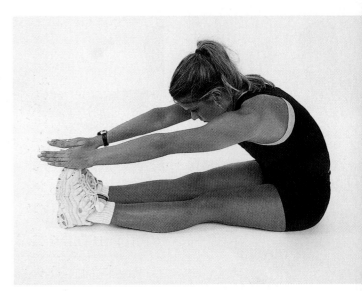

Static stretching is recommended for most people.

PNF Stretching

PNF stretching, or *proprioceptive neuromuscular facilitation*, utilizes and integrates the nervous and muscular systems to enhance flexibility. As mentioned earlier, Gogli tendon organs are located in the tendons that connect muscle to bone. They are sensitive to rapid forceful contraction and respond by causing the muscle to relax. In PNF stretching, you take advantage of the way Golgi tendon organs work and use them to enhance flexibility (Holcomb, 2000). You do this by causing a muscle to contract and then relaxing the muscle. The forced contraction aids in getting the muscle to relax.

An example of PNF stretching is the contract-relax-contract method. In this method, you first maximally contract an agonist (prime mover; for example, the biceps). The agonist muscle then relaxes. This is followed by contraction of the antagonist (resistor, triceps) muscle. The initial forceful contraction involves Golgi tendon organ feedback. The relaxation phase and subsequent contraction of the antagonist muscle further enhances the degree of relaxation felt in the agonist muscle.

There is some evidence that PNF may bring superior results compared with the other types of exercises done to increase flexibility (ACSM, 1998; Holcomb, 2000). However, it usually takes a greater degree of training to perform PNF safely and effectively. Static stretches, therefore, are commonly used, and for many individuals represent a safer and still-effective compromise (ACSM, 2006).

> **Ballistic stretching** Fast, momentum-assisted, pulsing movements used to stretch muscles.
>
> **PNF stretching** Proprioceptive neuromuscular facilitation; utilization and integration of the nervous and muscular systems to enhance flexibility.
>
> **Passive stretching** A natural stretch of the muscle and tendon with no additional force applied.
>
> **Active stretching** Taking a muscle beyond its normal range of motion with assistance.

Passive and Active Stretching

Two additional concepts that are related to stretching exercises and flexibility are the concepts of passive and active stretching. **Passive stretching** occurs when the individual allows the muscle and tendon to stretch naturally, without additional force being applied. This is a safer method of stretching than active stretching; however, gains in flexibility are usually not as large.

Active stretching involves taking a muscle beyond its normal range of motion with assistance. This may be facilitated by having a partner move the limb segment to the end of its normal range of motion, or by contracting antagonists to further stretch an agonist muscle. It takes a skilled partner to help you perform active stretching safely; if the muscle is moved too far, you may injure yourself.

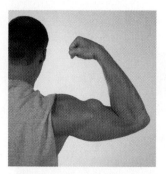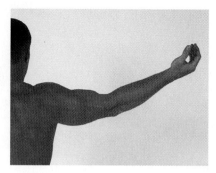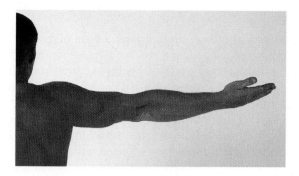

Contract, relax, antagonist-contract method of PNF stretching.

Guidelines for improving flexibility suggest stretching a muscle and holding the position for 10 to 30 seconds.

Flexibility Guidelines

Flexibility guidelines vary based on individuals and their needs. Generally, however, you can improve your flexibility by following some common suggestions. First of all, flexibility exercises should be just one part of an overall physical activity program. The focus of the flexibility component of your physical activity program should be to develop and maintain a healthy range of motion. Exercises that stretch the major muscle groups should be performed a minimum of 2 to 3 days per week, and ideally 5 to 7 days per week (ACSM, 2006). Any of the previously described techniques (static, ballistic, PNF) may be used to enhance flexibility if they are performed properly.

Frequency, Intensity, and Duration

It is generally suggested that slow rates of stretching allow greater stress relaxation and generate lower tensile force on the tendon. For this reason, it is recommended that you hold a position that places a muscle on stretch for 10 to 30 seconds at the point of mild discomfort (ACSM, 2006). If you perform PNF stretches, they should involve a 6-second contraction followed by a 10- to 30-second assisted stretch (ACSM, 1998). Exercises that stretch multiple muscle groups are typically suggested because they allow you to stretch more muscles, more thoroughly, and in a shorter period of time. It appears that two to four repetitions of a stretching activity produce the best results (ACSM, 2006).

When to Stretch

It is best to make stretching a daily part of your physical activity program. Stretching exercises can take place any time, any place. They can be performed first thing in the morning or the last thing at night. Stretching activities can be performed while watching the news or a favorite television show. In fact, you can even perform stretching exercises while you work.

As part of your workout routine, it is advisable to perform low-intensity stretching exercises before moving to more vigorous physical activity. This will help prepare your body for the activity that is to follow and decrease your chance for injury. After performing your preferred physical activity, additional stretching exercises should be done. It is during this cool-down from physical activity that the greatest improvements in flexibility are obtained. Remember that a warmer muscle stretches better and your muscle will be its warmest immediately following physical activity.

Assessment of Flexibility

Before beginning any flexibility program, it is smart to do some assessment. This will help you to determine which muscle groups require the most work. Generally, it is recommended that you perform an overall stretching program that focuses on the major muscle groups and then supplement with additional activities that focus on the muscles that need more work.

When discussing the assessment of flexibility, it is important to use standardized terminology. Physical therapists often distinguish between active range of motion (unassisted) and passive range of motion (therapist assisted) in assessing static flexibility (Knudson, Magnusson, & McHugh, 2000). The type of test you perform will influence the results of the test. When results are compared, you need to know what type of flexibility was measured.

Single-joint flexibility tests are considered better measurements of flexibility than multiple-joint tests because they isolate specific muscles better and are less affected by limb segment length variations (Knudson et al., 2000). Goniometers are generally used to make single-joint flexibility measurements.

Multiple-joint flexibility assessments like the sit-and-reach test are utilized by most fitness professionals (Knudson et al., 2000). In addition to the sit-and-reach, the shoulder and trunk lifts are common multiple-joint tests.

Common Stretching Exercises

There are numerous stretching exercises from which you can choose. These range from such exotic movements as those found in yoga and tai chi to those practiced regularly by the recreational exerciser.

When selecting the stretching exercises that are right for you, remember to choose those that stretch the major muscle masses of the body. Multiple-joint stretches, which allow you to stretch many muscles at once, are efficient. There are a number of muscles that cross more than one joint, so they can be targeted by multiple-joint stretching exercises. These include the hamstring (back of thigh) muscles, the quadriceps (front of thigh) muscles, and the calf muscles.

Sample Stretching Program

Flexibility is specific to each joint in your body. You may have good flexibility in one region and poor flexibility in another (Knudson et al., 2000). We suggest that you focus a segment of your stretching program on each of the following: the arms, legs, shoulders, upper and lower trunk, neck, and hips. We also suggest that you perform static stretching because it is the easiest and safest method for improving flexibility (ACSM, 2006). **FIGURE 12.2** through **FIGURE 12.26** illustrate suggested stretching exercises.

When performing these activities, it is recommended that you first warm your muscles with some low-intensity aerobic movement (walking). Then, take the muscle you wish to stretch to a position of mild discomfort and hold that position for 10 to 30 seconds. You should perform each stretch three to four times. Flexibility exercises should be performed a minimum of 2 to 3 days per week, although 5 to 7 days per week would be ideal (ACSM, 2006).

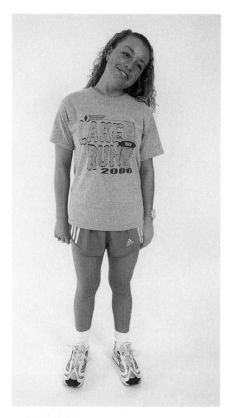

FIGURE 12.2 **Neck Stretch.** Ear to shoulder.

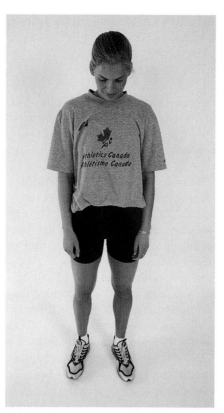

FIGURE 12.3 **Neck Stretch.** Chin to chest.

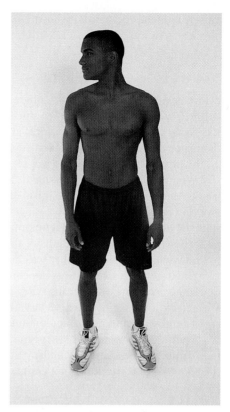

FIGURE 12.4 **Neck Stretch.** Look right and left.

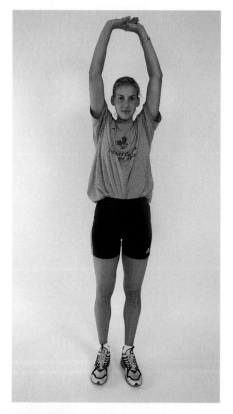

FIGURE 12.5 **Shoulder, Chest, and Upper-Back Stretch.** Reach up.

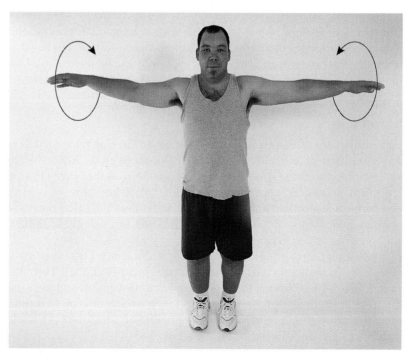

FIGURE 12.6 **Shoulder, Chest, and Upper-Back Stretch.** Slow arm circles.

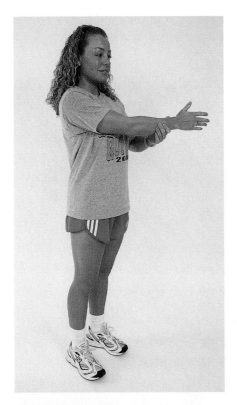

FIGURE 12.7 **Shoulder and Chest Stretch.** Arm across chest.

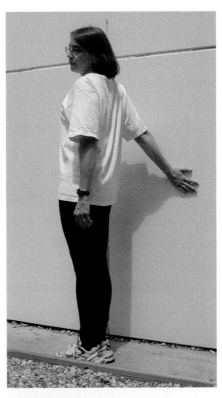

FIGURE 12.8 **Shoulder and Chest Stretch.** Wall chest stretch.

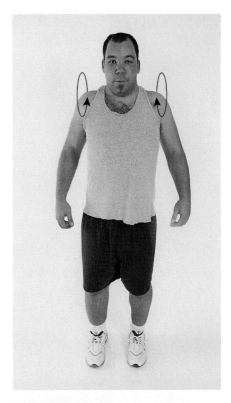

FIGURE 12.9 **Shoulder, Chest, and Upper-Back Stretch.** Shoulder roll.

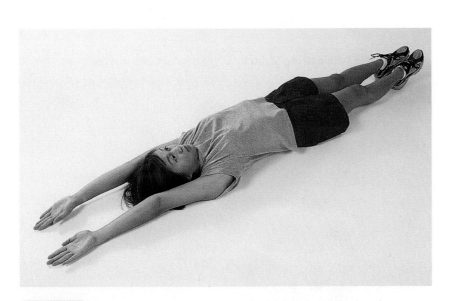

FIGURE 12.10 **Shoulder, Chest, and Abdominal Stretch.** Rack stretch.

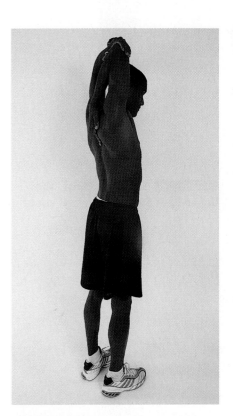

FIGURE 12.11 **Shoulder, Chest, and Upper-Back Stretch.** Back scratch.

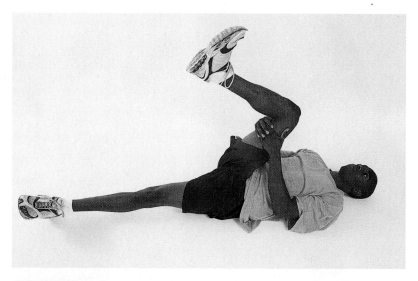

FIGURE 12.13 **Hamstring Stretch.** Single bent-leg vertical.

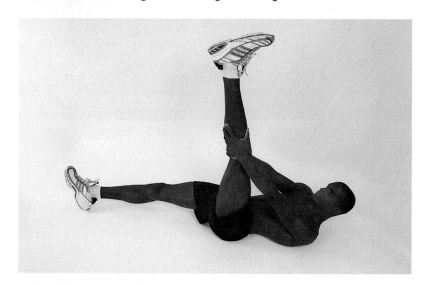

FIGURE 12.14 **Hamstring Stretch.** Single straight-leg vertical.

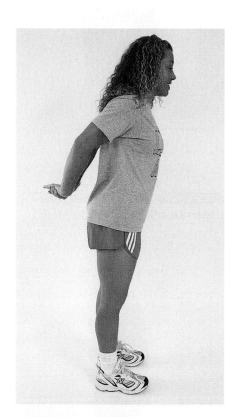

FIGURE 12.12 **Shoulder, Chest, and Upper-Back Stretch.** Handcuff stretch.

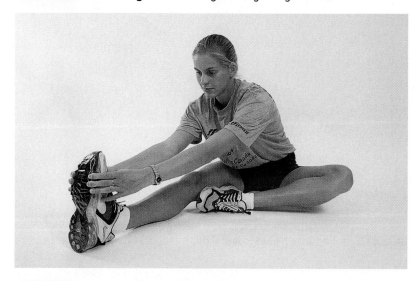

FIGURE 12.15 **Hamstring and Groin Stretch.** Modified hurdler stretch.

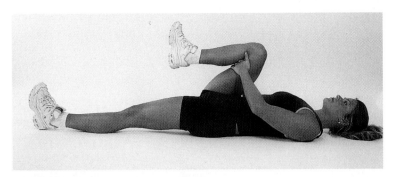

FIGURE 12.16 **Lower-Back and Hamstring Stretch.** Single knee to chest.

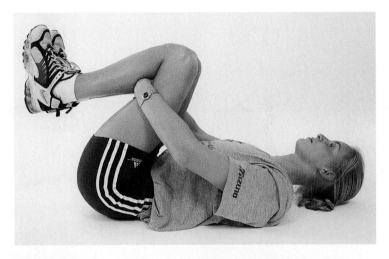

FIGURE 12.17 **Lower-Back and Hamstring Stretch.** Double knee to chest.

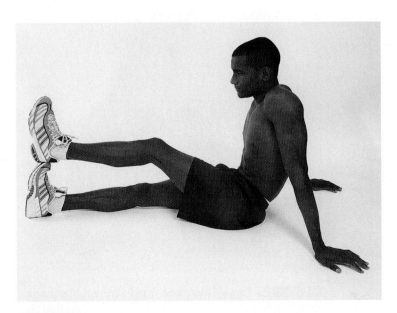

FIGURE 12.18 **Calf Stretch.** Seated toe stretch.

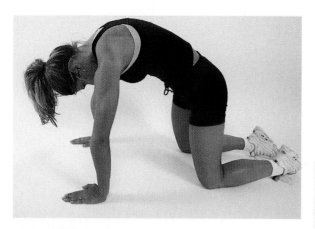

FIGURE 12.19 **Lower-Back Stretch.** Cat and camel.

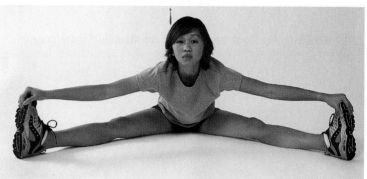

FIGURE 12.20 **Lower-Back, Groin, and Hamstring Stretch.** V-sit stretch.

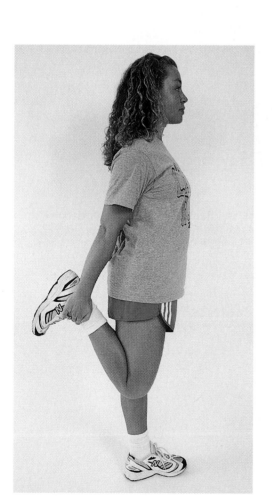

FIGURE 12.21 **Quad Stretch.** Standing heel-to-buttock stretch.

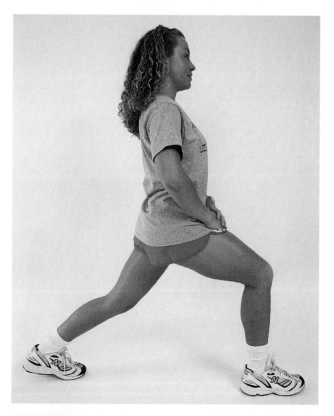

FIGURE 12.22 **Inner-Thigh and Quad Stretch.** Standing lunge stretch.

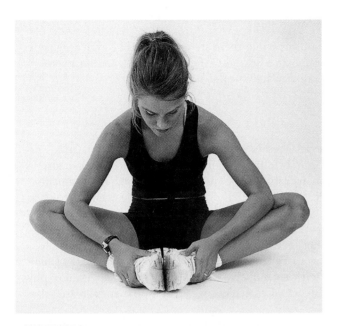

FIGURE 12.23 **Inner-Thigh and Quad Stretch.** Butterfly stretch.

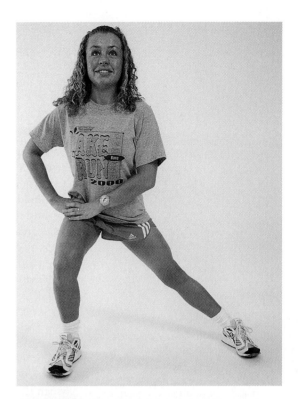

FIGURE 12.24 **Inner-Thigh, Quad, and Hip Stretch.** Side-lunge (skater) stretch.

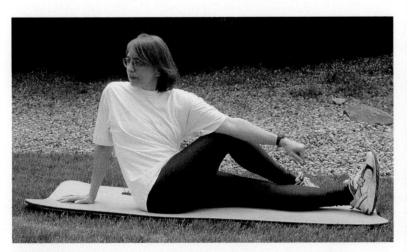

FIGURE 12.25 **Gluteal and Trunk Stretch.** Elbow-to-knee stretch.

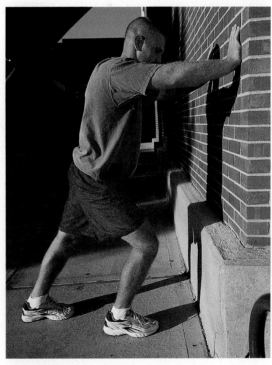

FIGURE 12.26 **Calf Stretch.** Wall lean.

Alternative Flexibility Activities

Although beyond the scope of this book, there are other forms of stretching activities that you can perform to enhance flexibility. Yoga and tai chi are but two of many popular alternative flexibility activities.

Improper Stretching

When we perform activities designed to improve flexibility, it is important to remember that the primary goal is to improve muscle compliance. We can also increase the range of motion available at a joint by overstretching the ligaments that hold the joints together. Overstretching can occur when ligaments are taken beyond their normal range of motion. Ligaments connect bone to bone and do not have great elastic properties. When ligaments are stretched, they do not regain their original shape. Over time, activities that stretch the ligaments may lead to joint laxity. *Joint laxity* means that the ligaments can no longer provide the stability necessary to hold the joint together properly. This is a negative adaptation to physical activity, wherein the joint actually becomes weaker and has an increased risk for joint injury.

The positions with the greatest likelihood of causing joint laxity are those that place the joint in positions well beyond its normal range of motion. Typically these positions involve some degree of **hyperextension** or **hyperflexion**. Hyperextension occurs when a joint is extended beyond its normal range; an example would be when the leg starts in a straight or extended position and then is forced backward at the knee. Hyperflexion occurs when a joint is flexed beyond its normal range; an example would be when an individual performs a squat and bends too low, forcing the angle at the knee below 90 degrees. Ballistic (rapid forceful) movement into or out of a hyperextended or hyperflexed position, with the addition of a load or external force being applied, further increases the risk for joint damage.

Movements that place an individual at risk for joint injury are referred to as *contraindicated* exercises, or exercises that we should avoid (**FIGURE 12.27** through **FIGURE 12.31**).

Hyperextension Moving beyond a normal extended position at a joint.

Hyperflexion Moving beyond a normal flexed position at a joint.

FIGURE 12.27 **Contraindicated Exercise.** Fully squat. Knees at risk.

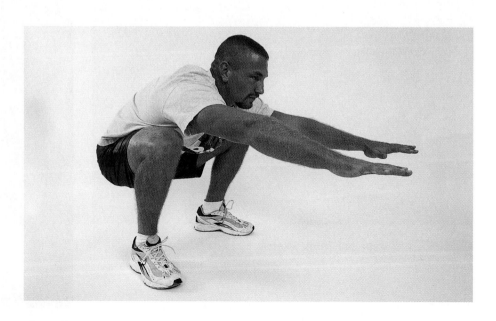

FIGURE 12.28 **Contraindicated Exercise.** Plough. Neck at risk.

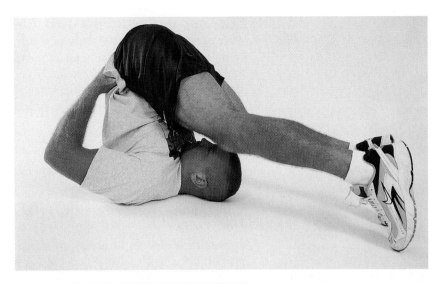

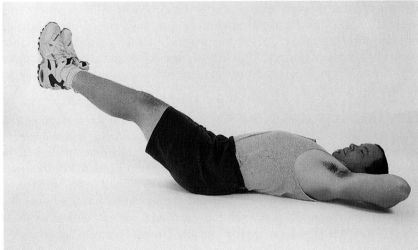

FIGURE 12.29 **Contraindicated Exercise.** Double-leg raises. Low back at risk.

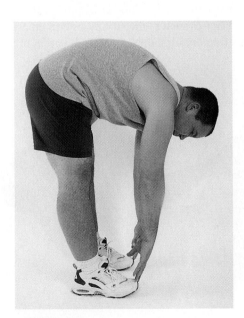

FIGURE 12.30 **Contraindicated Exercise.** Standing toe touch. Low back at risk.

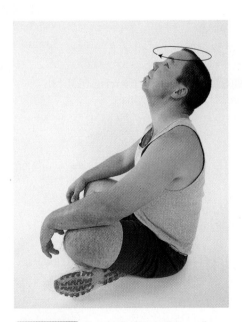

FIGURE 12.31 **Contraindicated Exercise.** Full neck circles. Neck at risk.

Changes in Flexibility with Age

As we age, we naturally lose some of the elasticity and compliance in our muscles and tendons. The degree and rate of loss are related to how active we are during the aging process. People who live sedentary lifestyles and those who don't perform any stretching activities lose muscle and tendon elasticity and compliance more rapidly than those who are active. A loss of elasticity and compliance will result in inflexibility and a reduction in joint range of motion (ACSM, 1998). A substantial loss of flexibility can significantly impair an individual's ability to accomplish daily activities and perform exercise (ACSM, 1998).

Role of Flexibility in Injury Prevention

Normal levels of static flexibility are needed for a low risk of injury in most vigorous physical activities, while very high or low levels of static flexibility may represent an increased risk of injury (Knudson et al., 2000). If a muscle is constantly tightened, either through inactivity or too much activity, without proper attention to stretching, the muscle may strain or tear. A strained muscle occurs when a tight muscle is overstretched rapidly to the point where damage to the connective tissue occurs. If a strain is extreme, muscle fibers and connective tissues will rupture. If muscles are not fit, such a rupture can occur while simply performing the activities of daily living.

FLEXIBILITY AND LOW-BACK PAIN   Low-back pain is a complaint common to many individuals. It is estimated that 80 percent of all Americans will experience some degree of low-back pain over the course of their lifetime. Inadequate flexibility is an important factor in the development of low-back pain. Regular stretching can both prevent and rehabilitate chronic low-back pain (ACSM, 2006).

If you develop low-back pain, your first step should be to contact your physician. With physician approval, or as a preventive measure, you may wish to try the following activities. The muscle groups most involved in low-back pain are the abdominals, hamstrings, hip flexors, and back extensors. A combination of muscles that are inflexible and muscles that are weak may contribute to low-back pain. Usually the abdominal muscles are too weak, so exercises such as the curl-up or crunch are recommended (FIGURE 12.32). The hamstring muscles, through a combination of too

Good flexibility protects against injury, enhances your ability to be physically active, and helps maintain an independent lifestyle.

Most low-back pain is caused by poor muscular fitness.

FIGURE 12.32 **Low-Back Exercise.** Curl-up. Tightens abdominals.

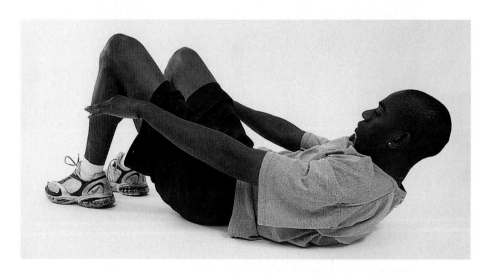

much sitting and not enough stretching, can become too inflexible. Exercises such as the knee to the chest (FIGURE 12.33) or the seated toe touch (FIGURE 12.34) are suggested to counteract this problem. The hip flexors tend to be too tight, so exercises like the lunge stretch are recommended (FIGURE 12.35). The back extensors may be both weak and inflexible, so both stretching and strengthening are recommended. To stretch the back extensors, use the cat-and-camel stretch (FIGURE 12.36); to strengthen the back extensors, do the modified chest lift (FIGURE 12.37).

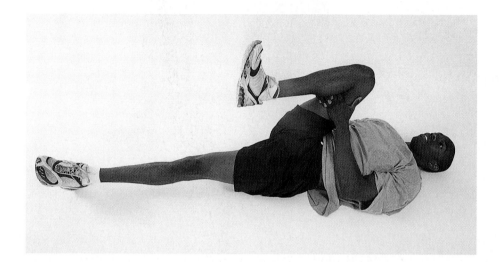

FIGURE 12.33 **Low-Back Exercise.** Knee to chest. Stretches hamstrings.

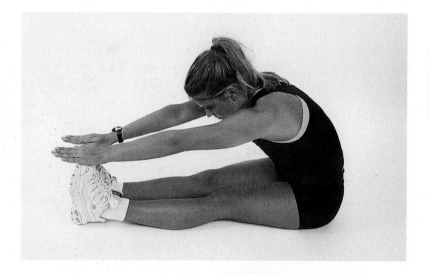

FIGURE 12.34 **Low-Back Exercise.** Seated toe touch. Stretches hamstrings.

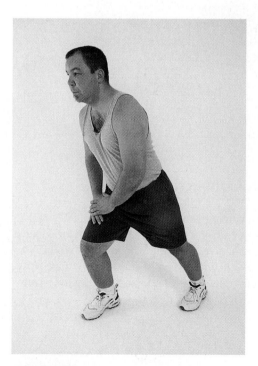

FIGURE 12.35 **Low-Back Exercise.** Lunge stretch. Stretches hip flexors.

FIGURE 12.36 **Low-Back Exercise.**
Cat and camel. Stretches low back.

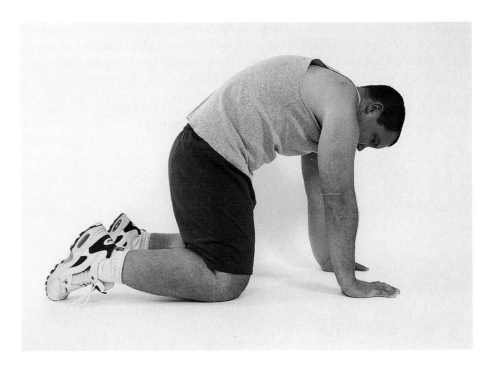

FIGURE 12.37 **Low-Back Exercise.**
Modified chest lift. Strengthens low back.

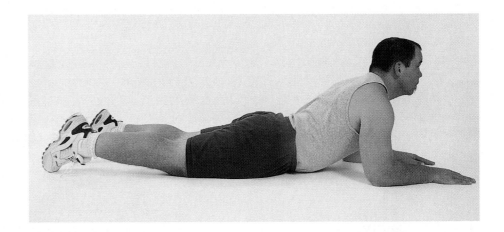

Physical Activity and Health Connection
....

Flexibility exercises are important in enhancing your range of motion. They make muscles more pliable and resistant to injury. Good flexibility helps to guard against the development of low-back pain and enhances sport performance. Flexibility is also important in helping maintain an independently active lifestyle. By improving your flexibility, you can maintain a higher degree of functional mobility over your lifetime.

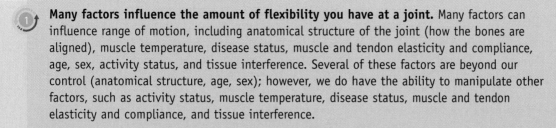

concept connections

1. Many factors influence the amount of flexibility you have at a joint. Many factors can influence range of motion, including anatomical structure of the joint (how the bones are aligned), muscle temperature, disease status, muscle and tendon elasticity and compliance, age, sex, activity status, and tissue interference. Several of these factors are beyond our control (anatomical structure, age, sex); however, we do have the ability to manipulate other factors, such as activity status, muscle temperature, disease status, muscle and tendon elasticity and compliance, and tissue interference.

2. Sense receptors located in your muscles and tendons play an important role in developing good flexibility. Muscle spindles and Golgi tendon organs are sense receptors that play an important role in muscle function. They control response to rapid movement. Muscle spindles cause muscles to contract in response to rapid forceful stretching. Golgi tendon organs cause muscles to relax in response to rapid forceful contractions.

3. Three common categories of flexibility exercises are static, ballistic, and PNF. *Static* stretching involves putting a muscle into a stretched position and holding that position for 10 to 30 seconds. *Ballistic* stretching involves using pulsing or bouncing movements to stretch a muscle. *PNF* involves the use of sense receptors and forceful agonist and antagonist contractions to stretch a muscle.

4. Guidelines for improving flexibility suggest stretching a muscle and holding the position for 10 to 30 seconds. Static stretches held for 10 to 30 seconds provide a safe and effective way to enhance your flexibility. Perform each stretch four times for optimal benefit.

5. Good flexibility protects against injury, enhances your ability to be physically active, and helps maintain an independent lifestyle. Maintaining a good range of motion decreases the likelihood of injury, reduces the risk of low-back pain, and enhances physical performance. Sore, inflexible muscles decrease your ability to move efficiently and increase the risk of muscle strain.

6. Most low-back pain is caused by poor muscular fitness. Low-back pain is most commonly the result of poor flexibility in the hamstrings, hip flexors, and back extensors. Poor muscular strength and endurance of the abdominal muscles are contributing factors. By regularly performing stretching activities that focus on the lower back, you can reduce your risk for developing low-back pain.

Terms

Elasticity, 256
Compliance, 256
Tissue interference, 256
Proprioceptors, 258
Muscle spindles, 258

Stretch reflex, 258
Golgi tendon organs, 258
Static stretching, 258
Ballistic stretching, 259
PNF stretching, 259

Passive stretching, 259
Active stretching, 259
Hyperextension, 268
Hyperflexion, 268

making the connection

Bob has now learned that flexibility is important to a healthy lifestyle. He spends some time daily working to improve his flexibility. Bob has also noticed that the low-back pain he was experiencing in the morning has disappeared. What he once thought unimportant in terms of his fitness plays a much more important role than Bob had realized.

Critical Thinking

1. In the vignette, Bob realized how important flexibility is to a healthy lifestyle and is spending time improving his flexibility. What types of exercises would you recommend for Bob to begin with and why? Once he has a routine in place, would you suggest that he add any flexibility exercises? If so, which ones and why?

2. Based on your current flexibility and your time commitments, identify three different types of stretching exercise you prefer and briefly explain why you selected these.

3. The last time you spoke with your parents they indicated that your grandfather was having problems getting around and that he was unable to bend over and pick things up off the floor, and he could not easily put on his shoes. Knowing what you know about flexibility diminishing when adults grow older, explain this process to your parents and make some flexibility exercise suggestions for your grandfather.

References

American College of Sports Medicine. (1998). The recommended quantity and quality of exercise for developing and maintaining cardiorespiratory and muscular fitness and flexibility in healthy adults. *Medicine and Science in Sports and Exercise* 30(6):975–991.

American College of Sports Medicine. (2006). *ACSM's Guidelines for Exercise Testing and Prescription*, 7th ed. Philadelphia: Lippincott, Williams & Wilkins.

Holcomb, W.R. (2000). Improved stretching with proprioceptive neuromuscular facilitation. *Strength and Conditioning Journal* 22(1):59–61.

Knudson, D.V., Magnusson, P., & McHugh, M. (2000). Current issues in flexibility fitness. *President's Council on Physical Fitness and Sports Research Digest* 3(10):1–8.

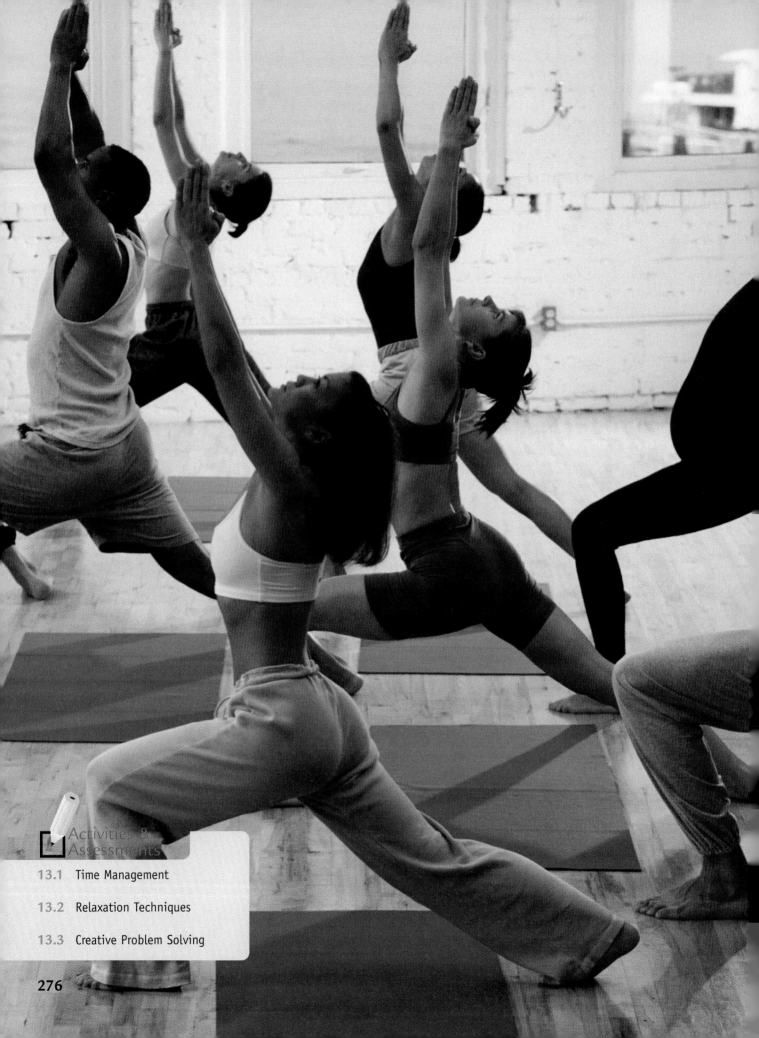

Activities & Assessments

13.1   Time Management

13.2   Relaxation Techniques

13.3   Creative Problem Solving

Understanding Mental Health, Stress, and Physical Activity

13

what's the connection?

Jesse felt anxious and tense as he rehearsed a speech in his dorm room. He had spent two weeks on this English class assignment and now, the day before he was to stand up in front of the class, he was having trouble remembering and delivering his speech. Three days ago he had no trouble reciting the 30-minute presentation in front of the mirror, but now he was fretting about presenting in front of his classmates and instructor. After a number of failed attempts, Jesse decided to take a break and go out for a 45-minute jog. Halfway through the jog, the anxiety and worrying subsided and he began to recite his speech easily in his mind. When Jesse returned to the dorm, his roommate Dave was there. Jesse asked Dave to listen to the speech before they went to the cafeteria for dinner. Jesse was able to deliver his speech flawlessly in front of Dave. He then showered and got dressed for dinner. As they walked to the cafeteria, Jesse told Dave that he planned to jog before presenting his speech because he felt that the exercise had helped him deliver it with a clear head.

concepts

1. People who are physically active tend to have better mental health.

2. Our mental and emotional health are central to the quality of our lives, and both influence our physical health.

3. Maintaining and optimizing our mental and physical health requires making countless adjustments to a variety of life's challenges.

4. The general adaptation syndrome describes the body's response to stress and the adaptability of the body to maintain homeostasis.

5. Stress is a natural process, and understanding its effects can help you use it to your own advantage.

6. The art of stress management is to keep yourself at a level of stimulation that is healthy and enjoyable.

http://physicalactivity.jbpub.com

The Web site for this book is a great source for supplementary physical health information for both students and instructors. Visit **http://physicalactivity.jbpub.com** to find a variety of useful tools for learning, thinking, and teaching.

People who are physically active tend to have better mental health.

Introduction

The positive relationship between physical activity and mental health has been well documented (Buckworth & Dishman, 2003; Biddle, Fox, & Boutcher, 2000). The scientific consensus linking physical activity to mental health has resulted in recommendations that exercise should be used for the promotion and maintenance of mental health and in the management of mental health problems (Biddle & Mutrie, 2001). The consensus is that people who are physically active score higher on important mental health factors such as self-esteem, self-concept, self-worth, body image, and cognitive functioning than sedentary people (Fox, 2000). Furthermore, physical activity has been shown to be effective in treating people who report symptoms of anxiety, depression, and stress (Fontaine, 2000).

Improved mental health and its conservation are topics of immense interest among health professionals due to the continuing commonness of mental illness (Satcher, 2000). If you survey the U.S. population during any 12-month span, one in four adults (25 percent) will meet the criteria for having a mental illness, and fully one-fourth of those will have a "serious" disorder that significantly disrupts their ability to function day to day (Kessler et al., 2005). These prevalence data are based on four major categories of mental illness: anxiety disorders (such as panic and post-traumatic stress disorders), mood disorders (such as major depression and bipolar disease), impulse control disorders (such as attention-deficit/hyperactivity disorder), and substance abuse. In addition, it has been estimated that almost 5 of every 10 people (46 percent) experience a significant mental disorder at some point in their lifetime (Kessler et al., 2005). Add to this the fact that fewer than half of those in need get treated and you soon realize the scope of the problem. Those who do seek treatment usually do so after a decade or more of delays, during which time they have suffered needlessly.

Another point of interest is that although mental stress is not considered an illness, it can cause specific medical symptoms that are often serious enough to require medical care. In fact, nearly half of all adults suffer adverse health effects from stress, and 60 to 90 percent of all physician office visits have stress-related components (Benson & Proctor, 2003).

Mental illness can afflict anyone, no matter their age, gender, race, or economic status. A mental illness is a disease that causes mild to severe disturbances in thinking, perception, and behavior. If these disturbances significantly impair a person's ability to cope with life's ordinary demands and routines, then he or she should immediately seek proper treatment with a mental health professional. With the proper care and treatment, a person can recover and resume normal activities. As with other chronic conditions, medical science has made incredible progress over the last couple of decades in helping us to understand, cure, and eliminate the causes of mental illness (Satcher, 2000).

Mental health care resources and expenditures for treatment are important considerations when addressing mental illness and its consequences. However, it has been pointed out that, similar to other health problems in which major advances have come from prevention rather than treatment, *preventing* mental health problems is inherently better than having to treat the illness after its onset (Institute of Medicine, 1994). Although there continues to be an insufficient understanding of all of the biological, psychological, and sociocultural effects on mental health and illness, some successful strategies have materialized. A meaningful one includes the choice of a lifestyle that incorporates regular physical activity. Physical activity has the potential to not only enhance mental functioning but also to serve as a protective factor against, as well as provide a treatment modality for, a number of mental disturbances along the mental health continuum (**FIGURE 13.1**).

Emotional health includes temporary feelings of sadness and disappointment.

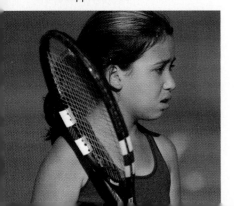

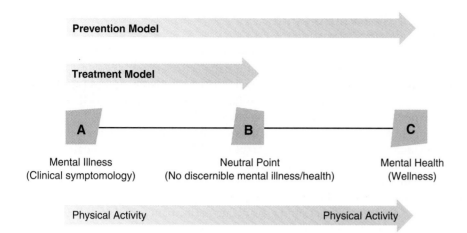

FIGURE 13.1 **The Physical Activity and Mental Health Continuum.** Physical activity has the potential to not only enhance mental functioning but also to serve as a protective factor against, as well as provide a treatment modality for, a number of mental disturbances along the mental health continuum.

Many theories have been proposed to explain the positive research findings related to physical activity and mental health along the mental health continuum. To address completely these explanations related to mind and body functioning, we must first begin by looking at mental and emotional health and how they are central to the quality of our lives.

Mental and Emotional Health

Defining mental health is not easy because it encompasses a broad group of values across different cultures and subgroups (Fletcher-Janzen, Strickland, & Reynolds, 2000). The U.S. Department of Health and Human Services (USDHHS) defines **mental health** as a "state of successful performance of mental function, resulting in productive activities, fulfilling relationships with other people, and the ability to adapt to change and to cope with adversity" (USDHHS, 1999). Evident from the definition is that mental health doesn't just occur; we need to pay attention to our mental needs just as we do our physical needs.

Mental health involves such factors as a sense of coherence and insight, moods, self-esteem, and coping ability. It allows us to make informed selections between alternate courses of action. We must use our cognitive abilities to make wise choices based on both previous experience and a willingness to undergo new experiences. An important part of mental health is learning to fully understand and trust the decisions we make. Mental health involves having a mind open to new ideas and concepts. Mental health embodies factors not only of intellect but also of emotions, and of their relationships.

Emotional health calls for understanding our emotions and coping with changes that arise in everyday life (Chapter 1). Emotional health encompasses mental states that include feelings or subjective experiences in response to changes in our environment. Joy, disappointment, fear, anxiety, guilt, love, sadness, anger, jealousy, trust, empathy, and compassion describe subjective experiences that are real to us. These emotions play an important role in our overall health.

Everything you think and feel reflects who you are. An *emotion* is a thought linked to a sensation. The thought is usually about the past or the future, but the sensation is in the present. Your mind quickly links this sensation with involuntary and immediate changes in your body function. Our minds and our emotions are interrelated and interdependent. Mental functions do not exist separately from our emotions, and our emotions affect our mental state. Therefore, we will speak of mental and emotional health interchangeably in this chapter.

Our mental and emotional health are central to the quality of our lives, and both influence our physical health.

Mental health A "state of successful performance of mental function, resulting in productive activities, fulfilling relationships with other people, and the ability to adapt to change and to cope with adversity" (USDHHS, 1999).

Emotional health Encompasses mental states that include feelings or subjective experiences in response to changes in our environment.

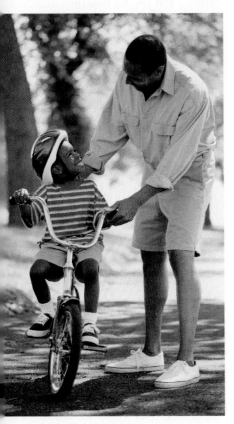

Emotional health also includes feelings of joy and love.

Mind-Body Relationship

Much research related to physical activity has centered on its relationship to physical health. However, holistic health perspectives emphasize mind-body unity and include the complex relationship between mental and physical function as well as the continuum between health and illness (Buckworth & Dishman, 2002). Because of this view, there is currently a great deal of interest in the study of physical activity as it relates to mental health. The line between psychology and biology is becoming increasingly blurred. The physiological parameters of our bodies are constantly eavesdropping on our thoughts and being changed in the process. Similarly, research is now able to substantiate the proposed mental and emotional benefits of habitual physical activity, which include improved intellectual functioning, academic performance, and moods (Biddle, Fox, & Boutcher, 2000). The old paradigm that distinguished between mental and physical health is thus somewhat unsound, in the sense that we now know mental and physical health to be highly integrated. Indeed, the U.S. Department of Health and Human Services asserted that it is important to adopt the paradigm that mind and body are inseparable and eliminate the old idea that the mind and body are separate and independent from each other (USDHHS, 1999). The mind-body dualism we speak of today is founded in the classical connection made by the Greeks 24 centuries ago when they considered physical activity and mental health simultaneously.

Mens Sana in Corpore Sana

The Greeks long believed in the mental benefits derived from physical activity. They deemed that a healthy and fit body was positively associated with increased mental and emotional wellness. This was best exemplified by the phrase attributed to Homer: "*Mens* (mind, intellect) *sana* (sound, healthy, sane), *in corpore* (body) *sana*," which translates into "In a sound body is a sound mind." The Greeks maintained that physical activity made the mind more rational and perceptive. During the Golden Age of Greece, regular and vigorous physical activity was engaged in for its contribution to mental as well as physical health.

Former President John F. Kennedy underscored the Greek ideal of *mens sana in corpore sana* when he said:

> Physical fitness is not only one of the most important keys to a healthy body, it is the basis of dynamic and creative intellectual activity. Intelligence and skill can only function at the peak of their capacity when the body is strong. Hardy spirits and tough minds usually inhabit sound bodies.

Many studies on the effects of physical activity on the mental health of physically active versus physically inactive people generally show positive effects (Galper et al., 2006; Goodwin, 2003). The invariable findings are that the higher the level of an individual's physical activity, the higher the level of good mental health. Mental health is defined in these studies as feelings of general well-being, positive moods, and fewer bouts of anxiety and depression. The studies conclude that physical activity may indeed play a role in maintaining or promoting positive mental health. We have seen that adequate and enhanced mental and emotional states can be associated with physical activity of the body. Is the reverse true? Can poor mental health states lead to deterioration of the body? A number of research studies seem to indicate that poor mental and emotional states can have an effect on our physical health (Biddle, Fox, & Boutcher, 2000).

Psychosomatic Disease

Psychosomatic disease describes bodily symptoms caused by mental or emotional disturbance. The word *psychosomatic* comes from the Greek words *psyche* (the mind) and *soma* (the body). Numerous studies have confirmed that being emotionally distressed from a number of negative emotions, including chronic anxiety or depression, can lead to physical health problems such as headaches, ulcers, high blood pressure, altered insulin needs, and a suppressed immune system. These physical problems can lead to an increased risk of heart disease, stroke, cancer, and infections. The prevalence of many of these underlying emotions that begin the disease sequence is associated with life-stress circumstances (Wein, 2000). Emotionally, stress can lead to feelings of depression, anxiety, and decreased mental health (McEwen & Stellar, 1993).

Mental Illness

Mental illness encompasses all diagnosable mental disorders (USDHHS, 1999). These mental disorders are quantified by changes in our thinking, mood, or behavior that lead to impaired functioning. Our focus here will be limited to mental health concerns related to anxiety, depression, and stress. These mental problems are the most common experienced by Americans and are influenced by physical activity both as a protective factor and a therapeutic modality.

ANXIETY   **Anxiety** is one of the most easily understood and responsive symptoms of mental disorders. Everyone feels anxious from time to time. Anxiety is a normal feeling that each of us experiences when a fear-eliciting situation arises in our environment. These fearful situations can be real or imagined, and the natural physiological response is "fight or flight." Anxiety is inflated worry and tension that sets off the fight-or-flight response. Most of us have felt the pounding of our heart when we think the teacher will call on us for an answer we do not know, or the muscle tension we feel when we think our parents are going to be angry with us over something we have done or not done, or that feeling of lightheadedness before calling someone for a first date (TABLE 13.1). A certain level of anxiety is good because it can spur us on to action. However, it is important that we be able to regulate anxiety, or it may materialize in mood disturbances (depression) and pathological physiological activity (disease).

Experiencing heightened arousal or fear over a sustained period of time can lead to **anxiety disorders**, which are debilitating and disruptive to our health. Anxiety disorders are the most common mental disorders in the United States; they

> **Psychosomatic disease** Bodily symptoms caused by mental or emotional disturbance.
>
> **Mental illness** Diagnosable mental disorders that change our thinking, mood, or behavior and lead to impaired functioning.
>
> **Anxiety** Normal response when a fear-eliciting situation arises.
>
> **Anxiety disorders** Mental disorders caused by heightened arousal or fear over a sustained period of time.

TABLE 13.1	Common Signs of Acute Anxiety

Feelings of fear or dread

Trembling, restlessness, and muscle tension

Rapid heart rate

Lightheadedness or dizziness

Perspiration

Cold hands/feet

Shortness of breath

SOURCE: U.S. Department of Health and Human Services. (1999). *Mental Health: A Report of the Surgeon General*. Rockville, MD: U.S. Department of Health and Human Services, 40.

Generalized anxiety disorder (GAD) Experiencing exaggerated worrying, inability to relax, and insomnia for 6 months or more.

Depression A mental disorder notable for negative alteration in mood.

Depressive reactions Normal depressed feelings such as sadness and hopelessness.

Dysthymia Chronic form of depression.

Major depression Serious condition that leads to inability to function and possibly suicide.

Stress Response that includes both a mental reaction (stressor) and a physical reaction (stress response).

Maintaining and optimizing our mental and physical health requires making countless adjustments to a variety of life's challenges.

Coping and adapting to the demands of everyday life stressors in an effective manner is of great importance for one's health.

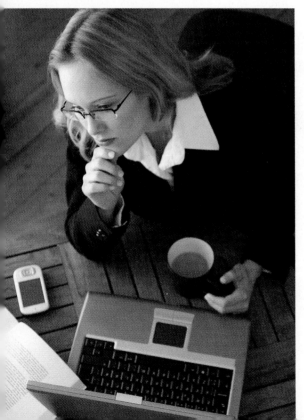

include **generalized anxiety disorder (GAD)**, panic disorder, obsessive-compulsive disorder, post-traumatic stress disorder (PTSD), and phobias (USDHHS, 2000). Of these, GAD represents a more extended and unfounded version of anxiety.

Generalized anxiety disorder is most often experienced as exaggerated worrying, inability to relax, and insomnia for a sustained period lasting 6 months or more. In many GAD cases, there is no immediate external situation that sets off the physiological response. Many people with GAD endure physical symptoms such as fatigue and headaches. If a physician determines your symptoms are due to an anxiety disorder, the next step is referral to a mental health professional for treatment.

DEPRESSION   **Depression** illustrates a mental disorder mainly noted by alterations in mood. Depression often accompanies GAD and other anxiety disorders (Barbee, 1998). Like anxiety disorders, depression can vary in severity and duration. All of us have experienced **depressive reactions** because of a disturbing event in our lives. *Depressive reactions* encompass the normal depressed feelings, such as sadness, hopelessness, rejection, and worthlessness, that arise because of a specific life situation. Fortunately, these deviations do not last long, and they lessen over time. However, when symptoms last for an extended period of time or feature one or more major depressive episodes, the condition may be serious.

Dysthymia is a chronic form of depression. *Dysthymia* is similar to *depressive reactions* in its symptoms except that the degree of suffering from its unrelenting, seething attack can lead to depressive illness, as well as increasing the susceptibility to **major depression**. *Major depression* is a serious condition that leads to an inability to function, or even to suicide. Whereas the symptoms in *dysthymia* are less intense, fewer in number, and longer lasting, *major depression* is marked by one or more major depressive episodes over a 2-week period. Many treatments are available for depression and vary according to the cause and severity. Most people seeking help for depression visit their primary care physician.

Maintaining our mental health requires making countless adjustments to life's challenges. How successfully we adjust depends largely on how we view and adapt to life's challenges. Life's challenges may be viewed as **stress**. Stress includes both a mental reaction (stressor) and a physical reaction (stress response).

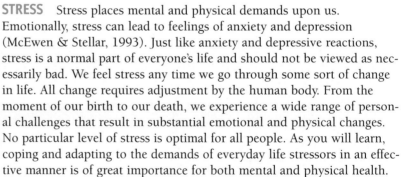

STRESS   Stress places mental and physical demands upon us. Emotionally, stress can lead to feelings of anxiety and depression (McEwen & Stellar, 1993). Just like anxiety and depressive reactions, stress is a normal part of everyone's life and should not be viewed as necessarily bad. We feel stress any time we go through some sort of change in life. All change requires adjustment by the human body. From the moment of our birth to our death, we experience a wide range of personal challenges that result in substantial emotional and physical changes. No particular level of stress is optimal for all people. As you will learn, coping and adapting to the demands of everyday life stressors in an effective manner is of great importance for both mental and physical health.

Understanding Stress

Decades ago, it was pointed out that "the states of health or disease are the expressions of the success or failure experienced by the human body in its efforts to respond adaptively to environmental challenges" (Dubos 1965, p. xvii). Those who developed many of today's concepts of stress correctly understood that different life stressors could induce helpful (**eustress**; *eu* is Greek for "good") and harmful (**distress**) outcomes. That is, good health requires the presence of eustress and also the limitation of distress to a level to which the human body can adapt (Selye, 1976). A stressor sets into motion a sequence of chemical and nervous system changes that is the same regardless of the type of stressor that initiates it. This sequence has been referred to as the general adaptation syndrome.

General Adaptation Syndrome

Hans Selye, a pioneer in stress research, is generally recognized as the father of stress physiology and stress education. Selye coined the word *stress*, which he defined as the "nonspecific response of the body to any demand made upon it" (Selye, 1976). The key concept in Selye's definition is that there is a nonspecific response by the body to readjust itself following any demand made on it. Selye termed this nonspecific response the **general adaptation syndrome (GAS)**. This syndrome is based on the principle that your body is constantly attempting to maintain homeostasis (*homeo* = similar, and *stasis* = position), or an internal balance. Maintaining homeostasis requires energy. Any situation or force that disturbs the body's homeostasis, or equilibrium, is a stressor. Adapting to stressors requires the body to provide the right amount of energy at the right time.

The GAS describes the body's response to stress and the adaptability of the body to maintain homeostasis. Selye's (1976) research provided evidence that the body goes through a predictable three-stage physiological response to any kind of stressor: (1) the alarm reaction, when the adrenal glands are activated in an attempt to mobilize the body's energy resources for physical action, (2) the stage of resistance, in which the readjustment occurs, and (3) if the readjustment is not complete, the stage of exhaustion may follow, leading to illness and possibly death (FIGURE 13.2). The demand or stimulus that elicits the GAS stress response is referred to as a **stressor**.

Stressors

The stressor itself does not actually create the body's response; it is the individual's reaction to the stressor. The stress reaction is triggered by our perception of a physical or emotional danger. It is important to underscore that it is our *perception* of each demand or stressor that makes it stressful or not stressful. What is considered a stressor for one person may not be a stressor for another. For example, the

The general adaptation syndrome describes the body's response to stress and the adaptability of the body to maintain homeostasis.

Eustress Helpful or good stress.

Distress Harmful or bad stress.

General adaptation syndrome (GAS) The body's response to stress and the adaptability of the body to maintain homeostasis.

Stressor The demand or stimulus that elicits the general adaptation syndrome.

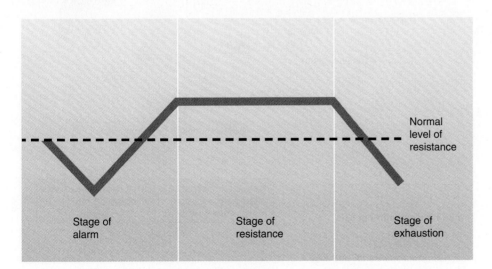

FIGURE 13.2 **The Three Phases of the General Adaptation Syndrome.** In the alarm stage, the body readies itself for action, lowering resistance. In the resistance stage, the body adapts and returns to homeostasis. In the stage of exhaustion, the body's ability to resist the stressor becomes exhausted and resistance is compromised.

person who loves to mediate disputes and moves from job site to job site would be stressed in a job that was stable and routine, whereas the person who thrives under stable conditions would very likely be stressed on a job where the duties were highly varied. Each individual will have a different response to the same stressor.

Stressors tend to be different not only for different types of people but also for different ages. As we progress through life, each stage is accompanied by its own distinctive sources of stressors.

Our reactions to stressors can be both psychological and physiological. The psychological changes may present themselves as changes in the ways we express our emotions. One of the most frequent undesirable emotional changes is chronic worrying. Worrying too much can lead to variations in mood; you may become depressed, anxious, or irritable. These moods work against you, making finding a solution more difficult. Psychological responses to stressors can be difficult to predict. Your physiological response to stress is much more predictable.

Alarm Reaction

The **alarm reaction** is our immediate response to a stressor and is triggered by any threat to our physical or emotional well-being. The reason for this reaction is simple. When a danger or challenge is present, our body reacts in certain ways in order to protect ourselves. This reaction is part of our human biological makeup. The body follows a typical physiological pattern when reacting to a stressor. When a threat to our well-being is perceived, a small area of the brain known as the hypothalamus is activated (**FIGURE 13.3**). The hypothalamus stimulates a number of physiological changes, involving activity in both the **autonomic nervous system** (nerve pathways) and the **endocrine system** (hormonal pathways). These two systems, acting in concert, alter the functioning of almost every part of the body to prepare for vigorous muscle activity. This response to stressors that challenge the body to respond physically, mentioned earlier, is referred to as the **fight-or-flight response**.

Alarm reaction Immediate response to a stressor that is triggered by any threat to our physical or emotional well-being.

Autonomic nervous system The part of the nervous system that controls smooth muscle, cardiac muscle, and glands; subdivided into sympathetic and parasympathetic.

Endocrine system The hormone-secreting cells of the body; this system is influenced in part by the nervous system.

Fight-or-flight response Response to stressors that challenge the body to respond physically.

FIGURE 13.3 **The Stress Response.** The physiological response to stress activates both the pituitary-adrenal axis and the sympathoadrenal pathway.

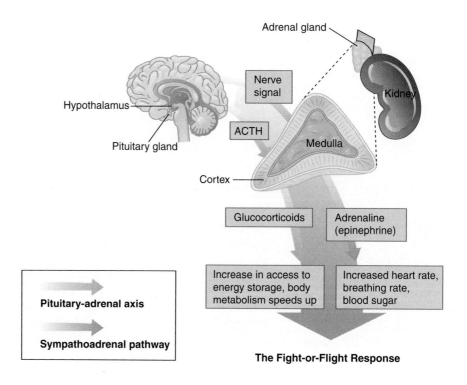

FIGHT-OR-FLIGHT RESPONSE   The action of the sympathetic nervous system that prepares the body for intense physical activity is aptly referred to as the fight-or-flight response. The fight-or-flight response occurs when the adrenal glands are activated. The paired adrenal glands are located above each kidney and are composed of an outer adrenal cortex (layer) and an inner adrenal medulla (core). The initial pattern of the fight-or-flight response is called the **pituitary-adrenal axis** (see Figure 13.3). The hypothalamus stimulates the pituitary gland, the master gland of the endocrine system, to increase the release of adrenocorticotropic hormone (ACTH) into the bloodstream. ACTH activates the outer layer of the adrenal gland, which results in the increased production of **glucocorticoids**. Glucocorticoids are chemicals responsible for speeding up the body's metabolism and increasing its access to energy storage.

Simultaneous to the activation of the pituitary-adrenal axis, the second pattern of the fight-or-flight response, called the **sympathoadrenal system**, is set in motion. The nerve impulses from the sympathetic branch of the autonomic nervous system reach the core of the adrenal glands, resulting in the increased release of **epinephrine** and **norepinephrine**. Epinephrine is referred to as the "fear hormone" and helps supply glucose to be used for increased muscle and nervous system activity. Norepinephrine is referred to as the "anger hormone" and helps speed up the heart rate and raises blood pressure in an attempt to provide more oxygen for the body. The effects of epinephrine and norepinephrine are similar to those produced by the sympathetic nervous system, except that the effects of the hormones last about 10 times longer.

The sum of the increased activation of the pituitary-adrenal axis and sympathoadrenal patterns (the fight-or-flight response) is to provide chemicals and hormones that permit the person to perform far more strenuous physical activity. If your reaction to the fight-or-flight response is physical activity (to fight or flee), the chemicals and hormones you have generated will be metabolized right away. If your reaction is to "sit tight" and not be physically active, the excess chemicals and hormones released in the body may cause unnecessary wear and tear. This damage, if repeated over time, may result in a number of diseases, including heart disease, stroke, and ulcerative colitis.

Stage of Resistance

Your body responds to all stress, both positive and negative, by trying to get back to normal. After the alarm reaction and the fight-or-flight responses, a stage of resistance occurs. During the resistance stage, the body attempts to adapt to the stressor and return to homeostasis. Readjustment occurs as resistance to stress rises and body functions return to normal. Physiologically, the parasympathetic nervous system is the counterpart to the sympathetic nervous system. The effects of the **parasympathetic nervous system** are the opposite of the effects of the sympathetic nervous system (TABLE 13.2). When no danger is perceived, the parasympathetic nervous system releases acetylcholine, a chemical that plays an inhibitory role on the effects of sympathetic stimulation of organs. This is commonly known as the **relaxation response** (FIGURE 13.4). The actions of both divisions of the autonomic nervous system must be balanced in order to maintain homeostasis.

Even though the body may adapt successfully to stressors in the short term, if continual major adaptation is required, or a number of adaptations are required over time, this may exact a serious toll on the body, particularly on the neuroendocrine and immune systems. The ongoing level of demand for adaptation in an individual is called **allostatic load** (*allo* = all, *static* = equilibrium) on that person, and it may be an important contributor to many chronic diseases (McEwen & Stellar, 1993). The continual setting off of the alarm stage and the resultant efforts

Pituitary-adrenal axis The first pattern of the fight-or-flight response.

Glucocorticoids Chemicals responsible for speeding up the body's metabolism and increasing access to energy storage.

Sympathoadrenal system The second pattern of the fight-or-flight response.

Epinephrine The "fear hormone"; helps supply glucose for increased muscle and nervous system activity.

Norepinephrine The "anger hormone"; helps speed the heart rate and raises blood pressure to provide more oxygen for the body.

Parasympathetic nervous system The counterpart to the sympathetic nervous system.

Relaxation response The opposite of the fight-or-flight response to stressful or threatening situations.

Allostatic load The ongoing level of demand for adaptation in an individual.

TABLE 13.2	Effects of the Autonomic Nervous System on Various Visceral Effector Organs	

Effector Effect	Sympathetic Effect	Parasympathetic Effect
Eye		
Iris (pupillary dilator muscle)	Dilation of pupil	—
Iris (pupillary sphincter muscle)	—	Contraction (for near vision)
Glands		
Lacrimal (tear)	—	Stimulation of secretion
Sweat	Stimulation of secretion	—
Salivary	Decreased secretion; saliva becomes thick	Increased secretion; saliva becomes thin
Stomach	—	Stimulation of secretion
Intestine	—	Stimulation of secretion
Adrenal medull	Stimulation of hormone secretion	—
Heart		
Rate	Increased	Decreased
Conduction	Increased rate	Decreased rate
Strength	Increased	—
Blood vessels	Mostly constriction; affects all organs	Dilation in a few organs (e.g., penis)
Lungs		
Bronchioles (tubes)	Dilation	Constriction
Mucous glands	Inhibition of secretion	Stimulation of secretion
Gastrointestinal tract		
Motility	Inhibition of movement	Stimulation of movement
Sphincters	Closing stimulated	Closing inhibited
Liver	Stimulation of glycogen hydrolysis	—
Adipocytes (fat cells)	Stimulation of fat hydrolysis	—
Pancreas	Inhibition of exocrine secretions	Stimulation of exocrine secretions
Spleen	Stimulation of contraction	—
Urinary bladder	Muscle tone added	Stimulation of contraction
Arrector pili muscles	Stimulation of hair erection, causing goosebumps	—
Uterus	If pregnant, contraction If not pregnant, relaxation	
Penis	Ejaculation	Erection (due to vasodilation)

of resistance to reestablish equilibrium in the body are increasingly becoming the focal point of research on illness and disease. Repeated alarms can lead to the stage of exhaustion in which the symptoms of the alarm reaction return.

Stage of Exhaustion

The mobilization of forces during the alarm reaction, and the return to homeostasis during the resistance stage, requires a substantial amount of energy. The stage of exhaustion occurs when the body's resources become depleted and fatigued. Prolonged exposure to a stressor can cause the body organs to become weakened and increase the susceptibility to illness (**FIGURE 13.5**). If stress is unrelenting, and

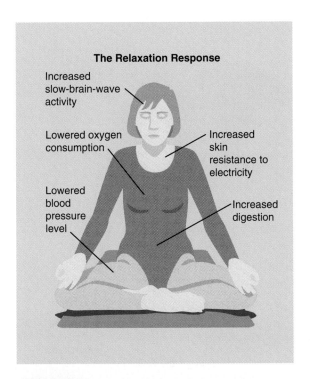

FIGURE 13.4 **The Relaxation Response.** The relaxation response is important because it allows the body to return to homeostasis following the fight-or-flight response.

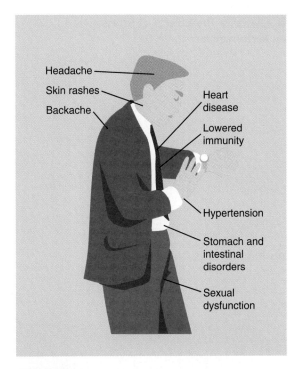

FIGURE 13.5 **The Physical Toll of Stress.** Unrelieved stress can cause a number of physical symptoms.

present long enough, it can produce permanent physical deterioration. Physical indicators reflecting high stress include the following (McEwen, 1998):

- Increases in blood pressure
- Suppressed immunity
- Increased fat around the abdomen
- Bone loss
- Increases in blood sugar
- Increases in levels of cortisol
- Weaker muscles
- Increases in blood cholesterol levels

Each person has a breaking point for dealing with stress. In addition to chronic or extended stress, stress research also indicates the cumulative adjustments required from intermittent and sequential stressors may affect the body over time. Selye (1976) observed that the number of stress responses and readjustments increases the wear and tear on the body, accelerating degenerative disease processes.

Stress and Performance

Stress is a natural process, and understanding its effects can help you use it to your own advantage. Stress researchers have long recognized that some stress or stimulation is needed for optimal performance. Yerkes and Dodson described a phenomenon, known today as the **Yerkes-Dodson law**, of an inverted U-shaped function between stress and performance (Benson & Proctor, 2003). The Yerkes-Dodson law

> **Yerkes-Dodson law** Predicts an inverted U-shaped function between stress and performance.

> Stress is a natural process, and understanding its effects can help you use it to your own advantage.

FIGURE 13.6 The Effects of Stress on Performance.

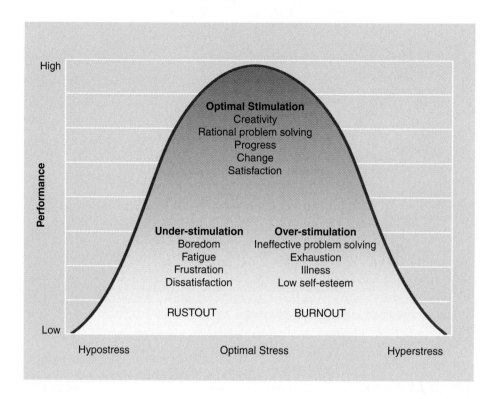

Hypostress Too little stress or stimulation.

Hyperstress Too much stress; the body begins to decrease in its level of performance.

theorizes about the ways health and performance are affected as stress increases. Although the relationship between stress and performance varies from person to person, the general pattern can be expressed by viewing the curve in **FIGURE 13.6**.

The curve is divided into three sections. The far left of the curve represents **hypostress**, not enough stress, which occurs when we lack stimulation. This area is often referred to as *rustout*. Rustout is a result of decreased drive and motivation and is caused by lack of challenges in our lives. The middle of the curve represents an area of optimal productivity. This amount of increased stress or stimulation in your life can fuel creativity, create excitement, or physically energize you for important events in your life. This moderate amount of stress can be a motivator toward change and growth that brings forth good results related to our mental and physical health. Moving to the right side of the curve, we find **hyperstress**, or stress beyond that which is optimal. This condition is called *burnout*, a point where the body begins to decrease in its level of performance. Stress becomes unmanageable and out of control at this point, and we experience impaired mental and physical capabilities.

Again, no single level of stress is optimal for all people. We are all individual beings with unique requirements. There is no way to predict conclusively how an individual will respond to different stressors. Individual differences in responding to the challenge of stress are products of our experiences, our developmental and environmental influences, and our genetics (McEwen & Stellar, 1993). Some people may cope well with stress, rising to meet the challenge, and others may be more adversely affected, responding with mental and physical fatigue. And, even when we agree that a particular event is distressing, we are likely to differ in our physiological and psychological responses to it.

It has been found that most illness is related to hyperstress and unrelieved stress. When your resistance resources are overworked, your exhausted body stops functioning smoothly. The signs of hyperstress are so pervasive in our culture that people often fail to recognize them as signs of distress. The signs may show up

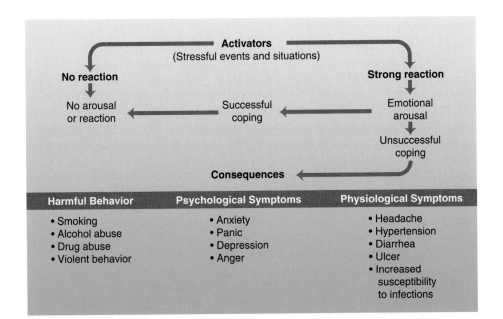

psychologically, physically, or behaviorally (FIGURE 13.7). Psychological signs may include inappropriate anger or intolerance, diminished ability to make priorities and decisions, an inability to concentrate, and a sense of hopelessness or frustration. Physical symptoms may include headaches, aching neck and back, upset stomach, and indigestion. Behavioral signs may include grinding the teeth, biting the fingernails, and overreacting to minor problems.

Maintaining and optimizing our mental and physical health requires making countless adjustments to a variety of life's challenges. Life's challenges are viewed as stress. Stress places certain physical and mental demands upon us, and how we adapt to these challenges significantly influences our mental and physical health. Your mind and body are connected, and during stressful times it is important to understand the relationship that exists between them.

Stress Management

The art of stress management is to keep yourself at a level of stimulation that is healthy and enjoyable. Life without stimulus would be dull and boring. Life with too many stimuli becomes unpleasant and tiring. The primary purpose for developing stress management techniques is to reduce the potential psychological and physical illnesses that result from too much stress. There are many specific strategies available for managing hyperstress. The specific strategies can be categorized into three basic approaches: (1) the environmental engineering, or "controlling your circumstances," approach; (2) the mind engineering, or "mind over matter," approach; and (3) the physical engineering, or the "stress-fit," approach.

These three basic stress approaches can be used singly or in any combination. Different approaches work for different stressors. Additionally, approaches vary among individuals. Before you begin reading about the three basic solutions, it may be helpful for you to have at hand a list of sources of stress in your life. You can then apply a basic approach to your source of stress and select from the wide variety of specific strategies presented at the end of the chapter.

The art of stress management is to keep yourself at a level of stimulation that is healthy and enjoyable.

Environmental engineering Stress management approach that attempts to avoid it in the first place.

Mind engineering Stress management approach concerned with reducing the intensity of our emotional responses to stressors.

Environmental Engineering

The **environmental engineering**, "control your circumstances," approach deals with the stressor by attempting to avoid it in the first place. This approach advocates controlling as many environmental circumstances as you can. To accomplish this, you need to analyze the situations in your environment that may lead to foreseeable stressful situations. Keeping a stress diary is a helpful way of finding out what causes you stress and when and where the event occurs. After a few weeks you should be able to analyze this information and be able to better plan a change in your environment to avoid the stressor.

For example, lately you have been feeling unprepared and tired for your Friday 8 A.M. economics class, an important class in your major field. Your journal reveals that you have routinely stayed out late with your friends on Thursday evenings and thus not studied for your economics class. You decide to take positive action by changing these circumstances; you make time to study on Thursday evening and get to bed at a reasonable hour. This new course of action leaves you feeling prepared and rested for your economics class.

Recognizing what stressors you can avoid by eliminating interaction with them is a good solution for dealing with a number of stressors. This strategy requires being able to plan ahead so that you can have the forethought to avoid the stressor. However, when a stressor is not foreseeable or avoidable, you must apply another approach to manage stress.

Mind Engineering

Mind engineering, "mind over matter," refers to how we deal with a stressor through the mind-body relationship. The mind and body are inseparable. Mind engineering reduces the intensity of our responses to stressors. Your mind activates your body's stress response. When your mind is healthy, your body can better resist illness. Similarly, when your mind is unhealthy, your resistance to illness decreases. The success of mind engineering depends on your attitude because the attitude you carry into a particular situation will greatly influence your perceptions of any stressor or event.

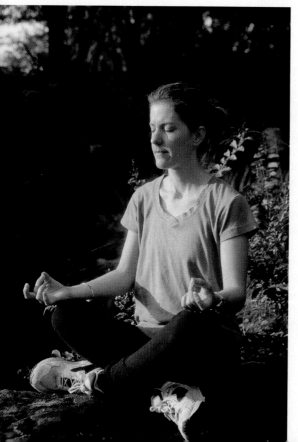

Meditation is a form of mind engineering. Mediation uses a rhythmic activity such as breath awareness to focus the mind, lifting you out of your ordinary level of consciousness into a state of "passive awareness" where the body can deal with stress problems.

Attitude is the by-product of our thoughts. We have explicit control over our own attitudes (see Chapter 3). It is in our attitudes that we discover strength or weakness, patience or anxiety, determination or frustration, when faced with a stressor. Our attitude about what we believe we should be, and the imagined punishment if we fail, determines how we see and react to stressors. When we view stressors positively, we are secure in our knowledge that we can make them beneficial to our growth if we choose. When we view stressors negatively, we are uncertain about our abilities to deal with them effectively and consequently feel that we are not in control.

Are you viewing your stressors in exaggerated terms—taking a challenging situation and making it a disaster? Positive thinking is everything when it comes to managing stress. Most people carry on a silent conversation with themselves, which is referred to as *self-talk* (see Chapter 3). Positive self-talk offers many stress-reduction benefits. If you think "I know I can ace my chemistry exam," you will have a better chance of success and will have made the stressor a positive one. If you engage in negative self-talk, "I can't pass that chemistry exam," you increase your chances of failure and the stressor becomes negative. As any sailor knows, "It is not the direction of the wind that determines our course so much as how we set our sails"; in sailing parlance, this is known significantly as the *attitude*.

STRESS RESISTANCE   Although it is not possible to become totally immune to stressors, you can "inoculate" yourself against stress—make it more tolerable and reduce its intensity—by learning to resist its harmful effects. Some people are better equipped to handle and manage stress than others because they have a "risk taker" attitude. Risk takers view new situations and responsibilities as challenges for further growth rather than as opportunities for failure. They want to try something new and enjoy the thrill. They need to feel the emotion of the situation.

Physical Engineering

The **physical engineering**, "stress-fit," approach is predicated on the fact that it is easier to deal with the stress response when your body is healthy from regular physical activity. Regular physical activity is useful in removing the by-products that occur due to the stress response and in reducing the physiological reactivity of the body to stressors.

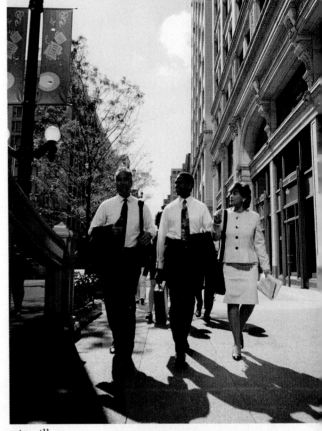

An excellent form of physical engineering to reduce stress is to take a walk.

EXPENDING EXCESS ENERGY AND BIOCHEMICALS   When the body experiences the fight-or-flight reaction, it provides us with energy via stress hormones and chemicals. The result is that our bodies go into a state of high energy, but there is often nowhere for this energy to be expended, so our bodies stay in a state of arousal for hours. Additionally, the biochemicals that initiated this high state of energy are left to circulate in the body and have the capability for causing illness. During times of high stress, we can benefit from a physical outlet. Physical activity is the most logical way to expend excess energy and throw off its biochemical by-products. When our bodies are in a high state of energy, it is healthful to expend this energy in a brisk walk or run. In addition to enjoying the available energy, the exercise is ridding the body of stress hormones and flushing the excessive biochemical buildup.

Studies show that those who experience stress-related illness, or symptoms of stress, can best reduce or eliminate those symptoms with a program of stress management that includes physical activity. Physical activity reduces many of the physical symptoms associated with stress and illness. A regular physical activity program lowers the resting heart rate and blood pressure and protects against fatigue, reduces digestive problems, and relaxes muscles.

> **Physical engineering** Stress management approach using regular exercise to optimize your stress responses.

PHYSIOLOGICAL REACTIVITY   The second part of the physical engineering approach deals with the theoretical assumption that higher levels of aerobic fitness are associated with less physiological reactivity to psychosocial stressors. This stress-buffering or inoculation effect occurs as a result of improved physiological functioning of the body. The improved cardiovascular adaptation from aerobic exercise appears to mediate and decrease an individual's physiological reactivity in response to a number of psychosocial stressors (Taylor et al., 2004). In other words, since physical activity provides an almost identical physiological response to that which occurs with mental stress, strengthening the body to react to physical activity will strengthen the body's response to mental stress. Long-term physical activity may adjust the brain's responsiveness to chemicals associated with stress, allowing the brain to deal with stress more efficiently.

The Mental Health Benefits of Physical Activity

You have just read about how physical activity can be therapeutic when it comes to managing stress. Interestingly, the psychological benefits from physical activity across all areas of mental well-being are advocated. There is much speculation, however, about the mechanisms by which physical activity improves mental health. What follows is a brief overview of the most frequently discussed mechanisms. Although these explanations are discussed independently, it is important to understand that they may operate interactively.

Cognitive Behavioral Theory

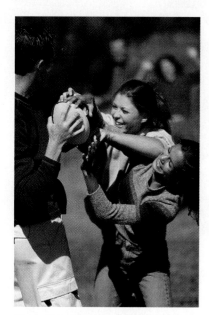

Physical activity with friends can improve mental and emotional well-being.

This explanation maintains that, as a person engages in physical activity and experiences bodily changes, self-efficacy increases. That is, participating in and mastering a specific physical task creates positive feelings because individuals perceive that they can perform activity even in tough situations. This is related to one's self-efficacy (see Chapter 3), in which the strength of a belief is enhanced by continued successful execution of a behavior. Feelings of mastery and control are incompatible with negative thoughts (anxiety, depression). Additionally, self-esteem is fostered when you realize that you are doing something that will ultimately benefit you. Participating in physical activity has a positive social value attached to it because it is a health-enhancing activity.

Social Interaction Theory

The buffering effects of social support are well documented when it comes to physical activity (see Chapters 2 and 3). Physical activities that are done with friends and colleagues, or in social settings, can have a net effect of improving mental health. This mental health effect is much more noticeable in groups in which people feel a collective sense of achievement and accomplishment.

Distraction Theory

The solitude experienced when performing physical activities that require a fairly consistent, repetitive motion (bicycling, jogging, hiking) can alter your state of consciousness. The regular breathing and movement associated with these activities may act as a mantra that induces feelings of calmness and tranquility similar to those obtained while practicing meditation. Physical activity provides a distraction, or time-out, from the daily worries of a stressful society. Furthermore, physical activity provides an opportunity for introspective thinking that can stimulate creativity in problem solving.

The Endorphin Hypothesis

Endorphins Body chemicals responsible for enhancing emotions and providing pain relief.

The endorphin hypothesis represents the most popular biological explanation, despite questionable evidence. The term **endorphins** is a general classification for important body chemicals that are responsible for enhancing emotions (euphoric feelings) and providing pain relief (analgesic effect). The neurochemical reaction from endorphin release has been shown to increase following physical activity of 20 minutes or more.

The Thermogenic Hypothesis

During physical activity the body temperature rises (see Chapter 8). This body-warming effect has been shown to reduce muscle tension, thereby countering the tension that may build up in muscles from stress (neck, lower back).

The therapeutic benefits of regular physical activity are without rival when it comes to reducing stress and maintaining mental health. The form of physical activity you choose should be enjoyable, noncompetitive, and personally satisfying. Choose activities you like, or they will feel like a chore and you will begin to avoid them. It is also beneficial to have a variety of physical activity outlets.

Quick Relaxation Techniques

Other ways to reduce stress in the body are through certain disciplines that fall under the heading of relaxation techniques. The term *relaxation training* is used in the health literature to refer to various techniques that stimulate the relaxation response (see Figure 13.4). The relaxation response is the opposite of the fight-or-flight response to stressful or threatening situations. Just as we are all capable of heightening and sustaining a stress reaction, we have also inherited the ability to put our bodies into a state of relaxation. In this state, all the physiological events in the stress reaction are reversed: breathing and pulse slow, blood pressure declines, and muscles relax. It has been found that relaxing for just 20 minutes each day can be beneficial to both your physical and mental health. Unlike the stress reaction, which is automatic, *the relaxation response needs to be induced by intention*. Fortunately, there are many simple ways to do this. The following relaxation techniques can be practiced by anyone at any time during the day and provide instant relief from stress.

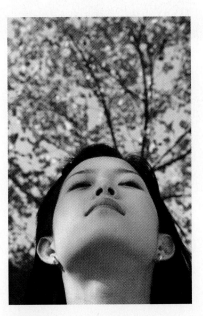

Finding a quiet place where you feel relaxed and can focus on one peaceful thought is important in using visualization.

Deep Breathing

Deep breathing is a countermeasure to stress. When stressed, your breathing becomes rapid and shallow, causing an insufficient amount of oxygen to reach your lungs. The goal in deep breathing is to slow and increase the volume of air inhaled, thus providing extra oxygen to the blood. Slowly inhale through your nose, expanding your abdomen before allowing air to fill your lungs. Reverse the process by constricting your stomach and exhaling through your mouth, making a quiet, whooshing sound as you blow out calmly. Continue to take long, slow, deep breaths, focusing on the sound and feeling of breathing. After a few minutes you should become more relaxed. You may want to perform this technique a couple times a day. Deep breathing is a very effective method of relaxation and is the most basic technique used in relaxation training.

Visualization

Visualization is using your imagination to reduce stress. Find a quiet place where you feel comfortable. Sit down and close your eyes, breathing slowly. Next, try focusing on one peaceful thought, or on a goal you want to attain. If your mind strays back to the problem causing stress, make yourself return to the peaceful thought for a couple of minutes. Another variation of visualization is to create a picture in your mind of a beautiful place and imagine yourself there, using as many of your senses as you can.

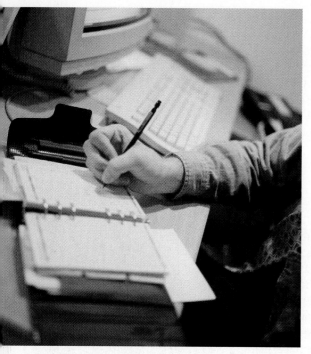

Keeping a daily log of how you spend your time is a helpful technique in time management.

Progressive Muscle Relaxation

Progressive muscle relaxation (PMR) is a simple technique used to induce neuromuscular relaxation by creating an awareness of the difference between muscular tension and a relaxed state. Progressive muscle relaxation is a two-step process. First, each muscle or muscle group is tensed from 5 to 10 seconds and then relaxed for 15 to 25 seconds. Repeat this procedure at least once; if the area remains tense, repeat up to five times.

Time Management

A major contributor to stress is inadequate time management skills. Despite an image of college life being carefree and fun-filled, college life will probably require more careful and effective utilization of time than a student has ever needed to achieve before. A typical student schedules 15 or more classroom hours a week and is expected to average about 2 hours of preparation for each hour in the classroom. This means that students have at least a 45-hour work week, equivalent to a full-time job. In addition, many students find that they must balance their academic responsibilities with part-time jobs, family, and social responsibilities. Thus, it is not surprising that a common concern among college students is not having enough time to get everything accomplished. The job of being a college student, like most other jobs, can be carried out more effectively with the use of time management techniques that increase your productivity.

Assess Current Time Use

A good place to begin is to keep track of how you currently use your time. Assess how you spend your time each day for a week by faithfully keeping a daily log of how you spend your waking hours.

Setting Priorities

Write down your goals and priorities. Divide your goals into essential, important, and trivial. Having a record of how you spend your time allows you to compare your current use of time to essential and important goals and priorities. You need to be spending virtually all of your time on essential and important priorities.

Time Scheduling

One of best techniques for developing more efficient time-use habits is to prepare a schedule. The following is a flexible way to help establish long-term, intermediate, and short-term goals. A long-term schedule consists of your fixed commitments. These include only obligations you are required to meet every week: classes, job, physical activity, church, organizational meetings. Your immediate schedule consists of a short list of major tasks to be accomplished in the next week: quiz on Monday, ballgame on Wednesday, read 60 pages in history by Friday. Finally, each evening before going to bed, write down on a small card what you must accomplish the next day. Carry this card with you during the day and cross out each item after you accomplish it.

Physical Activity and Health Connection

Our mental and emotional health is essential to the quality of our lives and influences our physical health. The relationship between regular physical activity and mental wellness has been established. Much is known about the physical health benefits of physical activity as it relates to fitness, weight management, and control of a number of chronic disease conditions. Now we can also look at physical activity as an important contributor to mental health and comprehensive stress management strategies. Stress management experts increasingly regard physical activity as one the most healthful ways to reduce stress. People who are physically active tend to have better mental health. Being regularly active increases general feelings of well-being and positive moods, and decreases bouts of anxiety and depression. By engaging your body regularly in physical activity, you prepare it to deal with the physiological strains associated with emotional crises. Your body becomes better able to handle stress and the chemicals that are released during stressful situations. A sound mind and a sound body are equally important to our overall health.

concept connections

1. **People who are physically active tend to have better mental health.** The consensus is that people who are physically active have higher scores on important mental health factors such as self-esteem, self-concept, self-worth, body image, and cognitive functioning than sedentary people. Furthermore, physical activity has been shown to be effective in treating people who report symptoms of anxiety, depression, and stress.

2. **Our mental and emotional health are central to the quality of our lives, and both influence our physical health.** Holistic health perspectives emphasize mind-body unity and include the complex relationship between mental and physical functioning as well as the continuum between health and illness.

3. **Maintaining and optimizing our mental and physical health requires making countless adjustments to a variety of life's challenges.** Life's challenges are perceived internally as stress. Stress places certain physical and mental demands upon us, and how we adapt to these challenges significantly influences our mental and physical health. Your mind and body are connected, and during stressful times it is important to understand the relationship that exists between them.

4. **The general adaptation syndrome describes the body's response to stress and the adaptability of the body to maintain homeostasis.** Selye's research provided evidence that the body goes through a predictable three-stage physiological response to any kind of stressor: (1) the alarm reaction, when the adrenal glands are activated in an attempt to mobilize the body's energy resources for physical action; (2) the stage of resistance, in which the readjustment occurs; and (3) if the readjustment is not complete, the stage of exhaustion may follow, leading to illness and possibly death.

5. **Stress is a natural process, and understanding its effects can help you use it to your own advantage.** Stress researchers have long recognized that some stress (stimulation) is needed for optimal performance. Yerkes and Dodson described a phenomenon that is known today as the Yerkes-Dodson law, which predicts an inverted U-shaped function between stress and performance. The Yerkes-Dodson law theorizes about the ways health and performance are affected as stress increases.

The art of stress management is to keep yourself at a level of stimulation that is healthy and enjoyable. Life without stimulus would be dull and boring. Life with too much stimulus becomes unpleasant and tiring. The primary purpose for developing stress management techniques is to reduce the potential psychological and physical illnesses that result from too much stress.

Terms

Mental health, 279
Emotional health, 279
Psychosomatic disease, 281
Mental illness, 281
Anxiety, 281
Anxiety disorders, 281
Generalized anxiety disorder (GAD), 282
Depression, 282
Depressive reactions, 282
Dysthymia, 282
Major depression, 282
Stress, 282

Eustress, 283
Distress, 283
General adaptation syndromes(GAS), 283
Stressor, 283
Alarm reaction, 284
Autonomic nervous system, 284
Endocrine system, 284
Fight-or-flight response, 285
Pituitary-adrenal axis, 285
Glucocorticoids, 285
Sympathoadrenal system, 285
Epinephrine, 285

Norepinephrine, 285
Parasympathetic nervous system, 285
Relaxation response, 285
Allostatic load, 285
Yerkes-Dodson law, 287
Hypostress, 288
Hyperstress, 288
Environmental engineering, 290
Mind engineering, 290
Physical engineering, 291
Endorphins, 292

making the connection

Jesse now knows that research supports the idea that physical activity can enhance mental health and well-being. Therefore, his impulse to jog before he had to give the speech for English class was a good idea. The jog likely provided a distraction, or time-out, from the anxiety he was experiencing about delivering his speech.

Critical Thinking

1. Jesse was able to determine that exercising helped relieve the speech anxiety he was having. Review Figures 13.5 and 13.6. Are you experiencing any of the harmful stress symptoms listed? If so, do you think stress is the cause? If yes, what are the specific stressors? What physical activities might you do to help relieve these stressors?

2. Review your list of life stress sources. Next to each source, list whether you would use environmental engineering, mind engineering, or physical engineering to manage the stressor. Would more than one strategy be useful? Do you see physical activity helping to manage the stress in your life? Why or why not?

3. Stressors can be a result of situations present on your campus or campus community. Community stressors may be problems such as crime, pollution, lack of recreation facilities, and overcrowded classrooms or residence halls. Identify what you consider to be a major stressor in your campus community. How would you go about changing this stressor?

References

Barbee, J.G. (1998). Mixed symptoms and syndromes of anxiety and depression: Diagnostic, prognostic, and etiologic issues. *Annuals of Clinical Psychiatry* 10:15–29.

Benson, H., & Proctor, W. (2003). *The Breakout Principle: How to Activate the Natural Trigger That Maximizes Creativity, Athletic Performance, Productivity and Personal Well-Being*. New York: Simon & Schuster.

Biddle, S.J.H., Fox, K.R., & Boutcher, S.H. (2000). *Physical Activity and Psychological Well-Being*. London: Routledge.

Biddle, S.J.H., & Mutrie, N. (2001). *Psychology of Physical Activity Determinants, Well-Being and Interventions*. London: Routledge.

Buckworth, J., & Dishman, R.K. (2002). *Exercise Psychology*. Champaign, IL: Human Kinetics.

Dubos, R. (1965). *Man Adapting*. New Haven, CT: Yale University Press.

Fletcher-Janzen, E., Strickland, T.L., & Reynolds, C.R., eds. (2000). *Handbook of Cross-Cultural Neuropsychology*. New York: Kluwer Academic/ Plenum Publishers.

Fontaine, K.R. (2000). Physical activity improves mental health. *The Physician and Sports Medicine* 28(10):83–84.

Fox, K.R. (2000). Physical activity and mental health promotion: The natural partnership. *International Journal of Mental Health Promotion* 2(1):4–19.

Galper, D., Trivedi, M., Barlow, C., Dunn, A., & Kampert, J. (2006). Inverse association between physical inactivity and mental health in men and women. *Medicine and Science in Sports and Exercise* 38(1):173–178.

Goodwin, R.D. (2003). Association between physical activity and mental disorders among adults in the United States. *Preventive Medicine* 36(6):698–703.

Institute of Medicine. (1994). *Reducing the Risk for Mental Disorders: Frontiers for Preventive Intervention Research*. Washington, DC: National Academy Press.

Kessler, R.C., Demler, O., Frank, R.G., Olfson, M., Pincus, H.A., Walters, E.E., Wang, P., Wells, K.B., & Zaslavsky, A.M. (2005). Prevalence and treatment of mental disorders, 1990 to 2003. *New England Journal of Medicine* 352:2515–2523.

McEwen, B.S. (1998). Protective and damaging effects of stress mediators. *New England Journal of Medicine* 338(3):171–179.

McEwen, B.S., & Stellar, E. (1993). Stress and the individual. *Archives of Internal Medicine* 153:2093–2101.

Satcher, D. (2000). Mental health: A report of the surgeon general—executive summary. *International Journal of Psychosocial Rehabilitation* 31(1):5–13.

Selye, H. (1976). *The Stress of Life*. New York: McGraw-Hill.

Taylor, M.K., Pietrobon, R., Pan, D., Huff, M., & Higgins, D.L. (2004). Healthy People 2010 physical activity guidelines and psychological symptoms: Evidence from a large nationwide database. *Journal of Physical Activity and Health* 1(2):114–130.

United States Department of Health and Human Services. (1999). *Mental Health: A Report of the Surgeon General*. Rockville, MD: Author.

United States Department of Health and Human Services. (2000). *Healthy People 2010: Understanding and Improving Health*, 2nd ed. Washington, DC: U.S. Government Printing Office.

Wein, H. (2000). Stress and disease: New perspectives. *The NIH Word on Health*. Online: http://www.nih.gov/news/WordonHealth/oct2000/story01.htm.

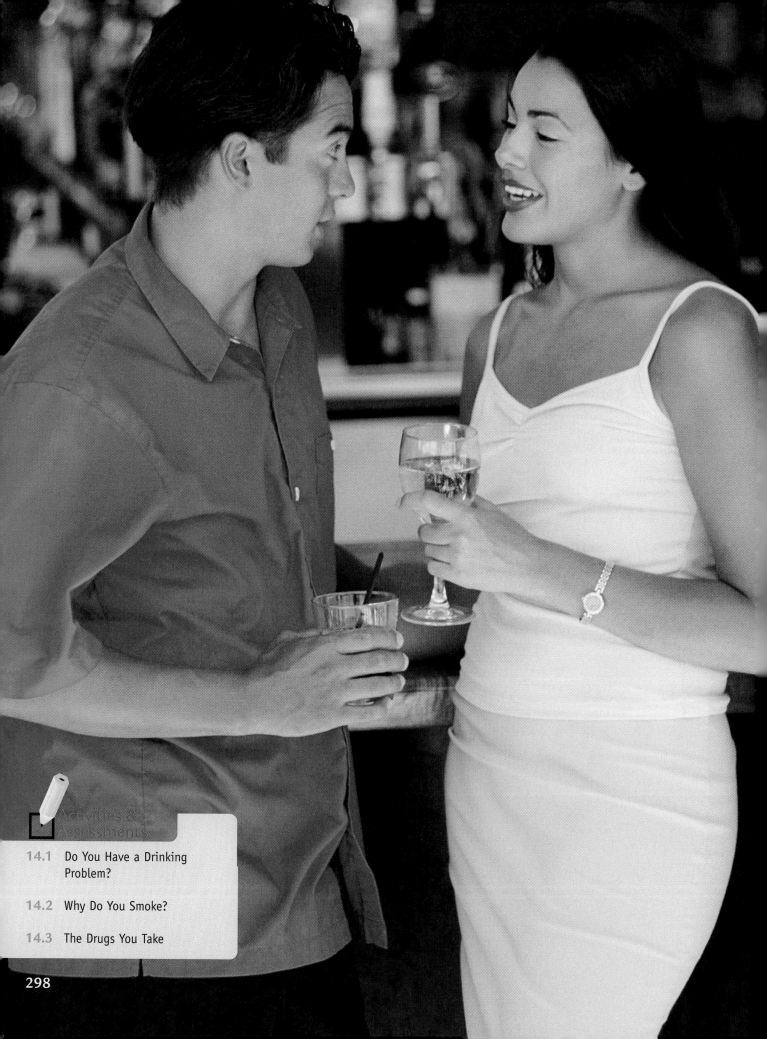

Activities & Assessments

14.1 Do You Have a Drinking Problem?

14.2 Why Do You Smoke?

14.3 The Drugs You Take

Making Informed Decisions About Substance Use

Recently, Jim has realized that his friend and roommate Bill is not handling his drinking of alcohol very well. Whenever they go out to a bar or a club, Bill drinks to get drunk. Furthermore, Jim recognizes that even when they do not go out, Bill still needs to have a few drinks every evening. This has caused Bill to miss class and work due to his drinking, as well as to get into trouble with his family and friends. This is making Jim worry about whether Bill has a problem with his drinking and how to approach Bill about this. Jim wonders, "Where can I go for help?"

concepts

1. College students face a conscious choice on whether to drink alcohol, smoke cigarettes, or use other psychoactive drugs while they pursue their degree.

2. Chronic substance use can disrupt the body's normal balance, or homeostasis.

3. Making wise substance use decisions is important.

4. Alcohol misuse and abuse is one of the most significant health-related drug problems in the United States.

5. Cigarette smoking is the most preventable cause of premature death in the United States.

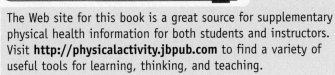

http://physicalactivity.jbpub.com

The Web site for this book is a great source for supplementary physical health information for both students and instructors. Visit **http://physicalactivity.jbpub.com** to find a variety of useful tools for learning, thinking, and teaching.

College students face a conscious choice on whether to drink alcohol, smoke cigarettes, or use other psychoactive drugs while they pursue their degree.

Introduction

Most students are in college for a number of reasons: for an education, to succeed academically, and to get a degree. Students are in college because they are intelligent, certainly smart enough to get into a college and, if they so choose, smart enough to stay there. However, when some students leave school early, it's not because they struggled in the classroom; it may be because they struggled with their choices with psychoactive substance use. Their psychoactive substance use may have resulted in missing classes, performing poorly on tests and assignments, disciplinary issues, or other problems (National Institute on Alcohol Abuse and Alcoholism [NIAAA], 2005).

Nearly all college students face a conscious choice on whether to drink alcohol, smoke marijuana or cigarettes, or use other psychoactive drugs while they pursue their degree. What they choose to do is related to a host of factors, including wanting to have a good time, to fit in or feel more comfortable socially and be accepted, to regulate moods and feelings, to forget about problems or numb out, to relieve emotional or physical pain, or to have a mind-altering experience. However, the use of many psychoactive drugs often creates the opposite effect. Psychoactive drug use can impair alertness and achievement by distorting sensory perception, interfering with memory, and causing a loss of self-control. For example, even occasional use of marijuana affects cognitive development and short-term memory. The major problem with psychoactive drugs is that when people take them, they focus on the immediate desired mental and emotional effects and ignore the potentially damaging mental and physical side effects that can occur. One way or another, the use of psychoactive substances alters the normal functioning of the human body, and in the long run they can cause serious damage.

TABLE 14.1 lists the major types of drugs that affect brain functioning and provides examples of each. Later in the chapter we cover two commonly used and abused psychoactive drugs—alcohol and tobacco. Before we begin our discussion of these drugs, we examine some general terminology and concepts related to drugs.

Drug Terminology

The word **drug** has many different meanings. For the purpose of this chapter, we define a *drug* as any absorbed substance, other than food, that changes or enhances any physical or psychological function in the body. This comprehensive definition of a drug includes a variety of substances that many people use for medical or nonmedical purposes. **Substance use** or drug use is the taking of a drug for its intended purpose in an appropriate amount, frequency, strength, and manner. The many wonders of modern medicine are based on **drug therapeutics**, the proper use of drugs in treating and preventing diseases and preserving health. For example, a physician prescribes a medication to help fight an infection, reverse a disease process, or restore normal body function, and you follow the directions exactly (TABLE 14.2).

Substance misuse or drug misuse is the unintentional or inappropriate use of prescribed or nonprescribed medicine resulting in the impaired physical, mental, emotional, or social well-being of the user. Continuing with the preceding medication example, taking the medication at the wrong times, not taking all of the medication, or taking too much at one time is drug misuse. As a result, you may not recover as expected, or your condition may worsen.

Drug Any absorbed substance, other than food, that changes or enhances any physical or psychological function in the body.

Substance use The taking of a drug for its intended purpose in an appropriate amount, frequency, strength, and manner.

Drug therapeutics The proper use of drugs in treating and preventing diseases and preserving health.

Substance misuse The taking of a substance for its intended purpose, but not in the appropriate amount, frequency, strength, or manner.

| TABLE 14.1 | Psychoactive Drugs: Effects on the Body |

Drug Category	Trade or Other Names	Physical Dependence	Psycho-logical Dependence	Tolerance	Possible Side Effects	Overdose Effects	Withdrawal Effects
Stimulants	Caffeine, cocaine (snow, Big C), methampheta-mine, crystal meth (crystals), Preludin, Ritalin, Dexadrine or "dex," black beau-ties, black hollies	Possible	High	Yes	Alertness, eupho-ria, increased pulse rate and blood pressure, sleeplessness, lack of appetite	Fever, hallucinations, convulsions, death	Prolonged sleep, irritabili-ty, depression, anxiety, moodi-ness, headaches
Depressants	Alcohol, barbitu-rates (goofballs), Valium, Halcion, Quaalude, GHB, GBL, "roofies" (Rohypnol)	Varies	Varies	Yes	Slurred speech, drunken behavior	Depressed breathing, dilated pupils, coma, death	Depression, anxiety, sleep-lessness, con-vulsions, death
Opiates	Heroin (China white), morphine, codeine-contain-ing products, methadone, Demerol, OxyContin, Vicodin, Darvon, Percodan	Moderate to high	Moderate to high	Yes	Euphoria, sleepi-ness, depressed breathing, nausea	Slowed breathing, convulsions, coma, death	Teary eyes, watery nose, yawning, tremors, anxi-ety, abdominal cramps
Marijuana (cannabis)	Pot, hash, hashish oil, Acapulco gold, blunts, buds, Columbo, weed	Unknown	Moderate	Possible	Euphoria, relax-ation, increased appetite, distort-ed time percep-tion	Anxiety, paranoia	Anxiety, depression
Hallucinogens	LSD blotters, mescaline, STP, psilocybin, high doses of PCP, pey-ote, psychedelic mushrooms, keta-mine	None (LSD and mescaline); others: unknown	Unknown	Yes	Euphoria, halluci-nations, poor time perception	Anxiety, psychotic behavior	None reported
Inhalants	Gasoline, paint thinners and removers, freon, aerosols, butyl nitrate	None	Possible	No	Euphoria, sleepi-ness, confusion, slurred speech	Brain, kidney, or liver damage; headaches; death	Anxiety
Drugs with mixed effects	Nicotine, PCP, MDMA (Ecstasy)	Unknown	High (PCP); unknown (MDMA)	Yes	Hallucinations and altered perception	Psychosis, possible death (PCP)	Unknown

SOURCES: U.S. Department of Justice, Drug Enforcement Administration. (1996). *Drugs of Abuse*. Washington, DC: Author; Goldberg, R. (1997). *Drugs Across the Spectrum*. Englewood, CO: Morton Publishing; and Hanson, G.R., Venturelli, P.J., & Fleckenstein, A.E. (2004). *Drugs and Society*, 8th ed. Sudbury, MA: Jones and Bartlett.

TABLE 14.2	Tips for Taking Medicines

Whether prescription or over-the-counter (OTC), no medicine is without risk. Besides benefits, medicines may cause side effects, allergic reactions, and interactions with foods, drinks, or other drugs. For prescription drugs, a patient's first step to safe and effective treatment is to ask the doctor questions with each new prescription.

For example:

What is the medicine's name, and what is it supposed to do?

How and when do I take it, and for how long?

While taking this medicine, should I avoid:

- certain foods or dietary supplements?
- caffeine, alcohol, or other beverages?
- other medicines, prescription and OTC?
- certain activities, such as driving or smoking?

Will this new medicine work safely with prescription and OTC medicines I'm already taking? Are there side effects, and what do I do if they occur?

Will the medicine affect my sleep or activity level?

What should I do if I miss a dose?

Is there written information available about the medicine? (At the very least, ask the doctor or pharmacist to write out complicated directions and medicine names.)

It's wise to write down the answers to these questions immediately, to make sure you'll remember all the details.

SOURCE: U.S. Food and Drug Administration. (2001). Tips for taking medication. Online: http://www.fda.gov/fdoc/reprints/medtips.html.

This information is not intended to be a substitute for professional medical advice. You should not use this information to diagnose or treat a health problem or disease without consulting with a qualified health care provider. Please consult your health care provider with any questions or concerns you may have regarding your condition.

Substance abuse The deliberate use of a substance for other than its intended purpose, in a manner that can damage health or ability to function.

Psychoactive drug A chemical substance that alters one's thinking, perceptions, feelings, and behavior.

Substance dependence A chronic, progressive, and relapsing disorder that applies to all situations in which drug users develop either a psychological or physical reliance on a drug.

Substance abuse or drug abuse is a pattern of substance (drug) use leading to significant problems such as failure to attend school, substance use in dangerous situations (driving a car or risky sexual behavior), substance-related legal problems, or continued substance use that negatively affects friends, family, and society. People are more likely to abuse psychoactive drugs than other drugs because of their effects on the mind. A **psychoactive drug** is a chemical substance that alters one's thinking, perceptions, feelings, and behavior (see Table 14.1). Such drugs include both legal and illegal substances. According to many, alcohol is the most commonly abused psychoactive drug in the United States today (National Institute on Drug Abuse [NIDA], 2005).

Substance dependence is used to describe continued use of drugs even when significant problems related to their use have developed. Signs include an increased tolerance or need for increased amounts of substance to attain the desired effect, withdrawal symptoms with decreased use, unsuccessful efforts to decrease use, increased time spent in activities to obtain substances, withdrawal from social and recreational activities, and continued use of the substance even with awareness of physical or psychological problems encountered because of the extent of substance use (American Psychological Assoication [APA], 2000; NIDA, 2005). TABLE 14.3 lists the diagnostic criteria for substance dependence.

It is generally assumed that no one starts using drugs with the goal of misusing, abusing, or becoming dependent on them; however, it is possible to drift from

TABLE 14.3	Criteria for Substance Dependence Diagnosis

Diagnostic and Statistical Manual IV

A maladaptive pattern of substance use leading to clinically significant impairment or distress as manifested by three (or more) of the following, occurring at any time in the same 12-month period:

- Substance is often taken in larger amounts or over longer period than intended
- Persistent desire or unsuccessful efforts to cut down or control substance use
- A great deal of time is spent in activities necessary to obtain the substance (e.g., visiting multiple doctors or driving long distances), use the substance (e.g., chain smoking), or recover from its effects
- Important social, occupational, or recreational activities given up or reduced because of substance abuse
- Continued substance use despite knowledge of having a persistent or recurrent psychological or physical problem that is caused or exacerbated by use of the substance
- Tolerance, as defined by either:
  a. need for greater amounts of the substance in order to achieve intoxication or desired effect; or
  b. markedly diminished effect with continued use of the same amount
- Withdrawal, as manifested by either:
  a. characteristic withdrawal syndrome for the substance; or
  b. the same (or closely related) substance taken to relieve or avoid withdrawal symptoms

International Classification of Diseases 10

[ICD-10 research criteria differ from the clinical diagnostic guidelines listed here.] Three or more of the following must have been experienced or exhibited at some time during the previous year:

- Difficulties in controlling substance-taking behavior in terms of its onset, termination, or levels of use
- A strong desire or sense of compulsion to take the substance
- Progressive neglect of alternative pleasures or interests because of psychoactive substance use; increased amount of time necessary to obtain or take the substance or to recover from its effects
- Persisting with substance use despite clear evidence of overtly harmful consequences, depressive mood states consequent to heavy use, or drug-related impairment of cognitive functioning
- Evidence of tolerance, such that increased doses of the psychoactive substance are required in order to achieve effects originally produced by lower doses
- A physiological withdrawal state when substance use has ceased or been reduced, as evidenced by the characteristic withdrawal syndrome for the substance, or use of the same (or a closely related) substance with the intention of relieving or avoiding withdrawal symptoms

SOURCE: National Institute on Drug Abuse. (2004). Criteria for substance dependence diagnosis. Online: http://www.nida.nih.gov/Drugpages/DSR.html.

responsible use to misuse, abuse, or dependence for a number of commonly used drugs. It is also clear that many chronic users eventually do experience problems with drugs and may eventually suffer negative health consequences. Addressing or treating chronic users in terms of their level of involvement is essential in forestalling a number of detrimental health effects. Therefore, it is critical to understand the processes that one's body and mind undergo with chronic drug use.

Chronic substance use can disrupt the body's normal balance, or homeostasis.

Tolerance Adaptation of the body to a drug in such a way that repeated exposure to the same dose results in less effect on the body.

Chronic Drug Use

Chronic drug use often unsettles the body's normal balance, or homeostasis. The person who continues to use a drug moves to a level of risk one step beyond, because each exposure carries with it the possibility that the body's chemical pathways will change to adapt to repeated exposure to the drug. This can be a difficult idea to grasp, but within it lies the foundation for *tolerance, psychological dependence, physical dependence*, and *withdrawal illness*. The following sections define each of these key terms and explain how they are related to the gradual distress of the body. This continuum of involvement with drugs is essential for people to consider as they honestly examine their own drug use and evaluate its possible long-range consequences in terms of quitting or changing drug-related behaviors.

Tolerance

Tolerance, a homeostatic response, is the adaptation of the body to a drug in such a way that repeated exposure to the same dose results in less effect on the body. To counteract the tolerance phenomenon, the individual requires increasing doses to produce the original effect. These increased doses may be dangerous to certain parts of the body, since all body parts do not become equally tolerant to the drug. For example, a higher blood alcohol concentration is thought to be required to diminish a chronically heavy drinker's physical performance as compared with a moderate drinker's performance because the central nervous system is less depressed in the heavy drinker due to the nerve tissue's having become more tolerant of alcohol. Similarly, the brain and stomach do not adapt well to higher concentrations of alcohol—are not as tolerant to its toxicity—which results in blackouts (not remembering events) and acute stomach irritation and inflammation.

Another example of tolerance occurs with the chemical nicotine, found in cigarettes. Nicotine produces pleasurable feelings that make the smoker want to smoke more; it also acts as a depressant by interfacing with the flow of information between nerve cells. As the nervous system adapts to nicotine, smokers tend to increase the number of cigarettes they smoke and hence the amount of nicotine in their blood. After a while, the smoker develops a tolerance for the drug, which leads to an increase in smoking over time. Eventually, the smoker reaches a certain level and then smokes to maintain this level. Tolerance has been proposed as an important component in understanding substance dependence.

Substance Dependence

Substance dependence, commonly known as drug addiction, is a chronic, progressive, and relapsing disorder that applies to all situations in which drug users develop either a psychological or physical reliance on the drug. **FIGURE 14.1** lists health experts' ratings of how easy it is to become addicted and how difficult it is to stop using various psychoactive drugs. Substance dependence is a strong dependence on a drug typified by three factors: (1) tolerance to a given dose or the need for more and more of the substance, (2) severe withdrawal symptoms, and (3) the loss of control, or the need to consume the substance at all costs. This drug dependence is characterized by a *compulsive and continued use* in spite of adverse health consequences. Substance dependence is based on the concepts of psychological and physical dependence.

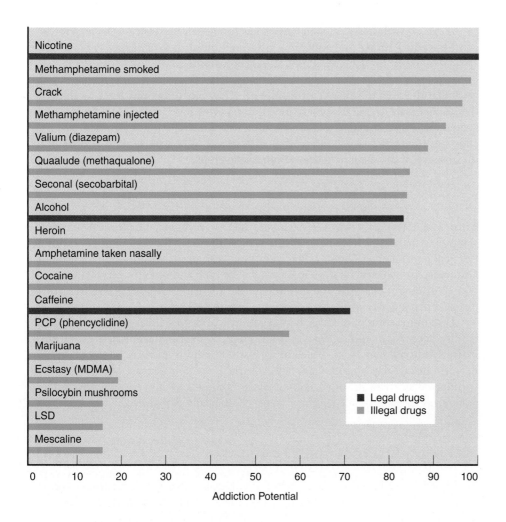

FIGURE 14.1 Addiction Potential of Various Drugs. The chart shows health experts' ratings of the addiction potential of various drugs, with 100 being the highest addiction potential. Note that both legal and illegal drugs can be highly addictive.

Psychological Dependence

Psychological dependence, or behavioral dependence, is a craving for a drug for primarily psychological or emotional reasons. The person begins to rely on a drug as a solution to a variety of emotional problems ranging from boredom to relief of anger or frustration. A good example of psychological dependence can be seen in cigarette smokers. Some smokers use the habit to enhance their moods and feelings of competency, whereas others use the habit to reduce their feelings of distress and anxiety. Smoking becomes a means of emotional and psychological support for many smokers and a necessary way of dealing with life. Once this happens, any attempt to quit or reduce smoking results in psychological distress. Psychological cravings for drugs may last for years after quitting.

Physical Dependence

Physical dependence is the biological adaptation to a drug by the body, in which the drug has become necessary to maintain a balance related to certain body processes. Physical dependence studies investigate the motivational properties of physical withdrawal reactions. At some point the body becomes so completely adapted to the drug that it is a necessity for physiological function. The discomfort experi-

Psychological dependence Craving for a drug for primarily psychological or emotional reasons.

Physical dependence The body's biological adaptation to a drug, in which the drug has become necessary to maintain a balance in certain body processes.

enced during withdrawal of some drugs has long been presumed to be a factor in continued drug intake and addiction. Although physical dependence is not a necessary condition for drug addiction, it may contribute to the total reinforcing impact of some drugs. For example, in many dependent smokers, evidence suggests that the urge to smoke correlates with a low blood nicotine level, as though the smoker were trying to achieve a certain nicotine level and avoid withdrawal symptoms. Thus, smokers may be smoking to achieve the reward of nicotine effects or to avoid the pain of nicotine withdrawal. When the body has to adapt to the absence of the drug, withdrawal illness develops.

Withdrawal Illness

Withdrawal illness, or *abstinence syndrome*, displays recognizable physical signs and symptoms that result from drug abstinence. Withdrawal illness is a direct result of physical dependence. The signs and symptoms can occur within hours of drug abstinence or take several days to develop. The type and severity vary with the type of drug. For example, the nicotine found in cigarette smoke is a significant physical dependency-producing drug (see Figure 14.1).

Discontinuation of nicotine may result in withdrawal illness symptoms—irritability, depression, and dizziness—within hours. The physical distress of the abstinence syndrome may be of sufficient intensity to require medical intervention; it may last from 1 day up to several days (nearly 1 week in the case of alcohol). Once withdrawal sickness subsides, individuals are thought no longer to be physically dependent; however, they still may be psychologically dependent.

Making Substance Use Decisions

We have reviewed several levels of drug involvement that can occur from chronic drug use. The choice of which drug to use, the amount, and how long to use it are all important individual decisions and should not be made thoughtlessly. Therefore, it is important for an individual to practice decision-making skills related to taking drugs so that an appropriate response may be made when choosing to use drugs. Following is a six-stage decision-making strategy that you can use to evaluate your individual drug use (Engs, 2001):

1. Think about the situation and try to understand your reasons for using the drug.
2. Consider all the alternatives to using the drug by examining the reasons and thinking about alternatives for achieving your goals.
3. Attempt to identify potential difficulties associated with each of the alternatives.
4. Consider each alternative in the context of your situation, and select the one that seems best for you.
5. Take action on the alternative you have selected.
6. Assess the results, so that you may have more information available to you the next time you are faced with a similar situation.

Commonly Used and Misused Psychoactive Drugs

The following sections examine some of the most familiar and frequently used and misused psychoactive drugs in our society. We believe it is important for you to understand the pharmacology of these drugs. **Pharmacology** is the study of drugs, their sources, how they enter the body, how the body reacts to them, and their

---

Withdrawal illness Recognizable physical signs and symptoms that result from withdrawing drug use.

Pharmacology The study of drugs, their sources, how they enter the body, how the body reacts to them, and their short-term and long-term effects on the body.

Making wise substance use decisions is important.

Cigarette smoking is the leading cause of preventable death in the United States.

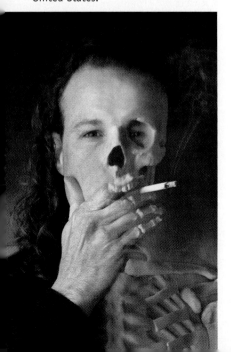

short-term and long-term effects on the body. By understanding the positive and negative effects these common drugs have on your body, you will be able to make better-informed decisions related to their use as part of your lifestyle.

Alcohol and Society

Alcohol is the most widely used *psychoactive*, or mood-changing, social drug in the United States. Approximately 55 percent of U.S. adults (18 years and older) consume alcoholic beverages on a regular basis, while 45 percent do not drink any alcohol (Substance Abuse and Mental Health Services Administration [SAMHSA], 2005). People drink to relax, reduce self-consciousness and anxiety, celebrate, and have fun, and for social companionship—psychological or emotional benefits that may improve health and well-being (Little, 2000). Research also suggests that drinking small to moderate amounts of alcohol can lower the risk of cardiovascular disease and certain other diseases in comparison with nondrinkers (Ellison, 2002). On the other hand, the risk of excessive alcohol intake is well known, and heavy drinkers should decrease their intake or stop drinking. Ten percent of adult Americans, or an estimated 18 million adults in the United States, have significant alcohol-related problems due to heavy drinking. All in all, adult consumers of alcohol in this country contribute to some astounding statistics. It is estimated that alcohol is involved in 100,000 deaths annually (NIDA, 2005). Half of all traffic crash deaths are alcohol related. There are more than one million annual alcohol-related hospital discharges. Newborns are also affected, because maternal consumption of alcohol contributes to alcohol-related birth defects in 36,000 children every year.

Alcohol has long been the drug of choice among college students aged 18 to 25. Although it is illegal for anyone under the age of 21 to purchase, possess, and consume alcohol, many college students under age 21 drink alcoholic beverages. College students have notably high rates of heavy drinking compared with the general population. Data from several national surveys indicate that about four in five college students drink and that nearly half of college student drinkers engage in heavy episodic consumption of alcohol. The consequences of excessive and underage drinking affect virtually all college students, campuses, and college communities, whether they choose to drink or not (NIAAA, 2005). TABLE 14.4 lists the consequences of high-risk college drinking.

It is easy to understand why alcohol misuse and abuse is one of the most significant health-related drug problems in the United States. Public health campaigns traditionally urge people to avoid or cut back on their drinking, and appropriately so, since misuse or abuse of alcohol costs the United States $150 billion in health and social expenditures (NIDA, 2005). Therefore, personal decisions about your alcohol consumption and the associated risks and benefits should be reviewed periodically as part of your health lifestyle strategy.

Measures of Alcohol Consumption

The consumption of alcoholic beverages can have helpful or harmful effects depending on the amount consumed; the pattern of drinking, age, and other characteristics of the person consuming the alcohol; and the specifics of the situation (U.S. Department of Health and Human Services [USDHHS] & U.S. Department of Agriculture [USDA], 2005).

SOCIAL DRINKING **Social drinking** is use of alcohol that consists of an occasional drink or two in the company of friends: a glass of champagne at a wedding or

Alcohol misuse and abuse is one of the most significant health-related drug problems in the United States.

Social drinking Use of alcohol that consists of an occasional drink or two in the company of friends.

| TABLE 14.4 | A Snapshot of Consequences of High-Risk College Drinking* |

- **Death:** 1700 college students between the ages of 18 and 24 die each year from alcohol-related unintentional injuries, including motor vehicle crashes (Hingson et al., 2005).
- **Injury:** 599,000 students between the ages of 18 and 24 are unintentionally injured under the influence of alcohol (Hingson et al., 2005).
- **Assault:** More than 696,000 students between the ages of 18 and 24 are assaulted by another student who has been drinking (Hingson et al., 2005).
- **Sexual abuse:** More than 97,000 students between the ages of 18 and 24 are victims of alcohol-related sexual assault or date rape (Hingson et al., 2005).
- **Unsafe sex:** 400,000 students between the ages of 18 and 24 had unprotected sex, and more than 100,000 students between the ages of 18 and 24 report having been too intoxicated to know if they consented to having sex (Hingson et al., 2002).
- **Academic problems:** About 25 percent of college students report academic consequences of their drinking, including missing class, falling behind, doing poorly on exams or papers, and receiving lower grades overall (Engs, Diebold, & Hanson, 1996; Presley et al., 1996a, 1996b; Wechsler et al., 2002).
- **Health problems/Suicide attempts:** More than 150,000 students develop an alcohol-related health problem (Hingson et al., 2002), and between 1.2 and 1.5 percent of students indicate that they tried to commit suicide within the past year due to drinking or drug use (Presley, Leichliter, & Meilman, 1998).
- **Drunk driving:** 2.1 million students between the ages of 18 and 24 drove under the influence of alcohol in 2001 (Hingson et al., 2002).
- **Vandalism:** About 11 percent of college student drinkers report that they have damaged property while under the influence of alcohol (Wechsler et al., 2002).
- **Property damage:** More than 25 percent of administrators from schools with relatively low drinking levels and over 50 percent from schools with high drinking levels say their campuses have a "moderate" or "major" problems with alcohol-related property damage (Wechsler et al., 1995).
- **Police involvement:** About 5 percent of 4-year college students are involved with the police or campus security as a result of their drinking (Wechsler et al., 2002), and an estimated 110,000 students between the ages of 18 and 24 are arrested for an alcohol-related violation such as public drunkenness or driving under the influence (Hingson et al., 2002).
- **Alcohol abuse and dependence:** 31 percent of college students met criteria for a diagnosis of alcohol abuse and 6 percent for a diagnosis of alcohol dependence in the past 12 months, according to questionnaire-based self-reports about their drinking (Knight et al., 2002).

*High-risk college student drinking includes the following: (1) underage drinking, (2) drinking and driving or other activities where the use of alcohol is dangerous, (3) drinking when health conditions or medications make use dangerous, and (4) binge drinking, that is, five drinks in a row per occasion for males and four for females. (*Moderate drinking by persons of legal age is defined as no more than two standard drinks per day for men and one drink per day for women.*)

SOURCE: College Drinking Prevention. A snapshot of annual high-risk college drinking consequences. Online: http://www.collegedrinkingprevention.gov/StatsSummaries/snapshot.aspx.

Moderate drinking Drinking that causes no problems, either for the drinker or for society; quantified as no more than one drink a day for most women, and no more than two drinks a day for most men.

special occasion, a glass of wine with a special meal, a cold beer after a softball game. This small, infrequent amount of drinking is extremely low risk for harming any body tissue or organ.

MODERATE DRINKING   **Moderate drinking** may be defined as drinking that does not generally cause problems, either for the drinker or society (TABLE 14.5). It should be understood that a given dose of alcohol affects different people differently. Therefore,

TABLE 14.5	Criteria for Moderate and At-Risk Alcohol Use

Moderate Drinking

Men: ≤2 drinks/day*

Women: ≤1 drink/day

Over 65 (men and women): ≤1 drink/day

At-Risk Drinking

Men: >14 drinks/week, or >4 drinks/occasion

Women: >7 drinks/week, or >3 drinks/occasion

Alcohol Abuse

Significant impairment or distress in a 12-month period, including

- Failure to meet obligations at work, school, or home
- Recurrent use of alcohol in hazardous situations
- Legal problems related to alcohol
- Continued use despite alcohol-related social or interpersonal problems

Alcohol Dependence

Significant impairment or distress in a 12-month period, including

- Tolerance to alcohol
- Withdrawal symptoms with abstinence from alcohol
- Use of larger amounts over a longer period than intended
- Persistent desire for alcohol (craving)
- Unsuccessful attempts to cut down or control use
- Important social, occupational, or recreational activities given up because of drinking
- Use despite knowledge of alcohol-related problems (denial)

*One drink = 12 g of alcohol, which is the equivalent of 180 ml (6 oz) of wine, 360 ml (12 oz) of beer, or 45 ml (1.5 oz) of 90-proof distilled spirits.

SOURCE: U.S. National Institute on Alcohol Abuse and the American Psychiatric Association.

individuals making the decision to drink must be aware that they are assuming a small inherent risk.

Current recommendations by the *Dietary Guidelines for Americans 2005* state that "those who choose to drink alcoholic beverages should do so sensibly and in moderation—defined as the consumption of up to one drink per day for women and up to two drinks per day for men" (USDHHS & USDA, 2005). A standard drink contains approximately 0.5 ounce, or 12 grams, of alcohol. A standard drink is generally considered to be 12 ounces of beer, 5 ounces of wine, or 1.5 ounces of distilled spirits (FIGURE 14.2). This current advice about moderate drinking by the *Dietary Guidelines* should be acknowledged with the understanding that the guidelines also make two key recommendations about who should not drink alcoholic beverages (USDHHS & USDA, 2005):

- Alcoholic beverages should not be consumed by some individuals, including those who cannot restrict their alcohol intake, women of childbearing age who may become pregnant, pregnant and lactating women, children and adolescents, individuals taking medications that can interact with alcohol, and those with specific medical conditions.
- Alcoholic beverages should be avoided by individuals engaging in activities that require attention, skill, or coordination, such as driving or operating machinery.

FIGURE 14.2 **Alcohol Beverages.**
Ethyl alcohol is a common psychoactive drug in all alcoholic beverages. One drink—defined as a
12-ounce beer, a 5-ounce glass
of wine, or a 1.5-ounce shot of
distilled spirits—contains about
0.5 ounce of ethyl alcohol.

Count as a Drink . . .

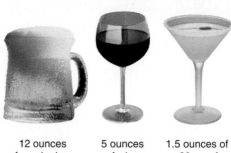

12 ounces	5 ounces	1.5 ounces of
of regular beer	of wine	80-proof
		distilled spirits

Binge drinking For males, having
five or more drinks in a row at one
sitting, and for females, having
four or more drinks in a row at
one sitting.

Problem drinking The consumption of alcohol that results in
significant risk of health consequences, social problems, or both.

You may be wondering why the recommendation for women is less than that
for men. First, women generally have a smaller body size and a lower proportion
of water content in which to dilute any alcohol consumed. Second, women have
less of a protective stomach enzyme (alcohol dehydrogenase) that breaks down
(oxidizes) a portion of alcohol before it enters the bloodstream. Therefore, women
will absorb more alcohol into the bloodstream than males of the same weight who
have drunk an equal amount of alcoholic beverages. We look further into the
chemical properties and metabolism of alcohol in the alcoholic beverage section.

BINGE DRINKING   Binge drinking differs from social and moderate drinking in
terms of the amount of alcohol consumed and the pattern of drinking. Binge
drinkers often drink to get drunk and believe that heavy drinking is appropriate
and desirable in social situations. The binge is usually planned and will not continue for more than one day. **Binge drinking** is defined for males as consuming five or
more drinks in a row at one sitting, and for females as consuming four or more in
a row. This amount of alcohol is approximately the amount of alcohol needed to
raise the average-sized person's blood alcohol concentration to about 0.10 percent.
In other words, it is the amount of alcohol consumption that would lead to the
presumption of intoxication (drunkenness). Every state considers a person intoxicated and incapable of operating a vehicle safely at this level of intoxication.
Furthermore, this high level of intoxication increases the risk for hangovers,
fatigue, headaches, shakiness, bloodshot eyes, nausea and vomiting, injuries from
accidents, severe impairment of driving, unprotected sex, seizures, brain damage,
and death from alcohol overdose.

Most binge drinkers do not feel that they are problem drinkers because they
do not drink daily. After a binge, the person will be able to go for days, weeks, or
months with little or no drinking before another binge occurs. It is a myth that
only daily drinkers have an alcohol problem. Binge drinking is more likely in situations where people drink in groups, where they serve themselves, or where drinking games are involved. Binge drinking is most common in college students aged
18 to 24 years, possibly in response to increased freedom in their lives. In the past
decade, approximately half (44 percent) of college students were considered binge
drinkers (Wechsler et al., 2002).

PROBLEM DRINKING   **Problem drinking** is the consumption of alcohol that results
in significant risk of health consequences, social problems, or both (Table 14.5 and
 TABLE 14.6). Chronic abuse of alcohol can lead to a number of serious health conditions (see the section on long-term effects of alcohol), as well as to dependence
or alcoholism. *Alcohol dependence*, or *alcoholism*, refers to a disease that is characterized by abnormal alcohol-seeking behavior that leads to impaired control over

TABLE 14.6	How Do You Know If You Are Drinking Too Much?

If you are drinking too much, you can improve your life and health by cutting down.

How do you know if you drink too much?

Read these questions and answer yes or no:

- Do you drink alone when you feel angry or sad?
- Does your drinking ever make you late for work?
- Does your drinking worry your family?
- Do you ever drink after telling yourself you won't?
- Do you ever forget what you did while you were drinking?
- Do you get headaches or have a hangover after you have been drinking?

If you answered yes to any of these questions, you may have a drinking problem. Check with your doctor to be sure. Your doctor will be able to tell you whether you should cut down or abstain. If you are alcoholic or have other medical problems, you should not just cut down on your drinking—you should stop drinking completely. Your doctor will advise you about what is right for you.

SOURCE: National Institute on Alcohol Abuse and Alcoholism. (1996). How to cut down on your drinking. Online: http://pubs.niaaa.nih.gov/publications/handout.htm.

drinking. Many factors contribute to alcohol dependence, including personality characteristics, stress, family environment, heredity, and the addictive nature of alcohol. Many alcoholics become able to drink ever-larger quantities of alcohol before feeling or appearing drunk. Alcohol users commonly medicate themselves with alcohol, using it, often daily, to help them relax, as a confidence booster, or in order to avoid withdrawal symptoms.

Alcoholic Beverages

Ethyl alcohol is the common psychoactive ingredient in all alcoholic beverages. It is a direct central nervous system depressant that causes a decreased level of consciousness and decreased motor function. At high concentrations, ethyl alcohol is toxic. It is an anesthetic and can cause autonomic dysfunction leading to death from respiratory depression and cardiovascular failure.

Ethyl alcohol is one of several chemicals in the alcohol family, and is a thin, clear, colorless fluid with a mild, aromatic odor and pungent taste. It is capable of being mixed with water in all proportions and is diffusible through body membranes. Ethyl alcohol contained in beverages is created by fermentation, a process in which the yeast fungus feeds on the sugars or starches in certain plants such as barley or grapes and excretes alcohol along with carbon dioxide. From the cheapest beer to the most expensive wine or after-dinner liqueur, all alcohol is made with the same fermentation process. The different colors, tastes, potencies, and flavors come from the different fruits or vegetables used as well as the additives, byproducts, and diluting substances of the fermentation process. The three basic types of alcohol beverages are beer, wine, and distilled spirits (see Figure 14.2).

Beer is made from fermented grains and has an alcohol content of approximately 5 percent. Light ("lite") beer, or reduced-calorie beer, has the same percentage of alcohol as regular beer. Wine is made from fermented fruits and has an alcohol content of approximately 12 percent. Some wine drinks, such as wine coolers, have lower alcohol content because of the fruit juice and sugar added to them. Fortified wines, such as port, have alcohol added to them, raising the alcohol content above 12 percent. Finally, distilled spirits, so named because liquid distillation

Ethyl alcohol A direct central nervous system depressant that causes a decreased level of consciousness and decreased motor function; the common psychoactive ingredient in all alcoholic beverages.

after sugar fermentation increases their alcohol content, originate from sources of starch or sugar, including cereals, molasses from sugar beets, grapes, potatoes, cherries, plums, and other fruits. Distilled spirits (gin, rum, vodka, whiskey) produce a drink that usually contains 40 to 50 percent alcohol. The alcohol content in distilled spirits is sometimes indicated by degrees of proof, which in the United States is a figure that is twice the percentage of alcohol by volume in a beverage. Thus, 70-proof liquor is 35 percent alcohol. In general, a 12-ounce bottle of beer, a 5-ounce glass of wine, and a 1.5-ounce shot of liquor all contain the same amount of alcohol (0.5 ounce) and therefore have an identical psychoactive effect on the drinker when it comes to intoxication (see Figure 14.2).

ALCOHOL AND WEIGHT Pure alcohol contains about 7 calories per gram, which makes it nearly twice as fattening as carbohydrates or protein (both contain about 4 calories per gram) and only just under the caloric value for fat (9 calories per gram). These calories are considered "empty" calories because they supply no energy value or nutrients. That is, alcohol calories are useless in meeting your body's nutrient needs (TABLE 14.7). Unlike starches and sugars that are converted to glucose, glycogen, or fat, alcohol is denatured—mostly in the liver—into carbon dioxide and water. Since an estimated 95 percent of all alcohol we consume is catabolized (the other 5 percent is eliminated through the breath, skin, urine, and feces), it has no direct caloric or nutrient significance. However, many argue that alcoholic beverages indirectly cause a stimulus in appetite, decreased physical activity, suppression of the basal metabolic rate, and increased consumption of nonalcohol calories from high-calorie unhealthy snacks—all contributing to weight gain. This means that if you want to lose weight, reduce excess body fat, and become physically fit, alcohol is not a good choice.

Alcohol Absorption

When a person drinks alcohol, the alcohol is absorbed primarily by the stomach (20 percent) and small intestine (80 percent) (FIGURE 14.3). Since alcohol molecules are small, they are readily absorbed into the blood without being digested. Once the alcohol has been absorbed, it is rapidly carried throughout the body by the blood. A

TABLE 14.7	**Calories in Selected Alcoholic Beverages**		
Beverage	Approximate Calories per 1 Fluid Ounce[a]	Example Serving Volume	Approximate Total Calories[b]
Beer (regular)	12	12 oz	144
Beer (light)	9	12 oz	108
White wine	20	5 oz	100
Red wine	21	5 oz	105
Sweet dessert wine	47	3 oz	141
80-proof distilled spirits (gin, rum, vodka, whiskey)	64	1.5 oz	96

[a]Data are from Agricultural Research Service Nutrient Database for Standard Reference, Release 17. Online: http://www.nal.usda.gov/fnic/foodcomp/index.html. Calories are calculated to the nearest whole number per 1 fluid oz.

[b]The total calories and alcohol content vary depending on the brand. Moreover, adding mixers to an alcoholic beverage can contribute calories in addition to the calories from the alcohol itself.

SOURCE: U.S. Department of Agriculture. (2005). *Dietary Guidelines for Americans.*

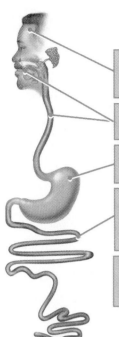

FIGURE 14.3 Alcohol Absorption.
How alcohol is absorbed and
metabolized.

As BAC rises, motor skills, judgment, and reaction times are impaired. If BAC reaches 0.5%, central nervous system function is depressed and coma or death may result.

Small amounts of alcohol are absorbed in the mouth and esophagus as it is swallowed.

Alcohol is readily absorbed in the stomach (approximately 20%), but food will dilute the alcohol and delay its passage into the small intestine.

The small intestine efficiently absorbs most of the alcohol consumed (about 80%). The alcohol is then carried through the bloodstream to all the body's tissues and organs and eventually reaches the liver, where it is metabolized.

The portion of alcohol that is not excreted (about 95%) through sweat, urine, or breath is metabolized by the liver. The liver detoxifies alcohol at a rate of about 1/2 ounce per hour.

balance occurs such that blood at all points in the system contains approximately the same amount of alcohol. The amount of alcohol in your blood is expressed as **blood alcohol concentration (BAC)**. Blood alcohol concentration is measured in percentages. A simple way to estimate your BAC is shown in TABLE 14.8.

Blood alcohol concentration (BAC) The amount of alcohol in the blood.

Alcohol Elimination

The body readily recognizes alcohol in the bloodstream as a toxic substance and begins to remove it from the blood as soon as it reaches the liver. The liver is responsible for eliminating 95 percent of ingested alcohol from the body though an active process of metabolism. The remainder of the alcohol is eliminated through excretion of alcohol in urine, sweat, and breath. Most of the metabolism of alcohol is performed by the enzyme alcohol dehydrogenase (ADH), which is found mostly in the liver. Alcohol dehydrogenase is also found in other tissues of the body, notably in the stomach lining, where it breaks down some of the alcohol before it ever reaches the bloodstream. The ADH enzyme is found in greater quantities and is more active in the stomachs of men than of women—meaning men break down more alcohol before it reaches their bloodstream. The liver can metabolize approximately 0.5 ounce (the equivalent of one drink) per hour. Nothing can be done to speed up this process; cold showers, exercise, black coffee, fresh air, or vomiting will not help. Only time will allow the liver to break down the alcohol in the bloodstream, and unprocessed alcohol circulates through the bloodstream until the liver can process it.

If a person drinks alcohol faster than it can be eliminated from the body, the BAC rises, increasing the toxic effects of ethyl alcohol on the body. There are several important factors that a person can control related to influencing BAC. These include controlling the amount of alcohol consumed and the rate of consumption, and eating before drinking.

AMOUNT OF ALCOHOL   As more drinks are consumed, more alcohol is readily available to be absorbed in the blood. It is important to understand the amount of

| TABLE 14.8 | Alcohol Impairment Chart—Never Drink and Drive! |

Men*

Approximate Blood Alcohol Percentage
Body Weight in Pounds

Drinks	100	120	140	160	180	200	220	240	
0	.00	.00	.00	.00	.00	.00	.00	.00	Only Safe Driving Limit
1	.04	.03	.03	.02	.02	.02	.02	.02	Impairment Begins
2	.08	.06	.05	.05	.04	.04	.03	.03	Driving Skills Significantly
3	.11	.09	.08	.07	.06	.06	.05	.05	Affected
4	.15	.12	.11	.09	.08	.08	.07	.06	
5	.19	.16	.13	.12	.11	.09	.09	.08	Possible Criminal Penalties
6	.23	.19	.16	.14	.13	.11	.10	.09	
7	.26	.22	.19	.16	.15	.13	.12	.11	Legally Intoxicated
8	.30	.25	.21	.19	.17	.15	.14	.13	
9	.34	.28	.24	.21	.19	.17	.15	.14	Criminal
10	.38	.31	.27	.23	.21	.19	.17	.16	Penalties

Women*

Approximate Blood Alcohol Percentage
Body Weight in Pounds

Drinks	90	100	120	140	160	180	200	220	240	
0	0.00	.00	.00	.00	.00	.00	.00	.00	.00	Only Safe Driving Limit
1	.05	.05	.04	.03	.03	.03	.02	.02	.02	Impairment Begins
2	.10	.09	.08	.07	.06	.05	.05	.04	.04	Driving Skills Significantly
3	.15	.14	.11	.10	.09	.08	.07	.06	.06	Affected
4	.20	.18	.15	.13	.11	.10	.09	.08	.08	
5	.25	.23	.19	.16	.14	.13	.11	.10	.09	Possible Criminal Penalties
6	.30	.27	.23	.19	.17	.15	.14	.12	.11	
7	.35	.32	.27	.23	.20	.18	.16	.14	.13	Legally Intoxicated
8	.40	.36	.30	.26	.23	.20	.18	.17	.15	
9	.45	.41	.34	.29	.26	.23	.20	.19	.17	Criminal
10	.51	.45	.38	.32	.28	.25	.23	.21	.19	Penalties

*Subtract .01% for each 40 minutes of drinking. One drink is 1.25 oz of 80-proof liquor, 12 oz of beer, or 5 oz of table wine.

SOURCE: The National Commission Against Drunk Driving. Online: http://www.ncadd.com/08_impairmentcharts.cfm.

alcohol in each of the three categories of alcoholic beverages. Some people attempt to distinguish among beer, wine, and liquor when explaining their drinking. But, a 12-ounce bottle of beer, a 5-ounce glass of wine, and a 1.5-ounce shot of liquor all contain the same amount of alcohol (0.5 ounce) and therefore have an identical effect on the drinker (see Figure 14.2). The three forms of alcohol have the same potential for intoxication and addiction.

RATE OF CONSUMPTION   The rate of drinking affects BAC due to a constant rate of alcohol metabolism or elimination by the body. Metabolism of alcohol occurs in the liver. The liver can process about 0.5 ounce (one drink) of alcohol every 1 to 1.5 hours. Because the body metabolizes alcohol at this constant rate, ingesting alcohol at a rate higher than the rate of elimination results in a cumulative effect of increasing BAC.

THE EFFECT OF FOOD   The absorption of alcohol is slowed if the stomach contains food. The major reason for this is that alcohol is absorbed most efficiently in the small intestine. The presence of food in the stomach keeps the alcohol from reaching the small intestine. The pyloric valve at the bottom of the stomach remains closed to allow for the digestion of the food in the stomach. Alcohol will still be absorbed through the stomach, but at a much slower rate.

Another factor that significantly influences BAC is body weight. In general, the less you weigh, the more you will be affected by a given amount of alcohol. This is because smaller people have less blood volume than larger people and, therefore, less blood in which to distribute the alcohol. In addition to body weight, body composition also affects the distribution of alcohol. Since alcohol dissolves much more freely in water, a well-muscled individual will be less affected than someone with a higher percentage of fat because fatty tissue does not contain as much water as muscle tissue.

Immediate Effects of Alcohol

The effects of any drug vary from person to person. The immediate effects of alcohol depend on how much you drink, whether you are used to drinking, your mood, and many other factors such as your weight, sex, and general health status.

Alcohol is considered a **depressant**. Depressants are drugs that produce a slowing of mental and physical activities. When alcohol is absorbed into the circulatory system, its effects are distributed throughout the body. The brain is remarkably sensitive to the effects of alcohol. Alcohol acts on the nerve cells deep in the brain, causing a suppressing effect on the central nervous system. The centers that control cognition, thought, judgment, and speech are depressed with the consumption of one or two drinks. As the blood alcohol concentration increases, depression occurs in the respiratory and spinal cord reflexes. An important correlation exists between the BAC and mental and physical behavior (**FIGURE 14.4**). Five drinks consumed in 2 hours may raise the blood alcohol concentration to 0.10 percent, high enough to be considered legally intoxicated in every state. Signs and symptoms of alcohol use and intoxication include irritability, euphoria, depression, loss of consciousness, impaired short-term memory, inappropriate or violent behavior, loss of balance, unsteady gait, and decreased functioning of the cardiorespiratory system.

> **Depressant** A drug that produces a slowing of mental and physical activities.

ALCOHOL, MEMORY, AND LEARNING   Alcohol inhibits a part of your brain called the hippocampus. This region of the brain is vital to the formation of new memories. If you have alcohol in your system while you are in class or studying, you are less likely to store information in your memory (White, 2003). Learning and storing memories are complex processes. You are working hard to turn the information you have learned into memories, even after you have stopped thinking about it. Drinking after spending a day in the library will likely negate your hard work.

ALCOHOL AND SLEEP   Sleep is as important for our health as diet and exercise. The average adult needs 8 hours of sleep each night. Yet, most Americans sleep less than 7 hours a night. In fact, one in three adults sleeps 6 or fewer hours each night during the workweek. As a result, many individuals are living with sleep deficits. As our sleep deficit increases, our health and safety decline proportionally. Sleep deprivation causes decreased mental function, reduced reaction time, increased irritability, and hormonal and metabolic changes that mimic the effects of aging. These problems, in turn, can cause driving accidents and on-the-job

FIGURE 14.4 Blood Alcohol Concentration and Physical and Mental Balance.

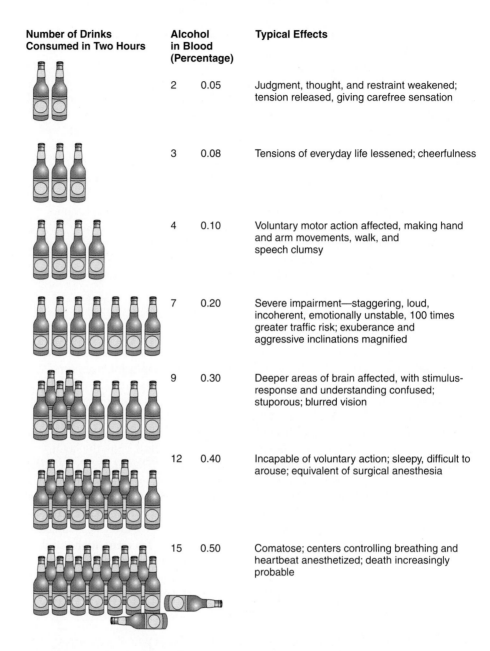

Number of Drinks Consumed in Two Hours	Alcohol in Blood (Percentage)	Typical Effects
2	0.05	Judgment, thought, and restraint weakened; tension released, giving carefree sensation
3	0.08	Tensions of everyday life lessened; cheerfulness
4	0.10	Voluntary motor action affected, making hand and arm movements, walk, and speech clumsy
7	0.20	Severe impairment—staggering, loud, incoherent, emotionally unstable, 100 times greater traffic risk; exuberance and aggressive inclinations magnified
9	0.30	Deeper areas of brain affected, with stimulus-response and understanding confused; stuporous; blurred vision
12	0.40	Incapable of voluntary action; sleepy, difficult to arouse; equivalent of surgical anesthesia
15	0.50	Comatose; centers controlling breathing and heartbeat anesthetized; death increasingly probable

injuries as a result of human error directly related to fatigue. A few simple lifestyle changes can often ensure better sleeping habits. Most important is getting 8 hours of uninterrupted sleep every night. To help with this, avoid drinking alcohol and caffeinated beverages in the evening. Alcohol consumed within 6 hours of sleep can lead to disruption of valuable rapid eye movement (REM) sleep and often leaves one feeling fatigued and irritable the next morning.

ALCOHOL AND SEXUAL FUNCTION Despite the fact that, at low doses, alcohol often has a stimulating effect and may help people unwind and socialize, alcohol can have a devastating effect on sexual performance and response. Dehydration from alcohol use leads to less lubrication in the vaginal canal, which increases the potential for painful intercourse and condom breakage. Men are not able to control premature ejaculations when consuming even small amounts of alcohol, and mod-

TABLE 14.9	Symptoms of Alcohol Poisoning

Binge drinking may result in an overdose of alcohol, or alcohol poisoning—a medical emergency that requires immediate attention. It's sometimes hard to tell if someone has only "passed out" or is in serious medical danger. Here are some symptoms of alcohol poisoning:

- Does not respond to being talked to or shouted at
- Does not respond to being pinched, prodded, or poked
- Cannot stand up
- Will not wake up
- Slow, labored, or abnormal breathing
- Skin has a purplish color
- Skin feels clammy
- Rapid pulse rate
- Irregular heart rhythm
- Lowered blood pressure

erate amounts of alcohol result in fewer or no orgasms, a decreased quality of orgasms, difficulty in forming and maintaining erections, and uncertain orgasms.

ALCOHOL POISONING The dangerous effects of alcohol use can be seen in people who consume large amounts of alcohol relatively quickly. College students frequently engage in this type of drinking behavior, usually in the form of binge drinking. The challenge to drink to your personal limit has become a celebrated observance of college life. In one of the most extensive reports on college drinking, it was found that the majority (52 percent) of students drink "to get drunk" (Wechsler et al., 2002). Many college students see being drunk as a primary way of socializing.

Drinking to intoxication may result in *alcohol poisoning*, which is a medical emergency that requires immediate attention. Experts estimate that excessive drinking is involved in thousands of student deaths annually. Deadly consequences from alcohol poisoning are usually the result of central nervous system and respiratory depression, or of choking to death on vomit after an alcohol overdose. Symptoms of alcohol poisoning are listed in TABLE 14.9 . People who have overdosed on alcohol are unable to help themselves, so it is up to their companions to get assistance. Call for medical attention immediately. Unfortunately, there are no hard and fast rules on how many drinks will result in alcohol poisoning. Generally, a drinker in alcohol poisoning will have a BAC that exceeds 0.25 percent.

UNINTENTIONAL INJURIES More than 40 percent of all automobile-related deaths (the leading cause of unintentional death in the United States) are related to alcohol. Even at low blood alcohol concentrations, alcohol impairs your judgment and dulls your reflexes. If you weigh 140 pounds, just two drinks are enough to increase your chances of having a driving accident. You should never operate any type of machinery if you have had alcohol.

Long-Term Effects of Alcohol

Heavy drinking over many years has major toxic effects on the liver, heart, brain, stomach, intestines, and pancreas. These effects increase the risk for developing a number of chronic diseases,

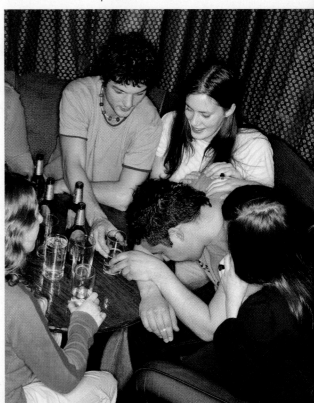

College students have notably high rates of drinking compared with the general population and therefore are at higher risk for alcohol-related problems.

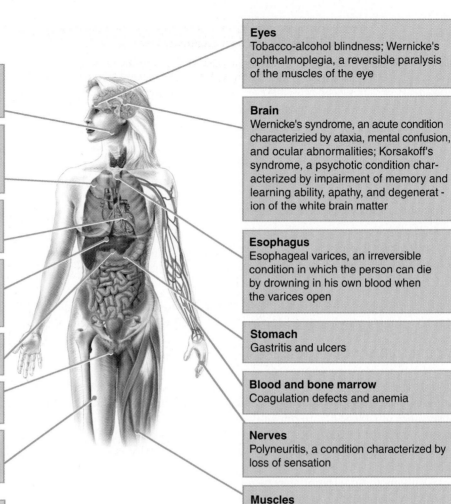

Pharynx
Cancer of the pharynx is increased tenfold for drinkers who smoke

Lungs
Lowered resistance is thought to lead to greater incidence of tuberculosis, pneumonia, and emphysema

Heart
Alcoholic cardiomyopathy, a heart condition

Liver
An acute enlargement of the liver, which is reversible, as well as irreversible cirrhosis of the liver

Pancreas
Acute and chronic pancreatitis

Rectum
Hemorrhoids

Osteoporosis
Heavy drinking contributes to bone loss, especially in older women

Testes
Atrophy of the testes

Eyes
Tobacco-alcohol blindness; Wernicke's ophthalmoplegia, a reversible paralysis of the muscles of the eye

Brain
Wernicke's syndrome, an acute condition characterizied by ataxia, mental confusion, and ocular abnormalities; Korsakoff's syndrome, a psychotic condition characterized by impairment of memory and learning ability, apathy, and degeneration of the white brain matter

Esophagus
Esophageal varices, an irreversible condition in which the person can die by drowning in his own blood when the varices open

Stomach
Gastritis and ulcers

Blood and bone marrow
Coagulation defects and anemia

Nerves
Polyneuritis, a condition characterized by loss of sensation

Muscles
Alcoholic myopathy, a condition resulting in painful muscle contractions

FIGURE 14.5 **Long-Term Effects of Alcohol Use.** Because excess alcohol reaches all parts of the body, it causes a wide array of physical problems.

including liver disease and cirrhosis, cardiomyopathy and stroke, permanent brain damage, ulcers, pancreas inflammation, and certain forms of cancer (USDHHS, 2000) (**FIGURE 14.5**).

Alcohol and Physical Activity

There are some people who believe that physical activity and exercise will offset any detrimental effects of alcohol use. Although moderate drinking the night before physical activity does no real harm, it may limit in a number of ways how well you are able to perform the next day.

Alcohol has various acute and chronic metabolic and physiological effects. You need energy to work out, but the calories from alcohol are unique in that they cannot be stored in the muscles as energy; claims that alcohol provides substantial carbohydrates or energy are false. Alcohol is also a diuretic (it stimulates the production of urine). This increase in urination leads to dehydration and the loss of valuable electrolytes, such as magnesium, calcium, and potassium. These diuretic effects severely impair muscle contraction.

Drinking alcohol the day before or after a workout can also impede one's workout performance. Alcohol depletes an important chemical called human growth hormone (HGH). HGH is part of the muscle-building and repair process, and is the body's way of saying that muscle needs to grow. Because of its effects on sleep patterns, alcohol can decrease sleep-related HGH release by as much as 70 percent. Therefore, drinking before or after a workout essentially cancels out most of one's hard work.

Tobacco Use: An Enduring Health Threat

Although the United States has made significant progress in reducing the number of adult smokers over the last couple of decades, people are still not giving up the habit quickly enough for the country to meet its health goals. Since the U.S. surgeon general's report in the 1960s about smoking and heart disease, cancer, chronic lower respiratory disease, and other health problems, the nation's smoking rate has fallen dramatically. In the mid-1960s, male smoker rates were well above 50 percent, and approximately one in three women (33 percent) smoked. Currently, only one in five adults (20.9 percent) smoke cigarettes (males, 23 percent; females, 18 percent) (Centers for Disease Control and Prevention [CDC], 2005). Although this progress is outstanding, the United States still has a way to go to reach the *Healthy People 2010* goal of reducing smoking to fewer than one in eight adults or 12 percent.

Tobacco is still the number one cause of preventable death in the United States. Smoking damages nearly every organ in the body. Annually, approximately 438,000 Americans die as a result of diseases caused by or made worse by smoking, including coronary heart disease (see Chapter 5), lung cancer and at least nine other cancers (see Chapter 6), chronic respiratory disease, and stroke (FIGURE 14.6).

Most smokers have a general sense that cigarette smoking is harmful to their health but have difficulty understanding the magnitude of the risk when it comes to the myriad of diseases with which smoking is associated. For many of these people it is important to understand that quitting has an almost immediate impact on a smoker's health. Within minutes, blood pressure and heart rate return to normal.

Cigarette smoking is the most preventable cause of premature death in the United States.

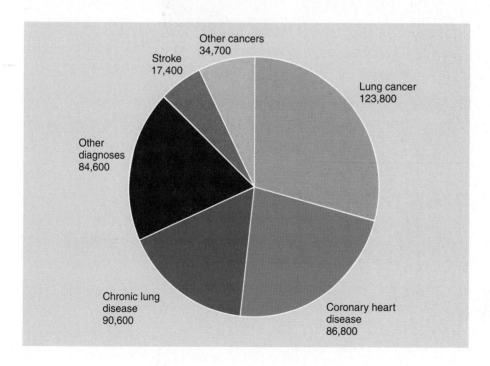

FIGURE 14.6 **About 438,000 Annual Deaths Attributable to Cigarette Smoking Each Year in the United States.** SOURCE: Centers for Disease Control and Prevention. (2005). *Morbidity and Mortality Weekly Report.* 54(25):625–628.

Other cancers
34,700

Stroke
17,400

Lung cancer
123,800

Other diagnoses
84,600

Chronic lung disease
90,600

Coronary heart disease
86,800

After a few hours, harmful levels of carbon monoxide drop and beneficial levels of oxygen in the blood improve. Within a few weeks or months, respiratory lung function and shortness of breath improve. Over the course of a few years, former smokers can expect to reduce their risk of coronary heart disease, stroke, and cancer.

But cigarette smoking is a tough habit to beat because it is not just a habit but a full-blown addiction to the psychoactive drug **nicotine** (see Figure 14.1). In most cases, the decision to start smoking cigarettes is not made by an adult, but rather by a teenager or preteen. Most adult smokers start smoking before reaching the age of 19 (**FIGURE 14.7**). Currently one in five high school students of all ages (22 percent) are smokers (CDC, 2004). The good news is that recent trends indicate a reduction in the daily use by eighth, tenth, and twelfth graders (**FIGURE 14.8**).

Smoking is particularly dangerous for teenagers because shortly after initiating the behavior, regular use and dependency can develop. This dependence on smok-

Nicotine A dynamic psychoactive stimulant.

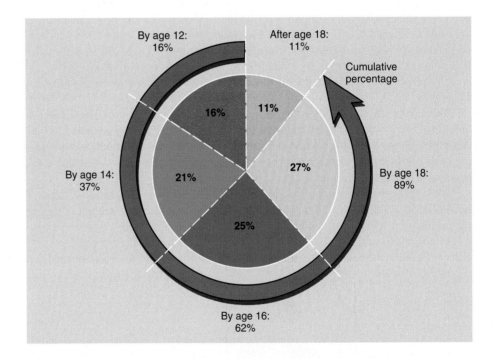

FIGURE 14.7 **Age at Which Adults Say They Started Smoking.** Most smokers started this habit when they were in their teens or preteens. SOURCE: Alters, S., & Schiff, W. (2003). *Essential Concepts for Healthy Living*, 3rd ed. Boston: Jones and Bartlett, 207.

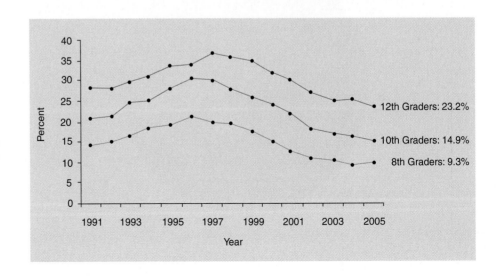

FIGURE 14.8 **Cigarettes: Trends in Daily Use for Eighth, Tenth, and Twelfth Graders, 1990 to 2005.** SOURCE: Johnston, L., O'Malley, P., Bachman, J., & Schulenberg, J. (2005). *The future national results on adolescent drug use: Overview of key findings, 2004.* Bethesda, MD: National Institutes of Health, National Institute on Drug Abuse.

ing can occur in a relatively short time: nicotine addiction can start within a few days of smoking and after just a few cigarettes. Most teenagers believe they will not become dependent or addicted—that they will be able to stop smoking whenever they wish. Their continuation of smoking behavior into adulthood is maintained by a variety of psychological and physiological mechanisms, including familiarity with the act and the events in which it occurs, as well as addiction to nicotine.

The younger a person starts smoking, the more that person will smoke and the longer he or she will do it, all of which leads to greater impairment. Smoking cigarettes doesn't do any part of the body any good, at any time, under any conditions. Although all organs and tissues can be damaged by the toxic chemicals present in cigarette smoke, the developing bodies of teenagers are at particular risk for chemical damage (TABLE 14.10).

Over the past couple of decades, nonsmokers have become increasingly aware that inhaling tobacco smoke from another person's cigarette, cigar, or pipe (secondhand smoke) can pose serious health risks. The process of smoking a cigarette produces three different types of tobacco smoke. The first is mainstream smoke, the smoke directly inhaled through the burning cigarette by the smoker. Second is exhaled mainstream smoke, the smoke breathed out by the smoker from his or her lungs. The composition of mainstream and exhaled mainstream smoke is likely to differ, with some of the compounds in smoke being retained by the smoker or otherwise altered by the process. Third is sidestream smoke, the smoke that drifts from the end of the lit cigarette. **Secondhand smoke**, or environmental tobacco smoke (ETS), consists of exhaled mainstream smoke and sidestream smoke. Prolonged and repeated exposure to secondhand smoke means you are more likely to develop secondhand smoke diseases, including lung cancer, coronary heart disease, asthma, reduced lung function, bronchitis, and pneumonia.

Secondhand smoke Exhaled mainstream smoke and sidestream smoke from another person's cigarette, cigar, or pipe. Also known as environmental tobacco smoke (ETS).

TABLE 14.10	Facts on Youth Smoking, Health, and Performance

Among young people, the short-term health effects of smoking include damage to the respiratory system, addiction to nicotine, and the associated risk of other drug use. Long-term health consequences of youth smoking are reinforced by the fact that most young people who smoke regularly continue to smoke throughout adulthood.* (p. 15)

Smoking hurts young people's physical fitness in terms of both performance and endurance—even among young people trained in competitive running.* (p. 28)

Smoking among youth can hamper the rate of lung growth and the level of maximum lung function.* (p. 17)

The resting heart rates of young adult smokers are two to three beats per minute faster than those of nonsmokers.* (p. 28)

Among young people, regular smoking is responsible for cough and increased frequency and severity of respiratory illnesses.* (p. 9)

The younger people start smoking cigarettes, the more likely they are to become strongly addicted to nicotine.* (p. 9)

Teens who smoke are three times more likely than nonsmokers to use alcohol, 8 times more likely to use marijuana, and 22 times

more likely to use cocaine. Smoking is associated with a host of other risky behaviors such as fighting and engaging in unprotected sex.* (pp. 36, 104)

Smoking is associated with poor overall health and a variety of short-term adverse health effects in young people and may also be a marker for underlying mental health problems, such as depression, among adolescents. High school seniors who are regular smokers and began smoking by grade nine are

- 2.4 times more likely than their nonsmoking peers to report poorer overall health

- 2.4 to 2.7 times more likely to report cough with phlegm or blood, shortness of breath when not exercising, and wheezing or gasping

- 3.0 times more likely to have seen a doctor or other health professional for an emotional or psychological complaint.

(Arday DR, Giovino GA, Schulman J, Nelson DE, Mowery P, Samet JM. Cigarette smoking and self-reported health problems among US high school seniors, 1982–1989. *Am J of Health Promotion*, 1995;10(2):111–116.)

*CDC. (1994). Preventing tobacco use among oung people—a report of the surgeon general.

SOURCE: Centers for Disease Control and Prevention. CDC's tips on youth smoking, health, and performance. Online: http://www.cdc.gov/tobacco/research_data/youth/ythsprt.htm.

Other forms of tobacco use are not safe alternatives to smoking cigarettes. Many people believe that cigar smoking is a safe choice. Large cigars, cigarillos, and little cigars are the three major types of cigars sold in the United States (Maxwell, 2004). Dangerously, some cigar manufacturers claim (falsely) that cigar smokers experience little or no increased disease risk. These beliefs, along with the growing status symbolism of cigars, have contributed to a trend toward greater cigar use over the past decade. The number of new cigar smokers more than doubled in the past decade (SAMHSA, 2004). Cigars contain the same toxic and carcinogenic compounds found in cigarettes and are not a safe alternative to cigarettes (Baker et al., 2000).

The smallest group of tobacco consumers uses smokeless tobacco ("spit" tobacco) in the form of snuff or chewing tobacco. Nationally, an estimated 3 percent of adults are current smokeless tobacco users (SAMHSA, 2005). Smokeless tobacco use is much higher among men (6 percent) than women (0.3 percent). Smokeless tobacco causes a number of severe health problems, including cancer of the month, leukoplakia, inflammation of the gums, heart disease, and tooth loss.

Few behaviors have as many—and as harmful—effects upon a person's health as tobacco use. We will now examine the composition of tobacco as a drug, the damaging effects of tobacco on users, why it is habit forming, and how this habit can be defeated.

Constituents of Tobacco Smoke

Tobacco comes from the dried leaves of the native American tobacco plant *Nicotiana tabacum*. Tobacco, in its unprocessed form, contains a number of hazardous chemicals that become increasingly dangerous as it is processed into cigarettes, cigars, or smokeless tobacco forms. The smoke from burning tobacco is the most hazardous to our health. Smoke from burning tobacco consists of a mixture of approximately 4000 chemical substances that are dangerous to living tissue. Within this immense amount of harmful matter, scientists have identified more than 40 chemicals in cigarette smoke that cause cancer. Tobacco smoke is primarily composed of droplets of **tars**, which form 40 percent of the smoke; nicotine, a drug that is poisonous and has addicting qualities; and a dozen gases, including **carbon monoxide**.

TARS   Tars are the yellowish-brown solid, sticky materials that are inhaled as part of tobacco smoke. A person who smokes a pack of cigarettes a day will accumulate about 4 ounces of tar in his or her lungs annually. Many tars are deposited on the bronchi, contributing to chronic bronchitis and smoker's cough. Research has shown tobacco tars to be *carcinogenic*, or cancer causing (see Chapter 6). Other chemicals in tobacco tars are co-carcinogens, or stimulate the growth of cancer when combined with other carcinogens.

NICOTINE   Nicotine is a dynamic psychoactive stimulant. **Stimulants** are drugs that increase central nervous system activity. Nicotine is quickly absorbed into the blood, immediately affecting the brain and the spinal cord as well as the peripheral central nervous system. Nicotine causes a short-term increase in heart rate and blood pressure, and a narrowing or constricting of the peripheral blood vessels and bronchial airways, all of which contribute to an increased workload on the heart.

Nicotine is a powerfully addictive drug (see Figure 14.1). This means that the use of nicotine causes changes in the brain that force people to want to use more of the drug. The pharmacological and behavioral processes that reinforce tobacco addiction are similar to those for other addictive drugs. These characteristics include physical dependence and tolerance for the drug, highly controlled or com-

Tars The yellowish-brown solid, sticky materials that are inhaled as part of tobacco smoke.

Carbon monoxide One of the most abundant and poisonous gases in cigarette smoke.

Stimulants Drugs that increase central nervous system activity.

pulsive use, use of the drug to restore psychoactive or physical effects, and predictable withdrawal symptoms when attempts are made to quit (APA, 2000).

CARBON MONOXIDE   Carbon monoxide (CO) is one of the most abundant and poisonous gases in cigarette smoke. Carbon monoxide is an odorless, tasteless, and colorless gas that impairs oxygen transportation to body tissues by competing with oxygen molecules for attachment to the red blood cells. Red blood cells are responsible for carrying oxygen from the lungs to the tissues. Carbon monoxide actually has far greater attachment properties when it comes to binding with the red blood cells than does oxygen. As a result, the capacity of the blood to carry oxygen to the brain, heart, and muscles is diminished. Carbon monoxide also leads to damage of the inner walls of the arteries, a destruction that contributes to plaque buildup and arteriosclerosis (see Chapter 5).

Cigar Smoking

Americans consume over 5 billion cigars annually, compared with over 400 billion cigarettes annually. While cigarette sales have shown a recent decline, cigar sales are on the increase. This upward trend in cigar use has become a concern for many in public health. All available scientific evidence indicates that the magnitude of risk from cigar smoke is similar to that for cigarette smoke (Baker et al., 2000). The smoke from both cigars and cigarettes results largely from incomplete combustion of tobacco, and has the same toxic and carcinogenic constituents. This scientific evidence related to cigar smoking, along with the common misperception that cigar smoking may not be as dangerous as cigarette smoking, has led to the requirement that cigars sold in the United States carry health warnings. The 2000 agreement orders that cigar boxes, smaller packages, and individual cigars be labeled with one of the five different Surgeon General statements (TABLE 14.11). The warnings for cigars and cigar products go beyond those for cigarettes. They require a more prominent package display and include mention of the dangers of secondhand smoke. In truth, cigar smoking is bad for your health and is not a safe alternative to cigarettes.

TABLE 14.11   **Warning Labels on Cigar Products**

On June 26, 2000, the FTC announced a settlement with seven of the largest U.S. cigar companies requiring health warnings on cigar products. Health warnings must appear on the principal display panel to ensure warnings are easily seen. Each of the five required warnings must be displayed an equal number of times. The agreement also calls for warnings to be placed on various types of advertising, such as magazines and other periodicals, point-of-purchase displays, and catalogs.

Every cigar package and advertisement will require the following warnings on a rotating basis:

SURGEON GENERAL'S WARNING: Cigar Smoking Can Cause Cancers of the Mouth and Throat, Even If You Do Not Inhale.

SURGEON GENERAL'S WARNING: Cigar Smoking Can Cause Lung Cancer and Heart Disease.

SURGEON GENERAL'S WARNING: Tobacco Use Increases the Risk of Infertility, Stillbirth and Low Birth Weight.

SURGEON GENERAL'S WARNING: Cigars Are Not a Safe Alternative to Cigarettes.

SURGEON GENERAL'S WARNING: Tobacco Smoke Increases the Risk of Lung Cancer and Heart Disease, Even in Nonsmokers.

SOURCE: Centers for Disease Control and Prevention, Tobacco Information and Prevention Source. Online: http://www.cdc.gov/tobacco/sgr/sgr_2000/factsheets/factsheet_labels.htm.

Smoking and Physical Activity

Many studies have shown that smoking before or during exercise decreases performance, due to a number of factors. The undesirable effects of carbon monoxide become especially obvious during physical activity. Muscles require more oxygen during physical activity, but acquire less from the red blood cells because carbon monoxide has reduced the amount of oxygen the blood can carry. Consequently, muscles tire more quickly.

Smoking also puts an extra burden on the heart and circulatory system. Combined with the effects of decreased oxygen, nicotine's constricting effects on the blood vessels require the heart to work harder to deliver the oxygen. Breathing also becomes hindered as the lungs get irritated and accumulate more mucus from smoking, leading to increased airway resistance. Extra effort to get air in and out of the lungs occurs if a cigarette is smoked within an hour of physical activity. During heavy physical activity, the respiratory muscles are required to work twice as hard for chronic smokers as for nonsmokers.

Quitting Smoking

Quitting smoking is the single most important step that smokers can take to enhance the length and quality of their life (USDHHS, 2000). Moreover, the health benefits and physical activity benefits of quitting smoking are immediate and substantial for all smokers regardless of age, gender, disease state, or smoking history (TABLE 14.12).

Most people who have quit smoking state that they have done it on their own, without the help of a formal program. Most smokers quit a number of times before

TABLE 14.12	**Immediate and Long-Term Health Benefits of Stopping Smoking**

Within 20 minutes after you smoke that last cigarette, your body begins a series of changes that continue for years.

20 Minutes After Quitting
Your heart rate drops.

12 Hours After Quitting
Carbon monoxide level in your blood drops to normal.

2 Weeks to 3 Months After Quitting
Your heart attack risk begins to drop.
Your lung function begins to improve.

1 to 9 Months After Quitting
Your coughing and shortness of breath decrease.

1 Year After Quitting
Your added risk of coronary heart disease is half that of a smoker's.

5 Years After Quitting
Your stroke risk is reduced to that of a nonsmoker's 5–15 years after quitting.

10 Years After Quitting
Your lung cancer death rate is about half that of a smoker's.
Your risk of cancers of the mouth, throat, esophagus, bladder, kidney, and pancreas decreases.

15 Years After Quitting
Your risk of coronary heart disease is back to that of a nonsmoker's.

SOURCE: Centers for Disease Control and Prevention, Tobacco Information and Prevention Source. Online: http://www.cdc.gov/tobacco/sgr/sgr_2004/posters/20mins.htm.

TABLE 14.13 Quit Tips

1. Don't smoke any number or any kind of cigarette. Smoking even a few cigarettes a day can hurt your health. If you try to smoke fewer cigarettes, but do not stop completely, soon you'll be smoking the same amount again.

   Smoking "low-tar, low-nicotine" cigarettes usually does little good, either. Because nicotine is so addictive, if you switch to lower-nicotine brands you'll likely just puff harder, longer, and more often on each cigarette. The only safe choice is to quit completely.

2. Write down why you want to quit. Do you want

   to feel in control of you life?

   to have better health?

   to set a good example for your children?

   to protect your family from breathing other people's smoke?

   Really wanting to quit smoking is very important to how much success you will have in quitting. Smokers who live after a heart attack are the most likely to quit for good. They're very motivated. Find a reason for quitting before you have no choice.

3. Know that it will take effort to quit smoking. Nicotine is habit forming. Half of the battle in quitting is knowing you need to quit. This knowledge will help you be more able to deal with the symptoms of withdrawal that can occur, such as bad moods and really wanting to smoke. There are many ways smokers quit, including using nicotine replacement products (gum and patches), but there is no easy way. Nearly all smokers have some feelings of nicotine withdrawal when they try to quit. Give yourself a month to get over these feelings. Take quitting one day at a time, even one minute at a time—whatever you need to succeed.

4. Half of all adult smokers have quit, so you can, too. That's the good news. There are millions of people alive today who have learned to face life without a cigarette. For staying healthy, quitting smoking is the best step you can take.

SOURCE: Centers for Disease Control and Prevention, Tobacco Information and Prevention Source (TIPS). Quit tips. Online: http://www.cdc.gov/tobacco/quit/quittip.htm.

---

achieving long-term abstinence. If you are a present smoker who wants to quit, don't let another day go by (TABLE 14.13). Get help if you need it. Many groups offer programs and free materials to help smokers quit for good (TABLE 14.14). Your college or university health center may also be a good source for help and support.

STAYING TRIM AFTER QUITTING   Most people who quit smoking are concerned about gaining weight. Approximately four of every five people gain weight after

TABLE 14.14 National Groups Are Available to Help You Quit Smoking

Get help if you need it. Many groups offer written materials, programs, and advice to help smokers quit for good. The following national groups have toll-free telephone numbers for information and resources:

Agency for Health Care Policy and Research, Clinical Practice Guidelines on Smoking Cessation, Instant Fax 301-594-2800 [Press 1]; or call 1-800-358-9295 for physician materials and a "You Can Quit Smoking" consumer guide.

American Cancer Society, 1-800-ACS-2345

American Heart Association, 1-800-AHA-USA1

American Lung Association, 1-800-LUNG-USA

Office on Smoking and Health, 1-800-CDC-1311

National Cancer Institute, 1-800-4-CANCER

quitting smoking, with the average weight gain being about 5 pounds. Changes in eating habits and in the body's processing of food leads to this weight gain.

Smoking suppresses taste-bud awareness and reduces the taste value of food. When people quit smoking they notice an improvement in the taste of food, leading to selection of higher portions and increased helpings. Increasing food consumption may also be an alternate way to deal with stress or a behavioral substitute for the oral satisfaction of smoking.

Some researchers believe that the absence of nicotine influences weight gain. First, nicotine causes the liver to release glycogen, raising the blood-sugar level and making the smoker feel satiated; absence of nicotine may factor into ex-smokers' cravings for high-sugar and high-calorie foods. Second, nicotine increases the body's basic metabolic rate, making it easier for the body to expend calories and contributing to a lower body weight.

Research provides compelling evidence that people who participate in an intensive physical activity program are more likely to succeed at quitting smoking and less likely to gain weight than people who did not include physical activity as part of their cessation strategy (Marcus, 1999). This is because many people use cigarettes to help them manage their weight, moods, and stress. Clearly, physical activity is a more healthy way to deal with each of these concerns. Moreover, the health benefits derived from avoiding any tobacco use, and the subsequent risk of developing a number of debilitating chronic diseases, overwhelmingly outweigh any small weight gain.

Smokeless Tobacco

Smokeless tobacco forms include snuff and chewing tobacco. Snuff is a powdered tobacco that is generally put between the lower lip and gum. It can also be inhaled through the nose. Chewing tobacco is shredded or loose-leaf tobacco, treated with moisturizing and flavoring agents that is pressed into *plugs* and then placed inside the cheek. Both tobacco products stimulate saliva production, requiring users to spit frequently to clear the mouth of excess saliva and any tobacco that has lost its flavor. Some people refer to smokeless tobacco as "spit tobacco."

Smokeless tobacco contains over 2000 chemicals, many of which are potent carcinogens that lead directly to cancer. The strongest association is between smokeless tobacco and oral cancer. Oral cancer risk among regular smokeless tobacco users is *up to fifty times* that of nonusers. The use of smokeless tobacco products leads to nicotine dependence and addiction; the magnitude of nicotine exposure, and its absorption, distribution, and elimination, is similar to smoking cigarettes. Other health effects include gum recession, increased tooth decay, tooth discoloration, bad breath, and a decreased sense of taste, which leads to unhealthy eating habits.

Physical Activity and Health Connection

To develop a high level of physical activity and health in your life, you must address the issue of substance use. We live in a society that believes that some substance use is acceptable. This notion doesn't necessarily complement a physically active or healthy lifestyle. As you increased your understanding of the physical and psychological consequences of alcohol use and cigarette smoking, you came to better understand the many negative health consequences related to their use. Your path to being physically active can be significantly impaired by the use of drugs.

Before using any drug, remember that you have choices. By making responsible choices that support your goal of being physically active and healthy, you will not only enhance your present quality of life but also your future.

concept connections

1. **College students face a conscious choice on whether to drink alcohol, smoke cigarettes, or use other psychoactive drugs while they pursue their degree.** What they choose to do is related to a host of factors, including wanting to have a good time, to fit in or feel more comfortable socially and be accepted, to regulate moods and feelings, to forget about problems or numb out, to relieve emotional or physical pain, or to have a mind-altering experience. However, the use of many psychoactive drugs often creates the opposite effect. The major problem with psychoactive drugs is that when people take them, they focus on the immediate desired mental and emotional effects and ignore the potentially damaging mental and physical side effects that can occur.

2. **Chronic substance use can disrupt the body's normal balance, or homeostasis.** The person who continues to use a drug moves to a level of risk one step beyond, because each exposure carries with it the possibility that the body's chemical pathways will change to adapt to repeated exposure to the drug.

3. **Making wise substance use decisions is important.** The choices of which drug to use, how much, and how long are all important individual decisions and should not be made thoughtlessly. It is important for an individual to practice decision-making skills relating to potential substance use so that a well-prepared response is made.

4. **Alcohol misuse and abuse is one of the most significant health-related drug problems in the United States.** The consequences of excessive and underage drinking affect virtually all college students, campuses, and college communities, whether they choose to drink or not.

5. **Cigarette smoking is the most preventable cause of premature death in the United States.** Smoking damages nearly every organ in the body. Annually, approximately 438,000 Americans die as a result of diseases caused by or made worse by smoking, including coronary heart disease, lung cancer and at least nine other cancers, chronic respiratory disease, and stroke.

Terms

Drug, 300
Substance use, 300
Drug therapeutics, 300
Substance misuse, 300
Substance abuse, 302
Psychoactive drug, 302
Substance dependence, 302
Tolerance, 304
Psychological dependence, 305

Physical dependence, 305
Withdrawal illness, 306
Pharmacology, 306
Social drinking, 307
Moderate drinking, 308
Binge drinking, 310
Problem drinking, 310
Ethyl alcohol, 311

Blood alcohol concentration
  (BAC), 313
Depressant, 315
Nicotine, 320
Secondhand smoke, 321
Tars, 322
Carbon monoxide, 322
Stimulants, 322

•••• making the connection ••••••••••••••••••••••••••••••

Jim makes an appointment with both the college's Counseling and Psychological Services and Health Education Center to speak with professionals and obtain resources for his friend Bill. After learning the best way to approach Bill, Jim sits down Bill and discusses his concerns about Bill's drinking with him and convinces him to make an appointment with a counselor.

Critical Thinking

1. "I really don't like the taste of liquor that much, but after the first couple of shots, it doesn't taste all that bad. I know I shouldn't drink and I always have a hangover the next day but, hey, college is stressful and how else can I deal with the stress of getting the grades to keep my scholarship and making my parents happy?" What's your opinion of this person's attitude? Explain why you agree or disagree. If you disagree, how do you think this person can deal with the stress of getting good grades?

2. College campuses often accept money from companies that sell alcoholic beverages—to support athletic events, for example. By allowing these companies to advertise at campus events, the university makes considerable money to enhance the campus environment and provide quality education. What is your campus's policy on allowing alcohol companies to advertise or sponsor events on campus? Do you agree or disagree with this policy?

3. Purchase a popular magazine and count the number of cigarette ads in the issue. In reviewing each of the ads, respond to the following questions:
   a. Who is the ad targeting (young people, older adults, women)?
   b. How is the ad appealing to the target audience (fun, sex)?
   c. What does the ad seem to promise if you smoke their brand of cigarette?

References

American Psychological Association. (2000). *Diagnostic and Statistical Manual of Mental Disorders*, 4th ed., text revision. Washington, DC: Author.

Baker, F., Ainsworth, S.R., Dye, J., Crammer, M.M., Thun, M.J., Hoffman, D., et al. (2000). Health risks associated with cigar smoking. *Journal of the American Medical Association* 284:735–740.

Centers for Disease Control and Prevention. (2004). Cigarette smoking among high school students—United States, 1991–2003. *Morbidity and Mortality Weekly Report* 53(23):499–502.

Centers for Disease Control and Prevention. (2005). Cigarettes smoking among adults—United States, 2004. *Morbidity and Mortality Weekly Report* 54(44):1121–1124.

Ellison, R.C. (2002). Balancing the risks and benefits of moderate drinking. *Annals of the New York Academy of Sciences* 957:1–6.

Engs, R. (2001). *Clean Living Movements: American Cycles of Health Reform*. Westport, CT: Praeger.

Engs, R.C., Diebold, B.A., & Hanson, D.J. (1996). The drinking patterns and problems of a national sample of college students, 1994. *Journal of Alcohol and Drug Education* 41(3):13–33.

Hingson, R., Heeren, T., Zakocs, R.C., Kopstein, A., & Wechsler, H. (2002). Magnitude of alcohol-related mortality and morbidity among U.S. college students ages 18–24. *Journal of Studies on Alcohol* 63(2):136–144.

Hingson, R., et al. (2005). Magnitude of alcohol-related mortality and morbidity among U.S. college students ages 18–24: Changes from 1998 to 2001. *Annual Review of Public Health* 26:259–279.

Knight, J.R., Wechsler, H., Kuo, M., Seibring, M., Weitzman, E.R., & Schuckit, M. (2002). Alcohol abuse and dependence among U.S. college students. *Journal of Studies on Alcohol* 63(3):263–270.

Little, H.J. (2000). Behavioral mechanisms underlying the link between smoking and drinking. *Alcohol Research and Health* 36:24–30.

Marcus, B. (1999). Exercise helps smokers kick the habit. *Archives of Internal Medicine* 159:1169–1171.

Maxwell, J.C. (2004). *Cigar Industry in 2003*. Richmond, VA: The Maxwell Report.

National Institute on Alcohol Abuse and Alcoholism. (2005). A snapshot of annual high-risk college drinking. Online: http://www.collegedrinkingprevention.gov/StatsSummaries/snapshot.aspx.

National Institute on Drug Abuse. (2005). Understanding drug abuse and addiction. Online: http://www.nida.nih.gov/Infofacts/understand.html.

Presley, C.A., Leichliter, M.A., & Meilman, P.W. (1998). *Alcohol and Drugs on American Campuses: A Report to College Presidents. Third in a Series, 1995, 1996, 1997*. Carbondale, IL: Core Institute, Southern Illinois University.

Presley, C.A., Meilman, P.W., & Cashin, J.R. (1996a). *Alcohol and Drugs on American Campuses: Use, Consequences, and Perceptions of the Campus Environment, Vol. IV: 1992–1994*. Carbondale, IL: Core Institute, Southern Illinois University.

Presley, C.A., Meilman, P.W., Cashin, J.R., & Lyerla, R. (1996b). *Alcohol and Drugs on American Campuses: Use, Consequences, and Perceptions of the Campus Environment, Vol. III: 1991–1993*. Carbondale, IL: Core Institute, Southern Illinois University.

Substance Abuse and Mental Health Services Administration. (2004). *Results from 2003 National Survey on Drug Use and Health: National Findings*. Rockville, MD: Substance Abuse and Mental Health Services Administration, Office of Applied Studies. Online: http://www.oas.samhsa.gov/nhsda/2k3nsduh/2k3Results.htm#ch5.

Substance Abuse and Mental Health Services Administration. (2005). *Results from the 2004 National Survey on Drug Use and Health. Detailed Tables*. Rockville, MD: Substance Abuse and Mental Health Services Administration, Office of Applied Studies. Online: http://oas.samhsa.gov/nhsda/2k3tabs/Sect2peTabs1to56.htm#tab2.39b.

United States Department of Health and Human Services. (2000). *Healthy People 2010: Understanding and Improving Health*, 2nd ed. Washington, DC: U.S. Government Printing Office.

United States Department of Health and Human Services & United States Department of Agriculture. (2005). Dietary Guidelines for Americans 2005: Executive Summary. Online: http://www.health.gov/dietaryguidelines/dga2005/document/html/executivesummary.htm.

Wechsler, H., Lee, J. E., Kuo, M., Seibring, M., Nelson, T. F., & Lee, H. (2002). Trends in college binge drinking during a period of increased prevention efforts: Findings from 4 Harvard School of Public Health College Alcohol Study surveys, 1993–2001. *Journal of American College Health* 50:203–217.

Wechsler, H., Moeykens, B., Davenport, A., Castillo, S., & Hansen, J. (1995). The adverse impact of heavy episodic drinkers on other college students. *Journal of Studies on Alcohol* 56(6):628–634.

White, A. (2003). What Happened? Alcohol, Memory Blackouts, and the Brain. *Alcohol Research and Health* 27(2):186–196.

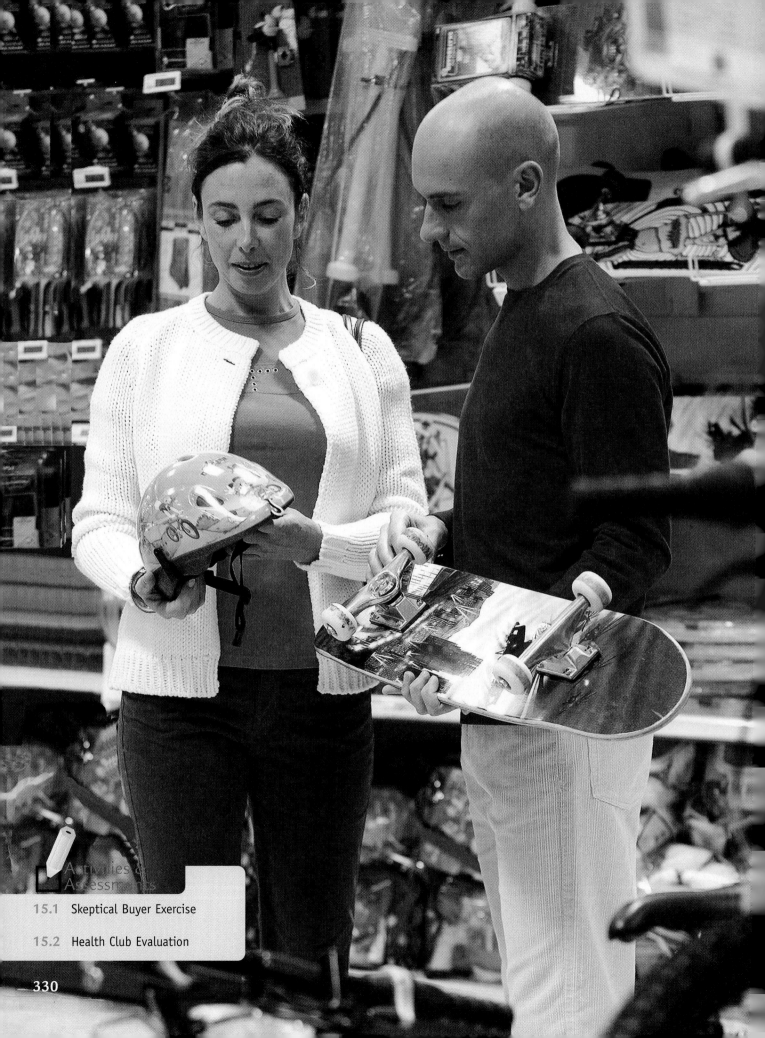

15.1   Skeptical Buyer Exercise

15.2   Health Club Evaluation

Exercise Consumerism

Janet's friend Kathy constantly asks her to try a new diet pill "guaranteed" to make her lose inches overnight. Kathy claims that the pill worked for her and pressures Janet into trying "just one." Janet is a bit skeptical and decides to investigate further. She asks Kathy for the ingredient list from the product and calls a registered dietitian in her town.

concepts

1. To develop a quality physical activity program, you must be a wise consumer of exercise information.

2. The physical activity industry suffers from a wide range of misinformation and fraudulent claims.

3. You need to be aware of some common misconceptions, frauds, and fallacies.

4. Being a critical consumer requires knowing where to turn for valid information.

5. There are several avenues you can take in seeking redress.

http://physicalactivity.jbpub.com

The Web site for this book is a great source for supplementary physical health information for both students and instructors. Visit **http://physicalactivity.jbpub.com** to find a variety of useful tools for learning, thinking, and teaching.

To develop a quality physical activity program, you must be a wise consumer of exercise information.

Introduction

This chapter provides information that will allow you to enhance your skills as an intelligent consumer of exercise information and products. It describes how to identify misinformation and fraud, and how to select the correct exercise equipment, products, and programs. It also provides suggestions on where to turn for factual information and how to seek redress if you think you have been a victim of fraud.

Scope of the Problem

Some people will go to any length, or take any shortcut, in the attempt to gain an edge. This statement is true in sport as well as in marketing. The exercise and fitness industry is rife with misleading advertising and fraudulent claims. Why are misleading products and statements, and even outright fraud, a problem for the consumer? First of all, misleading or fraudulent products make false promises that can lead you to develop a sense of mistrust and frustration. The result could be that you become too skeptical of all products and programs and you may miss out on the effective ones; you might decide to ignore all claims and just do nothing. Misleading claims and fraudulent products frequently turn people off from being physically active. They may also injure people. And finally, they indirectly steal money from legitimate fitness professionals. Money is spent on products that don't work rather than on programs that do work.

Ergogenic aid Any substance or phenomenon that enhances performance.

Ergolytic A substance that has a detrimental effect on performance.

Fraud Conscious promotion of unproven claims for profit.

Some consumers believe that certain products can make them more productive exercisers. These products are referred to as *ergogenic aids*. An **ergogenic aid** is any substance or phenomenon that enhances performance. Not all ergogenic aids are harmful. For example, endurance runners may eat a higher percentage of carbohydrates in the days leading up to a race. Carbo loading acts as an ergogenic aid by storing more fuel in your muscles. On the other hand, many bodybuilders falsely believe that the consumption of large amounts of protein will aid in muscle development. There is no scientific evidence to support the consumption of extra protein to develop larger muscles (Wilmore & Costill, 2004). In fact, excessive intake of protein may lead to kidney and liver dysfunction (Wilmore & Costill, 2004).

Some substances generally thought to be ergogenic might actually be *ergolytic*. Instead of enhancing performance, they actually diminish performance. An **ergolytic** substance is one that has a detrimental effect on performance (Wilmore & Costill, 2004). Alcohol was once thought by many to aid sport performance by calming the nerves, but we now know that alcohol adversely affects central nervous system function, coordination, and balance.

People try a wide variety of products in an attempt to enhance performance.

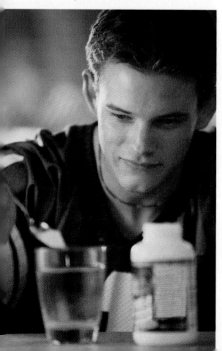

Many substances are used by people trying to gain an edge. If we add up the money spent on ergogenic aids and dietary supplements used by people in the belief that their performance will be enhanced, we would come up with a figure in the billions of dollars (Barrett, 2000). (TABLE 15.1) lists the most commonly used substances.

Fraud, Quackery, and Misinformation

To be an intelligent consumer of physical activity and fitness information, you need to know several terms. **Fraud** is a conscious promotion of unproven claims for profit. Most people hold an image of a fraudulent salesperson as one who sells watches out of a trench coat, or one who pedals snake oil on a shadowy corner. While there are certainly individuals who promote products knowing their claims cannot be true, many people promoting bad products may be unaware of the fraudulent intent of the manufacturer or distributor. Many promoters of fraudulent

TABLE 15.1 Ergogenic Aids and Performance Enhancing Substances

Ergogenic Aid	Purported Use	Effectiveness	Potential Problems
Amino acids	Increases rate of synthesis of muscle mass.	Amino acids are necessary to build and repair muscle tissue; however, taking additional amounts does not speed up this process.	Can get all necessary amino acids in a balanced diet. Much more expensive in powder, drink, or energy bar form.
Amphetamines	Improve alertness and cause weight loss.	Will enhance alertness if taken in reasonable dosage. Increases metabolism while on drug.	Addiction, cardiac arrhythmia, and sudden death are possible. Banned by many sport organizations.
Anabolic androgenic steroids	Decrease body fat, increase muscle mass, make more aggressive, increase strength.	Will do those things when combined with exercise, but with potentially severe negative side effects.	Side effects include testicular atrophy, gynecomastia, increased risk of joint injury, certain forms of cancer, and psychosis. Banned by most sport organizations.
Blood doping	Increase hemoglobin content and enhance oxygen delivery.	Enhances aerobic performance.	Banned by many sport organizations. May increase blood pressure. As with any injectible, risk of AIDS and hepatitis.
Caffeine	Improve alertness and enhance aerobic metabolism.	Some support in the research.	Nervousness. Large dosages banned by many sport organizations.
Chromium	Gain strength and muscle mass.	No evidence to support claims.	Side effects appear minimal. Waste of money since it does not work.
Creatine	Enhance muscle development by increasing stores of creatine phosphate.	Works in some individuals when combined with resistive training. Improves ability to work harder.	Reports of muscle and GI cramping. Does not work for all people.
Diuretics	Weight loss.	Will cause the loss of water weight.	Water weight regained when rehydrated. Doesn't increase fat loss. Dehydration negatively impacts sport performance.
Ephedra	Accelerate weight loss.	Can accelerate weight loss. Metabolic and cardiac stimulator.	Can cause sudden death. Banned by many sport organizations. Was banned by U.S. law, but currently under appeal.
Erythropoietin	Increase red blood cell production.	Apparently improves aerobic exercise performance.	Banned by many sport organizations. May increase blood pressure. As with any injectible, risk of AIDS and hepatitis.
Human growth hormone (Somatotropin)	Increased size, increased muscle mass, increased bone density.	Will do these things.	Acromegaly and hormone imbalance. Cardiomyopathy.
Nasal strips	Improve oxygen delivery.	Does not enhance oxygen delivery during aerobic or anaerobic exercise or during recovery.	No side effects other than spending money on a product that does not work.
Oxygen consumption	Improve oxygen delivery and recovery from exercise.	Does not enhance performance or recovery unless in oxygen-deprived environment (such as mountain climbing or underwater).	No side effects other than spending money on a product that does not work.

The physical activity industry suffers from a wide range of misinformation and fraudulent claims.

Quackery Overpromotion of a product in the field of health.

Misinformation Information that is not factual, but is passed off as being factual.

and misleading products are unwitting victims who themselves have been duped. They then share misinformation and personal experiences with others (Barrett & Jarvis, 2000). An example of fraudulent advertising is the "infrared body composition analyzer," which is discussed later in the chapter. **Quackery** is broadly defined as anything involving overpromotion of a product in the field of health (Barrett, 2000). This definition includes the promotion of questionable ideas as well as questionable products and services, regardless of the sincerity of their promoters (Barrett, 2000). An example of quackery would be the advertisements for "magnetic therapy," also discussed later.

Misinformation involves providing information that is not factual. In some cases, people actually believe that the products they support can produce the outcomes they are advertised to produce. They have been taken in by the marketing claims of a product and wish to share their "knowledge" with others. Friends, relatives, and neighbors who use the products and believe them to be effective typically introduce new customers to the product (Barrett & Jarvis, 2000). In these cases, there is no conscious effort to promote a useless product. Instead, misinformation is dispersed to a wider audience by people who think they know what a product can do. An example of misinformation is the common belief that shark cartilage can prevent cancer.

Common Marketing Techniques

Marketing usually involves an honest attempt to sell a product. However, we must be aware that the primary purpose of marketing is to persuade people to purchase products (Whitehead, 2000). This is true whether the person wants the product or not. There is a difference in the way products are marketed, based on the intent of the manufacturer. In some instances, marketing techniques rely on misinformation, deception, and fraud (Whitehead, 2000).

Those who seek to sell products through misleading ads, deception, or fraudulent practices use several common marketing techniques. Some examples include the misrepresentation of research, the use of testimonials ("It worked for me"), the promotion of unchallenged myths (excessive protein consumption for bigger muscles), and the quick fix (rapid weight loss, fitness is "easy"). Much of deceptive product marketing involves telling people something is bad for them (such as food additives) and selling a substitute, such as "organic" or "natural" food (Whitehead, 2000). Other common tactics can be found in TABLE 15.2.

It is not always easy to spot misleading and fraudulent products or advertising. Marketers often use scientific jargon that can fool people not familiar with the concepts being discussed (Barrett, 2000). Even health professionals sometimes have difficulty separating fact from fiction in fields unrelated to their expertise (Barrett, 2000).

People also rely on personal experience and testimonials in deciding if a product works. If you feel better after having used a product, you usually associate those sensations with the product (Barrett, 2000). However, many ailments resolve themselves, or have symptoms that change frequently. Even serious conditions can have day-to-day variation in intensity (Barrett, 2000). An unscrupulous person can take advantage of this and mislead you into believing a fraudulent product was responsible for the temporary cessation of symptoms (Barrett, 2000).

In addition, just taking some sort of action often produces temporary relief of symptoms (placebo effect). You feel better because you feel that you are taking control of the situation (Barrett, 2000). Though the placebo effect is a psychological response, the body's physical response is not merely imagined—it is quite real. We know that your mental state can be effective in altering your physical state (Barrett, 2000). For example, when we get anxious, our heart begins to beat more rapidly.

TABLE 15.2	Common Deceptive Marketing Tactics Used to Promote Products

Bait and switch   One product is focused on, but another is delivered.

False claims (symptom free)   The claim that there are no side effects or symptoms associated with the use of a product.

False expectations   The claim that the product will bring about results that sound too good to be true (they usually are!).

Play upon fears (scare tactics)   Desperation marketing. Most effective for people desperately seeking change.

Promise simple solutions to complex problems   "Take a pill and sleep away fat."

Redundancy   Persuade you to purchase a product that might actually bring about advertised results, but is not necessary to achieve those results. An example might be an abdominal assistance contraption. A simple curl-up performed properly will provide the same result for free.

Rarely provide scientific research to support claims (foreign research)   In America, the reference is to "European scientists" who have discovered some miracle product. In the rest of the world, it's "American scientists" who it is claimed have made the discovery.

Rely on testimonials   It worked for me, therefore you should believe that it will work for you. Many of the people giving testimonials are being paid by the company to do so, and their objectivity must be questioned.

Criticize the medical establishment (conspiracy)   Marketers tell you that the medical community doesn't want you to know about a product. They claim that there is a vast conspiracy being instigated by the medical community to withhold information from you.

Money-back guarantees   Companies offer money-back guarantees with the knowledge that most people won't take the time or effort to seek their money back. In some cases, it costs more to get your money back than the total amount of money you get back. Additionally, shipping and handling costs are not refunded, which can amount to a significant sum.

Cures or miracles   The manufacturer advertises their product in such a way as to imply that it will cure a disease or work miracles. Then, usually in small print and in a hard-to-find location, they issue a disclaimer that they don't intend to imply that the product cures any disease or causes the occurrence of a miracle.

Celebrity endorsements   Companies hire famous spokespersons who tout their product. The hope is that you will connect the product with the celebrity and in some way think that the product had something to do with making this person a celebrity.

Mass media marketing   The product is sold primarily through television, radio, newspaper, and magazine advertisements. You are saturated with ads pushing the product to the point that you come to associate the product with the advertising venue. Certain products are associated with certain TV shows. The intent is to get you to believe that the show (and/or actors) supports the product.

Buzzwords (e.g., secret, rapid)   The advertising companies use buzzwords to get your attention. They also try to focus your attention on the buzzwords rather than on the product.

Omission of facts   The marketers obscure or completely leave out certain facts that may keep you from purchasing their product. For instance, they may "forget" to tell you that there are certain side effects associated with use of the product. Another common example with weight loss products is when the companies forget to tell you that their product only works when combined with a regular physical activity program and proper nutrition.

For your eyes only   Advertising claims tell you that the product contains secret ingredients known only to a few people. This sometimes means that they don't know what is in the product, or they don't want you to know what is in the product. This method of advertising is meant to make you feel that you are being let in on the secret and are therefore special.

Highly pedigreed   Individuals with multiple degrees from well-known institutions tout a product. Background checks on these individuals sometimes show that the person may never have attended, let alone graduated from, the institution from which he or she claims to have a degree. Another example is where someone is listed as a doctor to lend credence to a marketing claim. In many cases, the doctor is not a medical doctor, or has an area of expertise completely unrelated to the product he or she is pushing. One prime example is of a doctor with training in anesthesiology passing himself off as an expert in nutrition.

Express mail   Many companies use express mail to deliver their product to you. One possible reason for doing this is because sending a fraudulent product through the U.S. mail constitutes mail fraud, which is a federal offense. By using express mail, the company skirts this law, since it does not apply to nongovernmental mailing agencies.

Sex!   It is well known that sex is used to sell just about everything. This is also true in the physical activity and fitness industry. Remember that the product will not enhance your sex life or make members of the opposite sex desire you more just because you use it.

Our own naiveté and gullibility often set us up for manipulation by misleading advertisers. People tend to believe what they hear often, and misleading information, particularly about nutrition, is everywhere (Barrett & Jarvis, 2000). As an example, the advertisements promoting the use of shark cartilage supplements to protect against cancer imply that sharks don't get cancer; so, if you take shark cartilage supplements, they claim you won't get cancer. In fact, sharks do get cancer and even get cancer of their cartilage.

Individuals who have serious or chronic diseases that make them feel desperate enough to try anything that offers hope are extremely susceptible to fraudulent advertising. Alienated people, some of whom may experience paranoia, form another victim group (Barrett & Jarvis, 2000). These people may be convinced that our food supply is unsafe; that drugs do more harm than good; and that doctors, drug companies, large food companies, and government agencies are involved in conspiracies and not interested in protecting the public (Barrett, 2000). Such beliefs make them vulnerable to those who offer foods and healing approaches alleged to be "natural" (Barrett & Jarvis, 2000). For these reasons, controlled scientific studies are needed to establish whether fitness and nutrition products actually work.

Facts, Fads, and Fallacies

You need to be aware of some common misconceptions, frauds, and fallacies.

It can be very difficult to separate fact from fiction. This section provides an overview of some of the more common fallacies surrounding physical activity, exercise, and fitness.

Common Myths in Physical Activity and Fitness

SPOT REDUCTION MYTH   The spot reduction myth implies that you can selectively reduce body fat in certain areas of your body by performing exercise that involves muscles in that area. The best example is performing sit-ups in an attempt to reduce abdominal fat. Spot reduction does not work. Your muscles receive energy (including energy from fat) from the bloodstream. Your body mobilizes fat from deposits throughout the body. Exercising a local muscle group does not cause your body to remove more fat from the deposits in that area. If spot reduction worked, everyone who chewed gum, or talked a lot, would have a lean face.

"CELLULITE" MYTH   The "cellulite" myth has convinced some people that cellulite is a special type of cell that can be treated through the use of pills, lotions, and/or massage. In fact, a quick look through any anatomy book will demonstrate that there is no specific cell in the body called *cellulite*. What people refer to as cellulite is nothing more than adipose tissue (fat) that is surrounded by stretched connective tissue. Rapid onset, or rapid loss, of adipose causes the dimpling look associated with "cellulite." The connective tissue running throughout and around the fat cells take some time to adjust to the fluctuations in fat stores and appears to be stretched. The reduction of "cellulite" requires the same procedures as the reduction of body fat: expend more calories than you consume.

MUSCLE STIMULATOR/PASSIVE EXERCISE MYTH   The muscle stimulator/passive exercise myth promotes weight loss and fitness gains without any effort by the person attempting to bring about these gains. The theory is that by applying muscle stimulators to a region of the body (for example, the abdominals) you can "get the equivalent of" a vigorous workout or a thousand sit-ups. Other devices that promote this myth are passive motion tables that claim that all you need to do is relax on the table while the table does the work, moving your limbs to provide an effective workout. The problem with both of these types of devices is that the device does the work. The energy expended comes from the electrical outlet in the wall and not from your cells. Therefore, you are not expending any energy to bring about fat loss. In addition, there is no training effect of your neuromuscular system because using these devices does not require you to stimulate your own muscles.

INSTANT GRATIFICATION MYTH   The instant gratification myth suggests that you can take a magic pill to lose fat or improve performance. This myth is appealing to those people who do not want to put the time or effort into a physical activity program. The reality is that it takes time and effort to bring about changes in fitness. The idea that someone can take a pill to bring about these changes is just an illusion. The systems of your body (cardiovascular, muscular, skeletal) respond to regular physical activity and become stronger. A pill will not cause this response to occur.

SHAKE, RATTLE, AND ROLL MYTH   The shake, rattle, and roll myth implies that you can vibrate, or massage away, unwanted fat. Adipose tissue (fat) is very resilient. Fat is designed to provide cushioning and shock absorption. In order to do this, fat must retain its structural characteristics when moved. Fat is also surrounded by connective tissue that has elastic properties allowing it to stretch and then regain its shape. In other words, fat bounces very well and is easily manipulated through massage. Shaking, rattling, or rolling fat will not make it disappear. To reduce body fat, you must expend more energy than you consume.

TORCH MYTH   The torch myth suggests that by increasing your body temperature you can melt away fat. You will see people wearing rubberized suits, extra layers of clothing, or working out in a hot, humid environment in an attempt to lose fat. Working out like this will cause you to lose weight, but the weight lost will be almost exclusively water weight. The water lost will be replaced as soon as fluids are consumed after exercise. Additionally, losing water puts you at risk for thermal stress (heat exhaustion, heat stroke). When dehydrated, you cannot work as hard, so your rate of energy expenditure is actually lower. You need to make sure you allow your body to sweat when active and you must allow the sweat to evaporate. It takes a great deal of heat to melt fat (see how hot your grill must get to cook the fat on a piece of steak). If it were possible to raise your body temperature high enough to melt fat, other tissues and organs would also melt.

BODY BEAUTIFUL MYTH   The body beautiful myth implies that if someone looks fit and attractive, they must be knowledgeable about physical activity and fitness. While this may be true in some instances, good genetics doesn't mean that the person has had the proper education to be an expert. Health clubs are full of people who are hired because they appear fit and because they can sell memberships. However, a brief conversation with some of these people will demonstrate that their knowledge of physical activity and fitness is extremely limited. Check to see that the person offering advice has a degree in exercise science or a related field from an accredited university. Check to see that they are certified by a reputable professional organization (e.g., American College of Sports Medicine, National Strength and Conditioning Association, American Council on Exercise).

APPLES AND ORANGES MYTH   The apples and oranges myth suggests that exercise can turn fat cells to muscle cells and inactivity can turn muscle cells to fat. Fat and muscle cells are two completely different types of cells. You cannot turn one into the other. You can cause them to shrink (atrophy) or enlarge (hypertrophy) by eating too much and being inactive (fat hypertrophy), or eating in a rational way and being physically active (muscle hypertrophy).

MAGICAL POTION MYTH   The magical potion myth promotes the rubbing of lotions on the skin to cause fat loss, remove lactic acid, or firm up your muscles. Fat will only be lost by expending more calories than you consume. The best way to do this is by eating wisely and maintaining a physically active lifestyle. Lactic acid is removed when oxygen becomes available in the muscle cells and bloodstream. This takes breathing and the delivery of oxygen to the cell. A good portion of the lactic acid is actually reconverted into pyruvic acid, which can then be used to supply energy to the cells (Wilmore & Costill, 2004). Lotions do not affect this process. Resistance training firms up muscles.

VANISHING ACT MYTH   A common claim made by misleading advertisers is that their product will cause you to lose inches. This vanishing act myth suggests that the loss of inches is directly related to the loss of fat. In fact, most of what is lost in lost-inches claims is water. The water is replaced once the restrictive piece of clothing is removed, or once the person drinks fluids after exercise. Watch what happens after you remove a pair of socks with good elastic at the top. Initially you notice indentations on your skin where the elastic compressed water out of the region, but within a very short period of time the water returns and the indentations disappear. Losing inches is not important. For most people the goal is to lose fat. Losing inches does not necessarily relate to a reduction in fat.

"ALL NATURAL" MYTH   The "all natural" myth claims that only "natural" products are good for you. These products claim that anything that contains chemicals is bad for you. In reality, your entire body is composed of chemicals, as is everything surrounding you. Does the *All Natural* label always indicate that a product is good for you? Several substances come to mind that are all natural and are not at all good for you—things you probably don't want to ingest, including botulism, aflatoxin, salmonella, *E. coli*, rattlesnake venom, poison ivy, nicotine, and cocaine (Whitehead, 2000).

Sources of Information

Being a critical consumer requires knowing where to turn for valid information.

To be a wise consumer of physical activity, exercise, and fitness information, it pays to be skeptical about advertising claims, statements made by celebrities, "information" from infomercials, and "breakthroughs" reported in the news media. You need to maintain a healthy degree of skepticism if you are to avoid misinformation and outright fraud.

To reduce the likelihood of becoming a victim of exercise and fitness fraud, it is important to develop the characteristics of intelligent consumer behavior. To become an intelligent consumer, you must learn to seek reliable sources of information.

Governmental Agencies

There are a number of places where you can get information on product safety and efficacy. The two agencies in the federal government directed to regulate product worthiness are the Food and Drug Administration (FDA) and the Federal Trade Commission (FTC). The FDA is one of our nation's oldest consumer protection agencies. It is housed within the Public Health Service, which in turn is a part of the Department of Health and Human Services. The FDA is charged with protecting American consumers by enforcing the federal Food, Drug, and Cosmetic Act and several related public health laws.

Among other things, the FDA oversees food, medicines, and medical devices. It monitors the manufacture, import, transport, storage, and sale of approximately $1 trillion worth of products each year. The FDA is also involved in testing products, assessing risks, and weighing risks against benefits. Additionally, the FDA tests drugs and devices after they have been put on the market to monitor for any unexpected adverse reactions.

A second governmental agency involved in product safety and regulation is the Federal Trade Commission (FTC). The Federal Trade Commission enforces a variety of federal antitrust and consumer protection laws. The role of the FTC is to ensure that the nation's markets function competitively and are vigorous, efficient, and free of undue restrictions. The FTC works to enhance the smooth operation of the marketplace by eliminating acts or practices that are unfair or deceptive.

The efforts of the FTC are directed toward stopping actions that threaten consumers' opportunities to exercise informed choice. The FTC also plays a major role in providing consumer education by making brochures available and by providing public service announcements.

Professional Health Organizations

You can also seek information from professional organizations such as the American College of Sports Medicine; the National Strength and Conditioning Association; the American Alliance for Health, Physical Education, Recreation and Dance; and the American Council on Exercise. These organizations offer publications and videos that provide the best information available to date. They are staffed by people who research and teach about physical activity, exercise, and fitness.

Community Experts

You can also check to see if there are any experts in your local community who might be able to provide assistance. Local colleges and universities are a good place to start. Look particularly to see if they have one or more specialists in exercise science.

In addition you might be able to find someone who can help in a YM/YWCA, or in a commercial health club. Remember to check on their training, background, and credentials. Most people working in community settings are fully capable of providing accurate information, but occasionally you may run across someone who lacks the background to be an accurate source for you.

The Internet

A final source of information is the Internet, which has some excellent sites providing reliable information. However, since the Internet lacks governmental regulation, you must be cautious in selecting your sources. A number of guides are available for evaluating the usefulness of websites (Kotecki & Siegel, 1998; Kotecki & Chamness, 1999).

Selecting a Physical Activity Program

Earlier chapters in this book have outlined the components of an effective physical activity program. If you decide to follow a "canned" activity program (one developed by someone and marketed as all-inclusive), make sure the program contains all of the

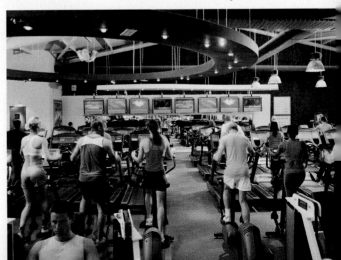

Not all fitness facilities are the same. Select one that meets your needs.

components covered in the preceding chapters. If you are thinking of using an exercise video, rent it first. Use caution and common sense. Don't attempt any activity that doesn't appear safe or logical.

Modify any program to fit your individual needs. If you are unsure about any claims or activities contained within the program, ask an expert to evaluate the product for you.

Selecting a Physical Activity and Fitness Facility

If you choose to carry out your physical activity program in a health club or exercise facility, it is wise to do some scouting before paying membership dues. A good place to start is to make sure you understand why some of the people who join health clubs eventually leave. A common reason that people stop attending a health club is that they did not make sufficient use of their membership (Orejan, 2000). They might have paid dues for a certain amount of time and realized that they did not attend frequently enough to make the dues cost-effective. Rather than spending more money, they just drop out.

A second reason may be that they have lost interest or motivation (Orejan, 2000). This may be due to personal factors on the part of the member, or it may be that the facility did not provide a varied and stimulating environment. A third reason could be that they did not like the atmosphere in the facility (Orejan, 2000). It sometimes takes a while before you can determine if the facility fits your needs. You need to get to know the management and staff, of course, but realize that other customers may influence your decision as well. If you don't feel safe or feel comfortable around the other people in the facility, your adherence rate will suffer. Additionally, the physical environment of the facility may begin to wear on you and add to your dissatisfaction.

Many people quit when they realize the dreams they had when they joined have not been met by reality (Orejan, 2000). If your goals are set too high and you cannot reach them, you may become frustrated and lose interest.

You can take several steps to enhance the likelihood that you will retain your membership. TABLE 15.3 outlines several suggestions for selecting a health club.

Once you have found a facility you like, don't hesitate to take advantage of everything it has to offer. Ask for instruction if you don't know how to use a piece of equipment. Make use of personal trainers if you need help designing a program. Exercise at your own pace; don't let someone else's pace put you at risk or act to de-motivate you (Orejan, 2000).

Examples of Misleading Products

When evaluating products for safety and efficacy, you must determine if the marketing claims made by the producer are scientifically plausible, valid, and reliable. The best way to make this determination is by investigating the scientific evidence provided through independent, rigorous research.

One example of misleading advertising concerns the use of magnets for health and fitness. The producers of "magnet therapy" would lead you to believe that magnets can improve your health and fitness. One theory proposed by the marketers of magnet therapy is that the blood contains iron (in hemoglobin), so wearing magnets will aid in circulation and in maintaining proper blood flow because the iron in the blood draws the blood in the direction of the magnets. A second is

TABLE 15.3	Guidelines for Selecting a Health Club

Prepare before you go.

- Identify your goals before joining a health club.
- Define your best workout environment.
- Set a budget.
- Determine the minimum amount of time you can devote to exercise and when you can do it.
- Shop around. Compare different health clubs. Take a trial membership.

Meet with the staff and get a thorough tour of the facility, its programs, and amenities.

- Participate in, or at least observe, a couple of the group exercise classes.
- Check out the cardio and weight equipment. Do they have what you want?
- Visit the club at a time that you would like to work out.
- Make lists of things you like or dislike.
- Ask current members what they like and what needs improvement.
- Check the helpfulness, knowledge, and friendliness of the staff.
- See if the club is clean and well maintained.
- Is the facility crowded? Will you need to wait to work out?
- Is there sufficient variety of programs and activities?
- Is there child care, if needed?
- Is there sufficient, well-lit parking?
- Do you feel safe and comfortable?
- Is the facility conveniently located?
- Does the club offer preactivity screening?
- Are members of the staff professionally qualified?

Understand the contract agreement.

- Make sure you read and understand everything before you sign.
- Opt for shorter-term memberships.
- Find out if there is a grace period in the contract in case you change your mind.
- Do not be pressured by an aggressive sales pitch.
- Ask what the specific rules are under which you can terminate a membership, such as permanent illness, medical condition or injury, or relocation to a place not served by the club.

SOURCES: J. Orejan. (2000). How to select a fitness center. *Fitness Management 16*(4):48; and American College of Sports Medicine. (2005, Spring). Selecting and effectively using a health-fitness facility. *ASCM Fit Society Page*: 9–10.

that our body needs to be exposed to magnetic fields for good health. No scientific evidence supports these claims.

We are told that concrete and pavement and other human structures supposedly block the earth's magnetic fields. However, magnetic fields are not blocked by concrete. Simple proof can be found by taking a compass into any structure. Any place a compass works, the earth's magnetic fields are present (Gessell, 1999).

Secondly, the iron in blood is not magnetic. If it were, the human body would explode in the magnetic resonance imaging (MRI) machines commonly used in hospitals (Gessell, 1999). If the advertiser's claims were true, you would also be able to make a drop of blood on a table follow a handheld magnet as it passed over the top of the droplet.

Finally, individuals who work with magnets in industrial and research settings are exposed to magnetic field strengths 6 to 10 orders of magnitude greater than that created by the magnets promoted by supporters of magnet therapy (Gessell, 1999). We also know that DC magnetic fields have no measurable effect on the human body at levels strong enough to bend steel bars (Gessell, 1999).

Another example of misleading advertising arose from so-called infrared technology; it purported to give valid and reliable measures of body composition. The claim was that accurate measures of body fat could be made with an infrared device, and the device was found to be anything but reliable and provided no valid results. After FBI and FDA investigations, the head of the company that makes the device was sentenced in district court to 4 months' home detention. He also was sentenced to 18 months' probation, a $3000 fine, and a $200 special assessment, plus settlements of $90,000 to the U.S. Customs Service and $50,000 to the U.S. Securities and Exchange Commission. The FDA's Office of Criminal Investigations received information that the clinical data used to validate the fat tester had been fabricated (Whitehead, 2000).

Dietary Supplement Health and Education Act of 1994

It has been estimated that 50 percent of the general population have used some form of dietary supplement, while 76 to 100 percent of athletes in some sports are reported to use them (Ahrendt, 2001). The nutritional supplement industry is an area frequently accused of fraud and deceptive advertising. For decades, the FDA regulated dietary supplements as foods. In most circumstances, this was done to ensure that they were safe and wholesome and that their labeling was truthful and not misleading. An important facet of ensuring safety was the FDA's evaluation of the safety of all new ingredients, including those used in dietary supplements, under the 1958 federal Food, Drug, and Cosmetic Act (FD&C Act).

However, with passage of the Dietary Supplement Health and Education Act of 1994 (DSHEA), Congress amended the FD&C Act to include several provisions

Many different products are marketed to underinformed consumers.

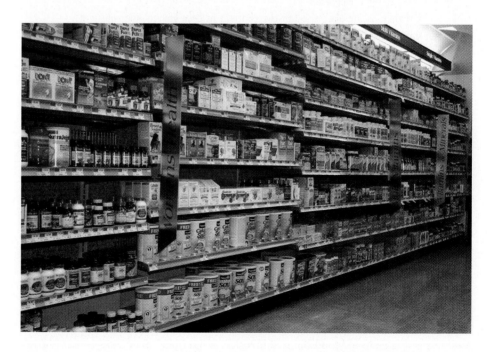

that apply only to dietary supplements and the dietary ingredients of dietary supplements (FDA, 1994). As a result of these provisions, dietary ingredients used in dietary supplements are no longer subject to the pre-market safety evaluations required of other new food ingredients or for new uses of old food ingredients.

Several concerns have arisen with respect to DSHEA. What was supposed to provide "health freedom" for consumers has instead provided "marketing freedom" for manufacturers (Whitehead, 2000). Since there is no FDA regulation of nutritional supplements, there is no guarantee of what is actually in a product and whether the ingredients are safe or effective. Rather than controlled testing in an independent laboratory, the consumer pays to be a guinea pig (Whitehead, 2000). Regulation takes place only after a product has been shown to cause harm in humans.

Examples include the nutritional supplements containing ephedra or ma huang. Ephedrine alkaloids act as an "all natural" speed. They are banned by many sports organizations, and their side effects have been documented to kill and injure people (Whitehead, 2000). However, manufacturers of products containing ephedra still defend its use. It can be found in many dietary supplements and decongestants and puts many consumers unknowingly at risk (Whitehead, 2000).

Seeking Redress

There are several avenues you can take in seeking redress.

When we are the victims of fraudulent or misleading advertising, we assume that we should "know better" and therefore deserve whatever we get as a consequence. This feeling is a major reason why journalists, law enforcement officials, judges, and legislators seldom give priority to combating misleading products (Barrett, 2000).

We also operate under the false assumption that someone else is going to be looking out for us. In reality, we are on our own most of the time.

When you are seeking help, you can consult one of the agencies listed in TABLE 15.4. Victims of fraud often have difficulty obtaining redress through the courts. Many are afraid of lawyers. Some are embarrassed at having been fooled. Too often the victim does nothing, simply dismissing the fraud as one of life's lessons (Barrett, 2000).

One way of fighting back is to lodge a complaint with the Federal Trade Commission if you suspect that you have been victimized by fraud. The FTC may begin an investigation in a number of ways. Letters from consumers or businesses, Congressional inquiries, or articles on consumer or economic subjects may trigger FTC action. Investigations are either public or nonpublic. (Generally, FTC investigations are nonpublic in order to protect both the investigation and the company.)

If the FTC believes a violation of the law occurred, it might attempt to obtain voluntary compliance by entering into a **consent order** with the company. A company that signs a consent order need not admit that it violated the law, but it must agree to stop the disputed practices outlined in an accompanying complaint. If a consent agreement cannot be reached, the FTC may issue an **administrative complaint**. If an administrative complaint is issued, a formal proceeding that is much like a court trial begins before an administrative law judge: evidence is submitted, testimony is heard, and witnesses are examined and cross-examined.

If a law violation is found, a **cease-and-desist order** may be issued. If the company violates the order, the commission may seek civil penalties or an injunction. In some circumstances, the FTC can go directly to court to obtain an injunction, civil penalties, or consumer redress. This usually happens in cases of ongoing

Consent order An agreement bringing about voluntary compliance without a judicial ruling.

Administrative complaint An action that brings about a formal proceeding; much like a court trial, it takes place before an administrative law judge.

Cease-and-desist order A legal order informing a company that it must no longer advertise or market a product.

| TABLE 15.4 | Agencies to Contact |

Problem	Agencies to Contact
False advertising	FTC Bureau of Consumer Protection or regional office State attorney general Editor or manager of media outlet where ad appeared
Product marketed with false or misleading claims	National or regional FDA office FDA Center for Drug Evaluation and Research State attorney general State health department Local Better Business Bureau Congressional representatives
Bogus mail-order promotion	Chief Postal Inspector, U.S. Postal Service Regional postal inspector State attorney general
Dubious telemarketing	State attorney general FTC Bureau of Consumer Protection or regional office
Improper treatment by licensed individual	Local district attorney State attorney general National Council Against Health Fraud Task Force on Victim Redress Quackwatch.com
Advice needed about questionable product or service	Quackwatch.com Local, state, or national professional or voluntary health groups
Internet-related consumer problem	eConsumer.gov (cross-border complaints) FDA Federal Bureau of Investigation Webguardian Internet Fraud Complaint Center
Junk e-mail, including health-related scams and chain letters	FTC's e-mail box

consumer fraud. By going directly to court, the FTC can stop the fraud before many consumers are injured. When issued, these rules have the force of law.

You can also seek to take legal action on your own. However, it is important to remember that health and nutrition fraud is not a specialty for most attorneys. Although the same general law applies, most lawyers have had no experience in dealing with such cases. Therefore dedicated, knowledgeable attorneys can be difficult to find (Barrett, 2000).

The National Council Against Health Fraud Task Force on Victim Redress helps victims of fraud obtain competent legal assistance. The services offered by this organization include providing help in deciding whether to take the company to court; making referral to suitable attorneys; and providing information on unproven, fraudulent, and potentially dangerous treatments (Barrett, 2000). The task force can also help with locating expert witnesses, providing information on defense witnesses, and supplying reports on cases adjudicated, settled, and in progress (Barrett, 2000).

The Food and Drug Administration is another avenue for seeking redress. The FDA is responsible for performing inspections and seeking legal sanctions. If a company is found to be violating any of the laws that the FDA enforces, the FDA can encourage the firm to correct the problem voluntarily or to recall a faulty product from the market. A recall is generally the fastest and most effective way to protect the public from an unsafe product.

When a company can't or won't voluntarily correct a public health problem with one of its products, the FDA can bring legal sanctions to bear. The FDA can force a company to stop selling a product, or it can have items already produced seized and destroyed. It can also seek criminal penalties, including prison sentences.

Finally, another free service that has been established to alert online consumers to prior complaints relating to products and services is the Fraud Bureau (http://www.fraudbureau.com/). This site allows you to search for complaints against companies and to file a scam complaint if you have had problems.

Separating Fact from Fallacy

Your best bet in separating fact from fallacy is to become an educated consumer. Staying abreast of the latest information about new products and techniques is a good way to get started. Learning to seek information from reliable sources and to question everything will make you less susceptible. Check out professional publications distributed by professional associations. Learn how to use information available from governmental (e.g., FDA, FTC) and business organizations (e.g., Better Business Bureau). Make sure that product claims are proven to you. Be a skeptic. See if the manufacturer's claims are documented by **peer-reviewed research**. Make sure the product stands the test of time. Don't depend on others for protection.

> **Peer-reviewed research** Research articles and presentations in which experts in the field of study review material for accuracy and validity before it is disseminated to the public.

There are certain things you can do to reduce the risk of being susceptible to misleading advertising. First, lead a healthy lifestyle. This will reduce your risk of becoming seriously ill and will lower your health care costs (Barrett, 2000). Living a healthy lifestyle also makes you less susceptible to desperation marketing (buying a product because you are desperate for change).

Understand the need for controlled scientific testing of products to ensure objectivity. Gather information as needed to determine which theories and practices are valid. Be wary of treatments that lack scientific support and a plausible rationale. Most treatments described as "alternative" fit the description of products whose claims have not been validated by carefully designed scientific research (Barrett, 2000).

Shop comparatively for equipment, exercise products, and nutritional aids. Report fraud, quackery, and other wrongdoing to appropriate agencies and law enforcement officials. Consumer vigilance is an essential ingredient of a healthy society (Barrett, 2000).

Understand the basic facts about physical activity. You must exercise to be fit. You must perform resistance training, secrete the proper hormones, and have good genetics to become strong and muscular. You must perform endurance exercise to obtain optimal cardiovascular fitness. You must combine regular exercise and sensible eating to maintain a healthy body composition. We are a product of our genetics, but we are also influenced by our environment. And finally, remember the credo of business: *Caveat emptor!* Let the buyer beware!

Physical Activity and Health Connection

Regular participation in physical activity is intricately interwoven with a healthy lifestyle. To make sure your physical activity program is safe and effective, you must be a wise consumer of activity, exercise, and fitness information and products. Many products are sold to consumers that are misleading at best and fraudulent at worst. Even though there is a certain degree of governmental oversight of products available to consumers, the best defense against misleading advertising and fraudulent products is an informed consumer. Certain products can be dangerous and can lead to ill health. It is important to be vigilant when purchasing activity, exercise, and fitness products.

concept connections

1. **To develop a quality physical activity program, you must be a wise consumer of exercise information.** You must learn to protect yourself and keep yourself up-to-date on the latest information regarding what works and what doesn't work.

2. **The physical activity industry suffers from a wide range of misinformation and fraudulent claims.** To avoid being misled, you need to be able to filter through advertiser claims and focus on what has been shown to work through independent research.

3. **You need to be aware of some common misconceptions, fraud, and fallacies.** Many misleading and fraudulent advertisers recycle the same old exercise and nutrition myths. By learning what these myths are and why they don't make sense, you can help to protect yourself from being victimized.

4. **Being a critical consumer requires knowing where to turn for valid information.** Turn to governmental agencies such as the FDA and FTC, or professional health and fitness organizations for the straight facts on exercise and fitness products. Look for peer-reviewed research that evaluates products objectively.

5. **There are several avenues you can take in seeking redress.** Prevention is the best cure. However, if you feel that you need to seek redress, several outlets are available to you to help you take the right steps.

Terms

Ergogenic aid, 332	Quackery, 334	Administrative complaint, 343
Ergolytic, 332	Misinformation, 334	Cease-and-desist order, 343
Fraud, 332	Consent order, 343	Peer-reviewed research, 345

Janet learns that the diet pill contains mostly useless ingredients and a good deal of caffeine. The registered dietitian explains that the caffeine would temporarily increase Janet's metabolic rate and make her feel nervous, but that the effect would not last long. The impact on Janet's metabolic rate would not result in the loss of body fatness and could be dangerous for some people. She also tells Janet that she would have difficulty sleeping after taking the pill. Armed with this information, Janet feels confident about telling Kathy "Thanks, but no thanks!"

Critical Thinking

1. Like Janet, we are constantly being bombarded with advertisements about a diet pill or drink that will *guarantee* losing X pounds per week. These advertisements are often seen on college and university campuses. As you walk to class, take a look around to see if you notice any of these advertisements. Record what you see. Also, review the most recent issue of your college or university newspaper. Are there any ads for fad diets or pills? If so, who are they targeting?

2. In a popular magazine, find an advertisement that you believe might be misleading or fraudulent. Determine which of the advertising approaches are used to convince readers to purchase the product. What argument would you present to counter the advertising claims?

3. Speculate about why people often fall victim to common physical activity and health misconceptions, frauds, or fallacies.

4. As a critical health consumer, where would you suggest peers go to find valid information on physical activity and health? Give three sources and explain how you determined they were valid.

References

Ahrendt, D. (2001). Erogenic aids: Counseling the athlete. *American Family Physician* 63:913–922.

Barrett, S. (2000). Quackwatch: Your guide to health fraud, quackery, and intelligent decisions. Online: http://www.quackwatch.com.

Barrett, S., & Jarvis, W.T. (2000). How quackery sells. *Nutrition Forum* 17(2):9–14.

Food and Drug Administration. (1994). Dietary Supplement Health and Education Act of 1994. Online: http://www.cfsan.fda.gov/~dms/dietsupp.html.

Food and Drug Administration. (2004). Sales of supplements containing ephedrine alkaloids (ephedra) prohibited. Online: http://www.fda.gov/oc/initiatives/ephedra/february2004/.

Gessell, D. (1999). Magnet therapy: Reader response. Online: http://www.quackwatch.com/04ConsumerEducation/QA/magnet.html.

Judge rules against FDA ban on ephedra. (2005, April 14). *The Washington Post*. Online: http://washingtonpost.com/wp-dyn/articles/A53586-2005Apr14.html.

Kotecki, J., & Chamness, B.E. (1999). A valid tool for evaluating health-related www sites. *Journal of Health Education* 30(1):56–59.

Kotecki, J., & Siegel, D.E. (1998). Using a critical thinking/questioning approach to evaluate www information. *American Journal of Health Behavior* 22(1):75–76.

Orejan, J. (2000). How to select a fitness center. *Fitness Management* 16(4):48.

Whitehead, J.R. (2000, March). *Exercise and Fitness Consumerism*. Presented at the American Alliance for Health, Physical Education, Recreation, and Dance conference, Orlando, Florida.

Wilmore, J.H., & Costill, D.L. (2004). *Physiology of Sport and Exercise*, 3rd ed. Champaign, IL: Human Kinetics.

Organizations to Contact For Help

Consumer Broadcast Group:
Online resource center for aggrieved consumers

Federal Trade Commission (FTC)
Bureau of Consumer Protection
Washington, DC 20580
Tel. (202) 326-2222

National Advertising Division
Council of Better Business Bureaus
845 Third Avenue, New York, NY 10022
Tel. (212) 753-1358

Food and Drug Administration (FDA)
5600 Fishers Lane, Rockville, MD 20857
Tel. (301) 295-8024

Chief Postal Inspector
U.S. Postal Service, Washington, DC 20260
Tel. (202) 268-4267

Consumer Health Information Resource Institute
300 E. Pinkhill Road, Independence, MO 64050
Tel. (816) 228-4595

Federal Bureau of Investigation (FBI)
935 Pennsylvania Avenue, N.W.,
Washington, DC 20535

National Council Against Health Fraud
P.O. Box 1276, Loma Linda, CA 92354
Tel. (909) 824-4690

Task Force on Victim Redress
Quackwatch.com
P.O. Box 1747, Allentown, PA 18105
Tel. (610) 437-1795

National Fraud Information Center
P.O. Box 65868, Washington, DC 20035
Tel. (800) 876-7060

For local or regional offices of federal agencies consult the telephone directory under U.S. Government.

Federal Government Agencies

Food and Nutrition Information Center
National Agricultural Library
10301 Baltimore Ave., Beltsville, MD 20705
(consumer inquiries)

Consumer Information Center
P.O. Box 100, Pueblo CO 81002
(free and low-cost publications)

Consumer Product Safety Commission
5401 Westbard Ave., Bethesda, MD 20207

Federal Trade Commission
6th & Pennsylvania Ave., N.W.
Washington, DC 20580

President's Council on Physical Fitness and Sports
450 E. 5th St., Washington, DC 20201

Voluntary and Professional Organizations

Most of the organizations listed below are voluntary groups that draw support and members from the general public as well as professionals. Some have a single national office, while others have chapters in various cities. Most of these organizations provide educational materials on request. Some raise and distribute funds for research. Some conduct educational programs for the public and encourage and develop local support groups. Some offer individual counseling.

Business and professional groups are composed exclusively or primarily of health professionals or other professionally trained individuals. Most of these groups publish a scientific journal and hold educational meetings for their members. Most of them also help the public by setting professional standards, disseminating information through the news media, and responding to inquiries from individual consumers.

Aerobics and Fitness Association of America
1520 Ventura Blvd., Sherman Oaks, CA 91403

American Alliance for Health, Physical Education, Recreation and Dance
1900 Association Drive, Reston, VA 22091

American College of Sports Medicine
P.O. Box 1440, Indianapolis, IN 46206

American Heart Association
7272 Greenville Ave., Dallas, TX 75231

SOURCE: Barrett, 2000.

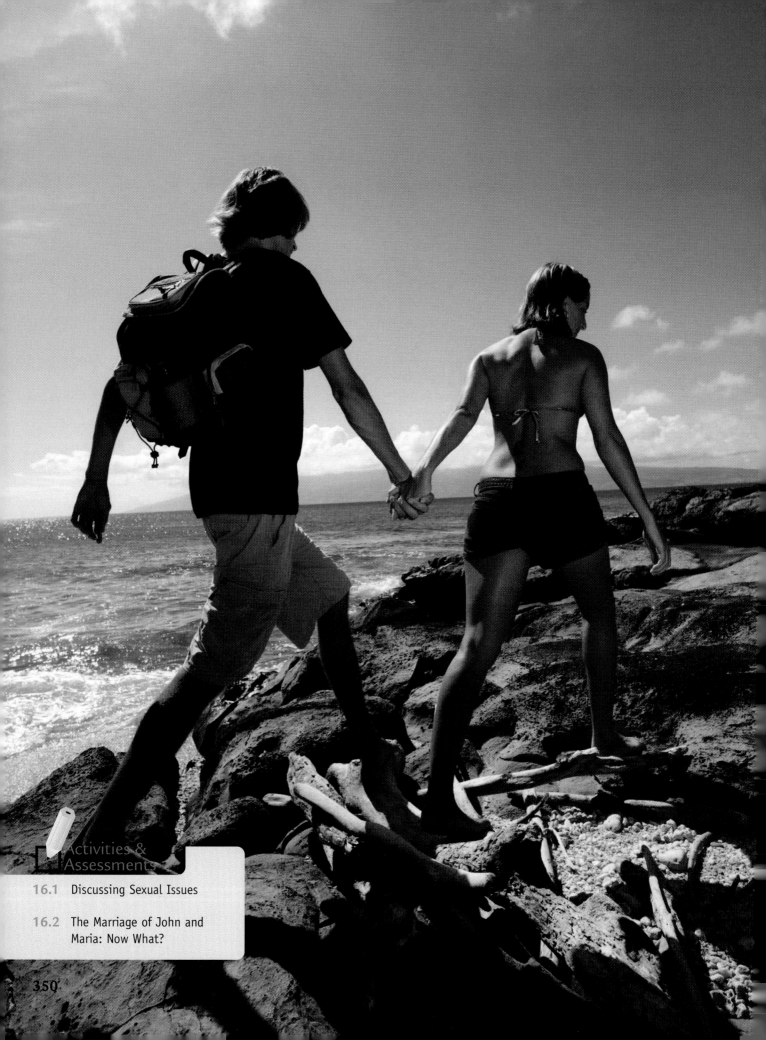

Activities &
Assessments

16.1   Discussing Sexual Issues

16.2   The Marriage of John and
        Maria: Now What?

Developing Healthy Sexual and Intimate Relationships

what's the connection?

Jeff and Susan have been dating for nearly a year—long enough to take each other for granted. This is most apparent at social gatherings with others. Jeff is very outgoing. He likes to "circulate," so he leaves Susan either with her friends or by herself, and he talks to his own friends or introduces himself to strangers. This bothers Susan because she would like to be included. But even more bothersome to her is that Jeff doesn't come back to spend time with her or include her in his conversations with others. Susan resents this. She has often told Jeff how she feels, but he says she is being unreasonable. Susan feels more angry and hurt each time Jim leaves her alone at social events. When this happens now she doesn't talk to him for a day or two.

concepts

1. *Sex* refers to a person's biological classification as male or female.

2. A person's sexual psychology is rooted in gender identity, which guides gender role behaviors.

3. A person's sexual biology is determined by genetic makeup, which in turn determines the nature of the sexual reproductive system.

4. Sexual response involves four phases.

5. Effective communication is critical for developing and maintaining relationships.

http://physicalactivity.jbpub.com

The Web site for this book is a great source for supplementary physical health information for both students and instructors. Visit **http://physicalactivity.jbpub.com** to find a variety of useful tools for learning, thinking, and teaching.

Introduction

Sexuality represents a truly holistic aspect of living, for it involves the simultaneous expression of mind, body, and spirit—the whole self. Although it is common to find sexuality represented in advertising and other media as having to do solely with physical gratification, most people are aware that sexuality involves much more than the stimulation of the body's sex organs. Sexuality involves thoughts, feelings, and identity. Sexuality is a powerful form of communication between people.

From the standpoint of physical activity and health, sexuality is an area over which you have considerable individual control. You choose when and with whom you wish to share sexual activity, and which feelings you wish to express in sexual ways. With some fundamental knowledge of sexual biology, you can conduct your sexual life responsibly, avoiding disease and freely choosing whether and when to have children. This chapter introduces the topic of sexuality and discusses the nature of the sexual self and of sexual expression.

Defining Sex and Sexuality

Understanding terminology is critical to good communication and relationships, including sexual relationships.

Sex

Sex can refer to (1) an individual's classification as male or female as determined by the presence of certain anatomical and physiological characteristics, (2) a set of behaviors, and (3) the experience of erotic pleasure.

At the most fundamental biological level, *sex* refers to the mating of two anatomically distinct individuals, a male and a female, each of whom manufactures specific cells, or **gametes**, which fuse to become the first cell of a new person. To facilitate the fusion process (called **fertilization**), males and females of a species possess specific organs and display certain behaviors that are intended to bring about the union of gametes.

Often the word *sex* is used to denote aspects of individuals' personal characteristics that are thought to derive from their biological classification. Thus, the biological property of femaleness is associated with the social quality of "femininity," and the biological property of maleness is associated with the social quality of "masculinity." Although most modern dictionaries still define sex as having to do with personality characteristics, this concept is more accurately referred to as *gender* to distinguish its origins in culture rather than biology.

Besides biological classification, sex is also associated with certain behaviors that are defined as **sexual**. These activities usually involve touching, in various ways, certain anatomical regions of the body, such as the genitalia and breasts, and sexual intercourse.

Sexuality

Sexuality, as distinct from sex, consists of the aspects of a person's sense of self that are used to create sexual experiences. Another term for sexuality is *the sexual self*, which has several dimensions:

1. The *physical dimension* refers to any region of the body to which an individual gives sexual meaning, including the organs and organ systems we employ to

Sex refers to a person's biological classification as male or female.

Sex (1) An individual's classification as male or female based on anatomical characteristics, (2) a set of behaviors, (3) the experience of erotic pleasure.

Gametes Sex cells, either sperm or ova, that fuse at fertilization; gametes carry a complete set of genetic information from each parent that is passed on to the child.

Fertilization The fusion of a sperm cell and an ovum.

Sexual Characterized by, or having, sex; opposed to asexual.

Sexuality A person's sense of self, which is used to create sexual experiences.

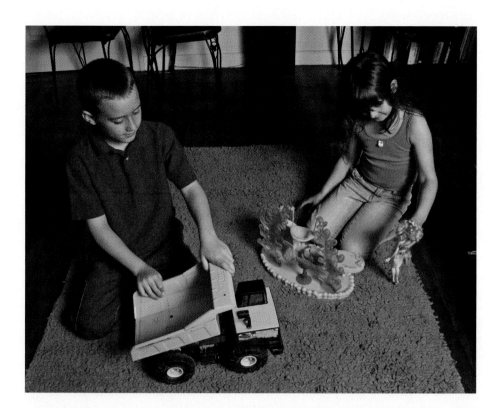

Young girls and boys learn their gender identities and roles at an early age.

create erotic experiences (the skin, the genitals). It also includes the physical features that define us to ourselves and others as a sexual being.

2. The *psychological dimension* refers to our emotions and our conscious and unconscious beliefs that guide the interpretation of experience. This aspect of sexuality generates strategies for actions that are intended to satisfy our wants and needs.

3. The *social dimension* refers to sexual attitudes and behaviors that affect our interactions with members of the social groups to which we belong.

4. The *orientation dimension* refers to the tendency to feel "naturally" attracted to people of a particular gender, and the ability to bond emotionally with them. About 85 to 90 percent of Americans have a **sexual orientation** to members of the opposite sex (**heterosexuals**); the rest of the population orients to individuals of either sex (**bisexuals**) or, more often, exclusively to members of the same sex (**homosexuals**). Individuals do not choose their sexual orientation; it develops as a fundamental aspect of a person's personality. Scientific studies have failed to uncover genetic, hormonal, metabolic, or psychological mechanisms underlying sexual orientation.

5. The *development dimension* is the evolution of our self throughout a lifetime. This evolution includes the body, the belief systems, and the ways sex is employed to create and maintain intimacy.

6. The *skill dimension* speaks to the physical and social skills that affect how well we meet our sexual wants and needs.

Sexual orientation Attraction toward and interest in members of one or both genders.

Heterosexuals People who are attracted to people of the opposite gender.

Bisexuals People who are attracted to members of both genders.

Homosexuals People who are attracted to people of the same gender.

A person's sexual psychology is rooted in gender identity, which guides gender role behaviors.

Gender identity Awareness and acceptance of being male or female.

Gender role Complex group of behaviors expected of males and females in a given culture.

A person's sexual biology is determined by genetic makeup, which in turn determines the nature of the sexual reproductive system.

Ova, ovum Eggs, egg.

Secondary sex characteristics Anatomical features appearing at puberty that distinguish males from females.

Ovaries A pair of almond-shaped organs in the female abdomen that produces egg cells (ova) and female sex hormones (estrogen and progesterone).

Fallopian tubes A pair of tube-like structures that transport ova from the ovaries to the uterus; the usual site of fertilization.

Uterus The female organ in which a fetus develops.

Vagina Female organ of copulation, and the exit pathway for the fetus at birth.

Cervix The lower and narrow end of the uterus.

Ovulation Release of an egg (ovum) from the ovary.

Clitoris Small, sensitive female organ located in front of the vaginal opening; center of sexual pleasuring.

Gender Identity and Gender Role

Although anatomy and physiology explain the biological basis of human sexuality, most people's sexual experiences also involve beliefs, thoughts, feelings, and social behaviors. How individuals come to think and behave sexually is almost entirely a product of what they learn as children about the kinds of behaviors that are expected of members of one sex or the other. The development of **gender identity** and the subsequent expression of sex-specific behaviors begins with the sex typing of newborn infants. When a child is born, almost the first thing noticed is its biological sex as determined by the appearance of its external genitals. If the infant is born with a penis, those attending the birth will exclaim "It's a boy!" Similarly, "It's a girl!" follows the observation of a newborn's female genitals.

Having been sex-typed at birth, the infant is thereafter treated by adults in a manner they think appropriate for a child of that sex, and eventually the infant incorporates into its self-image the awareness of being a male or a female. This awareness is called gender identity, and gender-specific behaviors are referred to as the **gender role**.

Sexual Biology

One of the fundamental roles of sexuality is biological reproduction. The reproductive role of the male is to produce reproductively capable sperm and to deposit them in the female reproductive tract during sexual intercourse. The reproductive role of the female is to provide reproductively capable eggs, called **ova**, and to provide a safe, nutrient-filled environment in which the fetus develops for the 9 months of pregnancy.

The genetic determination of sexual anatomy also specifies the pattern of male or female steroid hormone production, which in turn affects the **secondary sex characteristics** that distinguish adult males and females: the extent and distribution of facial and body hair, body build and stature, and the appearance of breasts (**FIGURE 16.1**).

Female Sexual Anatomy

A woman's internal sexual organs consist of two **ovaries**, which lie on either side of the abdominal cavity, the **fallopian tubes**, the **uterus**, and the **vagina**; together these structures make up a specialized receptacle and tube that goes from each ovary to the outside of the body (**FIGURE 16.2**). The function of the ovaries is to produce fertilizable ova as well as sex hormones, which control the development of the female body type, maintain normal female sexual physiology, and help regulate the course of a normal pregnancy. The fallopian tubes gather and transport the ova that are released from the ovaries (about one each month). The fallopian tubes connect to the uterus, an organ about the size of a woman's fist, which is situated just behind the pelvic bone and the bladder (**FIGURE 16.3**). The uterus is part of the passageway for sperm as they move from the vagina to the fallopian tubes to effect fertilization; after fertilization, it provides the environment in which the fetus grows. It is the inner lining of the uterus that is shed each month in menstruation.

The lower part of the uterus is the **cervix**, and the cavity of the uterus is connected to the vagina by means of a small opening called the cervical os. The cervix secretes mucus, which changes in consistency depending on the phase of the menstrual cycle. Some women learn to estimate the time of **ovulation** (ovum release) by examining their cervical mucus.

A woman's external genitals (**FIGURE 16.4**) consist of two pairs of fleshy folds that surround the opening of the vagina and the **clitoris**. The smaller, inner pair of

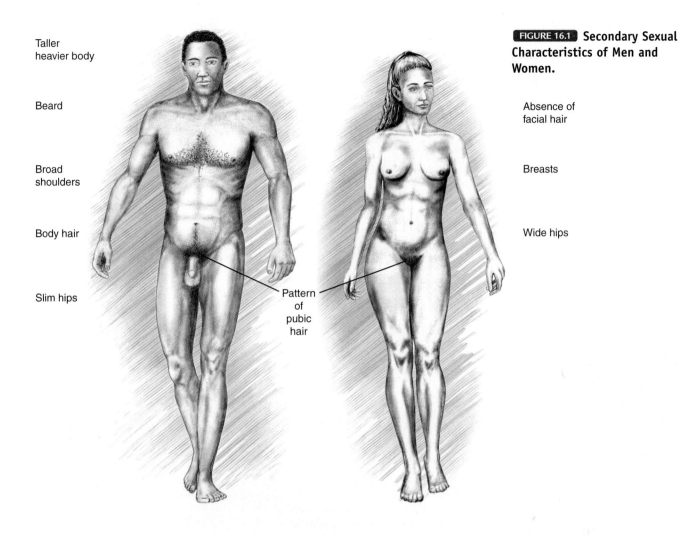

FIGURE 16.1 Secondary Sexual Characteristics of Men and Women.

Taller
heavier body

Beard

Broad
shoulders

Body hair

Slim hips

Pattern
of
pubic
hair

Absence of
facial hair

Breasts

Wide hips

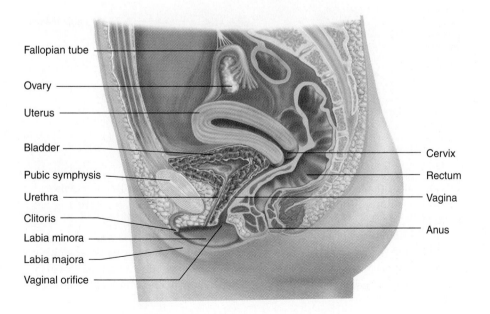

FIGURE 16.2 A Cross-section of the Female Sexual Reproductive System.

Fallopian tube

Ovary

Uterus

Bladder

Pubic symphysis

Urethra

Clitoris

Labia minora

Labia majora

Vaginal orifice

Cervix

Rectum

Vagina

Anus

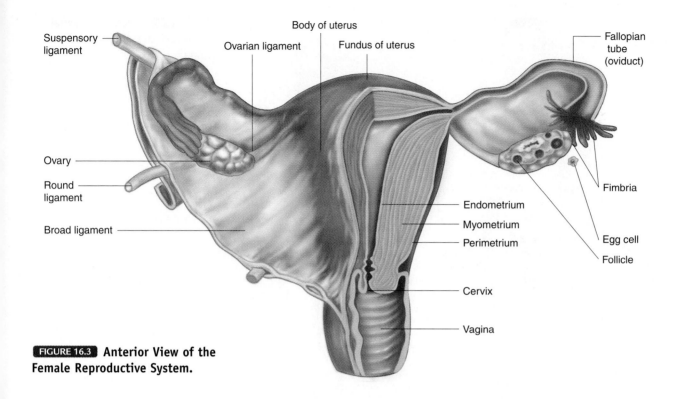

Suspensory ligament

Ovary

Round ligament

Broad ligament

Body of uterus

Ovarian ligament

Fundus of uterus

Fallopian tube (oviduct)

Fimbria

Egg cell

Follicle

Endometrium

Myometrium

Perimetrium

Cervix

Vagina

FIGURE 16.3 **Anterior View of the Female Reproductive System.**

FIGURE 16.4 **External Female Sexual Reproductive Organs.**

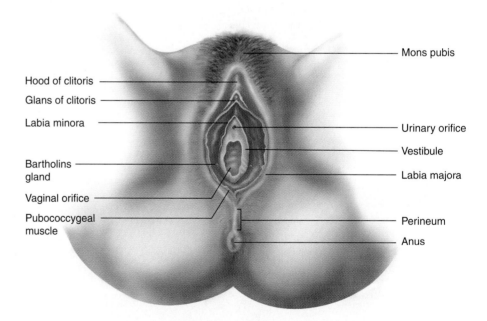

Hood of clitoris

Glans of clitoris

Labia minora

Bartholins gland

Vaginal orifice

Pubococcygeal muscle

Mons pubis

Urinary orifice

Vestibule

Labia majora

Perineum

Anus

Labia minora A pair of fleshy folds that cover the vagina.

Labia majora A pair of fleshy folds that cover the labia minora.

Breasts Network of milk glands and ducts in fatty tissue; secondary sex characteristic.

folds are called the **labia minora**, and the larger, outer pair are called the **labia majora**. The clitoris, a highly sensitive sexual organ, is situated above the vaginal opening.

In addition to the primary sex organs, women have secondary sex characteristics, including the **breasts**. The breasts are supplied with numerous nerve endings, which are important in the delivery of milk to a nursing baby. These nerves also make the breasts highly sensitive to touch, and many women find tactile stimulation to be sexually pleasurable. Sexual arousal, tactile stimulation, and cold temperatures can cause small muscles in the nipples to contract, resulting in erection of the nipples.

Male Sexual Anatomy

The principal reproductive role of male sexual organs is to make numerous viable sperm cells and to deliver them into the female reproductive tract during sexual intercourse. The male sexual and reproductive system consists of two **testes**, the sites of sperm and sex hormone production; a series of connected sperm ducts that originate at the testes, travel through the pelvis, and terminate at the urethra of the penis; glands that produce seminal fluid; and the **penis**, the organ of **copulation** (**FIGURE 16.5**).

The testes are located in a flesh-covered sac, the **scrotum**, which hangs outside the male body. In the embryo, the testes develop inside the body, but just before birth they descend into the scrotum. Inside the scrotum the testes are kept at a temperature a few degrees cooler than the internal body temperature, a condition that is apparently necessary for the production of reproductively capable sperm. One testis is usually a little higher than the other.

When a man ejaculates, sperm are propelled through the sperm ducts and out of the penis by contractions of the smooth muscles that line the ducts and the muscles of the pelvis. As they move out of the male body, the sperm mix with

Testes A pair of male reproductive organs that produce sperm cells and male sex hormones.

Penis The male organ of copulation and urination.

Copulation Sexual intercourse.

Scrotum The sac of skin that contains the testes.

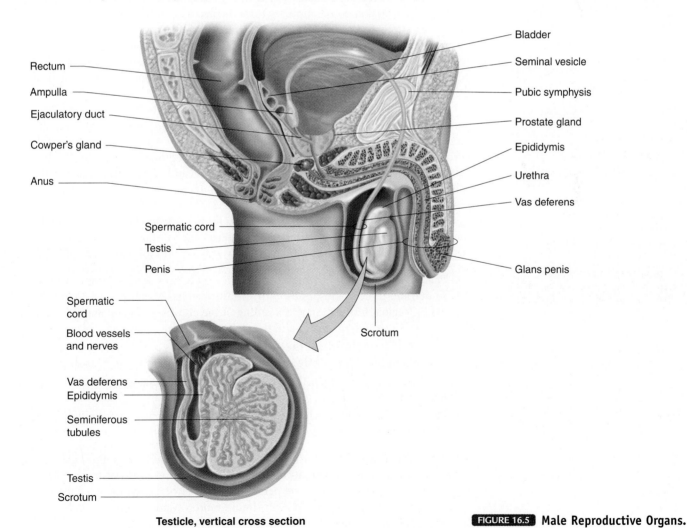

Rectum
Ampulla
Ejaculatory duct
Cowper's gland
Anus
Spermatic cord
Testis
Penis

Bladder
Seminal vesicle
Pubic symphysis
Prostate gland
Epididymis
Urethra
Vas deferens
Glans penis

Spermatic cord
Blood vessels and nerves
Vas deferens
Epididymis
Seminiferous tubules
Testis
Scrotum

Scrotum

Testicle, vertical cross section

FIGURE 16.5 Male Reproductive Organs.

Seminal vesicles Sac-like structures that secrete a fluid that activates the sperm.

Prostate gland Gland at the base of the male bladder that provides seminal fluid.

Cowper's glands Small glands that secrete drops of alkalinizing fluid into the urethra.

Semen A whitish, creamy fluid containing sperm.

Foreskin A fold of skin over the end of the penis.

Circumcision A surgical procedure to remove the foreskin from the penis.

Sexual response involves four phases.

Smegma Cheese-like substance that accumulates under the foreskin of the penis.

Myotonia Muscle tension.

Vasocongestion Engorgement of blood vessels in particular body parts in response to sexual arousal.

Sexual response cycle The physiological response in both men and women; described in four phases.

Orgasm The climax of sexual responses and the release of physiological and sexual tensions.

secretions of seminal fluid from the **seminal vesicles**, **prostate gland**, and **Cowper's glands** to form **semen**. The semen, which is the gelatinous milky fluid emitted at ejaculation, contains a mixture of 300 million sperm cells and about 3 to 6 milliliters of seminal fluid. The seminal fluid contributes 95 percent or more of the entire volume of semen.

The penis is normally soft, but when a male becomes sexually aroused, the internal tissues fill with blood and the penis enlarges and becomes erect. All men are born with a fold of skin, the **foreskin**, which covers the end of the penis. For centuries, Jewish and Moslem families have surgically removed the foreskin from male children for religious reasons. This procedure is called **circumcision**. Although there is no clear medical indication that circumcision is beneficial, removal of the foreskin does eliminate the buildup of **smegma**. The belief that circumcision leads to an increase in sexual arousal because it exposes the tip of the penis, and the related belief that circumcision produces an inability to delay ejaculation, are myths. For most men, circumcision has no effect on sexual arousal and sexual activity.

Sexual Response Cycle

When a person becomes sexually aroused, the brain and nervous system prepare the body for sexual activity. Impulses from the brain are transmitted by the spinal nerves to various parts of the body and cause physiological changes. These changes include the tightening of many skeletal muscles (**myotonia**); changes in the pattern of blood flow or **vasocongestion** (especially an increase in blood flow in the pelvis); increases in heart rate, blood pressure, and respiratory rate; increase in the general level of excitement; and increase in erotic feelings.

Increased pelvic blood flow in the male produces erection of the penis. The penis enlarges because the spongy tissues within it fill with blood. In the female, increased pelvic blood flow produces lubrication of the vagina and swelling of the clitoris and vaginal lips. Vaginal lubrication is produced by the release of fluids from the walls of the vagina. Swelling of the clitoris and vaginal lips is due to the filling with blood of spongy tissues within them. In some women the changes in blood flow due to sexual arousal also produce a swelling of the breasts.

Regardless of the type of sexual stimulation, the physiological response in both men and women is similar and follows a pattern called the **sexual response cycle**, which consists of four phases as identified by Masters and Johnson (**FIGURE 16.6**):

- *Phase 1.* Excitement, in which the person experiences sexual arousal from any source and the body responds with specific changes: erection of the penis in males; vaginal lubrication and swelling of the clitoris and genitalia in females; and sex flush in both males and females.
- *Phase 2.* Plateau, in which the physiological changes of the excitement phase level off, although subjective feelings of sexual arousal may increase.
- *Phase 3.* **Orgasm**, in which the tensions that build up during excitement and plateau are released.
- *Phase 4.* Resolution, in which the body returns to the physiologically nonstimulated state.

There is considerable variation in the extent and duration of the sexual response cycle among individuals of either sex. There is even variation in the nature of the response in the same person, for each sexual encounter is different. Years ago, Masters and Johnson (1966) found more variation in the sexual response cycle for women than for men.

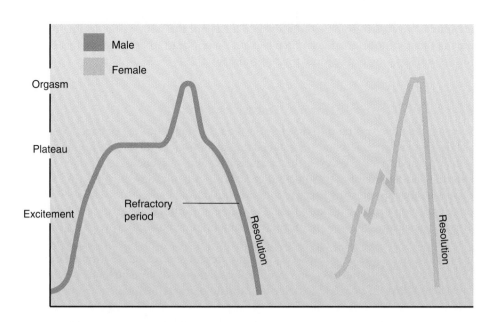

FIGURE 16.6 Sexual Response Cycle as Identified by Masters and Johnson.

Developing Positive Intimate Relationships

We all need intimacy—that feeling of closeness, trust, and openness with another person that tells us that our innermost self can be shared without fear of attack or emotional hurt and that we are understood in the deepest sense possible.

Intimate relationships can have an enormous impact on our sense of vitality and well-being. When an intimate relationship is flowing smoothly, it can produce rich emotional satisfaction unparalleled by any other experience. Those who are involved in genuinely supportive and caring relationships tend to feel unswervingly confident about the potential of life to be harmonious and beautiful. On the other hand, when an intimate relationship is not going well, those involved can be overwhelmed by moroseness, unable to think of anything but their misery. They can be angry, depressed, anxious, or distraught, sometimes to the point of being unable to function at work or at school.

What Intimacy Is

Many people mistakenly equate genuine intimacy with sexual intercourse. That happens because love and affection are feelings associated with intimacy, and in our culture there is much confusion about love and sex. But *intimacy is a feeling, not an act*. It is the *quality* of a relationship between two people—a shared experiencing of their personal lives. People who have an intimate relationship may or may not choose to express their closeness with sex.

Many kinds of intimacies are possible. There are intimacies between opposite-sex peers, same-sex peers, children and parents, members of a family, neighbors, close friends, and even coworkers. Each intimacy has its unique and distinctive quality depending on the people involved, the extent to which their personal histories are similar, and the facets of themselves they choose to share with each other.

Yet intimacies possess certain common characteristics. They are relationships of mutual consent. One person cannot be intimate with another unless both agree that that is what they want. Intimacies tend to grow deeper and richer over time; partners need to share meaningful experiences in order to establish genuine trust and caring. Intimacies also carry the feeling that the personalities of the intimates

Intimacy is a basic human need.

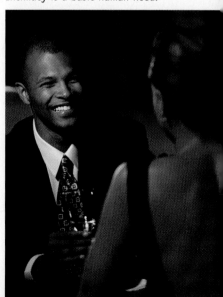

are interconnected in some complex way. This is not the same as the feeling of having their identities merge so they become "one," but rather that they feel both joined and separate at the same time in some way.

The Life Cycle of Intimate Relationships

Intimate relationships tend to develop through the stages of (1) selecting a partner, (2) developing intimacy, and (3) establishing commitment. Before an intimate relationship can develop, however, the partners have to be psychologically open to entering and maintaining it. Some individuals choose not to be involved in an intimate relationship, perhaps because they wish to devote energies to school, work, or self-development, or because they find intimate relationships to be distracting or psychologically threatening. In some instances, previous life experiences can leave an individual fearful of emotional closeness, which can block the establishment of intimacy. In some instances, there are repeated attempts to form relationships; however, without the element of intimacy, these relationships often fail.

Factors that influence the choice of intimate partners include:

- *Proximity.* People are most likely to become intimate with someone with whom they are in physical proximity.
- *Similarity.* Similar age, religion, race, education, and social background affect the possibility for intimacy in two ways: (1) they influence proximity, and (2) they reflect social norms for permissible peer intimacies. Note, for example, biases against interracial and older-younger intimacies. Colleges and universities provide students with relatively easy access to a pool of "eligibles" because they bring together individuals of similar age, religion, intelligence, expectations, and values.
- *Physical appearance.* Physical appearance provides cues that indicate who among the pool of eligibles is a desirable intimate partner. Those who are judged "attractive" tend to be thought of as kind, understanding, and affectionate ("what is beautiful is good"). In addition, pairing with someone who is considered physically attractive enhances an individual's social status and self-esteem.

Developing Intimacy

Most people want their intimate relationship to develop feelings of closeness, positive regard, warmth, and familiarity with the other's innermost thoughts and feelings. This deep knowledge of each other comes from sharing the most important and often secret aspects of our personality—our goals, aspirations, strengths, weaknesses, and physical and sexual desires. The sharing of such private information is called **self-disclosure**.

When relationships begin, little intimate information is disclosed. People talk about the weather, the stock market, or politics. They gossip about professors, students, or other people they know. And, they ask each other the classic leading questions: Where are you from? What do you do? What's your major? People face these questions so many times that they become adept at revealing as much or as little about themselves as feels comfortable. It is when they begin to talk about their personal history, current life problems, hopes and aspirations, and fears and personal failures that they disclose important information—important because disclosing it makes them feel vulnerable. Most people discuss their deepest feelings only with those in whom they have developed considerable trust.

Intimacy develops through a progressive, mutual revealing of innermost thoughts. Psychologists compare people's personalities to onions—having many

Self-disclosure The sharing of private information.

layers from an outer surface to an inner core. As acquaintances gain more and more knowledge about each other, they penetrate deeper and deeper through the layers of each other's personalities, which establishes their intimacy. Another view compares intimate development to the peeling of an artichoke. Resistance and barriers to sharing information about yourself are like the leaves of the artichoke; as intimacy progresses, intimates peel away the leaves to get to each other's "hearts."

Self-disclosure leads to the development of intimacy in two ways. First, you tend to be affected either positively or negatively by the information that is disclosed. If you make a positive judgment, you are likely to want to continue interacting with that person, for you believe that future interactions will be more positive. The same logic applies to negative assessments. If your reaction is unfavorable, you are likely to terminate the relationship, or perhaps maintain it on a lesser level of intimacy.

The second way that self-disclosure leads to intimacy is the *act of* self-disclosure, which, regardless of the information offered, often leads to reciprocal self-disclosure. By sharing important information, you communicate that you trust the other person, and usually that person accepts your trust and becomes more willing to disclose information. In this way intimacy progresses by a cycle of self-disclosure leading to trust, which brings about self-disclosure, which leads to more trust, and so on.

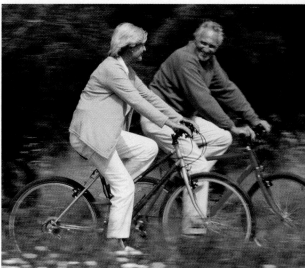

Relationships are key at every age.

Establishing Commitment

After a period of self-disclosure, individuals may sense that their relationship has progressed to a state of "us-ness," that it has become a special friendship, a love relationship, or a marital-type dyad. This state of "us-ness" is one of commitment, which has three aspects:

- *An action, pledge, or promise.* You make a promise and thus announce your intention explicitly, even if it is only to your partner. Various social values and norms regarding keeping promises and the guilt and loss of self-esteem that come with breaking promises are among the "push" factors that keep a person committed. If the promise involves a social ritual (marriage ceremony, getting pinned), then family, friends, and the state become additional "push" factors.

- *A state of being obligated or emotionally compelled.* This state involves a cluster of emotions such as love, comfort, caring, and relief from separation anxiety and loneliness.

- *An unwillingness to consider any partner other than the current one.* The rewards of the current relationship outweigh the costs of forgoing other opportunities for intimacy.

Endings

Everything in the universe (even the universe itself!) has a beginning and an end. Close relationships also have a beginning and an end. Sometimes a relationship lasts for only a few minutes; sometimes it lasts until one of the partners dies (and even then the relationship may still be "alive" in the imagination of the surviving partner). Sometimes the structure of a close relationship persists but the closeness and the dynamism wane, creating a "shell" relationship without vitality. Sometimes a relationship goes through cycles of birth and death within the structure of its ongoingness. When a close relationship ends, some or all of its structure, exchange of resources (love, caring, financial support) and feelings of attachment and emotional bondedness also end.

Endings occur for a variety of reasons. For example, partners' feelings of attachment and bondedness may be absent or weak. Life goals, values, and/or interests may no longer be shared. One or both partners may be unwilling or unable to invest personal resources, such as greater time shared with the partner, or to commit to an exclusive relationship. Whether partners continue in a relationship also is affected by their assessment of other options, such as another potential partner or singlehood. Without appealing alternatives, leaving a relationship may seem difficult, unwise, or impossible.

Another reason ongoingness stops is that the partners, either individually or as a dyad, are unable to move the relationship into its next stage. For example, some couples cannot navigate the transition from being idealistic, passionate lovers to realistic, compassionate lovers. In nonmarital close relationships, a partner may not be considered suitable as a potential marital partner, even in the presence of considerable love, attachment, and liking.

Another factor associated with endings is lack of support, or even hostility, from the partners' social network. Families may not accept a son's or daughter's choice of a partner. Interracial, mentally or physically challenged, and same-sex relationships are still heavily stigmatized in our society.

When a break-up does occur, individuals may feel tired, lethargic, lonely, sad, depressed, angry, resentful, and guilty. They may be unable to sleep or eat, may miss classes or be unable to work. They may withdraw from friends. They may find concentrating difficult, because they are continually thinking about the partner and what happened in the relationship. They may feel helpless ("What will become of me?") and hopeless ("I'll never find a true love"), or skeptical and cynical ("Love can never work out").

Some partners feel relaxed, hopeful, and relieved that what they identify as a bad or going-nowhere relationship has ended, and they are free to pursue personal goals or find a relationship partner who is better suited to them. Sometimes individuals feel euphoric and self-confident. They say that the separation was for the best, and they become more active and outgoing. This positive outlook may alternate with emotional distress.

Communicating in Intimate Relationships

Effective communication is critical for developing and maintaining relationships.

Communication is a symbolic process of creating and sharing meaning. At the heart of communication is an individual communication act, which involves imparting a message to another person to share information or feelings, to coordinate behavior with an individual or group of people, or to persuade someone to do something.

A communication act begins as a mental image—an idea, a wish, or a feeling (or some combination of all three). If humans were capable of mind reading, senders could impart mental images directly to receivers. Few people can read minds, however, so communication requires that thoughts be transformed into symbols that can carry information. Those symbols make up the message. The most common symbols in communication are:

- *Words:* spoken or printed
- *Visual images:* paintings, sculpture
- *Posture or body language:* gaze, touch, smile, physical proximity
- *Objects:* flowers, gifts, food
- *Behaviors:* doing a favor, giving a kiss, ignoring an appointment

The sender's encoding of mental images into the symbols that make up the message is only half of a communication act. The other half is the receiver's reactions, which involve taking in the symbols that make up the message and decoding them into her or his own mental images. Thus, a communication act requires two transformations: in the sender, the transformation of mental images into symbols; in the receiver, the transformation of symbols into mental images.

Consider this example of a communication act between Beth and Ron one morning. Beth hopes to meet Ron later in the day, so she decides to use spoken words as the symbols to encode her thoughts. Beth says, "What are you doing today?" Ron hears Beth's words, and decodes them into a mental image of his schedule for the day.

In this communication act Beth accomplished her goal. But a different outcome could have occurred if one or more of the steps in the communication act had been distorted, weakened, or blocked completely. For example, if Beth had said "What are you doing today?" in a tone of voice that Ron didn't appreciate, or if her words had been misunderstood, the communication process would have been distorted. Every communication act carries two types of message, or potential meaning. The first is the **literal message**, which is the message conveyed by the symbols themselves. The second is the **metamessage** (*meta* is Greek for "beyond," "additional," or "transcendent"), which carries implicit messages about the reason for the communication, how the message is to be interpreted, and the nature of the relationship of the sender and receiver. Most metacommunication occurs unconsciously.

When Beth said to Ron, "What are you doing today?" not only did she send a literal message about the day's events but she also sent several metamessages, including "I care about you" and "An expectation in our relationship that we are interested in each other's daily experiences."

After Beth had asked Ron about his plans for the day, if Ron had kissed Beth and said "Today's a real busy day, thanks for asking," he would have been responding to one of the metamessages in the communication. If Ron had interpreted the metamessage as, "Ron I need to know exactly what you are doing every minute of the day because I can't trust you"—even though Beth didn't intend to impart that message—Ron might have responded angrily with something like "Beth, do you always have to know everything I do!" Her feelings may then have been hurt, and possibly they would have had an argument. Acknowledging and responding to metamessages can sometimes be much more important than dealing with the literal ones.

Sending Clear Messages

A clear message is one in which the symbols represent the sender's intent as closely as possible. Clear messages are best delivered with **I-statements**; these are sentences that begin with (or have as the subject) the pronoun "I." I-statements clearly identify the sender as the source of a thought, emotion, desire, or act: I think. . . I feel. . . I want (need). . . I did (will do). . . .

You-statements, which begin with (or have as the subject) the pronoun "you," as in "You always. . . ," "You never. . . ," "You are. . . ," or the interrogatives, "Why don't you. . . ?" or "How could you. . . ?" often are put-downs or character assassinations. They imply that the receiver is not OK. Very often the not-OK message is explicit, as in "You're incompetent" or "You're stupid"—just about any negative adjective will do. People often respond to the metamessage in a you-statement, which is "I think you're no good," by feeling attacked, which can lead to hurt feelings and counterattacks or withdrawal.

Effective Listening

Effective communication requires both sending and receiving, both talking and listening. Effective listening is important because the receiver not only takes in the sender's message but also helps to establish the physical and emotional context for the com-

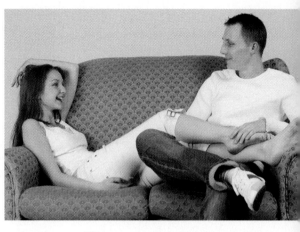

When you are in an intimate relationship, you should feel understood and accepted for who you are.

Literal message Message that is conveyed by symbols.

Metamessage Way the message is interpreted between sender and receiver.

I-statements Statements beginning with "I"; positive communication skill.

You-statements Statements beginning with "you"; negative communication skill.

Feedback Receiver response to a message, letting the sender know the message was received and what the message was.

munication. The listener also must communicate to the sender that the sender's message was received. This is called **feedback**. Some techniques for effective receiving are giving the sender your full attention, making eye contact, listening, being empathic, being open for receiving the message, giving verbal feedback, acknowledging the sender's feelings, praising the sender's efforts, and being unconditional.

Expressing Anger Constructively

Disagreements and conflicts are inevitable in any close relationship. The notion that people in intimate relationships shouldn't have to fight because love makes them see eye to eye on everything, or the idea that you can't possibly be angry with someone you love, is a romantic myth. By expressing anger constructively, intimates fight for the success of their relationship as well as for their individual needs.

Physical Activity and Health Connection

Participation in regular physical activity can make your body more attractive to others. As fitness improves, your self-image and self-concept also tend to improve. This can make you more self-confident. If you look good and feel good, others will find this attractive. From a physiological perspective, physical activity can also improve circulation and physical endurance, enhancing the sexual response.

concept connections

1. *Sex* **refers to a person's biological classification as male or female.** Beyond the biological classification, sex is associated with sexual behaviors. Sexuality is distinct from sex and consists of aspects of a person's sense of self that are used to create sexual experiences.

2. **A person's sexual psychology is rooted in gender identity, which guides gender role behaviors.** Gender identity is the sense of *being male* or *being female*.

3. **A person's sexual biology is determined by genetic makeup, which in turns determines the nature of the sexual reproductive system.** Female and male reproductive biology is genetically determined at conception. Secondary sex characteristics externally distinguish males and females from one another. Males: testes, sperm ducts, semen-producing glands, and penis. Females: ovaries, fallopian tubes, uterus, vagina, and external genitalia.

4. **Sexual response involves four phases.** *Excitement:* person experiences sexual arousal and physiological changes begin (penile erection, vaginal lubrication). *Plateau:* physiological changes begin to level off. *Orgasm:* sexual experience climaxes. *Resolution:* physiologically, the body returns to a nonaroused state.

5. **Effective communication is critical for developing and maintaining relationships.** Communication occurs between two people: a sender and a receiver. The messages we send (verbally and by our actions) are sometimes misread; therefore, it is critical that communication between two people be clear and that both the sender and receiver establish good listening habits.

Terms

Sex, 352
Gametes, 352
Fertilization, 352
Sexual, 352
Sexuality, 352
Sexual orientation, 353
Heterosexuals, 353
Bisexuals, 353
Homosexuals, 353
Gender identity, 354
Gender role, 354
Ova, ovum, 354
Secondary sex characteristics, 354
Ovaries, 354

Fallopian tubes, 354
Uterus, 354
Vagina, 354
Cervix, 354
Ovulation, 354
Clitoris, 354
Labia minora, 356
Labia majora, 356
Breasts, 356
Testes, 357
Penis, 357
Copulation, 357
Scrotum, 357
Seminal vesicles, 358
Prostate gland, 358

Cowper's glands, 358
Semen, 358
Foreskin, 358
Circumcision, 358
Smegma, 358
Myotonia, 358
Vasocongestion, 358
Sexual response cycle, 358
Orgasm, 358
Self-disclosure, 360
Literal message, 363
Metamessage, 363
I-statements, 363
You-statements, 363
Feedback, 364

making the connection

Jeff and Susan realized that their relationship was important to them and that they both needed to work on their communication skills. The communication skills they agreed to work on included sending clearer messages to one another by using I-statements and employing effective listening techniques like making eye contact, being empathic, acknowledging and praising the sender's message, and giving verbal feedback to one another.

Critical Thinking

1. Read the following scenario and identify several communication problems. How could Bob and Sandy have handled this differently?
Bob: Well, Sandy, you know that this weekend is the big reunion of all my fraternity brothers, and I'd like you to join me in celebrating our 100-year anniversary!
Sandy: Now you ask! I've already told my theater group that we would join them for their weekend outing.
Bob: Great, you didn't even ask me, you just went ahead and made plans for me this weekend!
Sandy: Ask you? You have been so busy lately with work and school, I haven't even had a chance to talk to you, let alone ask you if you wanted to spend the weekend with me and the theater group.
Bob: Oh great, now it is my fault that I've been working so hard and trying to get good grades. Go ahead, blame it on me!
Sandy: Okay! It's your fault we never spend any time together. I'm sick of this! What will it be, *your*

fraternity brothers or me?
Bob: Well, now I'm having to choose between you and my fraternity brothers. That's easy! My fraternity brothers any day—at least they understand how hard it is to work and go to school!

2. "An intimate relationship may be sexual, but a sexual relationship is not necessarily an intimate one." Discuss the difference(s) between an intimate relationship and a sexual relationship.

3. Identify ten terms that are gender-biased. Example: fireman.

4. Identify five television shows that have characters in stereotypical male or female roles. Identify the characters and briefly explain the role they play.

5. Do you and/or your partner wish to increase your level of communication? If so, what steps will you take to do so?

References

Masters, W., & Johnson, V. (1966). *Human Sexual Response*. Boston: Little, Brown.

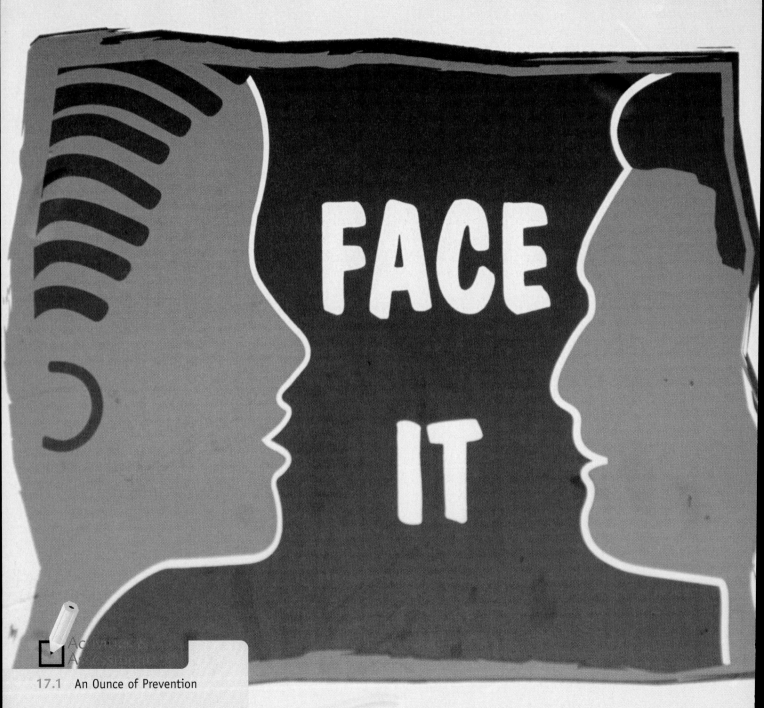

STOP AIDS

FACE IT

IT STARTS WITH YO

17.1 An Ounce of Prevention

17.2 Can You Be Assertive When You Need to Be?

Preventing Sexually Transmitted Diseases

Ken has a close friend, Amy, whom he loves very much. Ken has never been closer to anyone than he is to Amy. They attend the same college and get along well. Amy and Ken are best friends, and they have a close relationship, but Ken wants to take it to the level of sexual intimacy to show the depth of his love. Amy values the intimacy she has with Ken, but is not sure she is ready for sex, or that she even wants to include sexual intimacy and intercourse in their relationship. She feels uncomfortable discussing her feelings about these issues with Ken.

concepts

1. Sexually transmitted diseases are infections that are transferred from one person to another through sexual contact.

2. The United States has the highest rates of sexually transmitted diseases in the industrialized world.

3. Several factors increase the risk of contracting a sexually transmitted disease.

4. Common STDs include *Trichomonas* and *Gardnerella vaginalis* infections, chlamydia, gonorrhea, syphilis, herpes, genital warts, pubic lice, and scabies.

5. AIDS is caused by the human immuno-deficiency virus (HIV).

6. Preventing STDs requires health programs for education and treatment.

http://physicalactivity.jbpub.com

The Web site for this book is a great source for supplementary physical health information for both students and instructors. Visit **http://physicalactivity.jbpub.com** to find a variety of useful tools for learning, thinking, and teaching.

Introduction

Enjoying our sexuality is a normal and healthy part of our lives. Sexual behavior is an instinctive form of physical intimacy. It is most often performed for the purpose of expressing affection and enjoying oneself. When we decide to have sexual contact, we want it be satisfying for ourselves and our partner. We also need to understand what responsibilities our sexual behavior entails for both ourselves and our partner. For example, there are many types of infections that can be transferred from one person to another through sexual contact. These infections are called **sexually transmitted diseases (STDs)** or *sexually transmitted infections (STIs)*. Sexual responsibility related to STDs requires the disclosure of infection from or exposure to STDs. Each person must inform his or her partner about having or being exposed to an STD because of the serious health consequences. If you are infected, you must refrain from behaviors such as sexual intercourse, oral-genital sex, or other high-risk behaviors that may infect your partner.

Sexually transmitted diseases are more than humiliating and a nuisance. Some of these diseases may lead to major illness, particularly for women and their unborn babies. STDs can cause pelvic inflammatory disease, tubal pregnancy, sterility, certain types of cancer, or blindness. Some last a lifetime. There are more than 65 million people living with incurable STDs in the United States (Centers for Disease Control and Prevention [CDC], 2005). A few can be fatal. AIDS, genital warts, herpes, syphilis, and hepatitis have all been known to cause death. Sexually responsible people will take measures to reduce their risk of becoming infected with an STD. They will also reduce the risk of transmitting an STD to their sex partners. Each person is responsible for practicing safer sex. Therefore, education about the prevention of these diseases is important.

STD Statistics

Despite the fact that a great deal of progress has been made in STD prevention over the past couple of decades, the United States continues to have the highest rates of STDs in the industrialized world. Nearly 19 million new cases of STDs are reported each year in the United States, with almost half (48 percent) occurring in people 25 years or younger (Weinstock, German, & Cates, 2004). In fact, one in two sexually active youth will have contracted an STD by the age of 25.

STD Risk Factors

Most STDs are treatable; however, preventing an STD is easier than treating a disease once it occurs. Several factors increase the risk of contracting an STD. Understanding these factors can help you decrease your risk of infection.

Failure to Inform

From a personal and moral responsibility perspective, if a person knows that he or she is infected with an STD, it is that person's duty to inform his or her partner. Does this always occur in reality? No. Although failure to disclose the existence of an STD may result from shame or embarrassment or dishonesty, sometimes it is due to a person truthfully not knowing that he or she is infected, either because the individual has no symptoms or because he or she does not recognize the meaning of the symptoms. If a person has an incurable STD, the use of safer sex prac-

Sexually transmitted diseases are infections that are transferred from one person to another through sexual contact.

Sexually transmitted diseases (STDs) Diseases that are primarily contracted through sexual contact.

The United States has the highest rates of sexually transmitted diseases in the industrialized world.

Several factors increase the risk of contracting a sexually transmitted disease.

tices is even more essential. Safer sex practices are things one does not only to lower one's risk of getting an STD but also of transmitting it to another person.

Multiple Sexual Partners

There is a large pool in our society of unmarried, sexually active people because many individuals become active in late adolescence. This group consists of those who delay marriage until their mid- to late twenties and early thirties, or later, and those who are divorced or widowed and have subsequent sexual partners. One-third of unmarried, sexually active people report having more than one sexual partner in the previous year.

False Sense of Security

Using birth control pills tends to decrease the use of condoms and spermicides, both of which help prevent transmission of STDs. The availability of antibiotics has made many people less fearful of sexually transmitted diseases. They believe that as long as there is a cure for syphilis and gonorrhea, there is nothing to worry about.

Absence of Signs and Symptoms

Some STDs have very mild, or no, symptoms, which permits a worsening of the infection and the possibility of unknowingly passing it to others. Most people with chlamydia have no symptoms, for example. Approximately 80 percent of women who contract gonorrhea do not know it. People infected with the human immunod-eficiency virus (HIV) can have mild or no symptoms for years, yet still be infectious.

Untreated Conditions

Some individuals lack sufficient knowledge of the signs and symptoms of STDs to know that they are infected. Those who are not accustomed to seeking health care, or who cannot afford it, are less likely to seek treatment for an infection. Furthermore, many individuals with STDs do not comply with treatment regimens. When medications are not taken for the required length of time, an infection may not be completely eradicated even though symptoms may disappear, and people who do not complete treatment may still be infectious.

Impaired Judgment

The use of drugs, including alcohol, can increase the risk of transmitting STDs because people with impaired judgment do not stop to think about using con-doms. Also, people in this state may be more likely to have sex with someone they do not know; this also means they know nothing of their partner's sexual and drug history.

Lack of Immunity

Some STD-causing organisms, especially viruses, can escape the body's immune defenses, causing individuals to remain infected and to transmit the infection. This may permit reinfection and it also makes the development of vaccinations difficult to impossible.

Reactions to STDS

Many people who contract a sexually transmitted disease are embarrassed or ashamed to discuss it with their health care provider or partner. There are usually two reactions to a sexually transmitted disease: (1) it is shameful to have one, and (2) "It won't happen to me."

Value Judgments

Unlike nearly all other kinds of infections, STDs are associated with sinfulness, dirtiness, condemnation, shame, guilt, and disgust. These negative attitudes keep people from getting checkups, contacting partners when an STD has been diagnosed, and talking to new partners about previous exposures. In the nineteenth century, when syphilis was a scourge of Europe, rather than trying to prevent its spread (effective treatments had not yet been invented), countries blamed the disease on the weak character or immorality of their neighbors: the English referred to syphilis as the "French disease," and the French called it the "Spanish disease." This prejudice and scapegoating helped spread the disease.

Denial

With respect to contracting an STD, many people think "It can't happen to me" or "This person is too nice to have an STD" or "This isn't the type of person who would have an STD." Because there are no vaccinations against the infectious agents that cause sexually transmitted diseases, the only way to prevent them is for sexually active individuals who are not in *monogamous* (lifelong single-partner) sexual relationships to assume responsibility for protecting themselves and their partners. This means becoming aware of the signs and symptoms of the common STDs and seeking treatment when such signs occur. It means that sexually active people who have more than one partner within a year should obtain periodic (about every 6 months) STD checkups. It also means knowing about and practicing "safer sex."

Common STDs include *Trichomonas* and *Gardnerella vaginalis* infections, chlamydia, gonorrhea, syphilis, herpes, genital warts, pubic lice, and scabies.

Trichomonas vaginalis A protozoan that causes trichomoniasis, whose symptoms include a foul-smelling, foamy-white or yellow-green discharge that irritates the vagina.

Gardnerella vaginalis Bacterium that causes vaginal infection; symptoms of infection include vaginal irritation.

Common STDS

There are more than 25 diseases that are transmitted through sexual activity, the most common being genital warts (human papilloma virus, or HPV), trichomoniasis, chlamydia, herpes, gonorrhea, hepatitis B, syphilis, and HIV/AIDS (FIGURE 17.1 and TABLE 17.1). The major infectious agents and the diseases they cause are provided in TABLE 17.2 . Dealing directly and responsibly with STDs is not easy. However, we owe it to ourselves and the people we care about to do so.

Trichomonas and *Gardnerella Vaginalis* Infections

Referred to as a sexually related disease (SRD), vaginal infections caused by the protozoan ***Trichomonas vaginalis*** and the bacterium ***Gardnerella vaginalis*** are transmitted during intercourse. Symptoms tend to occur only in women (vaginal itching and a cheesy, odorous discharge from the vagina), but the organisms can survive in the urethra of the penis and under the penile foreskin. A man who harbors these organisms can infect other partners or even reinfect the partner who transmitted the organisms to him. Medications can eliminate these infections, and it is essential for both partners to undergo treatment.

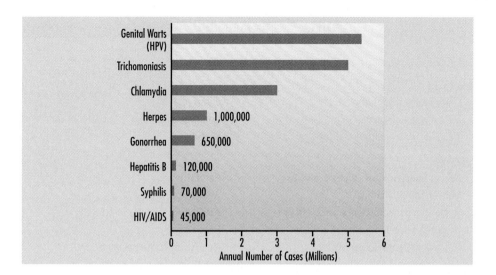

FIGURE 17.1 **Estimated Yearly Number of STDs in the United States.** SOURCE: Edlin, G., & Golanty, E. (2004). *Health and Wellness*, 8th ed. Boston: Jones and Bartlett, 217.

TABLE 17.1	Common Sexually Transmitted Diseases

STD	Symptoms	Treatment
HIV/AIDS	Flu-like symptoms followed by any of a number of diseases characteristic of immunodeficiency	New drugs may retard viral reproduction temporarily; opportunistic infections can be treated to some degree
Chlamydia	Usually occur within 3 weeks: Infected men have a discharge from the penis and painful urination; women may have a vaginal discharge, but often are asymptomatic	Antibiotics
Genital warts	Usually occur within 1 to 3 months: small, dry growths on the genitals, anus, cervix, and possibly mouth	Podophyllin
Gonorrhea	Usually occur within 2 weeks: discharge from the penis, vagina, or anus; pain on urination or defecation or during sexual intercourse; pain and swelling in the pelvic region; genital and oral infections may be asymptomatic	Antibiotics
Hepatitis B	Low-grade fever, fatigue, headaches, loss of appetite, nausea, dark urine, jaundice	Rest, proper nutrition; vaccination for hepatitis B
Genital herpes	Usually occur within 2 weeks: painful blisters on site(s) of infection (genitals, anus, cervix); occasionally itching, painful urination, and fever	None; acyclovir relieves symptoms
Molluscum contagiosum	Smooth, rounded, shiny, whitish growths on the skin of the trunk and anogenital region	Surgical
Pubic lice	Usually occur within 5 weeks: intense itching in the genital region; lice may be visible in pubic hair; small white eggs may be visible on pubic hair	Gamma benzene hexachloride
Scabies	Tiny, itchy lesions caused by mites burrowing into the skin	Topical insecticides
Syphilis	Usually occur within 3 weeks: a chancre (painless sore) on the genitals, anus, or mouth; secondary stage, skin rash (if left untreated); tertiary stage includes diseases of several body organs	Antibiotics
Trichomoniasis	Yellowish-green vaginal discharge with an unpleasant odor; vaginal itching; occasionally painful intercourse	Metronidazole

SOURCE: Edlin, G., & Golanty, E. (2004). *Health and Wellness*, 8th ed. Boston: Jones and Bartlett, 216.

TABLE 17.2	Agents That Cause Common STDs

Infectious agent	Disease
Bacteria	
Chlamydia trachomatis	Chlamydia
Neisseria gonorrhoeae	Gonorrhea
Treponema pallidum	Syphilis
Viruses	
Herpes simplex virus, types 1 and 2	Genital herpes
Human papillomavirus	Anogenital warts
Human immunodeficiency virus (HIV)	AIDS
Hepatitis virus B	Hepatitis
Molluscum contagiosum virus	Molluscum contagiosum
Protozoa	
Trichomonas vaginalis	Trichomoniasis (vaginitis)
Protozoa	
Phthirus pubis	Lice ("crabs")
Sarcoptes scabiei	Mites ("scabies")

SOURCE: Edlin, G., & Golanty, E. (2004). *Health and Wellness*, 8th ed. Boston: Jones and Bartlett, 218.

Chlamydia

Chlamydia Sexually transmitted disease caused by the bacterium *Chlamydia trachomatis*.

Epididymitis Inflammation of the epididymis (structure that connects the vas deferens and the testes).

Pelvic inflammatory disease (PID) Infection of the female reproductive organs; specifically, the uterus, fallopian tubes, and pelvic cavity.

Chlamydia is caused by the bacterium *Chlamydia trachomatis*, which specifically infests certain cells lining the mucous membranes of the genitals, mouth, anus, and rectum, the conjunctiva of the eyes, and occasionally the lungs. The chlamydial bacteria bind to their surfaces and induce the host cells to engulf them. After gaining entrance to the cell, these organisms resist a host cell's defenses and eventually "steal" from the host cell the biochemical compounds required for their own survival. The chlamydial organisms use the stolen nutrients to reproduce and multiply, and ultimately the host cells die. In as many as half of all cases, chlamydia occurs simultaneously with gonorrhea.

One reason that chlamydial infections are so prevalent is that infected individuals often have extremely mild or no symptoms. Thus, infected individuals can unknowingly transmit the infection to new sex partners. When symptoms do occur, they include pain during urination in both men and women (dysuria) and a whitish discharge from the penis or vagina. Symptoms generally appear within 7 to 21 days after infection.

An infection caused by chlamydia can be readily treated with antibiotics if diagnosed early. Left untreated, the chlamydial bacteria can multiply and cause inflammation and damage of the reproductive organs in both sexes. In men, untreated chlamydia can result in inflammation of the epididymis (**epididymitis**), characterized by pain, swelling, and tenderness in the scrotum, and sometimes by mild fever. In women, untreated chlamydia can lead to **pelvic inflammatory disease (PID)**.

Gonorrhea

Gonorrhea, also know as "the clap" or the "drip," is caused by the bacterium *Neisseria gonorrhoeae*. Gonorrheal organisms specifically infect the mucous membranes of the body, most often the genitals, reproductive organs, mouth and throat, anus, and eyes. *N. gonorrhoeae* cannot survive on toilet seats, doorknobs, bedsheets, clothes, or towels. Transmission in adults almost always occurs by genital, oral, or anal sexual contact; infection of the eyes occurs by hand (often through self-infection).

Although the bacteria causing them are quite different, the symptoms of gonorrheal and chlamydial infections are very similar. Like chlamydia, many people infected with gonorrheal organisms do not develop symptoms and their infections go unnoticed. If the infection progresses, men may develop epididymitis and women may develop infections of the uterus, fallopian tubes, and pelvic region. *Such infections may cause sterility.* When symptoms appear, they include painful urination in both sexes and a yellowish discharge from the penis or vagina. Occasionally there is pain in the groin, testes, or lower abdomen. The first symptoms of gonorrhea usually appear within 7 to 10 days after exposure.

Gonorrhea can be treated with antibiotics. However, new antibiotic-resistant strains of the organism are constantly evolving. In nearly half of all cases of gonorrhea, chlamydia also is present. Individuals undergoing diagnosis for gonorrhea should also be tested for chlamydia.

Syphilis

Syphilis is caused by a spiral-shaped bacterium called *Treponema pallidum*. These organisms are transmitted from person to person through genital, oral, and anal contact, as well as being acquired from blood. Syphilis can also be transmitted from a mother to her unborn fetus, perhaps as early as the ninth week of pregnancy.

The first noticeable sign of syphilis is a painless open sore called a **chancre** (pronounced "shanker"), which can appear any time between the first week and third month after infection. If the infection is not treated within that period, the chancre will heal and the disease will enter a secondary stage, characterized by a skin rash, hair loss, and the appearance of round, flat-topped growths on most areas of the body. Left untreated, the signs of the secondary stage also disappear, and the infection enters a symptomless (latency) period during which the syphilis organisms multiply in many other regions of the body. In the final, tertiary stage, the disease damages vital organs, such as the heart or brain, causing severe symptoms and leading to death. Syphilis can be treated with antibiotics at any stage of the infection.

Herpes

Herpes is caused by the herpes simplex virus, or HSV. Various strains of HSV can cause cold sores on the mouth ("fever blisters"), skin rashes, mononucleosis, and lesions on the penis, vagina, or rectum. Each year up to 500,000 adults acquire a genital herpes infection. As many as one of four American adults have already been infected with genital herpes.

Genital herpes infections are caused most frequently by the viral strain HSV-2. Oral herpes is caused most frequently by HSV-1. However, both HSV-2 and HSV-1 can cause genital and oral infections with virtually identical symptoms. Thus people with oral herpes can transmit the infection to partners via oral sex. Once a person has been infected, oral HSV-1 infections tend to recur much more frequently than do oral HSV-2 infections. Conversely, genital HSV-2 infections tend to recur

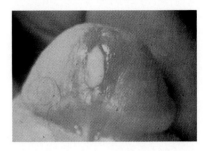
Gonorrheal discharge from the penis.

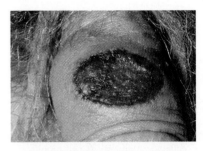
The first physical sign of a syphilis infection is an open lesion called a chancre.

Gonorrhea Sexually transmitted disease caused by the bacterium *Neisseria gonorrhoeae*.

Syphilis Sexually transmitted disease caused by spirochete bacteria (*Treponema pallidum*).

Chancre The primary lesion of syphilis, which appears as a hard, painless sore or ulcer, often on the penis or vaginal tissue; pronounced "shanker."

Herpes Sexually transmitted disease caused by herpes simplex virus, or HSV.

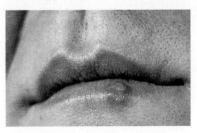
A cold sore is common among people infected by HSV.

more frequently than genital HSV-1 infections. Oral herpes can occur without sexual contact; however, genital herpes cannot occur without some form of sexual contact, either vaginal, anal, oral, or through masturbation.

A herpes lesion on the genitals usually appears within 2 to 20 days after contact with the virus. Transmission of the virus via bed linen, clothing, towels, toilet seats, and hot tubs is highly unlikely. The major symptoms of a genital herpes infection are the presence of one or more blisters, which eventually break to become wet, painful sores that last about 2 or 3 weeks; fever; and occasionally pain in the lower abdomen. Eventually these initial symptoms disappear, but the herpes virus remains dormant in certain of the body's nerve cells, permitting periodic recurrences of the symptoms, called "flare-ups," at or near the site(s) of the initial infection. Stress, anxiety, improper nutrition, sunlight, and skin irritation can bring on flare-ups.

There is no cure for herpes. Infected individuals remain so for life. The drug *acyclovir* can minimize the duration and severity of the symptoms of an initial infection or a flare-up.

Herpes is extremely contagious when a sore is present. People with open lesions should avoid sex with others until the lesions disappear. Even if no sore is present, transmission is possible, although much less likely, through the "shedding" of viral particles from the skin.

Because the herpes virus remains in the body, and because flare-ups are a persistent possibility, some people believe that infected persons can never be sexually active. This is not true. People with herpes can learn to manage the condition. In many instances, after one or two episodes, they can recognize an oncoming flare-up because they get a tingling sensation, itching, pain, or numbness at the site of the initial infection. This can be a signal to refrain from sexual contact. If used appropriately, this signal can protect against the spread of herpes.

Because genital herpes is associated with a risk of cervical cancer, women with herpes are especially urged to have annual Pap smears to ascertain the condition of the vagina and cervix.

Sexually Transmitted Warts

Sexually transmitted warts (*Condylomata acuminata*), also known as genital or venereal warts, are hard, cauliflower-like growths that appear in men on the penis, in women on the external genitals and cervix, and in both sexes in the anal region. Warts are caused by several of the approximately sixty varieties of **human papillomavirus (HPV)**. When HPV infects skin cells and cells of the genital tract, it causes them to multiply, thus forming the wart. Infection with many varieties of HPV is often more of a nuisance than it is dangerous.

Sexually transmitted warts usually appear about 3 months after contact with an infected person. They can be removed by coating the wart with a liquid containing podophyllin, which dries the wart. In severe cases, wart removal is accomplished by freezing the warts with liquid nitrogen or removing them with laser surgery.

Hepatitis B

Hepatitis B is a disease of the liver caused by the hepatitis B virus (HBV). Hepatitis B is transmitted sexually and in blood, similar to HIV transmission, whereas other types of hepatitis are transmitted in fecally contaminated food. Hepatitis B is more easily transmitted than HIV and it is estimated that worldwide there are 300 million people infected with HBV. You are at increased risk of contracting HBV if you are sexually active, have unsafe sex, have sex with more than one partner, have

Sexually transmitted warts Hard growths on the skin of the genitals or anus, caused by an infection with human papillomavirus, or HPV.

Human papillomavirus (HPV) Genus of viruses including those causing papillomas (small nipple-like protrusions of the skin or mucous membrane) and warts.

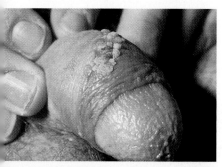
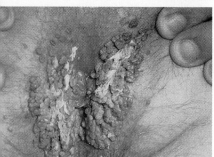

Genital warts on the penis (upper), and vaginal (lower) area.

another STD, work in health care, or share needles. You can also contract HBV if you are exposed to an infected person's blood via cuts or open sores. Although it is very rare in the United States, you can contract the hepatitis B virus through transfusions of infected blood or blood products.

There is no cure for HBV; however, an HBV vaccine is available, and everyone is advised to be vaccinated—especially children, health care workers, and others who are at high risk of exposure (sexually active). The CDC recommends HBV vaccination for infants and young adults before they become sexually active.

Pubic Lice

Pubic lice (*Phthirus pubis*), also known as "crabs," are barely visible insects that live on hair shafts primarily in the genital-rectal region and occasionally on hair in the armpits, beard, and eyelashes. The organisms' claws are specifically adapted for grasping hairs with the diameter of pubic and axillary hair, which differs in diameter from the shafts of scalp hair. Thus pubic lice are not usually found on the head (scalp hair is the ecological niche of the head louse, *Pediculus humanus capitis*).

Lice feed on blood taken from tiny blood vessels in the skin, which they pierce with their mouths. Some people are sensitive to the bites and may experience itching, which is often the main symptom of infestation. The lice can also be seen; they look like small freckles. The eggs of lice are enclosed in small white pods (called "nits"), which attach to hair shafts. The presence of nits is also a sign of infestation.

Transfer of lice is via physical—usually sexually—contact. They can also be transmitted via contact with objects on which eggs might have been laid, such as towels, bed linens, and clothes. An infestation of pubic lice can be eliminated by washing the pubic hair with liquids or shampoos containing agents that specifically kill lice (pyrethrins, piperonyl butoxide, and gamma benzene hydrochloride). All of an infected person's clothes, towels, and bed linens should also be washed with cleaning agents made specifically for killing lice.

Scabies

Scabies is an infestation of certain regions of the skin by extremely small (invisible to the naked eye) mites, *Sarcoptes scabiei*. The mites burrow into the skin, where they live and lay eggs. The tiny lesions produced by the mites often cause intense itching, which is the major sign of a scabies infection. The mites produce tiny burrows across skin lines, which often go unnoticed. Occasionally, an infestation will produce small round nodules. The mites tend to live in the webs between the fingers, on the sides of fingers, and on the wrists, elbows, breasts, abdomen, penis, and buttocks. Rarely do mites live on the face, neck, upper back, palms, or soles.

Scabies can be transmitted both sexually and nonsexually. All that is required is close personal contact. The itching and physical symptoms often take several weeks to appear. Scabies can be treated with topical agents that kill the mites and their eggs.

HIV Infection and AIDS

The acquired immunodeficiency syndrome (AIDS) was first recognized in 1981 and has since become a major worldwide pandemic. AIDS is caused by the **human immunodeficiency virus (HIV)**. By leading to the destruction or functional impairment of cells of the immune system, notably CD4+ T cells, HIV progressively destroys the body's ability to fight infections and certain cancers. An HIV-infected person is diagnosed with AIDS when his or her immune system is seriously compromised and manifestations of HIV infection are severe. The CDC currently

Pubic lice Small insects that live in hair in the genital-rectal region.

Scabies Infestation of the skin by microscopic mites (insects).

Human immunodeficiency virus (HIV) The virus that causes AIDS; it causes a defect in the body's immune system by invading and then multiplying within the white blood cells.

AIDS is caused by the human immunodeficiency virus (HIV).

defines AIDS in an adult or adolescent aged 13 years or older as the presence of one of 26 conditions indicative of severe immunosuppression associated with HIV infection, such as *Pneumocystis carinii* pneumonia (PCP), a condition extraordinarily rare in people without HIV infection (CDC, 1994). Most other AIDS-defining conditions are also opportunistic infections that rarely cause harm in healthy individuals. A diagnosis of AIDS also is given to HIV-infected individuals when their CD4+ T-cell count falls below 200 cells per cubic millimeter (mm³) of blood. Healthy adults usually have CD4+ T-cell counts of 600 to 1500 cells per mm³ of blood. In HIV-infected children younger than 13 years, the CDC definition of AIDS is similar to that in adolescents and adults, except for the addition of certain infections commonly seen in pediatric patients with HIV (CDC, 1994).

At the end of 2003, an estimated 1,039,000 to 1,185,000 persons in the United States were living with HIV/AIDS (Glynn & Rhodes, 2005). Approximately 40,000 new HIV infections occur each year in the United States, 73 percent of them among men and 27 percent among women (Glynn & Rhodes, 2005). Of the new infections among males, approximately 63 percent were from male-to-male sexual contact, and 17 percent from heterosexual contact (**FIGURE 17.2**). Of the new infections among females, 79 percent were from heterosexual contact, and 19 percent from injection drug use. Minority groups in the United States have also been disproportionately affected by the epidemic (**FIGURE 17.3**). African Americans,

FIGURE 17.2 **Exposure Categories of Adults and Adolescents Who Received a Diagnosis of HIV/AIDS, 2003.** The figure is based on data from 33 areas with long-term, confidential name-based HIV reporting. SOURCE: Centers for Disease Control and Prevention. (2005, June). A glance at the HIV/AIDS epidemic. Online: http://www.cdc.gov/hiv/pubs/Facts/At-A-Glance.htm.

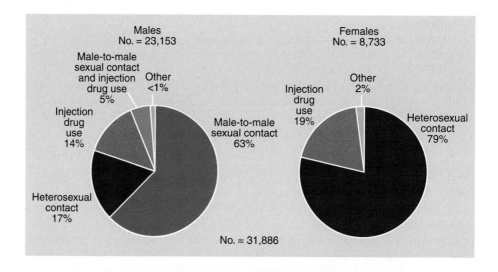

FIGURE 17.3 **Race/Ethnicity of Persons (Including Children) Who Received a Diagnosis of HIV/AIDS, 2003.** The figure is based on data from 33 areas with long-term, confidential name-based HIV reporting. It includes persons of unknown race or multiple races. SOURCE: Centers for Disease Control and Prevention. (2005, June). A glance at the HIV/AIDS epidemic. Online: http://www.cdc.gov/hiv/pubs/Facts/At-A-Glance.htm.

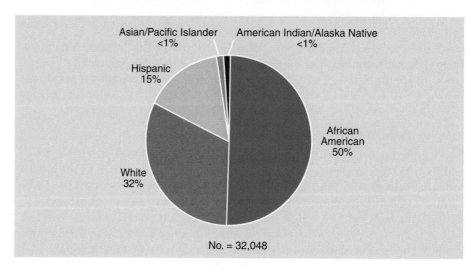

who make up approximately 12 percent of the population, accounted for half of the new HIV/AIDS cases diagnosed. As of 2003, an estimated 524,060 Americans had died of AIDS (CDC, 2004).

Worldwide, an estimated 40 million people are living with HIV/AIDS (Joint United Nations Program on HIV/AIDS [UNAIDS], 2005). About 80 percent of reported new cases now arise in developing countries where no funds are available for HIV/AIDS education and prevention programs. Sub-Saharan Africa has the highest number of cases, with approximately 26 million people living with HIV/AIDS. As of 2003, AIDS had killed more than 25 million people since it was first recognized in 1981, making it one of the most devastating epidemics in recorded history (UNAIDS, 2005).

METHODS OF TRANSMISSION   HIV is transmitted exclusively via blood, semen (which contains small amounts of blood), and vaginal fluids. The virus is not transmitted by touching the skin or clothes of an infected person, by saliva, by shared toilets or by air, food, or water that has been touched by an infected person. Indeed, hardly any HIV transmission has been found among family members who live in intimate contact with HIV-infected hemophiliacs who received the virus from HIV-contaminated blood products used to treat their hereditary bleeding disorder.

HIV is a **retrovirus**, which means that once it gains entry to a cell it incorporates itself into the host cell's DNA. This allows HIV to manufacture many copies of itself, which eventually infect neighboring cells. Because HIV incorporates itself into host cells, it cannot be eliminated from an infected person's body. HIV infections are lifelong.

> **Retrovirus** A type of virus (such as the one that causes AIDS) that can invade cells and integrate its own genetic information into chromosomes.

Within a few weeks of individuals' becoming infected with HIV, they usually experience flu-like symptoms from which they eventually recover. Their immune systems are still intact, and they produce copious antibodies to HIV. The mounting of an immune response in the early phases of an HIV infection provides the basis for HIV testing. Nearly all of the tests for HIV infection detect antibodies to HIV. A positive result ("seropositive") indicates that a person has been exposed to sufficient quantities of HIV particles to mount an immune response. The first stage of HIV infection is known as *silent infection*.

Some HIV-infected individuals will progress to the second stage of infection, *symptomatic infection*. The first signs of AIDS are usually mononucleosis-like symptoms (swollen lymph glands, fever, night sweats) and possibly headaches and impaired mental functioning caused by HIV infection of the brain. As the disease progresses, individuals often suffer weight loss, infections on the skin (shingles) or the throat ("thrush"), and one or more opportunistic infections, perhaps including cancer.

Because there is now no way to rid the body of HIV and hence cure AIDS, the best treatment available to infected individuals is to treat the opportunistic infections that result from immune suppression. In addition, there have been attempts to slow the replication of the virus. Because many viral diseases have been conquered by vaccination, much effort has gone into developing vaccines against HIV, so far without success. The only effective way to control the spread of AIDS is to prevent the transfer of HIV from person to person. This is accomplished by using condoms and spermicides (which destroy the virus), reducing exposure to infected individuals, and avoiding casual sex.

Preventing Sexually Transmitted Diseases

Preventing STDs requires that societies provide continuous, widespread public health programs and services for STD education and treatment. It is also crucial

Preventing STDs requires health programs for education and treatment.

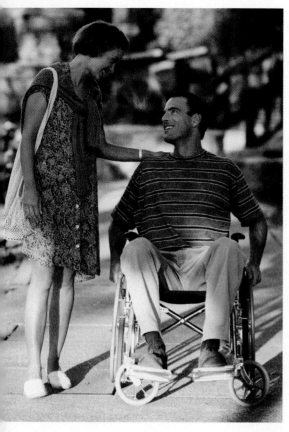

Everyone has a responsibility to practice safer sex.

that infected individuals seek prompt treatment, take responsibility for not infecting other individuals, and practice safer sex to lower their risk of infection.

The stigma associated with STDs is a great hindrance to prevention efforts. Viewing STDs in moral terms—that is, associating them with dirtiness and immorality—makes people reluctant to think and talk about them. It also makes society want to ignore STD epidemics. During World Wars I and II, American society supported massive gonorrhea and syphilis control programs; as a result, the incidence of these infections dropped tremendously. When the threat of a postwar STD epidemic seemed to wane, moralistic concerns thwarted the continuation of control efforts, and the incidence of STDs increased. Public health officials realize that ongoing efforts are the only way to control STDs.

Judgmental attitudes also make talking about STDs difficult. To have to tell a partner that you have an STD, or even to say that you once had an infection and are now perfectly OK, can bring feelings of guilt and shame, which can lead to avoiding the discussion altogether. Similarly, to ask about a partner's previous STDs may be interpreted as an accusation that the person is "loose" or immoral. To avoid feeling embarrassed or avoid the risk of offending a sexual partner, people are likely to dodge the topic of STDs. Prevention would be enhanced if sexually active individuals developed an open attitude about talking about STDs (and other aspects of sex) and acquired the necessary communication skills.

Practicing Safer Sex

The surest way to reduce the risk of acquiring a sexually transmitted disease is to abstain from sexual intercourse. This does not mean that you have to give up sexual interaction. There are many ways of giving and receiving sexual pleasure without engaging in sexual intercourse: touching, kissing, exchanging a massage, even sleeping together without intercourse.

Another way to reduce risk is to know a partner's sexual history, including all high-risk activities in which a partner may have engaged. Often this kind of information is difficult to gain early in a relationship, because exchanging information about sexual histories requires a level of trust that takes some time to develop.

Until you have this knowledge, it is essential to protect yourself by using condoms and spermicides when having sex, even if some other form of birth control is employed. *Birth control pills offer no protection against STDs.* Women and men who are sexually active should come to accept as standard practice with new partners the use of condoms and spermicides, even if the pill is used for birth control. Sexually active women and men should carry and be prepared to use condoms and spermicides whenever the possibility of sexual activity exists. This requires overcoming the gender-role stereotypes that women who admit to being sexual are "sluts" and men who behave the same way are "studs."

You may have noticed that the commonly heard term "safe sex" has been replaced in this chapter. Health practitioners have taught for decades that, no matter the precautions, *there is no such thing as completely safe sex for individuals who are sexually active with more than one partner.* Thus, these practitioners have suggested that the more accurate phrase is *safer sex.*

Some barriers to safer sex include the following:

* *Denying that there is a risk.* Many people assume that STDs happen only to "dirty," "promiscuous," and "immoral" people and, since they have sex only

with people who are "clean" and "nice," getting an STD is impossible. Another form of denial is to tell yourself "I eat right. I exercise. I can't get an STD."

- *Believing that the campus community is somehow insulated from STDs.* The truth is that about half of college students are sexually active before they enter college. As a result, students can arrive on campus already infected. Also, on many campuses, students in the same living groups and student organizations have sex with one another. One infected person can lead to a whole chain of infections.
- *Feeling guilty and uncomfortable about being sexual.* This prevents individuals from planning sex, so that they carry condoms and spermicides, and talking about possible risks with new partners.
- *Succumbing to social and peer pressure to be sexual.* These pressures encourage people to be sexual in situations that are potentially risky, such as one-night stands and brief relationships that are sexual virtually from the beginning. The risk of infection is lessened when individuals resist peer pressure to have sex with a relative stranger, and ask themselves instead "Is this the right relationship?" "Is this the right partner?" and "Am I going to feel OK about this afterwards?"

Physical Activity and Health Connection

Although there may not appear to be a direct link between physical activity and sexually transmitted diseases, regular participation in physical activity and the avoidance of STDs are both important components of living a healthy lifestyle. If you are physically active you generally have better self-esteem, which could provide you the ability to make more positive sexual health choices.

concept connections

1. **Sexually transmitted diseases are infections that are transferred from one person to another through sexual contact.** Sexually transmitted diseases are more than humiliating and a nuisance. Some of these diseases may lead to major illness, particularly for women and their unborn babies. STDs can cause pelvic inflammatory disease, tubal pregnancy, sterility, certain types of cancer, or blindness. Some last a lifetime. There are more than 65 million people living with incurable STDs in the United States (CDC, 2005). A few can be fatal. AIDS, genital warts, herpes, syphilis, and hepatitis have all been known to cause death. A sexually responsible person will take measures to reduce his or her risk of becoming infected with an STD.

2. **The United States has the highest rates of sexually transmitted diseases in the industrialized world.** Nearly 19 million new cases of STDs are reported each year in the United States, with almost half (48 percent) occurring in people 25 years or younger. In fact, one in two sexually active youth will have contracted an STD by the age of 25.

3. **Several factors increase the risk of contracting a sexually transmitted disease.** Not informing one's partner that one has an STD, having multiple sexual partners, not practicing safer sex precautions, not recognizing STD symptoms, not treating an STD, having impaired judgment because of alcohol or other drugs, and counting on the sense of security that "I won't get an STD" or that there is a cure for an STD if one is contracted all increase the chances of contracting an STD.

4 · **Common STDs include *Trichomonas* and *Gardnerella vaginalis* infections, chlamydia, gonorrhea, syphilis, herpes, genital warts, pubic lice, and scabies.** Sexually transmitted diseases, although widespread, can be prevented and treated before they are transmitted to someone else. Recognizing common signs and symptoms and understanding effective treatments will be useful in decreasing the incidence and prevalence of common STDs.

5 · **AIDS is caused by the human immunodeficiency virus (HIV).** By leading to the destruction or functional impairment of cells of the immune system, notably CD4⁺ T cells, HIV progressively destroys the body's ability to fight infections and certain cancers. An HIV-infected person is diagnosed with AIDS when his or her immune system is seriously compromised and manifestations of HIV infection are severe. The CDC currently defines AIDS in an adult or adolescent aged 13 years or older as the presence of one of 26 conditions indicative of severe immunosuppression associated with HIV infection.

6 · **Preventing STDs requires health programs for education and treatment.** Preventing STDs involves using health education to inform people about STD prevention and treatment. It also requires individuals to take personal responsibility for practicing safer sex and for seeking appropriate treatment if infected.

Terms

Sexually transmitted diseases (STDs), 368
Trichomonas vaginalis, 370
Gardnerella vaginalis, 370
Chlamydia, 372
Pelvic inflammatory disease (PID), 372

Epididymitis, 372
Gonorrhea, 373
Syphilis, 373
Chancre, 373
Herpes, 373
Sexually transmitted warts, 374

Human papillomavirus (HPV), 374
Pubic lice, 375
Scabies, 375
Human immunodeficiency virus (HIV), 375
Retrovirus, 377

making the connection

Ken and Amy both realize, after a number of heart- to-heart talks, that sexual intimacy does not necessarily need to include sexual intercourse. In deciding whether to engage in intimate sexual relations, including intercourse, they understand that they must consider psychological as well physical factors. They have learned that many people choose to abstain from sexual intercourse and that they can choose among varying levels of sexual intimacy. When they decide to become sexually intimate it will be a big step in their relationship, especially since having sex involves an emotional commitment as well as a physical one. Furthermore, the decision to become sexually intimate with one another must also be considered in light of HIV and the other sexually transmitted diseases that are prevalent among college students; many times infections may be asymptomatic, so someone may transmit the disease to another person unknowingly.

Critical Thinking

1. Ken and Amy have chosen to abstain from sexual intercourse. Describe for yourself the pros and cons of sexual abstinence. Have you been able to discuss your thoughts about sexuality with your current partner?

2. As more and more people become infected with HIV, more students attending universities and colleges are infected with HIV. Many universities have residence halls with living quarters that accommodate two to four people of the same gender. Is it necessary for universities to notify students in a residence hall if a person living there is HIV-positive? If so, why? If not, why not?

3. Herpes is a sexually transmitted disease that lasts a lifetime; however, herpes can be managed with medication. Explain, in detail, how you would go about telling your new partner that you have herpes.

4. You and your best college friend are talking, and your friend confides to you that about 2 months ago he may have had sexual intercourse with someone who could be HIV-positive, but your friend is not having any symptoms. What advice would you give him?

References

Centers for Disease Control and Prevention. (1994) Update: Trends in AIDS diagnosis and reporting under the expanded surveillance definition for adolescents and adults—United States, 1993. *Morbidity and Mortality Weekly Report* 43(45) 826–831.

Centers for Disease Control and Prevention. (2004). *HIV/AIDS Surveillance Report, 2003, Volume 15.* Atlanta, GA: U.S. Department of Health and Human Services, 1–46. Online: http://www.cdc.gov/hiv/stats/2003surveillancereport.pdf.

Centers for Disease Control and Prevention. (2005). *Sexually Transmitted Disease Surveillance, 2004.* Atlanta, GA: U.S. Department of Health and Human Services.

Glynn, M., & Rhodes, P. (2005). *Estimated HIV Prevalence in the United States at the End of 2003.* Presented at the National HIV Prevention Conference, Atlanta, GA. Abstract 595.

Joint United Nations Program on HIV/AIDS. (2005). *AIDS Epidemic Update: December 2005.* Online: http://www.unaids.org/epi/2005/index.asp.

Weinstock, H., Berman, S., & Cates, W. (2004). Sexually transmitted diseases among American youth: Incidence and prevalence estimates, 2000. *Perspectives on Sexual and Reproductive Health* 36(1):6–10.

Injury Prevention

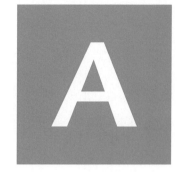

Introduction

While participating in most physical activity is safe, there is always a potential risk of injury. You can prevent most injuries by following a carefully planned activity program and by following the recommended prescreening suggestions found in this book. However, accidents occasionally happen and people do get injured. This appendix addresses what to do if you become injured.

Prevention Is the Best Medicine

Think safety! Many injuries can be avoided by preparing carefully for physical activity. Appropriate preparation includes the following:

- Warm-up, stretch out, and cool down.
- Wear proper clothing.
- Check shoes for signs of breakdown.
- Wear appropriate protective devices including helmets, padding and eyewear.

Then, check your activity environment to ensure that the exercise area is clear of obstacles. Regularly check equipment to make sure it has been maintained and is functioning properly. If you are unsure how to use a piece of equipment, seek instruction. Learning by trial and error usually means you will suffer through some error, which could cause injury. If you are active in a remote area (rock climbing or hiking), take a cell phone.

Take a first aid class and become certified in CPR. Learn how to contact emergency medical services (EMS). In most, but not all, communities dialing 911 is the quickest way to contact EMS.

Seek Professional Assessment

In all cases in which there is doubt, or when an injury presents more than just minor pain, you should seek advice from your physician. In many cases, injuries that appear minor may be more damaging than initially expected. It's better to be safe than sorry.

Emergency Action

If you need to call for help, for yourself or another, be prepared to tell EMS personnel the following information:

1. Where has the emergency occurred? Give the address or names of cross streets, roads, or other landmarks if possible.
2. Provide the telephone number from which you are calling.
3. What happened? Are you (or someone else) suffering from a heart attack, a fall, or some other emergency?
4. How many people need help?
5. What is the condition of the victim?
6. What is being done for the victim?

Remember to stay on the line. In a panic, you may forget to provide important pieces of information.

SOURCE: American Heart Association, 1987

Knowledge

You can also prepare yourself by learning a bit about injuries. Here are some of the signs of serious problems:

Signals of a Heart Attack

Is there persistent chest pain or discomfort? Does it increase with more activity?

Is breathing difficult (abnormal)?

Is there an abnormal change in pulse rate?

Does the skin appear pale or bluish in color?

SOURCE: American Red Cross, 1993

Signs of Internal Bleeding

Are there tender, swollen, bruised, or hard areas of the body, such as the abdomen?

Is there a rapid, weak pulse?

Does the skin feel cool or moist or look pale or bluish?

Are you suffering from excessive thirst?

Are you becoming confused, faint, drowsy, or unconscious?

SOURCE: American Red Cross, 1993

Signs of a Stroke

Is there sudden weakness or numbness of the face, arm, and leg on one side of the body?

Is there a loss of speech, or trouble speaking or understanding speech?

Are unexplained dizziness, unsteadiness, or falls occurring?

Is there dimness or loss of vision, particularly in one eye?

Was there any loss of consciousness?

SOURCE: American Heart Association, 1987

Common Injuries

You need to learn to identify and treat some common injuries. Remember, when in doubt, consult with your physician.

Tendinitis is an inflammation of a tendon. It is usually associated with overuse. Common areas affected by tendinitis include the Achilles' tendon, the elbow, and the ilio-tibial band. Tendinitis is usually treated by rest and anti-inflammatory medications.

Shin splints is a generic term that refers to any pain felt in the front portion of the lower leg. It may be caused by muscle imbalance, tendinitis, or being active on a new surface. Since this problem may be caused by a number of things, general suggestions for treatment are not possible. Occasionally stretching, cutting back on activity, and seeking better shoes may alleviate the problem. You may want to check with your physician to better define this condition.

Strains are injuries to the muscles caused by forcibly overstretching them. You can reduce the likelihood of strains by properly warming up your muscles prior to activity. Good muscular balance (symmetry) also reduces the likelihood of experiencing strains.

Sprains are injuries to the ligaments that are also caused by forceful overstretching. Sprains usually result from bending a joint into an unusual position. This can be caused by performing exercises incorrectly or by accident (sprained ankle).

Both sprains and strains are usually treated by R.I.C.E. (see below).

Fractures are broken bones. There are several degrees of fractures, from a hairline (small crack) to a compound fracture, in which the broken bone extends through the skin. If a fracture is suspected, try not to move the injured area and seek medical assistance.

Thermal stress is something those who are physically active need to learn to deal with. A few preventive steps can reduce your risk for suffering a thermal injury.

To prevent **heat injuries,** consider temperature and humidity. These two factors combine to provide a heat index. If possible, plan your activity for a climate-controlled environment. Many shopping malls will allow you to walk indoors on days with extreme temperatures. If you must be active outside on hot, humid days, wear breathable clothing, drink plenty of water, and plan your activity for the morning or evening. You might also want to lower your intensity. Wear sunscreen to reduce exposure to harmful rays.

To prevent **cold injuries,** consider temperature and wind chill. If possible, plan your activity for a climate-controlled environment. If you must be active outside on cold, windy days, wear multiple layers of clothing. You can shed layers as your body temperature rises, and you've got additional clothing to put on after your workout. Make sure you wear a hat, gloves or mittens, and protection for your nose.

SOURCE: Bristol-Myers Company, 1985

Immediate First Aid

When you suspect a muscle strain or ligament sprain, the R.I.C.E. procedure is followed for the first 72 hours: R = rest, I = ice, C = compression, E = elevation. After 72 hours, the application of heat will speed up the healing process. If a fracture is suspected, it is recommended that you immobilize the injured area and seek medical attention.

Caring for Bleeding

You can control bleeding by placing a clean covering, such as a sterile dressing, over the wound and applying pressure. Check for other injuries. If you don't find any broken bones, elevate the injured area. A bandage should be snugly applied over the dressing. If the bleeding cannot be stopped or reduced, put pressure on the nearby artery (pressure point). Always seek medical assistance for anything beyond minor bleeding.

>   SOURCE: American Red Cross, 1993

Follow Suggestions for Rehabilitation

To speed recovery time and to return to full health, it is critical that you follow the rehabilitation program that has been designed for you. Don't rush the program, skip steps, or fail to complete the entire rehab.

Don't Give Up the Ship

If you have an injury in one segment of your body, it doesn't mean you have to remain totally inactive. Check with your physician to see if there are any reasons you cannot be active in a modified way. For instance, if you have sprained an ankle and cannot walk comfortably, consider cycling or swimming.

References

American Red Cross. (1993). *Community First Aid & Safety.* Boston: Stay Well.

American Heart Association. (1987). *Heart Saver Manual.* Dallas.

Bristol-Myers Company. (1985). *Sports Injuries: An Aid to Prevention and Treatment.* Coventry, CT.

Caltoric Cost of Selected Activities

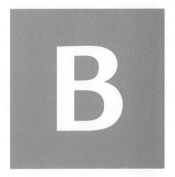

The following table shows some examples of activities and their corresponding caloric costs. You can use this information in the following ways:

- To determine level of estimated energy expenditure, multiply the figure in column three by the number of minutes you participate in the activity. (Please note that in this example the number in column three is for a person who weighs 150 pounds.)
- You can calculate your energy expenditure based on your weight in kilograms by multiplying the figure in column two by the minutes you are active and your weight in kilograms.

Activity	kcal/min/kg	kcal/min
Aerobics (medium intensity)	0.103	7.0
Basketball	0.138	9.4
Ballroom Dancing	0.051	3.5
Cycling		
Leisure (5.5 mph)	0.064	4.4
Golf	0.085	5.8
Jogging (9 min/mile)	0.193	13.1
Racquetball	0.178	12.1
Raking	0.054	3.7
Swimming (Breast Stroke)	0.162	11.0
Walking	0.08	5.4

A more detailed version of this chart follows in this appendix, taking into consideration variations in body weight.

APPENDIX B

Caloric Cost of Activities (cont.)

Activity	kcal·min⁻¹·kg⁻¹	50 110	53 117	56 123	59 130	62 137	65 143	68 150	71 157	74 163	77 170	80 176	83 183	86 190	89 196	92 203	95 209	98 216
Archery	0.065	3.3	3.4	3.6	3.8	4.0	4.2	4.4	4.6	4.8	5.0	5.2	5.4	5.6	5.8	6.0	6.2	6.4
Badminton	0.097	4.9	5.1	5.4	5.7	6.0	6.3	6.6	6.9	7.2	7.5	7.8	8.1	8.3	8.6	8.9	9.2	9.5
Bakery, general (F)	0.035	1.8	1.9	2.0	2.1	2.2	2.3	2.4	2.5	2.6	2.7	2.8	2.9	3.0	3.1	3.2	3.3	3.4
Basketball	0.138	6.9	7.3	7.7	8.1	8.6	9.0	9.4	9.8	10.2	10.6	11.0	11.5	11.9	12.3	12.7	13.1	13.5
Billiards	0.042	2.1	2.2	2.4	2.5	2.6	2.7	2.9	3.0	3.1	3.2	3.4	3.5	3.6	3.7	3.9	4.0	4.1
Bookbinding	0.038	1.9	2.0	2.1	2.2	2.4	2.5	2.6	2.7	2.8	2.9	3.0	3.2	3.3	3.4	3.5	3.6	3.7
Boxing																		
in ring	0.222	6.9	7.3	7.7	8.1	8.6	9.0	9.4	9.8	10.2	10.6	11.0	11.5	11.9	12.3	12.7	13.1	13.5
sparring	0.138	11.1	11.8	12.4	13.1	13.8	14.4	15.1	15.8	16.4	17.1	17.8	18.4	19.1	19.8	20.4	21.1	21.8
Canoeing																		
leisure	0.044	2.2	2.3	2.5	2.6	2.7	2.9	3.0	3.1	3.3	3.4	3.5	3.7	3.8	3.9	4.0	4.2	4.3
racing	0.103	5.2	5.5	5.8	6.1	6.4	6.7	7.0	7.3	7.6	7.9	8.2	8.5	8.9	9.2	9.5	9.8	10.1
Card Playing	0.025	1.3	1.3	1.4	1.5	1.6	1.6	1.7	1.8	1.9	1.9	2.0	2.1	2.2	2.2	2.3	2.4	2.5
Carpentry, general	0.052	2.6	2.8	2.9	3.1	3.2	3.4	3.5	3.7	3.8	4.0	4.2	4.3	4.5	4.6	4.8	4.9	5.1
Carpet sweeping (F)	0.045	2.3	2.4	2.5	2.7	2.8	2.9	3.1	3.2	3.3	3.5	3.6	3.7	3.9	4.0	4.1	4.3	4.4
Carpet sweeping (M)	0.048	2.4	2.5	2.7	2.8	3.0	3.1	3.3	3.4	3.6	3.7	3.8	4.0	4.1	4.3	4.4	4.6	4.7
Circuit Training																		
Hydra-Fitness	0.132	6.6	7.0	7.4	7.8	8.2	8.6	9.0	9.4	9.7	10.2	10.5	10.9	11.4	11.7	12.1	12.5	12.9
Universal	0.116	5.8	6.2	6.5	6.9	7.2	7.5	7.9	8.3	8.6	8.9	9.3	9.6	10.0	10.3	10.7	11.0	11.4
Nautilus	0.092	4.6	4.9	5.2	5.5	5.8	6.0	6.3	6.6	6.8	7.1	7.4	7.7	8.0	8.2	8.5	8.8	9.1
Free Weights	0.086	4.3	4.5	4.8	5.0	5.3	5.5	5.8	6.1	6.3	6.6	6.8	7.1	7.4	7.6	7.9	8.1	8.4
Cleaning (F)	0.062	3.1	3.3	3.5	3.7	3.8	4.0	4.2	4.4	4.6	4.8	5.0	5.1	5.3	5.5	5.7	5.9	6.1
Cleaning (M)	0.058	2.9	3.1	3.2	3.4	3.6	3.8	3.9	4.1	4.3	4.5	4.6	4.8	5.0	5.2	5.3	5.5	5.7
Climbing hills																		
with no load	0.121	6.1	6.4	6.8	7.1	7.5	7.9	8.2	8.6	9.0	9.3	9.7	10.0	10.4	10.8	11.1	11.5	11.9
with 5-kg load	0.129	6.5	6.8	7.2	7.6	8.0	8.4	8.8	9.2	9.5	9.9	10.3	10.7	11.1	11.5	11.9	12.3	12.6
with 10-kg load	0.140	7.0	7.4	7.8	8.3	8.7	9.1	9.5	9.9	10.4	10.8	11.2	11.6	12.0	12.5	12.9	13.3	13.7
with 20-kg load	0.147	7.4	7.8	8.2	8.7	9.1	9.6	10.0	10.4	10.9	11.3	11.8	12.2	12.6	13.1	13.5	14.0	14.4
Coal mining																		
drilling coal, rock	0.094	4.7	5.0	5.3	5.5	5.8	6.1	6.4	6.7	7.0	7.2	7.5	7.8	8.1	8.4	8.6	8.9	9.2
erecting supports	0.088	4.4	4.7	4.9	5.2	5.5	5.7	6.0	6.2	6.5	6.8	7.0	7.3	7.6	7.8	8.1	8.4	8.6
shoveling coal	0.108	5.4	5.7	6.0	6.4	6.7	7.0	7.3	7.7	8.0	8.3	8.6	9.0	9.3	9.6	9.9	10.3	10.6
Cooking (F)	0.045	2.3	2.4	2.5	2.7	2.8	2.9	3.1	3.2	3.3	3.5	3.6	3.7	3.9	4.0	4.1	4.3	4.4
Cooking (M)	0.048	2.4	2.5	2.7	2.8	3.0	3.1	3.3	3.4	3.6	3.7	3.8	4.0	4.1	4.3	4.4	4.6	4.7
Cricket																		
batting	0.083	4.2	4.4	4.6	4.9	5.1	5.4	5.6	5.9	6.1	6.4	6.6	6.9	7.1	7.4	7.6	7.9	8.1
bowling	0.090	4.5	4.8	5.0	5.3	5.6	5.9	6.1	6.4	6.7	6.9	7.2	7.5	7.7	8.0	8.3	8.6	8.8
Croquet	0.059	3.0	3.1	3.3	3.5	3.7	3.8	4.0	4.2	4.4	4.5	4.7	4.9	5.1	5.3	5.4	5.6	5.8
Cycling																		
leisure, 5.5 mph	0.064	3.2	3.4	3.6	3.8	4.0	4.2	4.4	4.5	4.7	4.9	5.1	5.3	5.5	5.7	5.9	6.1	6.3
leisure, 9.4 mph	0.100	5.0	5.3	5.6	5.9	6.2	6.5	6.8	7.1	7.4	7.7	8.0	8.3	8.6	8.9	9.2	9.5	9.8
racing	0.169	8.5	9.0	9.5	10.0	10.5	11.0	11.5	12.0	12.5	13.0	13.5	14.0	14.5	15.0	15.5	16.1	16.6

kg/lb shown in column headers (mass in kg over body weight in lb).

APPENDIX B | Caloric Cost of Activities (cont.)

kg/lb

Activity	$\text{kcal} \cdot \text{min}^{-1} \cdot \text{kg}^{-1}$	50/110	53/117	56/123	59/130	62/137	65/143	68/150	71/157	74/163	77/170	80/176	83/183	86/190	89/196	92/203	95/209	98/216
Dancing																		
Dancing (F)																		
aerobic, medium	0.103	5.2	5.5	5.8	6.1	6.4	6.7	7.0	7.3	7.6	7.9	8.2	8.5	8.9	9.2	9.5	9.8	10.1
aerobic, intense	0.135	6.7	7.1	7.5	7.9	8.3	8.7	9.2	9.6	10.0	10.4	10.8	11.2	11.6	12.0	12.4	12.8	13.2
ballroom	0.051	2.6	2.7	2.9	3.0	3.2	3.3	3.5	3.6	3.8	3.9	4.1	4.2	4.4	4.5	4.7	4.8	5.0
choreographed	0.168	8.4	8.9	9.4	9.9	10.4	10.9	11.4	11.9	12.4	12.9	13.4	13.9	14.4	15.0	15.5	16.0	16.5
"twist," "lambada"	0.103	5.2	5.5	5.8	6.1	6.4	6.7	7.0	7.3	7.6	7.9	8.2	8.5	8.9	9.2	9.5	9.8	10.1
Digging trenches	0.145	7.3	7.7	8.1	8.6	9.0	9.4	9.9	10.3	10.7	11.2	11.6	12.0	12.5	12.9	13.3	13.8	14.2
Drawing (standing)	0.036	1.8	1.9	2.0	2.1	2.2	2.3	2.4	2.6	2.7	2.8	2.9	3.0	3.1	3.2	3.3	3.4	3.5
Eating (sitting)	0.023	1.2	1.2	1.3	1.4	1.4	1.5	1.6	1.6	1.7	1.8	1.8	1.9	2.0	2.0	2.1	2.2	2.3
Electrical work	0.058	2.9	3.1	3.2	3.4	3.6	3.8	3.9	4.1	4.3	4.5	4.6	4.8	5.0	5.2	5.3	5.5	5.7
Farming																		
barn cleaning	0.135	6.8	7.2	7.6	8.0	8.4	8.8	9.2	9.6	10.0	10.4	10.8	11.2	11.6	12.0	12.4	12.8	13.2
driving harvester	0.040	2.0	2.1	2.2	2.4	2.5	2.6	2.7	2.8	3.0	3.1	3.2	3.3	3.4	3.6	3.7	3.8	3.9
driving tractor	0.037	1.9	2.0	2.1	2.2	2.3	2.4	2.5	2.6	2.7	2.8	3.0	3.1	3.2	3.3	3.4	3.5	3.6
feeding cattle	0.085	4.3	4.5	4.8	5.0	5.3	5.5	5.8	6.0	6.3	6.5	6.8	7.1	7.3	7.6	7.8	8.1	8.3
feeding animals	0.065	3.3	3.4	3.6	3.8	4.0	4.2	4.4	4.6	4.8	5.0	5.2	5.4	5.6	5.8	6.0	6.2	6.4
forking straw bales	0.138	6.9	7.3	7.7	8.1	8.6	9.0	9.4	9.8	10.2	10.6	11.0	11.5	11.9	12.3	12.7	13.1	13.5
milking by hand	0.054	2.7	2.9	3.0	3.2	3.3	3.5	3.7	3.8	4.0	4.2	4.3	4.5	4.6	4.8	5.0	5.1	5.3
milking by machine	0.023	1.2	1.2	1.3	1.4	1.4	1.5	1.6	1.6	1.7	1.8	1.8	1.9	2.0	2.0	2.1	2.2	2.3
shoveling grain	0.085	4.3	4.5	4.8	5.0	5.3	5.5	5.8	6.0	6.3	6.5	6.8	7.1	7.3	7.6	7.8	8.1	8.3
Field hockey	0.134	6.7	7.1	7.5	7.9	8.3	8.7	9.1	9.5	9.9	10.3	10.7	11.1	11.5	11.9	12.3	12.7	13.1
Fishing	0.062	3.1	3.3	3.5	3.7	3.8	4.0	4.2	4.4	4.6	4.8	5.0	5.1	5.3	5.5	5.7	5.9	6.1
Food shopping (F)	0.062	3.1	3.3	3.5	3.7	3.8	4.0	4.2	4.4	4.6	4.8	5.0	5.1	5.3	5.5	5.7	5.9	6.1
Food shopping (M)	0.058	2.9	3.1	3.2	3.4	3.6	3.8	3.9	4.1	4.3	4.5	4.6	4.8	5.0	5.2	5.3	5.5	5.7
Football	0.132	6.6	7.0	7.4	7.8	8.2	8.6	9.0	9.4	9.8	10.2	10.6	11.0	11.4	11.7	12.1	12.5	12.9
Forestry																		
ax chopping, fast	0.297	14.9	15.7	16.6	17.5	18.4	19.3	20.2	21.1	22.0	22.9	23.8	24.7	25.5	26.4	27.3	28.2	29.1
ax chopping, slow	0.085	4.3	4.5	4.8	5.0	5.3	5.5	5.8	6.0	6.3	6.5	6.8	7.1	7.3	7.6	7.8	8.1	8.3
barking trees	0.123	6.2	6.5	6.9	7.3	7.6	8.0	8.4	8.7	9.1	9.5	9.8	10.2	10.6	10.9	11.3	11.7	12.1
carrying logs	0.186	9.3	9.9	10.4	11.0	11.5	12.1	12.6	13.2	13.8	14.3	14.9	15.4	16.0	16.6	17.1	17.7	18.2
felling trees	0.132	6.6	7.0	7.4	7.8	8.2	8.6	9.0	9.4	9.8	10.2	10.6	11.0	11.4	11.7	12.1	12.5	12.9
hoeing	0.091	4.6	4.8	5.1	5.4	5.6	5.9	6.2	6.5	6.7	7.0	7.3	7.6	7.8	8.1	8.4	8.6	8.9
planting by hand	0.109	5.5	5.8	6.1	6.4	6.8	7.1	7.4	7.7	8.1	8.4	8.7	9.0	9.4	9.7	10.0	10.4	10.7
sawing by hand	0.122	6.1	6.5	6.8	7.2	7.6	7.9	8.3	8.7	9.0	9.4	9.8	10.1	10.5	10.9	11.2	11.6	12.0
sawing, power	0.075	3.8	4.0	4.2	4.4	4.7	4.9	5.1	5.3	5.6	5.8	6.0	6.2	6.5	6.7	6.9	7.1	7.4
stacking firewood	0.088	4.4	4.7	4.9	5.2	5.5	5.7	6.0	6.2	6.5	6.8	7.0	7.3	7.6	7.8	8.1	8.4	8.6
trimming trees	0.129	6.5	6.8	7.2	7.6	8.0	8.4	8.8	9.2	9.5	9.9	10.3	10.7	11.1	11.5	11.9	12.3	12.6
weeding	0.072	3.6	3.8	4.0	4.2	4.5	4.7	4.9	5.1	5.3	5.5	5.8	6.0	6.2	6.4	6.6	6.8	7.1
Furriery	0.083	4.2	4.4	4.6	4.9	5.1	5.4	5.6	5.9	6.1	6.4	6.6	6.9	7.1	7.4	7.6	7.9	8.1
Gardening																		
digging	0.126	6.3	6.7	7.1	7.4	7.8	8.2	8.6	8.9	9.3	9.7	10.1	10.5	10.8	11.2	11.6	12.0	12.3
hedging	0.077	3.9	4.1	4.3	4.5	4.8	5.0	5.2	5.5	5.7	5.9	6.2	6.4	6.6	6.9	7.1	7.3	7.5

APPENDIX B

Caloric Cost of Activities (cont.)

Activity	kcal · min⁻¹ · kg⁻¹	50 / 110	53 / 117	56 / 123	59 / 130	62 / 137	65 / 143	68 / 150	71 / 157	74 / 163	77 / 170	80 / 176	83 / 183	86 / 190	89 / 196	92 / 203	95 / 209	98 / 216
Gardening (cont.)																		
mowing	0.112	5.6	5.9	6.3	6.6	6.9	7.3	7.6	8.0	8.3	8.6	9.0	9.3	9.6	10.0	10.3	10.6	11.0
raking	0.054	2.7	2.9	3.0	3.2	3.3	3.5	3.7	3.8	4.0	4.2	4.3	4.5	4.6	4.8	5.0	5.1	5.3
Golf	0.085	4.3	4.5	4.8	5.0	5.3	5.5	5.8	6.0	6.3	6.5	6.8	7.1	7.3	7.6	7.8	8.1	8.3
Gymnastics	0.066	3.3	3.5	3.7	3.9	4.1	4.3	4.5	4.7	4.9	5.1	5.3	5.5	5.7	5.9	6.1	6.3	6.5
Horse-grooming	0.128	6.4	6.8	7.2	7.6	7.9	8.3	8.7	9.1	9.5	9.9	10.2	10.6	11.0	11.4	11.8	12.2	12.5
Horse-racing																		
galloping	0.137	6.9	7.3	7.7	8.1	8.5	8.9	9.3	9.7	10.1	10.6	11.0	11.4	11.8	12.2	12.6	13.0	13.4
trotting	0.110	5.5	5.8	6.2	6.5	6.8	7.2	7.5	7.8	8.1	8.5	8.8	9.1	9.5	9.8	10.1	10.5	10.8
walking	0.041	2.1	2.2	2.3	2.4	2.5	2.7	2.8	2.9	3.0	3.2	3.3	3.4	3.5	3.6	3.8	3.9	4.0
Ironing (F)	0.033	1.7	1.7	1.8	1.9	2.0	2.1	2.2	2.3	2.4	2.5	2.6	2.7	2.8	2.9	3.0	3.1	3.2
Ironing (M)	0.064	3.2	3.4	3.6	3.8	4.0	4.2	4.4	4.5	4.7	4.9	5.1	5.3	5.5	5.7	5.9	6.1	6.3
Judo	0.195	9.8	10.3	10.9	11.5	12.1	12.7	13.3	13.8	14.4	15.0	15.6	16.2	16.8	17.4	17.9	18.5	19.1
Jumping rope																		
70 per min	0.162	8.1	8.6	9.1	9.6	10.0	10.5	11.0	11.5	12.0	12.5	13.0	13.4	13.9	14.4	14.9	15.4	15.9
80 per min	0.164	8.2	8.7	9.2	9.7	10.2	10.7	11.2	11.6	12.1	12.6	13.1	13.6	14.1	14.6	14.6	15.6	16.1
125 per min	0.177	8.9	9.4	9.9	10.4	11.0	11.5	12.0	12.6	13.1	13.6	14.2	14.7	15.2	15.8	16.3	16.8	17.3
145 per min	0.197	9.9	10.4	11.0	11.6	12.2	12.8	13.4	14.0	14.6	15.2	15.8	16.4	16.9	17.5	18.1	18.7	19.3
Knitting, sewing (F)	0.022	1.1	1.2	1.2	1.3	1.4	1.4	1.5	1.6	1.6	1.7	1.8	1.8	1.9	2.0	2.0	2.1	2.2
Knitting, sewing (M)	0.023	1.2	1.2	1.3	1.4	1.4	1.5	1.6	1.6	1.7	1.8	1.8	1.9	2.0	2.0	2.1	2.2	2.3
Locksmith	0.057	2.9	3.0	3.2	3.4	3.5	3.7	3.9	4.0	4.2	4.4	4.6	4.7	4.9	5.1	5.2	5.4	5.6
Lying at ease	0.022	1.1	1.2	1.2	1.3	1.4	1.4	1.5	1.6	1.6	1.7	1.8	1.8	1.9	2.0	2.0	2.1	2.2
Machine-tooling																		
machining	0.048	2.4	2.5	2.7	2.8	3.0	3.1	3.3	3.4	3.6	3.7	3.8	4.0	4.1	4.3	4.4	4.6	4.7
operating lathe	0.052	2.6	2.8	2.9	3.1	3.2	3.4	3.5	3.7	3.8	4.0	4.2	4.3	4.5	4.6	4.8	4.9	5.1
operating punch press	0.088	4.4	4.7	4.9	5.2	5.5	5.7	6.0	6.2	6.5	6.8	7.0	7.3	7.6	7.8	8.1	8.4	8.6
tapping and drilling	0.065	3.3	3.4	3.6	3.8	4.0	4.2	4.4	4.6	4.8	5.0	5.2	5.4	5.6	5.8	6.0	6.2	6.4
welding	0.052	2.6	2.8	2.9	3.1	3.2	3.4	3.5	3.7	3.8	4.0	4.2	4.3	4.5	4.6	4.8	4.9	5.1
working sheet metal	0.048	2.4	2.5	2.7	2.8	3.0	3.1	3.3	3.4	3.6	3.7	3.8	4.0	4.1	4.3	4.4	4.6	4.7
Marching, rapid	0.142	7.1	7.5	8.0	8.4	8.8	9.2	9.7	10.1	10.5	10.9	11.4	11.8	12.2	12.6	13.1	13.5	13.9
Mopping floor (F)	0.062	3.1	3.3	3.5	3.7	3.8	4.0	4.2	4.4	4.6	4.8	5.0	5.1	5.3	5.5	5.7	5.9	6.1
Mopping floor (M)	0.058	2.9	3.1	3.2	3.4	3.6	3.8	3.9	4.1	4.3	4.5	4.6	4.8	5.0	5.2	5.0	5.5	5.7
Music playing																		
accordion (sitting)	0.032	1.6	1.7	1.8	1.9	2.0	2.1	2.2	2.3	2.4	2.5	2.6	2.7	2.8	2.8	2.9	3.0	3.1
cello (sitting)	0.041	2.1	2.2	2.3	2.4	2.5	2.7	2.8	2.9	3.0	3.2	3.3	3.4	3.5	3.6	3.8	3.9	4.0
conducting	0.039	2.0	2.1	2.2	2.3	2.4	2.5	2.7	2.8	2.9	3.0	3.1	3.2	3.4	3.5	3.6	3.7	3.8
drums (sitting)	0.066	3.3	3.5	3.7	3.9	4.1	4.3	4.5	4.7	4.9	5.1	5.3	5.5	5.7	5.9	6.1	6.3	6.6
flute (sitting)	0.035	1.8	1.9	2.0	2.1	2.2	2.3	2.4	2.5	2.6	2.7	2.8	2.9	3.0	3.1	3.2	3.3	3.4
horn (sitting)	0.029	1.5	1.5	1.6	1.7	1.8	1.9	2.0	2.1	2.1	2.2	2.3	2.4	2.5	2.6	2.7	2.8	2.8
organ (sitting)	0.053	2.7	2.8	3.0	3.1	3.3	3.4	3.6	3.8	3.9	4.1	4.2	4.4	4.6	4.7	4.9	5.0	5.2
piano (sitting)	0.040	2.0	2.1	2.2	2.4	2.5	2.6	2.7	2.8	3.0	3.1	3.2	3.3	3.4	3.6	3.7	3.8	3.9
trumpet (standing)	0.031	1.6	1.6	1.7	1.8	1.9	2.0	2.1	2.2	2.3	2.4	2.5	2.6	2.7	2.8	2.9	2.9	3.0

APPENDIX B   Caloric Cost of Activities (cont.)

Activity	kcal · min⁻¹ · kg⁻¹	50 / 110	53 / 117	56 / 123	59 / 130	62 / 137	65 / 143	68 / 150	71 / 157	74 / 163	77 / 170	80 / 176	83 / 183	86 / 190	89 / 196	92 / 203	95 / 209	98 / 216
Music playing (cont.)																		
violin (sitting)	0.045	2.3	2.4	2.5	2.7	2.8	2.9	3.1	3.2	3.3	3.5	3.6	3.7	3.9	4.0	4.1	4.3	4.4
woodwind (sitting)	0.032	1.6	1.7	1.8	1.9	2.0	2.1	2.2	2.3	2.4	2.5	2.6	2.7	2.8	2.8	2.9	3.0	3.1
Painting, inside	0.034	1.7	1.8	1.9	2.0	2.1	2.2	2.3	2.4	2.5	2.6	2.7	2.8	2.9	3.0	3.1	3.2	3.3
Painting, outside	0.077	3.9	4.1	4.3	4.5	4.8	5.0	5.2	5.5	5.7	5.9	6.2	6.4	6.6	6.9	7.1	7.3	7.5
Planting seedlings	0.070	3.5	3.7	3.9	4.1	4.3	4.6	4.8	5.0	5.2	5.4	5.6	5.8	6.0	6.2	6.4	6.7	6.9
Plastering	0.078	3.9	4.1	4.4	4.6	4.8	5.1	5.3	5.5	5.8	6.0	6.2	6.5	6.7	6.9	7.2	7.4	7.6
Printing	0.035	1.8	1.9	2.0	2.1	2.2	2.3	2.4	2.5	2.6	2.7	2.8	2.9	3.0	3.1	3.2	3.3	3.4
Racquetball	0.178	8.9	9.4	10.0	10.5	11.0	11.6	12.1	12.6	13.2	13.7	14.2	14.8	15.3	15.8	16.4	16.9	17.4
Running, cross-country	0.163	8.2	8.6	9.1	9.6	10.1	10.6	11.1	11.6	12.1	12.6	13.0	13.5	14.0	14.5	15.0	15.5	16.0
Running, horizontal																		
11 min, 30 s per mile	0.135	6.8	7.2	7.6	8.0	8.4	8.8	9.2	9.6	10.0	10.5	10.9	11.3	11.7	12.1	12.5	12.9	13.3
9 min per mile	0.193	9.7	10.2	10.8	11.4	12.0	12.5	13.1	13.7	14.3	14.9	15.4	16.0	16.6	17.2	17.8	18.3	18.9
8 min per mile	0.208	10.8	11.3	11.9	12.5	13.1	13.6	14.2	14.8	15.4	16.0	16.5	17.1	17.7	18.3	18.9	19.4	20.0
7 min per mile	0.228	12.2	12.7	13.3	13.9	14.5	15.0	15.6	16.2	16.8	17.4	17.9	18.5	19.1	19.7	20.3	20.8	21.4
6 min per mile	0.252	13.9	14.4	15.0	15.6	16.2	16.7	17.3	17.9	18.5	19.1	19.6	20.2	20.8	21.4	22.0	22.5	23.1
5 min, 30 s per mile	0.289	14.5	15.3	16.2	17.1	17.9	18.8	19.7	20.5	21.4	22.3	23.1	24.0	24.9	25.7	26.6	27.5	28.3
Scraping paint	0.063	3.2	3.3	3.5	3.7	3.9	4.1	4.3	4.5	4.7	4.9	5.0	5.2	5.4	5.6	5.8	6.0	6.2
Scrubbing floors (F)	0.109	5.5	5.8	6.1	6.4	6.8	7.1	7.4	7.7	8.1	8.4	8.7	9.0	9.4	9.7	10.0	10.4	10.7
Scrubbing floors (M)	0.108	5.4	5.7	6.0	6.4	6.7	7.0	7.3	7.7	8.0	8.3	8.6	9.0	9.3	9.6	9.9	10.3	10.6
Shoe repair, general	0.045	2.3	2.4	2.5	2.7	2.8	2.9	3.1	3.2	3.3	3.5	3.6	3.7	3.9	4.0	4.1	4.3	4.4
Sitting quietly	0.021	1.1	1.1	1.2	1.2	1.3	1.4	1.4	1.5	1.6	1.6	1.7	1.7	1.8	1.9	1.9	2.0	2.1
Skiing, hard snow																		
level, moderate speed	0.119	6.0	6.3	6.7	7.0	7.4	7.7	8.1	8.4	8.8	9.2	9.5	9.9	10.2	10.6	10.9	11.3	11.7
level, walking speed	0.143	7.2	7.6	8.0	8.4	8.9	9.3	9.7	70.2	10.6	11.0	11.4	11.9	12.3	12.7	13.2	13.6	14.0
uphill, maximum speed	0.274	13.7	14.5	15.3	16.2	17.0	17.8	18.6	19.5	20.3	21.1	21.9	22.7	23.6	24.4	25.2	26.0	26.9
Skiing, soft snow																		
leisure (F)	0.111	4.9	5.2	5.5	5.8	6.1	6.4	6.7	7.0	7.3	7.5	7.8	8.1	8.4	8.7	9.0	9.3	9.6
leisure (M)	0.098	5.6	5.9	6.2	6.5	6.9	7.2	7.5	7.9	8.2	8.5	8.9	9.2	9.5	9.9	10.2	10.5	10.9
Skindiving, as frogman																		
considerable motion	0.276	13.8	14.6	15.5	16.3	17.1	17.9	18.8	19.6	20.4	21.3	22.1	22.9	23.7	24.6	25.4	26.2	27.0
moderate motion	0.206	10.3	10.9	11.5	12.2	12.8	13.4	14.0	14.6	15.2	15.9	16.5	17.1	17.7	18.3	19.0	19.6	20.2
Snowshoeing, soft snow	0.166	8.3	8.8	9.3	9.8	10.3	10.8	11.3	11.8	12.3	12.8	13.3	13.8	14.3	14.8	15.3	15.8	16.3
Squash	0.212	10.6	11.2	11.9	12.5	13.1	13.8	14.4	15.1	15.7	16.3	17.0	17.6	18.2	18.9	19.5	20.1	20.8
Standing quietly (F)	0.025	1.3	1.3	1.4	1.5	1.6	1.6	1.7	1.8	1.9	1.9	2.0	2.1	2.2	2.2	2.3	2.4	2.5
Standing quietly (M)	0.027	1.4	1.4	1.5	1.6	1.7	1.8	1.8	1.9	2.0	2.1	2.2	2.2	2.3	2.4	2.5	2.6	2.6
Steel mill, working in																		
fetting	0.089	4.5	4.7	5.0	5.3	5.5	5.8	6.1	6.3	6.6	6.9	7.1	7.4	7.7	7.9	8.2	8.5	8.7
forging	0.100	5.0	5.3	5.6	5.9	6.2	6.5	6.8	7.1	7.4	7.7	8.0	8.3	8.6	8.9	9.2	9.5	9.8
hand rolling	0.137	6.9	7.3	7.7	8.1	8.5	8.9	9.3	9.7	10.1	10.6	11.0	11.4	11.8	12.2	12.6	13.0	13.4
merchant mill rolling	0.145	7.3	7.7	8.1	8.6	9.0	9.4	9.9	10.3	10.7	11.2	11.6	12.0	12.5	12.9	13.3	13.8	14.2
removing slag	0.178	8.9	9.4	10.0	10.5	11.0	11.6	12.1	12.6	13.2	13.7	14.2	14.8	15.3	15.8	16.4	16.9	17.4

APPENDIX B   Caloric Cost of Activities (cont.)

Activity	kcal · min⁻¹ · kg⁻¹	50 / 110	53 / 117	56 / 123	59 / 130	62 / 137	65 / 143	68 / 150	71 / 157	74 / 163	77 / 170	80 / 176	83 / 183	86 / 190	89 / 196	92 / 203	95 / 209	98 / 216
Steel mill, working in (cont.)																		
tending furnace	0.126	6.3	6.7	7.1	7.4	7.8	8.2	8.6	8.9	9.3	9.7	10.1	10.5	10.8	11.2	11.6	12.0	12.3
tipping molds	0.092	4.6	4.9	5.2	5.4	5.7	6.0	6.3	6.5	6.8	7.1	7.4	7.6	7.9	8.2	8.5	8.7	9.0
Stock clerking	0.054	2.7	2.9	3.0	3.2	3.3	3.5	3.7	3.8	4.0	4.2	4.3	4.5	4.6	4.8	5.0	5.1	5.3
Swimming																		
back stroke	0.169	8.5	9.0	9.5	10.0	10.5	11.0	11.5	12.0	12.5	13.0	13.5	14.0	14.5	15.0	15.5	16.1	16.6
breast stroke	0.162	8.1	8.6	9.1	9.6	10.0	10.5	11.0	11.5	12.0	12.5	13.0	13.4	13.9	14.4	14.9	15.4	15.9
crawl, fast	0.156	7.8	8.3	8.7	9.2	9.7	10.1	10.6	11.1	11.5	12.0	12.5	12.9	13.4	13.9	14.4	14.8	15.3
crawl, slow	0.128	6.4	6.8	7.2	7.6	7.9	8.3	8.7	9.1	9.5	9.9	10.2	10.6	11.0	11.4	11.8	12.2	12.5
side stroke	0.122	6.1	6.5	6.8	7.2	7.6	7.9	8.3	8.7	9.0	9.4	9.8	10.1	10.5	10.9	11.2	11.6	12.0
treading, fast	0.170	8.5	9.0	9.5	10.0	10.5	11.1	11.6	12.1	12.6	13.1	13.6	14.1	14.6	15.1	15.6	16.2	16.7
treading, normal	0.062	3.1	3.3	3.5	3.7	3.8	4.0	4.2	4.4	4.6	4.8	5.0	5.1	5.3	5.5	5.7	5.9	6.1
Table tennis (ping pong)	0.068	3.4	3.6	3.8	4.0	4.2	4.4	4.6	4.8	5.0	5.2	5.4	5.6	5.8	6.1	6.3	6.5	6.7
Tailoring																		
cutting	0.041	2.1	2.2	2.3	2.4	2.5	2.7	2.8	2.9	3.0	3.2	3.3	3.4	3.5	3.6	3.8	3.9	4.0
hand-sewing	0.032	1.6	1.7	1.8	1.9	2.0	2.1	2.2	2.3	2.4	2.5	2.6	2.7	2.8	2.8	2.9	3.0	3.1
machine-sewing	0.045	2.3	2.4	2.5	2.7	2.8	2.9	3.1	3.2	3.3	3.5	3.6	3.7	3.9	4.0	4.1	4.3	4.4
pressing	0.062	3.1	3.3	3.5	3.7	3.8	4.0	4.2	4.4	4.6	4.8	5.0	5.1	5.3	5.5	5.7	5.9	6.1
Tennis	0.109	5.5	5.8	6.1	6.4	6.8	7.1	7.4	7.7	8.1	8.4	8.7	9.0	9.4	9.7	10.0	10.4	10.7
Typing																		
electric	0.027	1.4	1.4	1.5	1.6	1.7	1.8	1.8	1.9	2.0	2.1	2.2	2.2	2.3	2.4	2.5	2.6	2.6
manual	0.031	1.6	1.6	1.7	1.8	1.9	2.0	2.1	2.2	2.3	2.4	2.5	2.6	2.7	2.8	2.9	2.9	3.0
Volleyball	0.050	2.5	2.7	2.8	3.0	3.1	3.3	3.4	3.6	3.7	3.9	4.0	4.2	4.3	4.5	4.6	4.8	4.9
Walking, normal pace																		
asphalt road	0.080	4.0	4.2	4.5	4.7	5.0	5.2	5.4	5.7	5.9	6.2	6.4	6.6	6.9	7.1	7.4	7.6	7.8
fields and hillsides	0.082	4.1	4.3	4.6	4.8	5.1	5.3	5.6	5.8	6.1	6.3	6.6	6.8	7.1	7.3	7.5	7.8	8.0
grass track	0.081	4.1	4.3	4.5	4.8	5.0	5.3	5.5	5.8	6.0	6.2	6.5	6.7	7.0	7.2	7.5	7.7	7.9
plowed field	0.077	3.9	4.1	4.3	4.5	4.8	5.0	5.2	5.5	5.7	5.9	6.2	6.4	6.6	6.9	7.1	7.3	7.5
Wallpapering	0.048	2.4	2.5	2.7	2.8	3.0	3.1	3.3	3.4	3.6	3.7	3.8	4.0	4.1	4.3	4.4	4.6	4.7
Watch repairing	0.025	1.3	1.3	1.4	1.5	1.6	1.6	1.7	1.8	1.9	1.9	2.0	2.1	2.2	2.2	2.3	2.4	2.5
Window cleaning (F)	0.059	3.0	3.1	3.3	3.5	3.7	3.8	4.0	4.2	4.4	4.5	4.7	4.9	5.1	5.3	5.4	5.6	5.8
Window cleaning (M)	0.058	2.9	3.1	3.2	3.4	3.6	3.8	3.9	4.1	4.3	4.5	4.6	4.8	5.0	5.2	5.3	5.5	5.7
Writing (sitting)	0.029	1.5	1.5	1.6	1.7	1.8	1.9	2.0	2.1	2.1	2.2	2.3	2.4	2.5	2.6	2.7	2.8	2.8

Data from Bannister, E.W. and Brown, S.R.: The relative requirements of physical activity, in H.B. Falls (ed): *Exercise Physiology*. New York, Academic Press, 1968: Howley, E.T. and Glover, M.E.: The caloric costs of running and walking one mile for men and women. *Medicine and Science in Sports* 6.235, 1974; Passmore, R. and Durnin, J.V.G.A.: Human energy expenditure. *Physiological Reviews* 35.801, 1955. Note: Symbols (M) and (F) denote experiments for males and females, respectively.

SOURCE: W.D. McArdle, F.I. Katch, and V.L. Katch. (1996). *Exercise physiology: Energy, nutrition, and human performance* (pp. 804–811). Baltimore, MD: Lippincott, Williams & Wilkins.

Nutrition and Health for Canadians

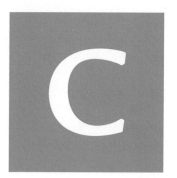

Canadian Guidelines for Nutrition

For more than 60 years, the government has worked to promote healthy and nutritious eating habits in Canadians. In 1987, Health and Welfare Canada began a major review of the system for guiding Canadians on their food choices. To perform the review, the government appointed two advisory committees—the Scientific Review Committee and the Communications and Implementation Committee.

After examining research evidence available on nutrition and public health, the Scientific Review Committee issued a report in 1990 called *Nutrition Recommendations*. The report included both updated Recommended Nutrient Intakes (RNI) and a scientific description of a healthy dietary pattern that would deliver adequate nutrients for health and reduce the risk of nutrition-related chronic diseases.

Meanwhile, the Communications and Implementation Committee translated these scientific findings into understandable guidelines and outlined implementation strategies in a report called *Action Towards Healthy Eating: Technical Report* (1990). This report suggested that Canada develop a "total diet approach" towards healthy eating. A total diet approach would give consumers a better idea of eating patterns associated with reducing the risk of developing chronic diseases.

In 1990, the government issued *Nutrition Recommendations: A Call for Action*, a summary report produced jointly by the Scientific Review Committee and the Communications and Implementation Committee.

A Revised Food Guide

In accordance with the recommendations of its two advisory groups, the Health Department undertook to revise *Canada's Food Guide*. In 1992, the agency launched *Canada's Food Guide to Healthy Eating* and an explanatory document called *Using the Food Guide*. This promoted dietary diversity, a reduction in total fat intake, and an active lifestyle. It also offers consumers a pattern for establishing healthy eating habits in their daily selection of foods.

Moreover, the guide introduced a number of new concepts. A range of servings from the four food groups accommodates the wide range of energy needs for different ages, body sizes, activity levels, genders, and conditions such as pregnancy and nursing. The wide range of servings in grain products, vegetables, and fruits is designed to give consumers a better idea of the type of diet that would help reduce the risk of developing nutrition-related chronic diseases.

The guide also introduced a category of "other" foods such as sweets, fats such as butter, and drinks like coffee, that, though part of the diets of many Canadians, would traditionally not have been mentioned in a food guide. The guide recommends moderation in the consumption of these foods and acknowledges their role, along with the wide range of servings in grains, vegetables, and fruits, as a "total diet approach" to healthy eating.

A Work in Progress

Some groups and organizations challenged specific aspects of the government's *Nutrition Recommendations*. In a typically Canadian twist, the government responded to challengers by including them in the development process. When the Canadian Pediatric Society, for example, queried the dietary recommendations on fat consumption in children, the Society was invited to join Health Canada in researching the issue. The result was *Nutrition Recommendations Update: Dietary Fat and Children* (1993), which adjusted the recommendation of appropriate levels of dietary fat for growing children. In 1995, Health Canada issued *Canada's Food Guide to Healthy Eating: Focus on Preschoolers* as a background paper for educators and communicators.

Health Canada also has positioned nutrition in a broader health context, which includes physical activity and a positive outlook on life. One result of this comprehensive approach was the *Vitality Leaders Kit* (1994), intended to help community leaders promote healthy eating, active living, and positive self- and body-image in an integrated way.

Looking Ahead

The job of keeping Canada's nutrition policy and consumer guidelines up-to-date is an ongoing task. New scientific research on nutrition and health continually uncovers new relationships and connections between them. Consumer tastes in foods vary in response to prevailing fashions and shifting demographics. Global trade also influences the food choices that appear on the Canadian dinner table.

The science underlying nutrition recommendations knows no borders. An increasingly complex knowledge base on nutrients, food and health, global trade, and international agreements requires international efforts. Scientists from Canada and the United States worked with the National Academy of Sciences to develop the Dietary Reference Intakes (DRIs), recommended nutrient intake levels for healthy people in the U.S. and Canada.

As a result of publication of the DRI values, Health Canada has undertaken an extensive review of Canada's dietary guidance. Current recommendations are presented in this appendix, but revised documents are expected to be published in late 2006. To keep abreast of the latest developments in Canada's nutrition policies, visit the Food and Nutrition area of the Health Canada Web site at: http://www.hc-sc.gc.ca/english/lifestyles/food_nutr.html or http://www.hc-sc.gc.ca/francais/vie_saine/nutrition.html.

Nutrient Intake Recommendations for Canadians

Health Canada has reviewed and made recommendations on nutrient requirements on a periodic basis since 1938. Known as the Recommended Nutrient Intakes, or RNI, these values were last published in 1990 as part of *Nutrition Recommendations: The Report of the Scientific Review Committee*. Since that time, there have been advances in science and by 1994, it was clear that it was time to initiate another review of the scientific data.

At the same time, the Food and Nutrition Board of the National Academy of Sciences was beginning a consultation process on the review of the Recommended Dietary Allowances, the nutrient recommendations used in the United States. Health Canada considered that participating in the U.S. review would offer several advantages to Canada. These were as follows:

- The science underlying nutrient requirements knows no borders and scientists everywhere are utilizing the same knowledge produced from studies conducted all over the world.
- The knowledge base on nutrients, foods, and health is increasing rapidly in scope and complexity. This increases the need for specialized expertise. Participating in the U.S. review permits Canada to expand the base of scientific expertise that could be utilized.
- International trade considerations, including NAFTA, suggest that the harmonization of the science base underlying nutrition policy will facilitate harmonization of such trade-related matters as nutrition labeling and food composition.

Canadian and American scientists establish DRIs through a review process overseen by the Food and Nutrition Board of the Institute of Medicine, National Academy of Sciences. The National Academy of Sciences is an American private nonprofit society of distinguished scholars engaged in scientific and engineering research, dedicated to the advancement of science and technology and to their use for the general welfare. The Academy has a mandate that requires it to advise the U.S. federal government on scientific and technical matters.

The Food and Nutrition Board (FNB) is a unit of the Institute of Medicine, part of the National Academy of Sciences. The Board is a multidisciplinary group of biomedical scientists with expertise in various aspects of nutrition, food sciences, biochemistry, medicine, public health, epidemiology, food toxicology, and food safety. The major focus of the FNB is to evaluate emerging knowledge of nutrient requirements and relationships between diet and the reduction of risk of common chronic diseases and to relate this knowledge to strategies for promoting health and preventing disease.

Nutrition Recommendations for Canadians

The scientific basis for current dietary guidance in Canada is provided by the *Nutrition Recommendations for Canadians*. These statements outline the desired characteristics of the Canadian diet and form the scientific basis for a dietary pattern that will supply recommended amounts of all essential nutrients while reducing the risk of chronic disease.

- The Canadian diet should provide energy consistent with the maintenance of body weight within the recommended range.
- The Canadian diet should include essential nutrients in amounts specified in the Recommended Nutrient Intakes.
- The Canadian diet should include no more than 30 percent of energy as fat (33 g/1,000 kcal or 39 g/5,000 kJ) and no more than 10 percent as saturated fat (11 g/1,000 kcal or 13 g/5,000 kJ).
- The Canadian diet should provide 55 percent of energy as carbohydrates (138 g/1,000 kcal or 13 g/5,000 kJ).
- The sodium content of the Canadian diet should be reduced.
- The Canadian diet should include no more than 5 percent of total energy as alcohol, or two drinks daily, whichever is less.
- The Canadian diet should contain no more caffeine than the equivalent of four cups of regular coffee per day.
- Community water supplies containing less than 1 mg/litre should be fluoridated to that level.

Healthy eating has been accepted as a significant factor in reducing the risk of developing nutrition-related problems, including heart disease, cancer, obesity, hypertension (high blood pressure), osteoporosis, anemia, dental decay, and some bowel disorders. Reducing risk means lowering the chances of developing a disease. It does not guarantee the prevention of a disease. Since the development of disease involves several factors, risk reduction usually involves several different strategies or approaches. Healthy eating is just one positive action that may help to avoid a potential problem.

The Nutrition Recommendations for Canadians listed above were released in 1990, and are currently under review. Revision will ensure that they continue to be scientifically sound and that they will continue to address those characteristics of the diet most relevant to the promotion of health and reduction of chronic disease. Updated Nutrition Recommendations will include recommendations with respect to Energy, Fat, Carbohydrates, and Essential Nutrients, and will be consistent with the findings and recommendations in the DRI reports. Keep in mind that these are scientific statements for use by health professionals and are not intended for use directly by consumers.

Canada's Guidelines for Healthy Eating

Following the release of the 1990 Nutrition Recommendations for Canadians, a committee of experts in communications and program planning worked with the committee of scientists and prepared the report Action Towards Healthy Eating. They adapted the Nutrition Recommendations into a more user-friendly set of statements called Canada's Guidelines for Healthy Eating. These Guidelines promote healthy eating in a general way:

- Enjoy a variety of foods.
- Emphasize cereals, breads, other grain products, vegetables, and fruits.
- Choose lower-fat dairy products, leaner meats, and foods prepared with little or no fat.
- Achieve and maintain a healthy body weight by enjoying regular physical activity and healthy eating.
- Limit salt, alcohol, and caffeine.

Based on the review and revision of the *Nutrition Recommendations, Canada's Guidelines for Healthy Eating* will also be reviewed, both from a scientific perspective and from a communications perspective to ensure that they remain the most appropriate key messages for Canadians.

Canada's Food Guide

Scientists have known for some time that adequate nutrition is essential for proper growth and development. More recently, healthy eating has been accepted as a significant factor in reducing the risk of developing nutrition-related problems, including heart disease, cancer, obesity, hypertension (high blood pressure), osteoporosis, anemia, dental decay, and some bowel disorders.

What "Reducing Risk" Means

Reducing risk means lowering the chances of developing a disease. It does not guarantee the prevention of a disease. Since the development of disease involves several factors, risk reduction usually involves several different strategies or approaches. Healthy eating is just one positive action that may help to avoid a potential problem.

Healthy Eating in Canada

The Food Guide is based on nutrition and food science. A key reference is *Nutrition Recommendations: The Report of the Scientific Review Committee*, published in 1990 by Health Canada. This report contains a review of nutrition research conducted by a committee of scientists and provides recommendations describing the desired characteristics of the Canadian diet. The *Nutrition Recommendations*, which are reviewed regularly, act as the foundation for all nutrition and healthy eating programs in the country.

Canada's Food Guide to Healthy Eating

Canada's Food Guide to Healthy Eating, released in 1992, takes *Canada's Guidelines for Healthy Eating* one step further and provides consumers with more detailed information for establishing healthy eating habits through the daily selection of food. The Food Guide is a basic nutrition education tool used:

- to help plan healthy meals for individuals or groups; and
- to evaluate a person's eating habits in a general way but not to assess nutritional status.

The Food Guide meets the nutritional needs of all Canadians four years of age and over and has been designed specifically for the general public with a reading level of grade seven. It is not appropriate for those under the age of four because the number of servings and the serving sizes are too large for toddlers and preschoolers. **FIGURE C.1** shows the current Food Guide.

A review of *Canada's Food Guide to Healthy Eating* was conducted beginning in 2002 to assess whether the current guidance continues to promote a pattern of eating that meets nutrient needs, promotes health, and minimizes the risk of nutrition-related chronic disease. This assessment concluded that the Food Guide continues to promote a diet that supplies nutrients in amounts that meet needs and contribute to reducing the risk of chronic diseases. But the assessment also showed that individuals may have a difficult time understanding and applying the Food Guide. Thus, Health Canada plans to make revisions to the Food Guide, which should be completed in late 2006.

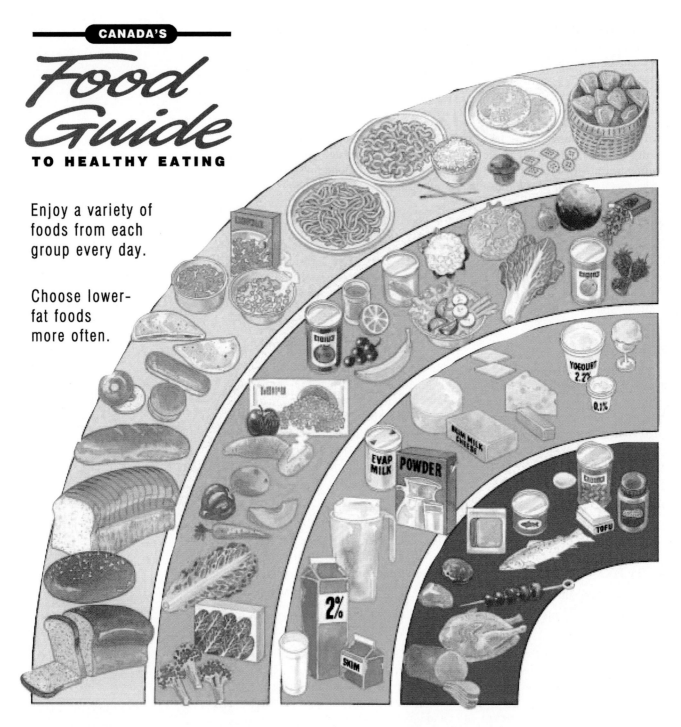

CANADA'S

Food Guide

TO HEALTHY EATING

Enjoy a variety of foods from each group every day.

Choose lower-fat foods more often.

Grain Products
Choose whole grain and enriched products more often

Vegetables & Fruit
Choose dark green and orange vegetables and orange fruit more often.

Milk Products
Choose lower-fat milk products more often

Meat & Alternatives
Choose leaner meats, poultry and fish, as well as dried peas, beans and lentils more often

FIGURE C.1 Canada's Food Guide to Healthy Eating, Public Health Agency of Canada. Reprinted with the permission of the Minister of Public Works and Government Services Canada, 2006.

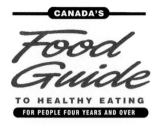

Different People Need Different Amounts of Food

The amount of food you need every day from the 4 groups and other foods depends on your age, body size, activity level, whether you are male or female and if you are pregnant or breast-feeding. That's why the Food Guide gives a lower and higher number of servings for each food group. For example, young children can choose the number of servings, while male teenagers can go to the higher number. Most other people can choose servings somewhere in between.

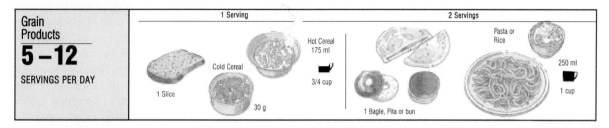

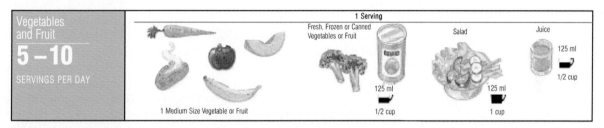

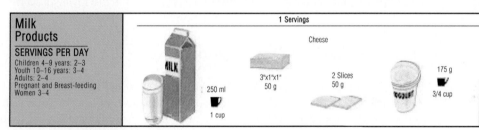

Other Foods

Taste and enjoyment can also come from other foods and beverages that are not part of the 4 food groups. Some of these foods are higher in fat or calories, so use these foods in moderation.

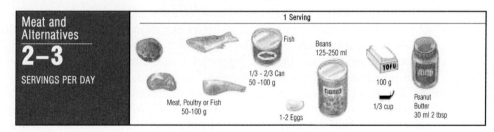

Enjoy eating well, being active and feeling good about yourself. That's *VITALIT*

©Minister of Supply and Services Canada 1992 Cat. No. H39-252/1992E No changes permitted. Reprint permission not required.
ISBN 0-662-19648-1

FIGURE C.1 Canada's Food Guide to Healthy Eating, Public Health Agency of Canada. Reprinted with the permission of the Minister of Public Works and Government Services Canada, 2006, continued.

Canada's Physical Activity Guide to Healthy Active Living

High levels of physical inactivity are a serious threat to public health in Canada. Nearly two-thirds of Canadians are not active enough to achieve optimal health benefits. These Canadians are at risk for heart disease, obesity, high blood pressure, adult-onset diabetes, osteoporosis, stroke, depression, and colon cancer. Although physical activity levels increased during the 1980s and early 1990s, the progress has stalled. Health Canada estimates that physical inactivity results in at least 21,000 premature deaths annually.

Canada's Physical Activity Guide to Healthy Active Living, produced by a joint effort of Health Canada and the Canadian Society for Exercise Physiology, provides the first set of Canadian guidelines for physical activity. It provides information to help Canadians understand how to achieve health benefits by being physically active. The guide complements the popular *Canada's Food Guide to Healthy Eating* and provides concrete examples of how to incorporate physical activity into daily life.

Designed for adults, the guide recommends 60 minutes of physical activity every day to stay healthy or improve your health. As a person progresses to more intense activity, they can cut down to 30 minutes, four days a week. The guide also suggests Canadians can add up their activities in periods of at least 10 minutes each, starting slowly and building up. **FIGURE C.2** shows the Physical Activity Guide.

Federal, provincial, and territorial governments are working to reduce the number of inactive Canadians. *Canada's Physical Activity Guide to Healthy Active Living* is a major step toward building the knowledge and awareness necessary for all Canadians to become more active. The healthy active living series now also includes *Physical Activity Guide to Healthy Active Living for Older Adults, Physical Activity Guide for Youth, Physical Activity Guide for Children,* and *Active Living at Work.*

Nutrition Labeling for Canadians

The nutrition label is one of the most useful tools in selecting foods for healthy eating (**FIGURE C.3**). The Food Guide outlines a pattern of healthy eating; the nutrition label supports the Food Guide by helping consumers to choose foods according to healthy eating messages.

Consumers can use labels to compare products and make choices on the basis of nutrient content. For example, consumers can choose a lower-fat product based on the fat content given on the labels.

Consumers also can use label information to evaluate products in relation to healthy eating. For instance, the *Nutrition Recommendations* advise Canadians to get 30 percent or less of their day's energy (kilocalories/kilojoules) from fat. This translates into a range of fat, in grams, that can be used as a benchmark against which individual foods and meals can be evaluated. The Food Guide covers a range of energy needs from 1,800 to 3,200 kilocalories (7,500 to 13,400 kilojoules) per day. A fat intake of 30 percent or less of a day's calories means a fat intake between 60 and 105 grams of fat.

Label Claims

A claim on a food label highlights a nutritional feature of a product. It is known to influence consumer's buying habits. Manufacturers often position label claims in a bold, banner-format on the front panel of a package or on the side panel along with the nutrition label. Since a label claim must be backed up by detailed facts relating to the claim, the consumer should look for the nutrition label for more information.

NUTRIENT CONTENT CLAIMS   A nutrient content claim describes the amount of a nutrient in a food. A food whose label carries the claim *high fibre* must contain 4 grams or more fiber per reference amount and serving of stated size. A "sodium-free" food must contain less than 5 mg of sodium per reference amount and serving of stated size.

DIET-RELATED HEALTH CLAIMS   Optional health claims highlight the characteristics of a diet that reduces the chance of developing a disease such as cancer or heart disease. They also tell how the food fits into the diet.

Characteristic of the Diet:	Reduced Risk of:
Low in sodium and high in potassium	High blood pressure
Adequate in calcium and vitamin D	Osteoporosis
Low in saturates and *trans* fats	Heart disease
Rich in fruits, and vegetables	Some types of cancer

For the latest information, visit the Nutrition Labeling area of the Health Canada Web site at: http:// www.hc-sc.gc.ca/hppb/nutrition/labels/index.html.

Canadian Diabetes Association's Meal Planning Guide

The Canadian Diabetes Association (CDA) works to promote the health of Canadians through diabetes research, education, service, and advocacy. In response to the introduction of new medications and new methods for the management of diabetes, CDA has revised its meal planning guide. Like the Exchange Lists, the CDA meal planning guide was designed to make it easier for people with diabetes to eat the right amount of food for their insulin supply. The system is based on two concepts: Most foods are eaten by people with diabetes in measured amounts, and foods within each of the system's eight food groups can be interchanged.

The new guide, *Beyond the Basics: Meal Planning for Diabetes Prevention and Management*, has several features. First, food items have been modified to reflect current thinking on heart health, glycemic index, and carbohydrate counting. A wider range of multicultural foods have also been added. Portion sizes have been adjusted to be more similar to the *Canada's Food Guide to Healthy Eating*, and to the Quebec and U.S. meal planning systems. The guide also used color coding to help consumers: green for "choose more often" or "everyday" foods and amber for "choose less often" or "special occasion foods." The listed portions of all carbohydrate-rich foods now contain 15 grams of available carbohydrate (total carbohydrate minus fiber and half of any sugar alcohols).

Beyond the Basics classifies foods into eight food groups:

- Grains & Starches
- Fruits
- Milk & Alternatives
- Other Choices
- Vegetables
- Meat & Alternatives
- Fats
- Extras

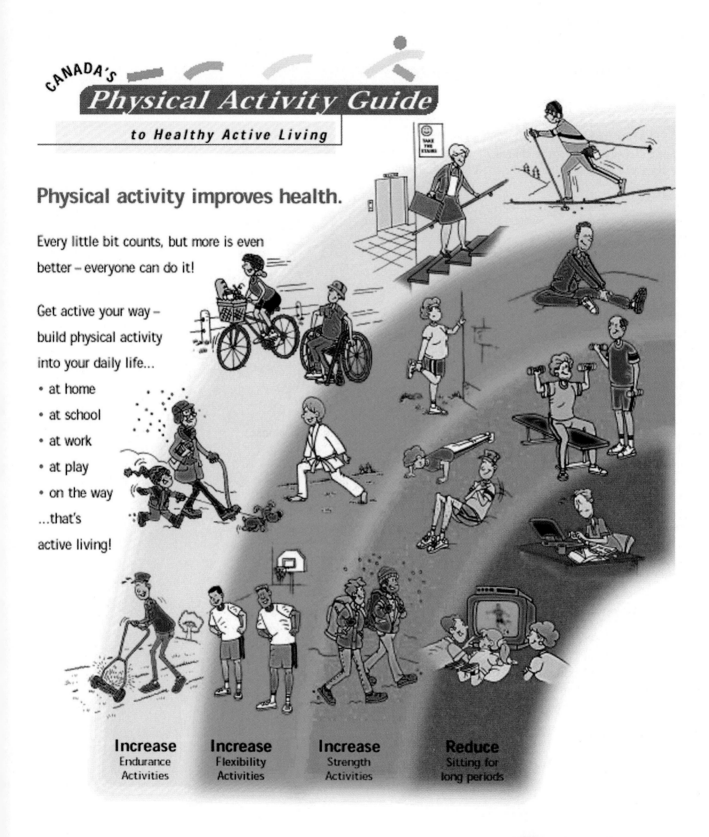

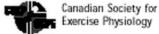

FIGURE C.2 Canada's Physical Activity Guide, Public Health Agency of Canada. Reprinted with the permission of the Minister of Public Works and Government Services Canada, 2006.

Choose a variety of activities from these three groups:

Endurance

4-7 days a week
Continuous activities for your heart, lungs and circulatory system.

Flexibility

4-7 days a week
Gentle reaching, bending and stretching activities to keep your muscles relaxed and joints mobile.

Strength

2-4 days a week
Activities against resistance to strengthen muscles and bones and improve posture.

Starting slowly is very safe for most people. Not sure? Consult your health professional.

For a copy of the *Guide Handbook* and more information:
1-888-334-9769, or
www.paguide.com

Eating well is also important. Follow *Canada's Food Guide to Healthy Eating* to make wise food choices.

Get Active Your Way, Every Day–For Life!

Scientists say accumulate 60 minutes of physical activity every day to stay healthy or improve your health. As you progress to moderate activities you can cut down to 30 minutes, 4 days a week. Add-up your activities in periods of at least 10 minutes each. Start slowly... and build up.

Time needed depends on effort

Very Light Effort	Light Effort *60 minutes*	Moderate Effort *30-60 minutes*	Vigorous Effort *20-30 minutes*	Maximum Effort
• Strolling • Dusting	• Light walking • Volleyball • Easy gardening • Stretching	• Brisk walking • Biking • Raking leaves • Swimming • Dancing • Water aerobics	• Aerobics • Jogging • Hockey • Basketball • Fast swimming • Fast dancing	• Sprinting • Racing

Range needed to stay healthy

You Can Do It – Getting started is easier than you think

Physical activity doesn't have to be very hard. Build physical activities into your daily routine.

- Walk whenever you can– get off the bus early, use the stairs instead of the elevator.
- Reduce inactivity for long periods, like watching TV.
- Get up from the couch and stretch and bend for a few minutes every hour.
- Play actively with your kids.
- Choose to walk, wheel or cycle for short trips.

- Start with a 10 minute walk – gradually increase the time.
- Find out about walking and cycling paths nearby and use them.
- Observe a physical activity class to see if you want to try it.
- Try one class to start – you don't have to make a long-term commitment.
- Do the activities you are doing now, more often.

Benefits of regular activity:

- better health
- improved fitness
- better posture and balance
- better self-esteem
- weight control
- stronger muscles and bones
- feeling more energetic
- relaxation and reduced stress
- continued independent living in later life

Health risks of inactivity:

- premature death
- heart disease
- obesity
- high blood pressure
- adult-onset diabetes
- osteoporosis
- stroke
- depression
- colon cancer

  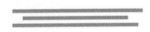 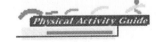

FIGURE C.2 Canada's Physical Activity Guide, Public Health Agency of Canada. Reprinted with the permission of the Minister of Public Works and Government Services Canada, 2006, continued.

The Nutrition Facts Box

The Nutrition Facts box allows consumers to make informed choices.

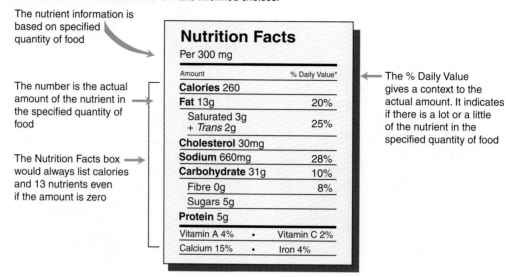

The nutrient information is based on specified quantity of food

The number is the actual amount of the nutrient in the specified quantity of food

The Nutrition Facts box would always list calories and 13 nutrients even if the amount is zero

Nutrition Facts
Per 300 mg

Amount	% Daily Value*
Calories 260	
Fat 13g	20%
Saturated 3g + *Trans* 2g	25%
Cholesterol 30mg	
Sodium 660mg	28%
Carbohydrate 31g	10%
Fibre 0g	8%
Sugars 5g	
Protein 5g	
Vitamin A 4% • Vitamin C 2%	
Calcium 15% • Iron 4%	

The % Daily Value gives a context to the actual amount. It indicates if there is a lot or a little of the nutrient in the specified quantity of food

FIGURE C.3 How to read a food label.

Within each group, food items are listed along with portions to show how much of one food is interchangeable with another food in the same group (**FIGURE C.4**). In the past, symbols for the meal planning guide food groups were used on food labels, but this has been phased out with the new food labeling regulations. However, CDA partnered with Dietetians of Canada to develop *Healthy Eating Is in Store for You*™, a nutrition labeling education program. For more information visit the CDA Web site:

http://www.diabetes.ca/Section_Professionals/btb.asp.

SOURCE: Insel, P., Turner, R. E., & Ross, D. (2006). *Discovering Nutrition,* 2nd ed. Sudbury, MA: Jones and Bartlett Publishers.

Ingredients List must be included by law and must list all of the ingredients used in the product. Ingredients are listed in the order of the amount used. The amount is based on the weight of an ingredient rather than its volume.

INGREDIENTS: Fructose Syrup (from Grapes, Corn, and Pears), Oat Bran, Maltodextrin (Complex Carbohydrate), Modified Milk Ingredients (Milk Protein with Lactose removed), Brown Rice, Almond Butter, Natural Berry Flavours, Carmine, Citric Acid, **VITAMINS AND MINERALS:** Dicalcium phosphate, Potassium bicarbonate, Ascorbic acid, Magnesium carbonate, Alpha tocopherol (vit. E), Zinc gluconate, Ferrous fumarate, Salt, Potassium iodide, Beta carotene (vit. A), Copper gluconate, Manganese sulfate, Calcium pantothenate, Pyridoxine hydrochloride (vit. B_6), Riboflavin (vit B_2), Niacin, Thiamin hydrochloride (vit. B_1), Cholecalciferol (vit. D), Folic acid, Biotin, Cyanocobalamin (vit. B_{12}).

INGRÉDIENTS: Sirop de fructose (de Raisin, de Maïs, et de Poire), Son d'avione, Maltodextrine (glucide complexe), Substances latières modifées (protéines du lait, lactose enlevé), Riz brun, Beurre d'amande, Arômes naturels de baie, Carmin, Acide citrique, **VITAMINES ET MINERAUX:** Phosphate bicalcique, Bicarbonate de potassium, Acide ascorbique, Carbonate de magnésium, Alpha tocophérol (vit. E), Gluconate de zinc Fumarate ferreux, Sel, Iodure de potassium, Bêta-carotène (vit. A), Gluconate de cuivre, Sulfate de manganèse, Pantothénate de calcium, Chlorhydrate de pyridoxine (vit. B_6), Riboflavine (vit. B_2), Niacine, Chlorhydrate de thiamine (vit. B_1), Cholécalciférol (vit. D), Acide folique, Biotine, Cyanocobalamine (vit. B_{12}).

FIGURE C.4 Ingredients list.

Calculations and Conversions

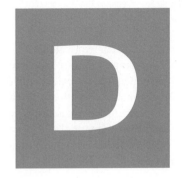

Energy from Food

grams carbohydrate $\times$ 4 kcal/g

grams protein $\times$ 4 kcal/g

grams fat $\times$ 9 kcal/g

grams alcohol $\times$ 7 kcal/g

total = energy from food

Example:		
Carbohydrate	**275 g $\times$ 4 kcal/g =**	**1,100 kcal**
Protein	**64 g $\times$ 4 kcal/g =**	**256 kcal**
Fat	**60 g $\times$ 9 kcal/g =**	**540 kcal**
Alcohol	**1 = g $\times$ 7 kcal/g =**	**105 kcal**
		TOTAL ENERGY 2,001 kcal

Calculating the percentage of calories for each:

Carbohydrate	**(1,100 kcal $\div$ 2,001 kcal) $\times$ 100 =**	**54.97% (55%)**
Protein	**(256 kcal $\div$ 2,001 kcal) $\times$ 100 =**	**12.79% (13%)**
Fat	**(540 kcal $\div$ 2,001 kcal) $\times$ 100 =**	**26.99% (27%)**
Alcohol	**(105 kcal $\div$ 2,001 kcal) $\times$ 100 =**	**5.25% (5%)**

   1 kilocalorie = 4.184 kilojoules
   1 kilojoule   = 0.239 kilocalories

Recommended Protein Intake for Adults

grams of recommended protein = weight in kilograms $\times$ 0.8 g/kg

Example:

A 70-kg (154-lb) person

grams of recommended protein = 70 kg $\times$ 0.8 g/kg = 56 grams protein, or

grams of recommended protein = (154 lb $\div$ 2.2) $\times$ 0.8 g/kg = 56 grams protein

Note: Endurance athletes involved in heavy training may require 1.2 to 1.4 grams of protein per kilogram of body weight per day.

Niacin Equivalents (NE)

Determining the amount of niacin from tryptophan:

NE = milligrams niacin

NE from tryptophan = grams excess protein $\div$ 6

NE from tryptophan = (grams dietary protein − protein RDA) $\div$ 6

Example:	**Assume dietary protein = 86 g and protein RDA = 56 g**
	NE from tryptophan = (86 g − 56 g) $\div$ 6
	NE from tryptophan = 5

Dietary Folate Equivalents (DFE)

Dietary folate equivalents account for differences in the absorption of food folate, synthetic folic acid in dietary supplements, and folic acid added to fortified foods. Food in the stomach also affects bioavailability. Folic acid taken as a supplement when fasting is two times more bioavailable than food folate. Folic acid taken with food and folic acid in fortified foods are 1.7 times more bioavailable than food folate.

1 μg DFE = 1 microgram of food folate

= 0.5 μg of folic acid supplement taken on an empty stomach

= 0.6 μg of folic acid supplement consumed with meals

= 0.6 μg of folic acid in fortified foods

1 μg folic acid as a fortificant = 1.7 μg DFE

1 μg folic acid as a supplement, fasting = 2.0 μg DFE

Example:

Food folate in cooked spinach	100 μg	= 100 μg DFE
Ready-to-eat cereal fortified with folic acid	100 μg	= 170 μg DFE
Supplemental folic acid taken without food	100 μg	= 200 μg DFE

Estimating DFE from Daily Value:

$$DFE = \%DV \times DV \times bioavailability\ factor$$

Example:

Assume that a serving of fortified breakfast cereal contains 10% of the Daily Value for folate

Daily Value = 400 μg folic acid

DFE = %DV × DV × bioavailability factor

DFE = 0.10 × 400 μg × 1.7

DFE = 68 μg, which can be rounded to 70 μg DFE

Retinol Activity Equivalents (RAE)

Retinol activity equivalents are a standardized measure of vitamin A activity that account for differences in the bioavailability of different sources of vitamin A. Of the provitamin A carotenoids, beta-carotene produces the most vitamin A.

1 μg RAE = 1 μg retinol

= 12 μg beta-carotene

= 24 μg of other vitamin A precursors

Although outdated, many vitamin supplements still report vitamin A content as International Units (IU).

1 μg RAE = 3.33 IU from retinol

= 10 IU from beta-carotene in supplements

= 20 IU from beta-carotene in foods

Vitamin D

Although outdated, many vitamin supplements still report vitamin D content as International Units (IU).

$$1\ IU = 0.025\ μg\ cholecalciferol$$

μg cholecalciferol = IU ÷ 40

Example:

A vitamin supplement contains 100 IU vitamin D

μg cholecalciferol = 100 ÷ 40 = 2.5

Vitamin E

Although outdated, many vitamin supplements still report vitamin E content as International Units (IU) rather than as milligrams of a-tocopherol. Two conversion factors are used to convert IU to milligrams of a-tocopherol. If the form of the supplement is "natural" or RRR-a-tocopherol (historically labeled as *d*-alpha-tocopherol), the conversion factor is 0.67 mg/IU. If the form of the supplement is *all rac*-a-tocopherol (historically labeled *dl*-a-tocopherol), the conversion factor is 0.4 = mg/IU.

Examples:

A multivitamin supplement contains 30 IU of *d*-a-tocopherol

30 IU × 0.67 = 20 μg a-tocopherol

A multivitamin supplement contains 30 IU of *dl*-a-tocopherol

30 IU × 0.4 = 513.5 μg a-tocopherol

Estimating Energy Expenditure

The Estimated Energy Requirement (EER) is defined as the dietary energy intake (in kilocalories per day) that is predicted to maintain energy balance in a healthy adult of a defined age, gender, weight, height, and level of physical activity consistent with good health.* The EER equations predict Total Energy Expenditure (TEE).

Adult men (age 19 and older):

$$EER = 662 - 9.53 \times Age\ [yr] + PA \times (15.91 \times Weight\ [kg] + 5 \times 9.6 \times Height\ [m])$$

PA is the Physical Activity coefficient that represents physical activity level

Sedentary	PA = 1.0
Low active	PA = 1.11
Active	PA = 1.25
Very active	PA = 1.48

Adult women (age 19 and older):

$$EER = 354 - 6.91 \times Age\ [yr] + PA \times (9.36 \times Weight\ [kg] + 726 \times Height\ [m])$$

PA is the Physical Activity coefficient that represents physical activity level

Sedentary	**PA = 1.0**
[Low activetab]PA = 1.12	
Active	**PA = 1.27**
Very active	**PA = 1.45**

Example: **A 21-year-old woman, 5′4[doubleprime] (1.6 m) tall, who weighs 120 pounds (54.5 kilograms), and is active.**

Example: **= 354 − 6.91 × 21 yr + 1.27 ×**

   (9.36 × 54.5 kg + 726 × 1.6 m)

   = 354 − 145.11 + 1.27 × (510.12 + 1,161.6)

   = 354 − 145.11 + 1.27 × 1,671.72

   = 354 − 145.11 + 2,123.08

   = 2,331.97

   = 2,332 kcal/day

*SOURCE: Institute of Medicine, Food and Nutrition Board. *Dietary Reference Intakes for Energy, Carbohydrate, Fiber, Fat, Fatty Acids, Cholesterol, Protein, and Amino Acids.* Washington, DC: National Academy Press; 2002.

Total energy expenditure can also be estimated by first estimating resting energy expenditure (REE) and then adding additional energy to account for physical activity and the thermic effect of food.

Resting Energy Expenditure (REE)

Harris-Benedict Equations

Adult men   REE = 66 + 13.7W + 5.0H − 6.8A

Adult women REE = 655 + 9.6W + 1.8H − 4.7A

(W = weight in kilograms, H = height in centimeters, A = age)

Note: Harris-Benedict equations may overestimate resting energy expenditure, especially for obese people.

Quick Estimate

Adult men   REE − weight (kg) × 1.0 kcal/kg × 24 hours

   REE = weight (kg) × 1.0 × 24

Adult women REE = weight (kg) × 0.9 kcal/kg × 24 hours

   REE = weight (kg) × 0.9 × 24

Physical Activity (PA)

Physical activity can be estimated as a percentage of the resting energy expenditure (REE) based on the frequency and intensity of physical activity.

Percentage of REE	Activity Level	Description
20–30%	Sedentary	Mostly resting, with little or no activity
30–45%	Light	Occasional unplanned activity (e.g., going for a stroll)
45–65%	Moderate	Daily planned activity, such as brisk walks
65–90%	Heavy	Daily workout routine requiring several hours of continuous exercise
90–120%	Exceptional	Daily vigorous workouts for extended hours; training for competition

Thermic Effect of Food (TEF)

The thermic effect of food can be estimated as 10% of the sum of REE + physical activity

Total energy expenditure (TEE) = REE + PA + TEF

Example using quick estimate of REE:

A 175-pound (79.5 kg), 30-year-old man engages in moderate activity (60% of REE).

REE	**= 79.5 kg × 1.0 kcal/kg/hr × 24 hr/day**
	= 1,908 kcal/day
PA	**= 60% of REE**
	= 0.60 × 1908 kcal/day
	= 1144.8 kcal/day
TEF	**= 10% of REE + PA**
	= 0.10 × (1908 + 1144.8 kcal/day)
	= 0.10 × 3052.8 kcal/day
	= 305.3 kcal/day
TEE	**= REE + PA + TEF**
	= 1908 + 1144.8 + 305.3 kcal/day
	= 3358 kcal/day

Body Mass Index (BMI)

U.S. Formula

BMI = [weight in pounds ÷ (height in inches)^2] × 703

Example: **A 154-pound man is 5 ft 8 inches (68 inches) tall**

BMI = [154 ÷ (68 in × 68 in)] × 703

BMI = (154 ÷ 4,624) × 703

BMI = 23.41

Metric Formula

BMI = weight in kilograms ÷ [height in meters]^2
    or
BMI = [weight in kilograms ÷ (height in cm)^2] × 10,000

Example: **A 70-kg man is 1.75 meters tall**

BMI = 70 kg ÷ (1.75 m × 1.75 m)
BMI = 70 ÷ 3.0625
BMI = 22.86

Metric Prefixes

giga-	G	1,000,000,000
mega-	M	1,000,000
kilo-	k	1,000
hecto-	h	100
deka-	da	10
deci-	d	0.1
centi-	c	0.01
milli-	m	0.001
micro-	m	0.000001
nano-	n	0.000000001

Length: Metric and U.S. Equivalents

1 centimeter	0.3937 inch
1 decimeter	3.937 inches
1 foot	0.3048 meter
1 inch	2.54 centimeters
1 meter	39.37 inches
	1.094 yards
1 micron	0.001 millimeter
	0.00003937 inch
1 millimeter	0.03937 inch
1 yard	0.9144 meter

Capacities or Volumes

1 cup, measuring	8 fluid ounces
	½ liquid pint
1 gallon (U.S.)	231 cubic inches
	3.785 liters
	0.833 British gallon
	128 U.S. fluid ounces
1 gallon (British Imperial)	277.42 cubic inches
	1.201 U.S. gallons

	4.546 liters
	160 British fluid ounces
1 liter	1.057 liquid quarts
	0.908 dry quart
	61.024 cubic inches
1 milliliter	0.061 cubic inches
1 ounce, fluid or liquid (U.S.)	1.805 cubic inches
	29.574 milliliters
	1.041 British fluid ounces
1 pint, dry	33.600 cubic inches
	0.551 liter
1 pint, liquid	28.875 cubic inches
	0.473 liter
1 quart, dry (U.S.)	67.201 cubic inches
	1.101 liters
	0.969 British quart
1 quart, liquid (U.S.)	57.75 cubic inches
	0.946 liter
	0.833 British quart
1 quart (British)	69.354 cubic inches
	1.032 U.S. dry quarts
	1.201 U.S. liquid quarts
1 tablespoon, measuring	3 teaspoons
	½ fluid ounce
1 teaspoon, measuring	⅓ tablespoon
	⅙ fluid ounce
1 kilogram	2.205 pounds
1 microgram (mg)	0.000001 gram

Food Measurement Equivalents

16 tablespoons = 1 cup
12 tablespoons = ¾ cup
10 tablespoons + 2 teaspoons = ⅔ cup
8 tablespoons = ½ cup
6 tablespoons = ⅜ cup
5 tablespoons + 1 teaspoon = ⅓ cup
4 tablespoons = ¼ cup
2 tablespoons = ⅛ cup
2 tablespoons + 2 teaspoons = ⅙ cup
1 tablespoon = ¹⁄₁₆ cup
2 cups = 1 pint
2 pints = 1 quart
3 teaspoons = 1 tablespoon
48 teaspoons = 1 cup

Food Measurement Conversions: U.S. to Metric

Capacity

⅕ teaspoon.......1 milliliter	1 cup ....237 milliliters
1 teaspoon ....5 milliliters	2 cups (1 pint) ......473 milliliters
1 tablespoon.....15 milliliters	4 cups (1 quart)....0.95 liter
1 fluid ounce ....30 milliliters	4 quarts (1 gal.) ....3.8 liters
⅕ cup ....47 milliliters	

Weight

1 ounce............28 grams
1 pound ....454 grams

Food Measurement Conversions: Metric to U.S.

Capacity	Weight
1 milliliter........⅕ teaspoon	1 gram ....0.035 ounce
5 milliliters.......1 teaspoon	100 grams.............3.5 ounces
15 milliliters.....1 tablespoon	500 grams.............1.10 pounds

Capacity	Weight
100 milliliters ...3.4 fluid oz	1 kilogram ....2.205 pounds
240 milliliters ...1 cup	.........................35 ounces
1 liter.............34 fluid oz	
..................4.2 cups	
..................2.1 pints	
..................1.06 quarts	
..................0.26 gallon	

Conversion Factors

To change	To	Multiply by
centimeters	inches	0.3937
centimeters	feet	0.03281
cubic feet	cubic meters	0.0283
cubic meters	cubic feet	35.3145
cubic meters	cubic yards	1.3079
cubic yards	cubic meters	0.7646
feet	meters	0.3048
gallons (U.S.)	liters	3.7853
grams	ounces avdp	0.0353
grams	pounds	0.002205
inches	millimeters	25.4000
inches	centimeters	2.5400
inches	meters	0.0254
kilograms	pounds	2.2046
liters	gallons (U.S.)	0.2642

liters	pints (dry)	1.8162
liters	pints (liquid)	2.1134
liters	quarts (dry)	0.9081
liters	quarts (liquid)	1.0567
meters	feet	3.2808
meters	yards	1.0936
millimeters	inches	0.0394
ounces avdp	grams	28.3495
ounces	pounds	0.0625
pints (dry)	liters	0.5506
pints (liquid)	liters	0.4732
pounds	kilograms	0.4536
pounds	ounces	16
quarts (dry)	liters	1.1012
quarts (liquid)	liters	0.9463

Fahrenheit and Celsius (Centigrade) Scales

°Celsius	°Fahrenheit
−273.15	−459.67
−250	−418
−200	−328
−150	−238
−100	−148
−50	−58
−40	−40
−30	−22
−20	−4
−10	14
0	32
5	41
10	50
15	59
20	68
25	77
30	86
35	95
40	104
45	113
50	122
55	131
60	140
65	149
70	158
75	167
80	176
85	185
90	194
95	203
100	212

Zero on the Fahrenheit scale represents the temperature produced by the mixing of equal weights of snow and common salt.

	°Fahrenheit	°Celsius
Boiling point of water	212°	100°
Freezing point of water	32°	0°
Normal body temperature	98.6°	37°
Comfortable room temperature	68–77°	20–25°
Absolute zero	2459.6°	2273.1°

Absolute zero is theoretically the lowest possible temperature, the point at which all molecular motion would cease.

To Convert Temperature Scales

To convert Fahrenheit to Celsius (Centigrade), subtract 32 and multiply by $5/9$.

$$°C = 5/9(°F - 32)$$

To convert Celsius (Centigrade) to Fahrenheit, multiply by $9/5$ and add 32.

$$°F = (9/5 \times °C) + 32$$

SOURCE: Insel, P., Turner, R. E., & Ross, D. (2006). *Discovering Nutrition*, 2nd ed. Sudbury, MA: Jones and Bartlett Publishers.

Glossary

Actin Thin protein filament found in muscle; plays an important role in muscle movement.

Action Stage of change in which the desired level of the new behavior has been reached and is consistently adhered to, although the individual has been doing it for less than 6 months.

Active stretching Taking a muscle beyond its normal range of motion with assistance.

Adaptation A long-term change in reaction to regular exposure to a stimulus (e.g., lower resting heart rate with increased fitness).

Adenosine triphosphate A highenergy phosphate that is the only useable form of energy in the human body.

Adipostat Brain mechanism that establishes a set point for a fixed amount of body fat.

Administrative complaint An action that brings about a formal proceeding; much like a court trial, it takes place before an administrative law judge.

Aerobic Metabolic process that relies on oxygen. For aerobic metabolism to take place, exercise intensity must be low to moderate.

Agonist Muscle that acts as the prime mover; the muscle most responsible for a movement.

Alarm reaction Immediate response to a stressor that is riggered by any threat to our physical or emotional well-being.

Allostatic load The ongoing level of demand for adaptation in an individual.

Amenorrhea Absence of menstrual periods.

Amino acid Complex chemical structure of protein, containing atoms of carbon, hydrogen, oxygen, and nitrogen.

Anaerobic Metabolic process that does not rely on oxygen. Anaerobic metabolism occurs at the start of physical activity and when intensity is very high.

Anemia Deficiency in red blood cells.

Angina pectoris Chest pain due to coronary heart disease.

Anorexia nervosa Eating disorder in which individuals incorrectly believe they are overfat; resultant excessive dieting leads to health problems.

Antagonist Muscle that resists the agonist; helps to maintain joint stability.

Anxiety Normal response when a fear-eliciting situation arises.

Anxiety disorders Mental disorders caused by heightened arousal or fear over a sustained period of time.

Aorta Large artery that receives blood from the heart's left ventricle and distributes it to the body.

Arteries Blood vessels that carry oxygenated blood from the heart to the body.

Arterioles Small, muscular branches of arteries; when they contract, they increase resistance to blood flow, and blood pressure increases.

Arteriosclerosis "Hardening of the arteries"; arterial walls thicken and lose elasticity.

Atherosclerosis A form of arteriosclerosis in which the inner layers of the artery become thick and irregular due to fatty deposits called plaque.

Atrophy Decrease in cell size, usually in reference to muscle or fat.

Autonomic nervous system The part of the nervous system that controls smooth muscle, cardiac muscle, and glands; subdivided into sympathetic and parasympathetic.

Autoregulation Self-regulation.

Ballistic stretching Fast, momentum-assisted, pulsing movements used to stretch muscles.

Basal metabolic rate (BMR) Basic energy requirement necessary to sustain life.

Behavioral factors Factors related to your behavior patterns that affect your adherence to an activity program.

Benign Not cancerous; does not invade nearby tissue or spread to other parts of the body.

Bicarbonate ions (HCO3) As a buffer, they prevent a change in blood pH.

Binge drinking Having five or more drinks at any one time.

Bioelectrical impedance Technique to measure body fat percentage that passes a harmless, low-level, single-frequency electrical current through the body using electrodes placed on the wrist and ankle.

Biological factors Factors related to your biology that affect your adherence to an activity program.

Bisexuals People who are attracted to members of both genders.

Blood alcohol concentration (BAC) The amount of alcohol in the blood.

Blood pressure The force blood applies to the walls of the blood vessels.

Blood pressure cuff (sphygmomanometer) Instrument that measures blood pressure.

Body composition The major chemical components of the body: fat mass, muscle mass, bone density, and water volume.

Body image The picture one has of one's body, what it looks like to one's self, and how one think it looks to others.

Bone mineral density (BMD) Usually expressed as the amount of mineralized tissue in the scanned area, it is a risk factor for fractures.

Breasts Network of milk glands and ducts in fatty tissue; secondary sex characteristic.

Bulimia nervosa Eating disorder in which individuals binge-eat and then force themselves to vomit.

Calorie Amount of heat it takes to raise the temperature of 1 gram of water 1 degree Celsius.

Cancer A term for diseases in which abnormal cells divide without control. Cancer cells can invade nearby tissues and spread through the bloodstream and lymphatic system to other parts of the body.

Capillaries Tiny blood vessels that circulate blood to all the body's cells.

Carbohydrates Organic compounds that contain carbon, hydrogen, and oxygen.

Carbon monoxide One of the most abundant and poisonous gases in cigarette smoke.

Cardiac output The amount of blood ejected from the heart each minute; calculated by multiplying heart rate by stroke volume.

Cardiorespiratory fitness The integration of the pulmonary and cardiovascular systems. The lungs, heart, and vascular network deliver key nutrients while removing waste products.

Cartilage Semi-rigid tissue that provides support.

Cease-and-desist order A legal order informing a company that it must no longer advertise or market a product.

Cerebral embolism Blood clot formed in one part of the body and then carried by the bloodstream to the brain, where it blocks an artery.

Cerebral hemorrhage Bleeding within the brain that results from a ruptured aneurysm or a head injury.

Cerebral thrombosis Blood clot in an artery that supplies the brain.

Cervix The lower and narrow end of the uterus.

Chancre The primary lesion of syphilis, which appears as a hard, painless sore or ulcer, often on the penis or vaginal tissue; pronounced "shanker."

Cholesterol Waxy substance that circulates naturally in the bloodstream; when levels are too high, it deposits in the walls of blood vessels.

Chronic diseases Illnesses that can develop early in life and last a long period of time.

Circuit weight training Method of training that involves moving from station to station, performing different exercises at each station.

Circumcision A surgical procedure to remove the foreskin from the penis.

Clitoris Small, sensitive female organ located in front of the vaginal opening; center of sexual pleasuring.

Chlamydia Sexually transmitted disease caused by the bacterium *Chlamydia trichomatis*.

Complex carbohydrates Called polysaccharides, these link three or more sugar molecules.

Concentric muscle action Muscle movement in which the muscle shortens while under tension.

Collagen The principle substance in connecting fibers and tissues, and in bones.

Compliance Ease with which amaterial is elongated or stretched; the opposite of stiffness.

Compound sets Consecutive performance of two sets of exercises that stress the same muscle group.

Consent order An agreement bringing about voluntary compliance without a judicial ruling.

Contemplation Stage of change that begins when the individual starts to think seriously about intending to make a long-term change in the near future (within 6 months).

Copulation Sexual intercourse.

Coronary heart disease Disease of the heart caused by atherosclerotic narrowing of the coronary arteries.

Cowper's glands Small glands that secrete drops of alkalinizing fluid into the urethra.

Creatine phosphate Fuel source used in the body to replenish ATP; stored in small amount, it depletes rapidly.

Decisional balance An individual's relative weighing of the pros and cons of changing.

Degeneration A gradual decrease in function.

Deoxygenated blood Blood returned to the heart, to be replenished with oxygen in the lungs.

Depressant A drug that produces a slowing of mental and physical activities.

Depression A mental disorder notable for negative alteration in mood.

Depressive reactions Normal depressed feelings such as sadness and hopelessness.

Diastolic pressure The lowest blood pressure measured in the arteries; occurs when the heart muscle is relaxed between beats.

Dietary fiber Diverse carbohydrate polysaccharides of plants that cannot be digested by the human stomach or small intestine.

Dietary Reference Intakes (DRIs) Umbrella term that includes Estimated Average Requirement, Recommended Dietary Allowance, Adequate Intake, and Tolerable Upper Intake Level.

Digestion Metabolizing of food through a series of complex mechanical and chemical reactions.

Disaccharide Two-sugar molecule.

Distress Harmful or bad stress.

Drug Any absorbed substance, other than food, that changes or enhances any physical or psychological function in the body.

Drug therapeutics The proper use of drugs in treating and preventing diseases and preserving health.

Dysthymia Chronic form of depression.

Eating disorder Refers to a wide range of harmful eating behaviors used in the attempt to lose weight or achieve a lean appearance.

Eccentric muscle action Muscle movement in which the muscle lengthens while under tension.

Elasticity Degree to which a material resists deformation and quickly returns to its normal shape.

Emotional health Encompasses mental states that include feelings or subjective experiences in response to changes in our environment.

Endocardium Thin, inner layer that lines the heart.

Endocrine system The hormonesecreting cells of the body; this system is influenced in part by the nervous system.

Endorphins Body chemicals responsible for enhancing emotions and providing pain relief.

Environmental engineering Stress management approach that attempts to avoid it in the first place.

Epidemiological studies Studies of diseases, their causes, and their spread.

Epididymitis Inflammation of the epididymis (structure that connects the vas deferens and the testes).

Epinephrine The "fear hormone"; helps supply glucose for increased muscle and nervous system activity.

Ergogenic aid Any substance or phenomenon that enhance performance.

Ergolytic A substance that has a detrimental effect on performance.

Essential amino acids The nine amino acids that the body cannot make.

Essential body fat Fat that is required for normal healthy functioning.

Essential fatty acids Support immune responses, form cell structures, regulate blood pressure, affect blood lipid concentration, and promote clot formation; must be obtained from food.

Essential nutrients Nutrients the body cannot make for itself; must be obtained from food.

Ethyl alcohol A direct central nervous system depressant that causes a decreased level of consciousness and decreased motor function; the common psychoactive ingredient in all alcoholic beverages.

Eustress Helpful or good stress.

Exercise A subset of physical activity that is a planned, structured, repetitive, and purposeful attempt to improve or maintain physical fitness.

Fallopian tubes A pair of tube-like structures that transport ova from the ovaries to the uterus; the usual site of fertilization.

Fats Members of a family of compounds called lipids.

Fat-soluble vitamins Vitamins A, D, E, K; must travel with dietary fats in the bloodstream to reach the cells.

Feedback Receiver response to a message, letting the sender know the message was received and what the message was.

Fertilization The fusion of a sperm cell and an ovum.

Fight-or-flight response Response to stressors that challenge the body to respond physically.

First law of thermodynamics Energy can neither be created nor destroyed.

Flexibility The range of motion available at a joint.

Foreskin A fold of skin over the end of the penis.

Fraud Conscious promotion of unproven claims for profit.

Functional foods Foods that contain significant levels of biologically active components that provide health benefits beyond basic nutrition.

Gametes Sex cells, either sperm or ova, that fuse at fertilization; gametes carry a complete set of genetic information from each parent that is passed on to the child.

Gardnerella vaginalis Bacterium that causes vaginal infection; symptoms of infection include vaginal irritation.

Gender identity Awareness and acceptance of being male or female.

Gender role Complex group of behaviors expected of males and females in a given culture.

General adaptation syndrome (GAS) The body's response to stress and the adaptability of the body to maintain homeostasis.

Generalized anxiety disorder (GAD) Experiencing exaggerated worrying, inability to relax, and insomnia for 6 months or more.

Glucocorticoids Chemicals responsible for speeding up the body's metabolism and increasing access to energy storage.

Glycogen Storage form of sugar energy for humans and animals.

Golgi tendon organs Sense receptors sensitive to rapid forceful contractions that cause a reflexive relaxation to occur within the muscle.

Gonorrhea Sexually transmitted disease caused by the bacterium *Neisseria gonorrhoera*.

Health A state of complete physical, mental, and social well-being and not merely the absence of disease or infirmity.

Health habit A health-related behavior that is firmly established and often performed automatically, without thought.

Healthy lifestyle A recurring pattern of health-promoting and disease-preventing behaviors undertaken to achieve wellness.

Heart rate The frequency at which the heart beats (contracts).

Heart rate reserve The difference between maximum heart rate and resting heart rate.

Hemoglobin The oxygen-carrying pigment of the red blood cells.

Hemorrhagic strokes Strokes caused by blood seeping from a hole in the wall of a blood vessel.

Heritability The amount genetics determines the differences between people.

Herpes Sexually transmitted disease caused by herpes simplex virus, or HSV.

Heterosexuals People who are attracted to people of the opposite gender.

Homosexuals People who are attracted to people of the same gender.

Hormones Substances secreted by the glands of the endocrine system that regulate cellular function.

Human immunodeficiency virus (HIV) The virus that causes AIDS; it causes a defect in the body's immune system by invading and then multiplying within the white blood cells.

Human papillomavirus (HPV) Genus of viruses including those causing papillomas (small nipple-like protrusions of the skin or mucous membrane) and warts.

Hyperextension Moving beyond a normal extended position at a joint.

Hyperflexion Moving beyond a normal flexed position at a joint.

Hyperglycemia Too much blood sugar.

Hyperstress Too much stress; the body begins to decrease in its level of performance.

Hypertension A chronic increase in blood pressure above its normal range.

Hypertrophy Increase in cell size. Adipose tissue (fat cells) hypertrophies when there is too much food; muscle cells hypertrophy when stressed through resistance training.

Hypoglycemia Not enough blood sugar.

Hypostress Too little stress or stimulation.

Incidence The frequency of occurrence of a particular disease, the number of new cases of a disease.

Independent risk factor A disease risk factor that stands alone; by itself, an independent risk factor can cause a disease.

Individualized Based on differing needs of different people.

Initial stage Early portion of a program in which you become accustomed to making physical activity a regular part of your life.

Insoluble fibers Dietary fibers not soluble in water or metabolized by the intestines; make feces bulkier and softer, promoting decreased passage time.

Intrinsic motivation Performing a behavior (being active) because you want to rather than because some outside influence is motivating you to do it.

Ischemia Decreased blood flow to an organ, usually due to constriction or obstruction of an artery.

Ischemic strokes Strokes caused by clots.

Isokinetic Form of resistance training in which the speed of movement is controlled.

Isometric Form of resistance training in which the muscle is stationary while under tension.

Isotonic Form of resistance training in which there is movement.

I-statements Statements beginning with "I"; positive communication skill.

Labia majora A pair of fleshy folds that cover the labia minora.

Labia minora A pair of fleshy folds that cover the vagina.

Lactic acid By-product of the anaerobic breakdown of carbohydrate; it upsets the acidbase balance in tissues and disrupts muscle function.

Lactovegetarian A vegetarian who includes milk in the diet.

Lipoproteins Lipid (fatty, insoluble substance in blood) surrounded by a protein; the protein makes it soluble in blood.

Literal message Message that is conveyed by symbols.

Low-density lipoproteins (LDL) Carriers of harmful cholesterol in the blood; "bad" cholesterol.

Macronutrients Raw fuel, in the form of protein, carbohydrates, and fats, for biological and mechanical energy requirements.

Maintenance Stage of change in which the behavioral practice is becoming habit.

Maintenance stage Stage of established regular physical activity designed to maintain current levels of fitness and health. Consolidation of gains and recovery from the progression stage.

Major depression Serious condition that leads to inability to function and possibly suicide.

Major minerals Mineral requirements that exceed 100 mg per day.

Malignant Cancerous; a growth with a tendency to invade and destroy nearby tissue and spread to other parts of the body.

Mental health A "state of successful performance of mental function, resulting in productive activities, fulfilling relationships with other people, and the ability to adapt to change and to cope with adversity" (USDHHS, 1999).

Mental illness Diagnosable mental disorders that change our thinking, mood, or behavior and lead to impaired functioning.

Metabolism Process whereby the body takes in energy, converts it to a useable form, stores what is needed, and eliminates what is not.

Metamessage Way the message is interpreted between sender and receiver.

Metastasis The spread of cancer from one part of the body to another. Cells in the metastic (secondary) tumor are the same as those in their original (primary) tumor.

Micronutrients Nutrients required in small amounts; includes vitamins and minerals.

Mind engineering Stress management approach concerned with reducing the intensity of our emotional responses to stressors.

Minerals Inorganic substances vital to many body functions.

Misinformation Information that is not factual, but is passed off as being factual.

Moderate drinking Drinking that causes no problems, either for the drinker or for society; quantified as no more than one drink a day for most women, and no more than two drinks a day for most men.

Monosaccharide One-sugar molecule.

Muscle spindles Sense receptors sensitive to rapid forceful stretching that cause a reflexive contraction of the muscle.

Muscular endurance The muscle's ability to generate force repeatedly.

Muscular strength The ability of the muscles to generate force.

Myocardial infarction (MI) Death of, or damage to part of, the heart muscle due to insufficient blood supply. Also known as a *heart attack*.

Myocardium Muscular middle layer that surrounds the heart.

Myosin Thick protein filament found in muscle; plays an important role in muscle movement.

Myotonia Muscle tension.

Neuromuscular adaptations Changes in the function of the nervous and muscular systems brought on by exposure to regular resistance training. These changes include the ability to selectively recruit motor units, to synchronize the recruitment of these units, and to maintain a state of equilibrium throughout the movement.

Neutralizer Muscle that prevents unwanted activity in muscles not directly involved in performing a movement.

Nicotine A dynamic psychoactive stimulant.

Nonessential nutrients Nutrients made by the body from the foods we eat.

Norepinephrine The "anger hormone"; helps speed the heart rate and raises blood pressure to provide more oxygen for the body.

Nutrient-calorie benefit ratio (NCBR) Amount of nutrient per energy unit, or the ratio of nutrients to calories.

Nutrients Elements in foods that are required for energy, growth, and repair of tissues and regulation of body processes.

Nutrition facts label Mandated food labeling designed to help consumers make appropriate choices.

Obesity A weight that exceeds the threshold of a health criterion standard to a greater degree than overweight.

Organ system A collection of specialized tissues that provide an important body function (musculoskeletal, cardiovascular).

Orgasm The climax of sexual responses and the release of physiological and sexual tensions.

Osteoblasts Bone-forming cells.

Osteoclasts A cell in developing bone concerned especially with the breaking down of unnecessary bone parts.

Osteocytes A bone cell responsible for the maintenance and turnover of the mineral content of surrounding bone.

Osteogenesis imperfecta A disease caused by abnormalities in the collagen matrix within the bone, resulting in a weak structure and the potential for multiple fractures.

Osteopenia Low bone mass.

Osteoporosis Literally means "porous bones"; a metabolic disease resulting in bone loss and bones that fracture easily.

Ova, ovum Eggs, egg.

Ovaries A pair of almond-shaped organs in the female abdomen that produces egg cells (ova) and female sex hormones (estrogen and progesterone).

Overfat Having body fat levels above recommended levels for good health.

Overload principle A body system (muscular, skeletal, cardiovascular) must be exposed to physical stress beyond that which is ordinary in order to adapt and improve function.

Overuse syndrome Condition in which too much exercise or physical activity causes the body to start to break down (symptoms: increased risk of injury, lethargy, loss of appetite, irritability, decreased motivation).

Overweight (chapter 8) Having a body weight above levels recommended for a certain height.

Overweight (chapter 9) A weight that exceeds the threshold of a health criterion standard.

Ovolactovegetarian A vegetarian who eats both eggs and milk products.

Ovovegetarian A vegetarian who includes eggs in the diet.

Ovulation Release of an egg (ovum) from the ovary.

Oxygenated blood Blood leaving the heart that is oxygen-rich.

Paget's disease A disease whose precise cause is unknown but that is a consequence of both genetic and environmental factors, such as a viral infection that triggers the osteoblasts to try to repair the damage (infection) by forming new bone. However, the new formation is disrupted, leading to weakness and deformities in the bone.

Parasympathetic nervous system The counterpart to the sympathetic nervous system.

Passive stretching A natural stretch of the muscle and tendon with no additional force applied.

Peer-reviewed research Research articles and presentations in which experts in the field of study review material for accuracy and validity before it is disseminated to the public.

Pelvic inflammatory disease (PID) Infection of the female reproductive organs; specifically, the uterus, fallopian tubes, and pelvic cavity.

Penis The male organ of copulation and urination.

Pericardium Thin, closed outer sac that surrounds the heart.

Periodization Form of resistance training in which a training program is subdivided into sections, or periods; the focus of training in each period varies, allowing for a greater overall adjustment to occur.

Pharmacology The study of drugs, their sources, how they enter the body, how the body reacts to them, and their short-term and long-term effects on the body.

Phospholipids Lipids made by the body and therefore not considered essential fatty acids.

Physical activity All energy expended by skeletal muscular movement.

Physical dependence The body's biological adaptation to a drug, in which the drug has become necessary to maintain a balance in certain body processes.

Physical engineering Stress management approach using regular exercise to optimize your stress responses.

Physical fitness A set of health-related attributes a person has, such as cardiorespiratory endurance, muscular strength and endurance, flexibility, and body composition, that contribute to one's capacity to do physical activity.

Pituitary-adrenal axis The first pattern of the fight-or-flight response.

Plaque A fatty deposit on the inner lining of the artery wall.

Plyometrics Form of resistance training that uses bounding-type exercises to overload muscles; recoil from bounding activity utilizes stored elastic energy in the connective tissue that runs through the muscle to improve performance.

PNF stretching Proprioceptive neuromuscular facilitation; utilization and integration of the nervous and muscular systems to enhance flexibility.

Precontemplation Stage of change during which individuals are not intending to make a long-term lifestyle change in the foreseeable future (usually the next 6 months).

Preparation Stage of change in which the individual intends to take action in the immediate future (usually in the next month).

Prevalence The predominance of a disease, the number of people who have the disease at one given point in time.

Primary hypertension Hypertension where the cause is unknown.

Primary prevention Actions that keep the disease process or health condition from becoming established in the first place by eliminating causes of disease or increasing resistance to disease.

Principle of individuality All people are different genetically and have different levels of potential physical development.

Principle of progression The logical and systematic application of the overload principle.

Principle of recovery An adequate rest period must be allowed for your body to adapt and become stronger.

Principle of reversibility All benefits gained through participation in a physical activity program will be lost if the activity is not continued.

Principle of specificity You must target activities to specific systems to improve their particular function.

Problem drinking The consumption of alcohol that results in significant risk of health consequences, social problems, or both.

Processes of change The mechanisms through which different techniques influence a person's behavior change.

Program factors Factors related to your physical activity program that affect your adherence to that program.

Progression stage Stage in which you stress your body so as to develop greater levels of conditioning and fitness. This stage is short due to high levels of stress on the body. Optimal levels of fitness are obtained.

Proprioceptors Sense receptors that provide feedback to our central nervous system.

Prostate gland Gland at the base of the male bladder that provides seminal fluid.

Protein An essential nutrient that the body uses in more ways than any other.

Protein filaments Strands of protein (actin and myosin) that give muscle its structure and functional ability.

Psychoactive drug A chemical substance that alters one's thinking, perceptions, feelings, and behavior.

Psychological dependence Craving for a drug for primarily psychological or emotional reasons.

Psychological factors Factors related to your state of mind that affect your adherence to an activity program.

Psychosomatic disease Bodily symptoms caused by mental or emotional disturbance.

Pubic lice Small insects that live in hair in the genital-rectal region.

Pulmonary system Pertaining to the lungs; includes pulmonary arteries and veins.

Pyramiding A gradual increase in the weight being lifted with a corresponding reduction in the number of repetitions until the one-repetition maximum is reached; this is followed by a gradual decrease in the resistance being lifted and an increase in the number of repetitions, until the exerciser returns to the initial load.

Pyruvic acid By-product of the breakdown of glucose metabolism. If oxygen is not present, pyruvic acid is converted into lactic acid. If oxygen is present, pyruvic acid is further broken down to provide energy for movement.

Quackery Overpromotion of a product in the field of health.

Relaxation response The opposite of the fight-or-flight response to stressful or threatening situations.

Remodeling The ongoing dual processes of bone formation and bone resorption after cessation of growth.

Reps Repetitions; a rep occurs each time a muscle action is performed.

Resorption The loss of substance (bone, in this case) through physiological or pathological means.

Response A short-term change in reaction to a stimulus (e.g., increased breathing rate after moving from inactive to active state).

Resting metabolic rate (RMR) A person's rate of energy use at rest.

Retrovirus A type of virus (such as the one that causes AIDS) that can invade cells and integrate its own genetic information into chromosomes.

Rickets A deficiency of vitamin D (usually seen in children), causing weak bones and deformation due to overgrowth of cartilage at the ends of the bones. In adults, this condition leads to softening of the bone, leading to fracture and deformity.

Sarcomere The functional unit of a muscle. The site where muscle movement takes place.

Scabies Infestation of the skin by microscopic mites (insects).

Scrotum The sac of skin that contains the testes.

Secondary hypertension Hypertension arising from another physical condition, such as kidney disease.

Secondary prevention Aims at early detection of asymptomatic disease through preventive screenings and tests.

Secondary sex characteristics Anatomical features appearing at puberty that distinguish males from females.

Secondhand smoke Exhaled mainstream smoke and sidestream smoke from another person's cigarette, cigar, or pipe. Also known as environmental tobacco smoke (ETS).

Self-changers Individuals who can manage and control their own lives.

Self-disclosure The sharing of private information.

Self-efficacy The confidence one has in one's ability to perform specific behaviors in specific situations.

Semen A whitish, creamy fluid containing sperm.

Seminal vesicles Sac-like structures that secrete a fluid that activates the sperm.

Semivegetarian A vegetarian who may eat fish and poultry, but not eat red meat.

Set point Level of resting metabolism that your body naturally prefers. Some research suggests that our metabolic rate will return to its set point even if we try to change our metabolism through modifying our diet.

Set point theory A theory that proposes that a regulatory system exists in the human body that is designed to maintain body weight at some fixed level.

Sets Groups of repetitions.

Sex (1) An individual's classification as male or female based on anatomical characteristics, (2) a set of behaviors, (3) the experience of erotic pleasure.

Sexual Characterized by, or having, sex; opposed to asexual.

Sexuality A person's sense of self, which is used to create sexual experiences.

Sexually transmitted diseases (STDs) Diseases that are primarily contracted through sexual contact.

Sexually transmitted warts Hard growths on the skin of the genitals or anus, caused by an infection with human papillomavirus, or HPV.

Sexual orientation Attraction toward and interest in members of one or both genders.

Sexual response cycle The physiological response in both men and women; described in four phases.

Simple carbohydrates Either one-sugar or two-sugar molecules.

Sinoatrial node The natural pacemaker of the heart.

Skinfold technique Measure of subcutaneous fat at various body sites using special calipers.

Smegma Cheese-like substance that accumulates under the foreskin of the penis.

Social drinking Use of alcohol that consists of an occasional drink or two in the company of friends.

Social factors Factors from your social environment that affect your adherence to an activity program.

Soluble fibers Dietary fibers soluble in water, metabolized in the large intestine; assist in removing cholesterol from the body.

Spiral model of change A relapse model that demonstrates that individuals move back and forth along the change continuum a number of times before attaining their behavioral goal and therefore views setbacks as positive because changers are learning something new every time they change.

Stages of change A variable process that is organized in a continuum according to the decision-making process that is required to effect change.

Starches Storage form of carbohydrates for plants.

Static contraction Muscle movement in which the muscle develops tension but does not move.

Static stretching Elongating a muscle and holding that position.

Storage fat Body fat, above essential levels, that accumulates in adipose tissue.

Stretch reflex Reflexive response to forceful rapid stretching that causes a muscle to contract.

Stress Response that includes both a mental reaction (stressor) and a physical reaction (stress response).

Stressor The demand or stimulus that elicits the general adaptation syndrome.

Stimulants Drugs that increase central nervous system activity.

Stroke Loss of muscle function, vision, or speech resulting from brain-cell damage caused by insufficient blood supply. Also known as *cerebrovascular accident* (CVA).

Stroke volume The amount of blood ejected with each contraction of the heart.

Subarachnoid hemorrhage Bleeding from a blood vessel on the surface of the brain into the space between the brain and the skull.

Substance abuse The deliberate use of a substance for other than its intended purpose, in a manner that can damage health or ability to function.

Substance dependence A chronic, progressive, and relapsing disorder that applies to all situations in which drug users develop either a psychological or physical reliance on a drug.

Substance misuse The taking of a substance for its intended purpose, but not in the appropriate amount, frequency, strength, or manner.

Substance use The taking of a drug for its intended purpose in an appropriate amount, frequency, strength, and manner.

Substrates Sources of energy that can be used by our bodies.

Supersets Consecutive performance of two sets of exercises that stress one muscle group and its antagonist without a rest period separating the sets.

Sympathetic nervous system Part of the autonomic nervous system; helps prepare the body for physical activity.

Sympathoadrenal system The second pattern of the fight-or-flight response.

Synergists Muscles that assist the agonist.

Syphilis Sexually transmitted disease caused by spirochete bacteria (*Treponema pallidum*).

Systolic pressure The highest blood pressure measured in the arteries; occurs as the heart contracts with each heartbeat.

Tars The yellowish-brown solid, sticky materials that are inhaled as part of tobacco smoke.

Termination Stage of change in which the individual's former problem behavior represents no threat or temptation; it denotes the concept of exiting the stages of change or the cycle of change.

Tertiary prevention Treatment after a person is already ill; typically offered by medical specialists.

Testes A pair of male reproductive organs that produce sperm cells and male sex hormones.

Thermic effect A warming effect; occurs when physically active, digesting food, or increasing energy expenditure in any other way.

Thermic effect of activity (TEA) The energy expended in skeletal muscle contraction and relaxation.

Thermic effect of food (TEF) The energy expended by our bodies in order to eat and process (digest, transport, metabolize, and store) food.

Tissue interference Occurs when either muscle or fat tissue physically blocks a movement, restricting a joint's full range of motion.

Tolerance Adaptation of the body to a drug in such a way that repeated exposure to the same dose results in less effect on the body.

Trace minerals Mineral requirements of less than 100 mg per day.

Trans fats Unsaturated fatty acids formed when vegetable oils are processed (hydrogenation) and made more solid.

Transtheoretical model of behavior change (TTM) A change model that is based on a time or temporal dimension (*trans*) using well-established psychological theories (*theoretical*) of behavior change.

Trichomonas vaginalis A protozoan that causes trichomoniasis, whose symptoms include a foul-smelling, foamywhite or yellow-green discharge that irritates the vagina.

Triglycerides Fatty acids that provide the body's largest energy store, act as insulation, transport fat-soluble vitamins, and contribute to satiety.

Tri-sets Consecutive performance of three sets of exercises that stress the same muscle group.

Tumors An abnormal mass of tissue that results from excessive cell division. Tumors perform no useful body function and can be benign or malignant.

Underfat Having body fat levels below what is recommended for good health.

Underwater weighing Technique to measure body fat percentage that requires weighing a person underwater as well as on land.

Underweight Having a body weight below levels recommended for a certain height.

Uterus The female organ in which a fetus develops.

Vagina Female organ of copulation, and the exit pathway for the fetus at birth.

Valsalva maneuver Condition that occurs when you hold your breath and exert force (grunting action); causes elevated blood pressure that increases the risk for stroke, heart attack, or hemorrhage.

Variability The differences among people.

Vasocongestion Engorgement of blood vessels in particular body parts in response to sexual arousal.

Vegan A strict vegetarian who eats no animal products.

Veins Blood vessels that return deoxygenated blood to the heart.

Venous return Blood returning through the veins to the heart.

Vitamins Essential organic substances needed by the body to perform highly specific metabolic processes in the cells.

VO$_2$ reserve The difference between maximal oxygen uptake (VO$_2$max) and resting oxygen consumption.

Water-soluble vitamins Vitamins that can be transported throughout the body by a watery medium.

Wellness A dynamic process of change and growth that is determined by the decisions one makes about how to live one's life.

Withdrawal illness Recognizable physical signs and symptoms that result from withdrawing drug use.

Yerkes-Dodson law Predicts an inverted U-shaped function between stress and performance.

You-statements Statements beginning with "you"; negative communication skill.

Photo Credits

p. 2, © Photos.com; p. 4, © Don Smetzer/PhotoEdit; p. 7, © Colin Paterson/Photodisc; p. 9, © Index Stock Imagery, Inc./Jupiterimages; p. 10 (top), © Doug Menuez/Photodisc, (bottom), © PhotoCreate/ShutterStock, Inc.; p. 15, © Lawrence M. Sawyer/Photodisc; p. 20, © Galina Barskaya/ShutterStock, Inc.; p. 24, © Botanica/Jupiterimages; p. 25, © Photodisc; p. 26, © David Buffington/Photodisc; p. 27 (top), © Javier Pierini/Photodisc, (bottom), © Photos.com; p. 33 (top), © Ryan McVay/Photodisc, (bottom), © Don Tremain/Photodisc; p. 34, © Joaquin Palting/Photodisc; p. 38, © Andy Sotiriou/Photodisc; p. 39, © Ian Wyatt/Photodisc; p. 41, © Ryan McVay/Photodisc; p. 43, © Photos.com; p. 46, © Comstock Images/Jupiterimages; p. 48, © AbleStock; p. 49, © Keith Brofsky/Photodisc; p. 50 (top), © Galina Barskaya/ShutterStock, Inc., (bottom), © Ryan McVay/Photodisc; p. 51, © Ryan McVay/Photodisc; p. 56, © Ryan McVay/Photodisc; p. 57, © EyeWire; p. 64, © image100/age footstock; p. 67, © Karl Weatherly/Photodisc; p. 68, © Jack Star/Photodisc; p. 71, © Rudi Von Briel/PhotoEdit; p. 78, © Brand X Pictures/Jupiterimages; p. 84, © W. Ober/Visuals Unlimited; p. 88, © Photos.com; p. 89, © Photodisc; p. 92, © Jeff Greenberg/Alamy Images; p. 96, © Bubbles Photolibrary/Alamy Images; p. 99, © Keith Brofsky/Photodisc; p. 100, © Creatas/Jupiterimages; p. 106, © Photos.com; p. 108 (top left), © Photodisc, (top right), © ShutterStock, Inc., (bottom left), © AbleStock, (bottom right), © LiquidLibrary; p. 113 (left), © Jess Alford/Photodisc, (middle), © Jules Frazier/PhotoDisc, (right), © PhotoLink/Photodisc; p. 114, Courtesy of National Cancer Institute; p. 116, © Mark Adams/SuperStock, Inc.; p. 123, © Don Farrall/Photodisc; p. 150, © Photos.com; p. 155, © Ryan McVay/Photodisc; p. 157, © Stockbyte Platinum/Alamy Images; p. 158, © Masterfile; p. 159, © SW Productions/Photodisc; p. 162, © E. Dygas/Photodisc; p. 163, © corfoto/ShutterStock, Inc.; p. 168, © Photodisc; p. 171 (left), © Peter Willi/SuperStock, Inc., (right), © Max Nash/AP Photos; p. 172 (top), © Galina Barskaya/ShutterStock, Inc., (bottom), Courtesy of Jesse Geraci; p. 182, © Anton Albert/ShutterStock, Inc.; p. 187, © Photodisc; p. 193, © Steve Mason/Photodisc; p. 195, © Gina Smith/ShutterStock, Inc.; p. 198, © PhotoLink/Photodisc; p. 199, © Jacob Yuri Wacherhausen/ShutterStock, Inc.; p. 201, © Jack Star/Photodisc; p. 206, © Philip Date/ShutterStock, Inc.; p. 210 (top), © Philip Date/ShutterStock, Inc., (bottom), © LiquidLibrary; p. 212, © Photodisc; p. 214, © Mitch Hrdlicka/Photodisc; p. 216, © Dr. Michael Klein/Peter Arnold, Inc.; p. 221 (top),

Index

A

abdomen
  exercises for, 242, 264
accommodating resistance, 234
Acquired Immune Deficiency Syndrome,
    375–377
ACSM (American College of Sports Medicine).
    See American College of Sports
    Medicine (ACSM).
actin, 228–229
action stage, 66
active stretching exercise, 259
activities, caloric cost of, 387–392
activity levels
  minimum requirements, 27–28
  moderate, 12, 26, 29
  sedentary, 26, 28–30
  vigorous, 26, 30
activity stage, 35
activity status. *See* activity levels.
adaptation, 23
adenosine triphosphate (ATP), 74, 154–155
Adequate Intake (AI), 128
adhering to a program. *See* program adherence.
adipose tissue, 155
adipostat, 191
advanced lift exercise, 245–248
aerobic exercise, 30
aerobic metabolism, 30, 156–157
affirmation, 57
age
  and cardiovascular disease, 85

flexibility, 257, 270
agonists, 231
AI (Adequate Intake), 128
AIDS, 375–377
alcohol
  and cardiovascular disease, 87
  absorption, 312–313
  binge drinking, 310
  blood alcohol concentration, 313, 314, 316
  college drinking, 307
  consumption, self-assessment, 311
  consumption patterns, 307–310
  depressant effects, 315–316
  and driving, 314, 317
  effects of food, 315
  effects on physical activity, 318–319
  elimination, 313–314
  ethyl alcohol, 311
  immediate effects, 315–317
  impairment charts, 314
  injuries caused by, 317
  long-term effects, 317–318
  moderate drinking, 308–309
  osteoporosis, 220
  people who should not drink, 309
  prevalence, 307
  problem drinking, 310–311
  properties of, 311
  psychoactive qualities, 315–316
  rate of consumption, 314–315
  self-assessment, 311
  social drinking, 307–308
  and societal problems, 307–308

alcohol abuse
  costs of, 307
  prevalence, 307
alcohol poisoning, 317
alcoholic beverages
  alcohol content, 309–310
  beer, 309–310
  caloric content, 312
  dietary guidelines, 130,309
  distilled spirits, 309–310
  wine, 309–310
"all natural" myth, 338, 357
allostatic load, 285
alpha-linoleic acid, 145–146
amenorrhea, 219
American Alliance for Health, Physical
    Education Recreation and Dance, 339
American College of Sports Medicine (ACSM)
  consumerism, 339
  resistance training guidelines, 235–236
American Council on Exercise, 339
amino acids, 113
anaerobic exercise, 30
anaerobic metabolism, 30, 156
android fat pattern, 161, 177
anemia, 123
anger, expressing, 364
angina pectoris, 81–82
anorexia nervosa, 164, 199–201
ANS (autonomic nervous system). *See* auto-
    nomic nervous system (ANS).
antagonists, 231
anxiety disorder, 281–282

aorta, 68
aortic valve, 68
appetite suppression, 196
apple-shaped fat pattern. *See* android fat pat-
    tern.
apples and oranges myth, 337
arm-across-chest exercise, 263
arteries
    atherosclerosis, 84
    definition, 68
    plaque, 84
arterioles, 68
arteriosclerosis, 84
assessment forms
    medical history questionnaire, 25
    PAR-Q questionnaire, 24
    pulse, checking, 73
    target heart rate, calculating, 31, 73
atherosclerosis, 84
ATP (adenosine triphosphate), 74, 154–155
atrophy
    definition, 23
    muscular, 158, 233
auto-regulation, 69
autonomic nervous system (ANS)
    definition, 284
    effects on organs, 286

B
back exercises
    lower back, 265–266, 271–272
    muscle development, 242–243
    upper back, 263–264
ballistic stretching exercise, 259
barriers to activity
    environmental factors, 39–40
    pain, 39
    psychological factors, 39, 40
    skill, 39
    social factors, 39–40
    time, 38
basal metabolic rate (BMR), 153, 188–189
beer, 309–310
behavior, health. *See* health behavior.
behavioral factors
    as cause of death, 9
    and program adherence, 40–41
    behavioral modification, and weight control,
        193
benign tumors, 96
bent-arm flies, 241
bent-arm pullover, 246
bent-over row, 243
bicarbonate ions, 69
binge drinking, 310
bingeing and purging. *See* bulimia nervosa.
biochemical factors of obesity, 191–192
bioelectrical impedance, 185
biological factors of program adherence, 40
bisexuality, 353
bleeding
    external, 385
    internal, 385
blood. *See also* cardiovascular function.
    bicarbonate ions, 69

circulation, 69
    deoxygenated, 68
    function of, 69
    hemoglobin, 69
    oxygenated, 68
    venous return, 69
blood alcohol concentration (BAC)
    definition, 313
    impairment charts, 314
    physical and mental balance, 316
blood clots, 84
blood pressure
    and cardiovascular disease, 85–86
    and metabolic syndrome, 162
    categories of levels, 83
    definition, 68
    high. *See* hypertension.
    measuring, 68
    and resistance training, 234, 238
blood pressure cuff, 68
    blood vessels, 66. *See also* cardiovascular
        function.
BMD (bone mineral density). *See* bone mineral
        density (BMD).
BMI (body mass index). *See* body mass index
        (BMI).
BMR (basal metabolic rate), 153, 188–189
body beautiful myth, 337
body composition
    abnormalities, 160
    definition, 36
body image
    definition, 198
    and eating disorders, 199
    and resistance training, 250
body mass index (BMI)
    calculation, 409–410
    measuring, 174–175
    weight control, 176
bone cells, 209
bone mass density T-scores, 220
bone mineral density (BMD)
    definition, 209
    test for osteoporosis, 220–221
bone robbers, 212
bones. *See also* osteoporosis
    caffeine, 212
    calcium, 211–212
    cartilage, 208
    collagen, 208
    formation, 209
    growth, 209
    length, and flexibility, 256–257
    and nutrition, 210–212
    osteoblasts, 208
    osteoclasts, 208
    osteocytes, 208
    and physical activity, 212–215
    physiology, 208–210
    protein, 212
    remodeling, 209–210
    salt, 212
    structure, 208
    vitamin C, 210
    vitamin D, 212
Borg, Gunnar, 74

brain, areas affected by stroke, 85
breast cancer
    description, 99
    early detection, 97
    frequency, 97
    and physical activity, 99–100
    risk factors, 98
breathing. *See also* cardiorespiratory.
    and relaxation, 293
    and resistance training, 238
bulimia nervosa, 164, 200–201
burnout, 288
butterfly exercise, 267

C
caffeine
    and bones, 212
calcium
    bone growth, 211–212
    nutritional role, 123
    requirements for, 211
    sources of, 211
calf, stretching exercise, 265, 267
calf raise, 245
caloric expenditure. *See also* calories, burning.
    chart of activities, 387–392
    definition, 74, 110
calories
    in alcoholic beverages, 312
    average daily consumption, 154
    burning, 188–189, 387–392. *See also* caloric
        expenditure.
    daily requirements, 134
    definition, 110
    sample food patterns, 135
Canadian health and nutrition, 393–405
Canada's Food Guide, 394, 397–399
Canada's Physical Activity Guide to Healthy
        Active Living, 400, 402–403
    nutrition labeling, 400—401, 404
cancer. *See* individual cancers.
    benign tumors, 96
    carcinomas, 97
    colon. *See* colorectal cancer.
    death rates, 96–97
    definition, 96
    early detection, 97
    lymphomas, 97
    malignant tumors, 96, 97
    melanomas, 97
    metastasis, 96
    rectum. *See* colorectal cancer.
    risk factors, 98
    sarcomas, 97
    by site and sex, 96–98
    tumors, 96–97
capillaries, 68
carbohydrates
    complex, 114–115
    definition, 114
    dietary fiber, 115
    dietary recommendations, 115
    disaccharides, 114
    fructose, 114
    function, 111

galactose, 115
glucose, 114–115, 155–156
glycogen, 115, 156
high-carbohydrate diets, 145
insoluble fibers, 116
lactose, 114–115
maltose, 114–115
metabolism, 155–156
monosaccharides, 114–115
polysaccharides, 114–115
simple, 114
soluble fibers, 116
source, 116
starches, 115
sucrose, 114–115
sugar, 114–115
carbon monoxide, in tobacco, 323
carcinomas, 97
cardiac. *See* cardiovascular.
cardiac output, 70
cardiorespiratory fitness, 30, 36, 70
    activities for, 31–32, 71
    assessing, 75
    cardiac output, 70
    cholesterol (HDL), 85, 162
    definition, 36
    heart rate, 31, 69, 71, 72–74
    high-density lipoproteins (HDL), 85, 86 162
    monitoring physical activity. *See also* target
        heart rate, physical activity.
    program design, 71
    stroke volume, 70
cardiovascular disease (CVD), 80, 82
    angina pectoris, 81–82
    arteriosclerosis, 84
    atherosclerosis, 84
    blood clots, 84
    as cause of death, 80, 82, 94
    cerebral embolism, 84
    cerebral hemorrhage, 84, 85
    cerebral thrombosis, 84
    cost of, 81
    hardening of the arteries. *See* atherosclerosis.
    hemorrhagic strokes, 84, 85
    hypertension, 83, 85–86
    ischemia, 82
    ischemic strokes, 84
    myocardial infarction, 82
    plaque, 84
    primary hypertension, 83
cardiovascular disease, risk factors
    age, 85
    cholesterol, definition, 86
    diabetes mellitus, 87, 94–96
    family history, 85
    gender, 85
    heredity, 85
    high-density lipoproteins (HDL), 86, 162
    hypertension, 83, 85–86
    independent, 80
    lipoproteins, 86
    low-density lipoproteins (LDL), 86
    modifiable, 85–87
    obesity, 87
    other, 87–88
    physical inactivity, 80, 87

saturated fats, 86
smoking, 86–87
sodium intake, 86
stress, 88
unmodifiable, 85
secondary hypertension, 83
stroke, 84
subarachnoid hemorrhage, 84, 85
cardiovascular function. *See also* heart.
    arteries. *See* arteries.
    arterioles, 68
    auto-regulation, 69
    blood circulation, 69
    blood function, 69
    capillaries, 68
    deoxygenated blood, 68
    diastolic pressure, 69
    neural control, 69
    oxygenated blood, 68
    and pulmonary system, 69
    systolic pressure, 68
    temperature control, 69
    thermoregulation, 69
    veins, 68
    venules, 68
career health, 7
cartilage, 208
cat and camel exercise, 266, 272
cease-and-desist orders, 343
cellulite, 336
cerebral embolism, 84
cerebral hemorrhage, 84, 85
cerebral thrombosis, 84
cerebrovascular accident (CVA). *See* stroke.
chest, exercises for, 241–242
chest, stretching exercise, 263–264
children
    and diabetes, 95
chin-to-chest exercise, 262
chlamydia, 372
Chlamydia trichomatis, 372
cholesterol, 119
    and cardiovascular disease, 80, 85–86
    definition, 119
    dietary guidelines, 119
    levels, 86
cholesterol (HDL), 85, 86, 162
chronic diseases. *See* diseases, chronic.
cigarettes. *See also* tobacco.
    as cause of death, 80, 319
    the decision to smoke, 320
    prevalence, 319
    rates, 87
    risk factor, 86
    vs. cigars, 323
cigars. *See also* tobacco.
    prevalence, 323
    risks, 323
    vs. cigarettes, 323
    warning labels, 323
circuit weight training, 228, 248–249
circulation, blood, 68–69
circulatory system, 66. *See also* cardiovascular
        function.
circumcision, 358
clap (STD), 373

clitoris, 354–355
cold injuries, 385
collagen, 208
college drinking, 307–308
colorectal cancer
    as cause of death, 97–98, 101
    description, 98
    early detection, 97
    and physical activity, 101
    risk factors, 98
commitment, 361
communication, 362–364
complex carbohydrates, 114
compliance, 256
compound sets, 248–250
compulsive overeating, 200–201
concentration curl, 247
concentric muscle action, 230–231
Condylomata acuminata, 374
consent orders, 343
consumer protection. *See* consumerism.
consumer protection agencies, 348
consumerism. *See also* program design.
    administrative complaints, 343
    "all natural" myth, 338
    American Alliance for Health, 339
    American College of Sports Medicine, 339
    American Council on Exercise, 339
    apples and oranges myth, 337
    body beautiful myth, 337
    cease-and-desist orders, 343
    cellulite, 336
    community experts, 339
    consent orders, 343
    consumer protection, 343–344
    consumer protection agencies, 348
    Dietary Supplement Health and Education
        Act of 1994, 342–343
    ergolytic 332
    fads, 336–338
    fallacies, 336–338
    fat/muscle cell conversion, 337
    Federal Trade Commission, 338–339
    Food and Drug Administration, 338, 345
    fraud, 332
    governmental agencies, 339
    health clubs, selecting, 340–341
    infrared technology, 342
    instant gratification, 337
    Internet resources, 339
    magic potions, 338
    magnet therapy, 340–341
    marketing techniques, 334–336
    massage, 337
    melting fat, 337
    misinformation, 332
    misleading advertising, 343–345
    misleading products, examples, 340–342
    muscle stimulators, 336
    myths, 336–338
    National Council Against Health Fraud Task
        Force on Victim Redress, 344
    National Strength and Conditioning
        Association, 339
    passive exercise, 336
    peer-reviewed research, 345

performance enhancers, 332
Physical Education, Recreation and Dance, 339
placebo effect, 334
product safety and efficacy, 339
professional health organizations, 339
quackery, 332
sources of information, 338
spot reduction, 336
torch myth, 337
vanishing acts, 338
vibration, 336–337
weight loss, 162, 337–338
contemplation stage, 51
contraction, muscular, 230–231
cool down stage, 35
copulation, 357
coronary heart disease. *See also* cardiovascular disease (CVD).
description, 81–82
preventive measures, 80
costs
alcohol abuse, 307
cardiovascular disease, 81
chronic diseases, 94
mental illness, 281
osteoporosis, 217
Cowper's glands, 357–358
crabs (pubic lice), 375
creatine phosphate, 155
criterion-referenced standards, 160–161
cross training, 35–36
curl-up exercise, 243, 270
CVA (cerebrovascular accident). *See* stroke.
CVD (cardiovascular disease). *See* cardiovascular disease (CVD).

D
dead lift, 246
death, causes of, 94
behavioral factors, 8–9, 48–49
breast cancer, 97, 99
cancer, 96–97
cardiovascular disease, 80, 85–88
chart of, 6
cigarettes, 319–321
colorectal cancer, 97
lifestyle factors, 8–9, 26, 48–49, 94
lung cancer, 97
men, 96–97
obesity, 163, 170–171
physical inactivity, 6
present day, 6
prostate cancer, 97
smoking, 319–321
stroke, 84
tobacco, 319–321
women, 96–97
decision-making process, 50–51
decline bench press, 246
deep breathing, 293
degeneration, 23
dehydration, 123, 145
deoxygenated blood, 68
depressive reactions, 282

diabetes mellitus
and cardiovascular disease, 85, 87
and physical activity, 96
as cause of death, 94
description, 94–96
high blood sugar. *See* hyperglycemia.
hyperglycemia, 95
hypoglycemia, 95
insulin-dependent. *See* Type 1 diabetes.
low blood sugar. *See* hypoglycemia.
non-insulin-dependent. *See* Type 2 diabetes.
Type 1, 95
Type 2, 95–96
diaries, writing, 56
diastolic pressure, 69
diet analysis records, 194
diet. *See also* dietary guidelines; eating; food; nutrition; weight control.
as cause of death, 108
and metabolic rate, 152–154
and obesity, 196–198
strategies for improving, 126–143
dietary fiber, 116
dietary guidelines. *See also* diet; eating; food; nutrition.
alcoholic beverages, 130
caloric requirements, 134
cholesterol, 119
energy balance equation, 157, 186–190
fats, 119–120
fitness goals, 29, 75
food groups, table of, 131–133
Food Guide Pyramid, vegetarian, 143–144
food labeling, 138–141
food safety, 130
fruits, 136
grains, 133
high-carbohydrate diets, 145
MyPyramid, 130–131
nutrient-calorie benefit ratio, 127
nutrient density, 127
nutrition facts label, 138–141
personal nutrition plan, 130
recommended number of servings, 141–143
salt, 130
sample food patterns, 135
saturated fat, 117–118
serving sizes, 141–143
sugars, 114–115
vegetables, 136
weight analysis, 128
weight goals, 128
Dietary Reference Intakes (DRIs)
Adequate Intake, 127
Estimated Average Requirement, 127
Recommended Dietary Allowances, 127–128
Tolerable Upper Intake Level, 128
Dietary Supplement Health and Education Act (DSHEA) of 1994, 342–343
dietary supplements, 143
digestion, 109
digestive system, anatomy of, 110
dip exercise, 242
disaccharides, 114
diseases. *See also* specific diseases.
caused by lifestyle, 9, 26, 94

caused by physical inactivity, 6, 80
cost of chronic diseases, 9, 94
and flexibility, 257
incidence, 94, 95
and metabolic abnormalities, 159
primary prevention, 48
secondary prevention, 48
tertiary prevention, 48
distilled spirits, 309–310
distraction theory, 292
distress, 283
double-knee-to-chest exercise, 265
double-leg press, 245
double-leg raise, 269
drinking. 307 *See* alcohol.
drip (STD), 373
DRIs (Dietary Reference Intakes). *See* Dietary Reference Intakes (DRIs).
driving and alcohol, 317
drug abuse, 302
drug misuse, 302
drug use
definition, 300
drugs. *See also* alcohol; caffeine; tobacco.
addiction, 304
addiction potential, 305
homeostasis, 304
pharmacology, 306
physical dependence, 305–306
psychological dependence, 305
tolerance, 304
withdrawal illness, 304
drunk driving, 314, 317
duration, exercise, 31, 75
dysthymia, 282

E
EAR (Estimated Average Requirement), 127
ear-to-shoulder exercise, 262
eating. *See also* diet; dietary guidelines; food; nutrition.
emotional, 197
speed, 198
style, 197
eating disorders, 163, 199
eccentric muscle action, 230–231
effective listening, 363–364
eggs (human), 354
elasticity, 256
elbow-to-knee exercise, 267
emergency action. *See* injury.
emotional eating, 197
emotional health, 7, 279
endocardium, 66
endocrine system, 284
endorphin hypothesis, 292
endurance
definition, 36, 228
muscular, 36
sample regimen, 239
training, 238
energy, from food, 109–110, 407
energy balance, 157, 186
energy balance equation
and body fatness, 157, 186

definition, 157, 186
  weight control, 193–194
energy expenditure, components of, 157, 188–189
energy storage, 156,186–187
energy transfer, 155
environmental engineering, 290
epidemiological studies, 160
epididymitis, 372
epinephrine, 285
ergogenic aids
  definition, 332
  table of, 333
ergolytic 332
essential amino acids, 113
essential body fat, 160, 183
essential fatty acids, 117–118
essential minerals, 122
essential nutrients, 112
Estimated Average Requirement (EAR), 127
Estimated Energy Expenditure (EER), 408–409
ethyl alcohol, 311
eustress, 283
exercise. *See also* physical activity; physical fitness; resistance training.
  definition, 10
  flexibility. *See* stretching exercises.
  muscle development. *See* muscle exercises.
  as stress management, 292
  stretching. *See* stretching exercises.
exercise and physical activity pyramid, 31–32

F
fads. *See* consumerism.
fallacies. *See* consumerism.
fallopian tubes, 354–355
fast-twitch fibers, 230
fat (body). *See also* fatness; obesity; weight control.
  adipose tissue, 155
  and disease, 170
  essential, 160, 183
  essential body fat, 160, 183
  healthy fat zones, 161, 183
  metabolism, 156
  nonessential, 160, 183
  overfat, 160, 183
  storage fat, 183
  subcutaneous, 176
  underfat, 160
  visceral, 161, 162, 177–178
fat/muscle cell conversion, 337
fat-soluble vitamins, 120
fatness. *See also* fat (body); obesity; weight control.
  bioelectrical impedance, 185
  energy balance equation, 157, 186–187
  healthy fat zones, 161
  healthy weight, 173–174
  measuring, 182–185
  men vs. women, 183
  regional distribution, 161, 176–179
  skinfold testing, 184
  underwater weighing, 184–185
fats (dietary)

alpha-linoleic acid, 117–118
and cardiovascular disease, 86
cholesterol, 119
dietary guidelines, 129
dietary recommendations, 119–120
essential fatty acids, 117–118
function, 118–119
hydrogenation, 119
linoleic acid, 117–118
monounsaturated, 117–118
phospholipids, 119
polyunsaturated, 117
saturated, 117
source, 116
trans fats, 119
triglycerides, 116
unsaturated, 117–118
FDA (Food and Drug Administration), 338–339
Federal Trade Commission (FTC), 338–339
feedback, 364
female athlete triad, 201–202
female muscle groups (illustration), 232
female sexual anatomy, 354–356
fertilization, 354
fight-or-flight response, 285
first aid. *See* injury.
first law of thermodynamics, 152
fitness. *See* cardiorespiratory fitness; exercise; physical activity; physical fitness.
flexibility. *See also* stretching exercises.
  aging, 257, 270
  assessment form, 261
  compliance, 256
  definition, 36, 256
  disease, 257
  elasticity, 256
  Golgi tendon organs, 258
  hamstrings, 256–257
  health-related, 36
  and injury prevention, 270–272
  joint laxity, 268
  length of bone, 256–257
  muscle spindles, 258
  muscle temperature, 257
  proprioceptors, 258
  sit-and-reach test, 256–257
  stretch reflex, 258
  tissue interference, 256–257
  women vs. men, 257
folate equivalents, 408
following a program. *See* program adherence.
food. *See also* diet; dietary guidelines; eating; nutrition.
  effects on alcohol, 315–317
  functional foods, 124–126
  functions of, 109–110
  intake, and weight control, 186–187
Food and Drug Administration (FDA), 338–339
food diary, 136
food groups, table of, 131–133
Food Guide Pyramid, vegetarian, 144
food labeling, 138–141
food safety, 130
foreskin, 358

fraud. *See* consumerism.
free weights vs. machines, 240
frequency, exercise, 30
fructose, 114
FTC (Federal Trade Commission), 338–339
full-neck-circle exercise, 269
full-squat exercise, 268
functional foods, 124–126

G
galactose, 114
gametes, 352
Gardnerella vaginalis, 370
gender, and cardiovascular disease, 85
gender identity, 354
gender roles, 354
General Adaptation Syndrome, 283
generalized anxiety disorder (GAD), 282
genetic
  factors, 33
  obesity, 190
  osteoporosis, 218
genetic predisposition, 158
glucocorticoids, 285
glucose, 114–115, 155–156
gluteals, stretching exercise, 267
glycogen
  definition, 115
  and metabolism, 155
goals and objectives, national
  adults, 13–14
  cancer screening, 97
  cancer reduction, 96
  children, 13
  muscular development, 13
  physical activity, 13
goals and objectives, personal
  for changing health behavior, 59–60
  choosing activities for, 28–30
  setting for physical activity, 32
Golgi tendon organs, 258
gonorrhea, 373
grains, 133–134
groin, exercises for, 244, 264
gynoid fat pattern, 161, 177

H
habits, health, 48–49
hamstring curl, 244
hamstrings
  exercises, 244, 264–265
  flexibility, 256–257
handcuff stretch exercise, 264
HBV (hepatitis B), 374–375
HDL-C. *See* high-density lipoproteins (HDL).
HDL (high-density lipoproteins). *See* high-density lipoproteins (HDL).
head lice, 375
health
  choosing activities for, 28–30
  definition, 6
  personal habits promoting, 8–9
health behavior, changing
  action stage, 51
  affirmation, 57

contemplation stage, 51
decision-making concept, 54
education, 55
experiential principles, 55
gradual increases, 53–54
increasing knowledge, 55
keeping a journal, 56–57
maintenance stage, 34, 51
motivation, 50
precontemplation stage, 51
preparation stage, 51
rational emotive technique, 56
readiness for change, 50–52
regression, 52–53
relapse, 52–53
reminders, 59
rewards, 57–58
self-contracts, 57–58
self-efficacy, 54–55
self-talk, 57
setting objectives, 59–60
social support, 58
spiral model of change, 52–53
techniques for, 55–59
termination stage, 52
health clubs, selecting, 340–341
health habits, 48–49
healthy weight, 173–174
heart. *See also* cardiovascular.
heart, anatomy of, 66–68
heart attack
definition, 82
warning signs, 83
heart disease. *See* cardiovascular disease
(CVD).
heart rate
definition, 71
monitoring, 72–74
regulating, 69
target, calculating, 31, 73
heart rate reserve (HRR), 72
heat injuries, 385
hemoglobin, 69
hemorrhagic strokes, 84, 85
hepatitis B (HBV), 374–375
heredity, and cardiovascular disease, 85
heritability, 33
herpes, 373–374
Herpes simplex (HSV), 373–374
heterosexuality, 353
high blood pressure. *See* hypertension.
high-carbohydrate diets, 145
high-density lipoproteins (HDL)
and cardiovascular disease, 85–86
and metabolic syndrome, 162
definition, 86
HIV (human immunodeficiency virus), 375
homeostasis, 304 315
homosexuality, 353 369
hormonal factors, osteoporosis, 219
hormones, 158
HPV (human papillomavirus), 374
HRR (heart rate reserve), 72
HSV (Herpes simplex), 373–374
human immunodeficiency virus (HIV), 375
human papillomavirus (HPV), 374

hunger, satiation, satiety cycle, 187
hydrogenation, 119
hyperextension, 268
hyperflexion, 268
hyperglycemia, 95
hyperinsulinemia, 162
hyperstress, 288
hypertension
and cardiovascular disease, 80, 83, 85–86
and metabolic syndrome, 162
measuring, 83
hypertrophy, 158–159, 232
hypoglycemia
definition, 95
and diabetes, 95
hypokinetic diseases, 26
hypostress, 288

I
I-statements, 363
imagining. *See* envisioning.
incidence, 94, 95
incline bench press, 245
individuality principle, 37
individualized programs, 28, 33
infrared technology, 342
initial stage, 34
injury. *See also* safety.
bleeding, internal, 384
cold injuries, 385
emergency action, 384–385
heart attack, 384
heat injuries, 385
from improper exercise, 43–44
internal bleeding, 384
prevention, 383
shin splints, 385
sprains, 385
strains, 385
stroke, 384–385
tendinitis, 385
thermal stress, 385
innervation, muscular, 230
insoluble fibers, 116
instant gratification, 337
insulin
and diabetes, 95
and metabolic syndrome, 162
intellectual health, 7
internal bleeding, 384
Internet resources, 339
intimacy, definition, 359
intimate relationships. *See also* sex.
choosing a partner, 360
commitment, 361
communication, 362–364
developing, 360–361
effective listening, 363
ending, 361
expressing anger, 364
feedback, 364
I-statements, 363
intimacy, definition, 359
life cycle of, 360
literal messages, 363

metamessages, 363
self-disclosure, 360
You-statements, 363
intrinsic motivation, 41
iron, 123
ischemia, 82
ischemic strokes, 84
isokinetic training, 234
isometric training, 234
isotonic training, 233–234

J
joint flexibility. *See* flexibility; stretching exercises.
joint laxity, 268
journals, writing, 56

K
kcals, 110
Kennedy, John F., on physical fitness, 280
kilocalories, 110
knee-to-chest exercise, 271

L
labia majora, 356
labia minora, 356
lactic acid, 156
lactose, 114–115
lactovegetarian diet, 143
lat pull down exercise, 242
LDL-C. *See* low-density lipoproteins (LDL).
LDL (low-density lipoproteins), 86
legs, exercises for, 244–245
leptin, 191
leukemia, 97
lifestyle
and hypokinetic disease, 26
as cause of death, 8–9, 26
definition, 8
diseases caused by, 9, 26, 94
and osteoporosis, 220
linoleic acid, 117
lipids. *See* fats.
lipoproteins, 86
literal messages, 363
look-right-and-left exercise, 262
low-density lipoproteins (LDL), 86
lower back, stretching exercise, 265–266,
271–272
lung cancer
as cause of death, 96
description, 98
risk factors, 98
and tobacco, 98
lunge exercise, 244, 271
lungs. *See* cardiorespiratory function.
lymphomas, 97

M
macronutrients, 111
magic potions, 338
magnet therapy, 340–341
maintenance stage, 34, 51
major depression, 282

major minerals, 120
male muscle groups (illustration), 232
male sexual anatomy, 357–358
malignant tumors, 96, 97
maltose, 114–115
mammography, 99
marketing techniques, 334–336
massage, 337
meal size and frequency, 197–198
measuring fatness, 182–186
medical history
    assessment form, 25
    preparing for physical activity, 24–26
meditation, 290
melanomas, 97
melting fat, 337
mens sana in corpora sana, 280
menstrual periods, absence of. *See* amenorrhea.
mental health. *See also* psychology; stress.
    anxiety disorder, 281–282
    cognitive behavioral theory, 292
    deep breathing, 293
    definition, 279
    depression reactions, 282
    distraction theory, 292
    dysthymia, 282
    effects of physical activity, 280
    emotional health, 279
    endorphin hypothesis, 292
    generalized anxiety disorder, 281
    major depression, 282
    mens sana in corpora sana, 280
    mind-body relationship, 280
    physical activity benefits, 23, 26, 278–279
    progressive muscle relaxation, 294
    psychosomatic disease, 281
    relaxation techniques, 293–294
    relaxation training, 293–294
    social interaction theory, 292
    sound body, sound mind, 280
    stress-fitness relationship, 291
    thermogenic hypothesis, 293
    time management, 294
    visualization, 293
mental illness
    costs of, 278
    definition, 281
metabolic rate
    basal metabolic rate, 153, 188–189
    and diet, 188–189
metabolic rate (continued)
    energy balance, 157, 186–188
    energy expenditure, how we use calories, 157, 188–189
    first law of thermodynamics, 152
    thermic effect of activity, 152–154
metabolic syndrome, 162–162
    risk factors, 162
metabolism
    adenosine triphosphate, 74, 155
    aerobic, 30, 156
    anaerobic, 30, 156
    and adipose tissue, 155
    atrophy, 158
    creatine phosphate, 155
    definition, 152

effects of resistance training, 250
    energy storage, 156
    energy transfer, 155
    essential (body) fat, 160, 183
    glycogen, 155
    hormones, 158
    hypertrophy, 158–159
    lactic acid, 156
    muscle mass, building, 158
    nonessential (body) fat, 160
    and physical activity, 157
    and physical inactivity, 80, 158
    pyruvic acid, 156
    set point, 154, 191
    subcutaneous fat, 176
    substrates, 152
    sympathetic nervous system, 154, 285
    visceral fat, 161, 162, 177–178
metabolism abnormalities
    android fat pattern, 161, 177
    anorexia nervosa, 164, 199
    body composition, 160
    bulimia nervosa, 164, 200
    compulsive overeating, 201
    criterion-referenced standards, 160–161
    and disease, 160–161
    eating disorders, 199
    fat (body), and disease, 160–162
    gynoid fat pattern, 161, 177
    metabolic syndrome, 162–162
    obesity, 163, 183
    overfat, 160, 173
    overweight, 160, 173
    underfat, 160
    underweight, 160, 174
metamessages, 363
metastasis, 96
METS (multiple of resting metabolism), 74
MI (myocardial infarction), 82
micronutrients, 111
mind-body relationship, 280
mind engineering, 290
mind-over-matter, 290
minerals
    calcium, 123, 211
    definition, 122
    dietary recommendations, 211
    essential, 122
    function, 123, 211
    iron, 123
    major, 120
    source, 121
    trace, 120
misinformation. *See* consumerism.
misleading advertising. *See* consumerism.
misleading products. *See* consumerism.
mitral valve, 67
mode, exercise, 31
moderate activity
    definition, 26
    starting a program, 32
moderate drinking, 308–309
modified chest lift exercise, 272
modified hurdler exercise, 264
monitoring physical activity
    caloric expenditure, 74–75

heart rate, 71, 72–74
    heart rate reserve, 72
    multiple of resting metabolism, 74
    pulse, checking, 73
    rating of perceived exertion, 74
    VO$_2$ max test, 70
    VO$_2$ reserve, 72
monitoring progress, 36
monosaccharides, 114
monounsaturated fats, 117–118
motivation
    changing health behavior, 50
    self-change approach, 49
motor units, 230
multiple of resting metabolism (METS), 74
muscle exercises. *See also* muscle training; resistance training.
    abdomen, 242
    advanced lifts, 245–248
    back, 242–243
    bent-arm flies, 241
    bent-arm pullover, 246
    bent-over row, 243
    calf raise, 245
    chest, 241–242
    concentration curl, 247
    curl-up, 243
    dead lift, 246
    decline bench press, 246
    dip, 242
    double-leg press, 246
    groin, 244
    hamstring curl, 244
    incline bench press, 245
    lat pull down, 242
    legs, 244–245
    lunge, 244
    neck, 241
    power clean, 247
    preacher curl, 247
    push-up, 241
    quad extensions, 244
    reverse bicep curl, 247
    sample program, 241–245
    seated press, 241
    seated row, 243
    shoulder shrug, 241
    shoulders, 241
    sit-up, 242
    snatch pull, 246
    squat, 244
    wall sit, 245
    wrist curl, 246
muscle/fat cell conversion, 337
muscle fibers, 230
muscle spindles, 258
muscle stimulators, 336
muscle training. *See also* muscle exercises; resistance training.
    accommodating resistance, 234
    circuit weight training, 228
    isokinetic training, 234
    isometric training, 234
    isotonic training, 233–234
    size, building, 232–233
    toning, 232–233

weight room etiquette, 248
muscles
    actin, 228–229
    agonists, 231
    anatomy, 228
    antagonists, 231
    atrophy, 233
    concentric muscle action, 230–231
    contraction, 230–231
    eccentric muscle action, 230–231
    fast-twitch fibers, 230
    female (illustration), 232
    hypertrophy, 159, 232
    innervation, 230
    male (illustration), 232
    mass, building, 158
    motor units, 230
    myosin, 228–229
    neuromuscular adaptations, 233
    neutralizers, 231
    physiology, 228
    protein filaments, 228–229
    sarcomeres, 228
    sliding filament theory, 228–229
    slow-twitch fibers, 230
    static contraction, 230–231
    synergists, 231
    temperature, and flexibility, 257
muscular endurance
    definition, 36, 228
    sample regimen, 239
    training, 238
muscular strength
    building, 232–233, 238–239
    definition, 36, 228
    sample regimen, 239
myocardial infarction (MI), 82
myocardium, 66
myosin, 228–229
MyPyramid, 130–135
myths. *See* consumerism.

N

National Council Against Health Fraud Task
    Force on Victim Redress, 344
National Institutes of Health (NIH), 80
    Consensus Statement, 80–81
National Strength and Conditioning
    Association, 339
NCBR (nutrient-calorie benefit ratio), 127
neck, exercises for, 241
neck, stretching exercise, 262
Neisseria gonorrheae, 373
neural control, 69
neuromuscular adaptations, 233
neutralizers, 231
nicotine, in tobacco, 322
nonessential (body) fat, 160
nonessential nutrients, 111–112
norepinephrine, 285
nutrient-calorie benefit ratio (NCBR), 127
nutrient density, 127
nutrients
    classes of, 111
    definition, 109

nutrition. *See also* diet; dietary guidelines; eat-
    ing; food.
    analysis,
    anemia, 123
    and bones, 210
    calories, definition, 110
    digestion, 109–110
    energy, 109–110
    essential nutrients, 111–112
    fats. *See* fats (dietary)
    macronutrients, 111
    micronutrients, 111
    nonessential nutrients, 111
    protein-sparing effect, 145
nutrition facts label, 138
nutrition labeling for Canadians, 400–401, 404
nutritional factors, osteoporosis, 210

O

obesity. *See also* fat (body); fatness; weight
    control.
    adipostat, 191
    biochemical factors, 191–192
    body fat distribution, 176
    and cardiovascular disease, 85, 87, 163, 177
    and disease, 162–163
    as cause of death, 163, 170
    causes of, 162, 190–192
    classifications of, 183
    definition, 196
    dietary factors, 196–197
    epidemic, 164
    genetic factors, 161, 190–191
    health problems of, 163, 170
    hunger, satiation, satiety cycle, 186–187
    leptin, 191
    measuring. *See* body mass index, body fat
        distribution.
    metabolic abnormality, 161, 177
    and physical inactivity, 80, 163, 192
    physiological factors, 191–192
    set point, 154, 191
    trends in the U.S., 164
occupational health, 7
omega-3 acid, 117
omega-6 acid, 117
one-sugar molecules. *See* monosaccharides.
organ systems, 23
orgasm, 358
osteoblasts, 208
osteoclasts, 208
osteocytes, 208
osteoporosis
    alcohol, 220
    amenorrhea, 219
    bone mass density T-scores, 220
    bone mineral density tests, 220–221
    cost of, 217
    definition, 215
    detection, 220
    female athlete triad, 220
    genetic factors, 218
    hormonal factors, 219
    lifestyle factors, 220
    nutritional factors, 220

    prevention, 220
    risk factors, 218–220
    smoking, 220
ova, 354
ovaries, 354–357
over-use syndrome, 42
overfat, 160
overload principle, 37
overtraining, 42
overweight. *See also* fat (body); fatness; obesity;
    weight control.
    by age, gender, and ethnicity, 173
    definition, 160, 173–174
    rise in, 164
ovolactovegetarian diet, 143
ovovegetarian diet, 143
ovulation, 354
ovum, 354
oxygenated blood, 68

P

pain, and physical activity, 39
PAR-Q questionnaire, 24
parasympathetic nervous system, 285
passive exercise, 336
passive stretching, 259
pear-shaped fat pattern. *See* gynoid fat pattern.
Pediculus humanus capittis, 375
peer-reviewed research, 345
pelvic inflammatory disease (PID),372
penis, 357
performance, choosing activities for, 30
pericardium, 66
periodization, 248
personal program
    equipment, selecting, 240
    exercises, selecting, 240
    free weights vs. machines, 240
    professional help, 239
    self-assessment, 25, 239
pharmacology, 306
phospholipids, 119
Phthirus pubis, 375
physical activities, choosing
    according to activity level, 28–30
    list of activities, 28
    for specific goals, 28–30
physical activity. *See also* exercise; physical
    fitness; physical inactivity.
    adaptation to, 23
    appetite suppression, 196
    barriers to. *See* barriers to activity.
    benefits of, 23, 26–27
    and bones, 212–215
    and breast cancer, 99
    burning calories, 195–196
    and caloric expenditure, 74–75
    and cancer
    and diabetes, 96
    definition, 10
    designing a program. *See* program design.
    and disease distribution, 80
    goals and objectives, national, 12–13
    guidelines, 27–30
    and heart rate, 71, 72–75

and heart rate reserve (HRR), 72
individualized programs, 28, 33
long-term effects, 23
loss of lean body mass, 196
mental health benefits, 292–293
monitoring.
and multiple of resting metabolism (METS), 74
and obesity-related diseases, 162–163, 195–196
and overall health, 11
preparing for. *See* preparing for physical activity.
pros and cons, 54
and prostate cancer, 100
psychological well-being, 196
pulse, checking, 73
rating of perceived exertion (RPE), 74
response to, 23
set point, lowering, 154, 196
short-term effects, 23
and women's health, 24
VO$_2$ max test, 70
VO$_2$ reserve, 72
physical activity levels. *See* activity levels.
physical activity, as prevention, 88
    cancer, 97
    duration of activity, 31, 75
    intensity levels, 72
    progression, 75
    selecting activities, 71
physical dependence, 305–306
Physical Education, Recreation and Dance, 339
physical engineering, 291
physical fitness. *See also* exercise; physical activity.
    choosing activities for, 28–32
    definition, 10
    dietary guidelines, 128–129
physical inactivity. *See also* physical activity.
    and cardiovascular disease, 80, 85, 87
    cardiovascular disease risk factor, 24, 80, 85
    cause of death, 6, 80
    causes, 6
    diseases caused by, 26, 80, 87
    hypokinetic diseases, 26
    injuries, 42–43
physical symptoms of, 287
physical health, 7
physiological factors of obesity, 163, 191
physiological reactivity, 291
PID (pelvic inflammatory disease), 372
pituitary-adrenal axis, 285
placebo effect, 334
plaque
    definition, 84
plough stretching exercise, 269
plyometrics, 248–249
PNF (proprioceptive neuromuscular facilitation) stretching, 259–260
polysaccharides, 114
polyunsaturated fats, 117
power clean, 247
preacher curl, 247
precontemplation stage, 51
preparation stage, 51

preparing for physical activity
    medical history, 24–26
    prescreening, 24–26
    self-assessment, 25–26
    setting goals, 32
prevalence, definition, 95
primary hypertension, 83
primary prevention, 81
principles of
    training. *See* training principles.
problem drinking, 310–311
product safety and efficacy. *See* consumerism.
professional health organizations, 339
program adherence, 40–41
program design. *See also* consumerism.
    activity stage, 35
    components of sessions, 35–36
    cool down stage, 35
    cross training, 35–36
    initial stage, 34
    maintenance stage, 34
    monitoring progress, 36
    preparation stage, 34–35
    principles of training, 37–38
    progression stage, 34
    stages of conditioning, 34–35
    transition stage, 35
program factors, and program adherence, 40–41
progression principle
    definition, 37
    resistance training, 235–236
progression stage, 34
progressive muscle relaxation (PMR), 294
proprioceptive neuromuscular facilitation (PNF) stretching, 259–260
proprioceptors, 258
prostate cancer
    description, 100
    early detection, 97
    frequency, 97
    and physical activity, 100
    PSA test, 100
    risk factors, 98
prostate gland, 358
prostate-specific antigens test. *See* PSA test.
protein filaments, 228–229
protein-sparing effect, 145
proteins
    amino acids, 113
    and bones, 212
    building muscle mass, 145
    description, 113
    dietary recommendations, 113
    essential amino acids, 113
    function, 113
    intake, for adults, 407
    metabolism, 155–156
    source, 113
PSA test, 100
psychoactive qualities of alcohol, 311
psychological dependence, 305
psychology. *See also* mental health.
    and physical activity, 39
    and program adherence, 39, 40
psychosomatic disease, 281

pubic lice, 375
pulmonary system, 69. *See also* cardiorespiratory function.
pulmonary valve, 67
pulse, checking, 73
push-ups, 241
pyramiding, 248
pyramids
    exercise and physical activity, 31–32
    Food Guide, vegetarian, 144
    MyPyramid, 130
pyruvic acid, 156

Q
quackery. *See* consumerism.
quad extensions, 244
quads, stretching exercise, 267
quitting smoking
    health benefits, 324–325
    support groups, 325
    tips for, 325
    weight control, 325–326

R
rack stretch exercise, 264
range of motion. *See* flexibility.
rating of perceived exertion (RPE), 74
rational emotive technique, 56
RDAs (Recommended Dietary Allowances), 127
reach up exercise, 263
Recommended Dietary Allowances (RDAs), 127
recovery principle
    definition, 38
    resistance training, 235–236
regional distribution of fat, 161, 176
relapse, 52–53
relaxation response, 285
relaxation techniques, 293–294
relaxation training, 293–294
reminders, 59
remodeling bones, 209–210
reps, 236
resistance training. *See also* muscle exercises; muscle training.
    American College of Sports Medicine guidelines, 236
    blood pressure increase, 234, 238
    and body image, 198
    breathing, 238
    circuit weight training, 228, 248–249
    compound sets, 248–250
    effect on metabolism, 251
    form and technique, 238
    free weights vs. machines, 240
    overload, 236–237
    periodization, 248–249
    plyometrics, 248–249
    principle of progression, 37, 236–237
    principle of recovery, 37, 236–237
    principle of specificity, 37, 236–237
    pyramiding, 248–249
    reps, 236
    sample workout, 236

sets, 236
    supersets, 248–250
    tri-sets, 248–250
    valsalva maneuver, 238
response, 23
Resting Energy Expenditure (REE), 409
Resting Metabolic Rate (RMR)
    definition, 153–154
    and physical activity, 157
retroviruses, 377
reverse bicep curl, 247
reversibility principle, 37
rewards, 57
risk factors. *See* specific diseases.
RMR (resting metabolic rate). *See* resting metabolic rate (RMR).
RPE (rating of perceived exertion), 74
rustout, 288

S
safer sex, 378–379
safety, 42. *See also* injury.
salt. *See* sodium.
sarcomas, 97
sarcomeres, 228
Sarcoptes scabiei, 375
saturated fats
    and cardiovascular disease, 87, 120
    chemical structure, 117
    dietary guidelines, 119
scabies, 375
scrotum, 357
seated press exercise, 241
seated row exercise, 243
seated-toe-stretch exercise, 265
seated-toe-touch exercise, 271
secondary hypertension, 83
secondary prevention, 81
sedentary activity
    definition, 26
    starting a program, 28–32
self-changers, 49
self-contracts, 58
self-disclosure, 366
self-efficacy
    definition, 54
self image. *See* body image.
self-talk, 57
Selye, Hans, 283
seminal vesicles, 358
semivegetarian diet, 143
servings
    recommended number of, 137
    sizes, 141
set point
    definition, 154, 191
    lowering, 154, 196
    obesity, 163, 183
sets, 236
sex. *See also* intimate relationships.
    biology of. *See* sexual anatomy.
    definition, 352
sexual, 352–353
sexual anatomy
    breasts, 355–356

cervix, 355–356
circumcision, 358
clitoris, 354–355
copulation, 357
Cowper's glands, 358
eggs, 354
fallopian tubes, 354–355
female sexual anatomy, 354–356
fertilization, 352
foreskin, 358
gametes, 352
labia majora, 356
labia minora, 356
male sexual anatomy, 357–358
myotonia, 358
orgasm, 358
ova, 354
ovaries, 354–355
ovulation, 354–355
ovum, 354
penis, 357
prostate gland, 357–358
scrotum, 357
secondary sexual characteristics, 354–355
seminal vesicles, 357–358
smegma, 358
testes, 357
uterus, 354–356
vagina, 354–356
vasocongestion, 358
sexual orientation, 353
sexual response cycle, 358–359
sexuality
    bisexuality, 353
    definition, 352
    gender identity, 354
    gender roles, 354
    heterosexuality, 353
    homosexuality, 353
    sexual orientation, 353
sexually transmitted diseases (STDs)
    absence of symptoms, 369
    AIDS, 375–377
    chlamydia, 372
    Chlamydia trichomatis, 372
    Condylomata acuminata, 374
    definition, 368
    denial, 370
    epididymitis, 372
    false sense of security, 369
    Gardnerella vaginalis, 370
    gonorrhea, 373
    head lice, 375
    hepatitis B, 374–375
    herpes, 373–374
    Herpes simplex, 373–374
    human immunodeficiency virus, 375–377
    human papillomavirus, 374
    impaired judgment, 369
    lack of immunity, 369
    multiple partners, 369
    Neisseria gonorrheae, 373
    Pediculus humanus capittis, 375
    pelvic inflammatory disease, 372
    Phthirus pubis, 375
    prevention, 377–379

pubic lice, 375
reactions to, 370
retroviruses, 377
safer sex, 378–379
Sarcoptes scabiei, 375
scabies, 375
sexually transmitted warts, 374
syphilis, 373
sexually transmitted diseases (STDs) (continued)
    table of, 371
    Treponema pallidum, 373
    Trichomonas vaginalis, 370
    untreated conditions, 369
    value judgments, 370
sexually transmitted warts, 374
shin splints, 385
shoulder roll exercise, 264
shoulder shrug, 241
shoulders, exercises for, 241, 263–264
side lunge exercise, 267
simple carbohydrates, 114
single bent-leg vertical exercise, 264
single knee-to-chest exercise, 265
single straight-leg vertical exercise, 264
sinoatrial node, 68–69
sit-and-reach test, 256–257
sit-up, 242
skater stretch exercise, 267
skeletal system, 22
skill, and physical activity, 39
skin cancer
    description, 98
    risk factors, 98
skinfold testing, 184
sliding filament theory, 228–229
slow-arm-circle exercise, 263
slow-twitch fibers, 230
smegma, 358
smokeless tobacco
    definition, 326
    oral cancer risk, 326
    prevalence, 326
smoking. *See also* tobacco.
    cardiovascular disease, 80, 86–87
    effects on physical activity, 324
    effects on young people, 321
    osteoporosis, 220
    prevalence, 323
    warning labels, 323
    and weight control, 325–326
snatch pull exercise, 246
snuff. *See* smokeless tobacco.
social drinking, 307–308
social factors
    physical activity, 39–40
    and program adherence, 40–41
social interaction theory, 292
social support, 58
social health, 7
sodium
    and bones, 212
    and cardiovascular disease, 86
soluble fibers, 116
sound body, sound mind, 280
specificity principle

definition, 37
    resistance training, 235–236
sphygmomanometer, 68
spiral model of change, 53
spiritual health, 7
spit tobacco. *See* smokeless tobacco.
sprains, 385
squat, 244
stages of
    activity sessions, 35
    change, 50
    conditioning, 34–35
standing heel-to-buttock exercise, 266
standing lunge exercise, 266
standing toe-touch exercise, 269
static contraction, 230–231
static stretching, 258
STDs (sexually transmitted diseases). *See* sexually transmitted diseases (STDs).
sticking to a program. *See* program adherence.
storage fat, 183
strains, 385
strength
    building, 232–233, 238–239
    definition, 36, 228
    muscular, 36
    sample regimen, 239
stress. *See also* mental health.
    allostatic load, 285
    and cardiovascular disease, 88
    autonomic nervous system, definition, 284
    autonomic nervous system, effects on organs, 285–286
    burnout, 288
    definition, 283
    distress, 283
    effects on performance, 288
    endocrine system, 284
    epinephrine, 285
    eustress, 283
    fight-or-flight response, 285
    General Adaptation Syndrome, 283
    glucocorticoids, 285
    hyperstress, 288
    hypostress, 288
    norepinephrine, 285
    ongoing demands, 285
    parasympathetic nervous system, 285
    physical symptoms of, 287
    physiological response, 284–285
    pituitary-adrenal axis, 284–285
    relaxation response, 287
    rustout, 288
    Selye, Hans, 283
    stage of alarm, 284–285
    stage of exhaustion, 286–287
    stage of resistance, 285–286
    stressors, 283–284
    sympathetic nervous system, 154, 284–285
    sympathoadrenal system, 284–285
    Yerkes-Dodson law, 287
stress-fitness relationship, 291
stress management
    environmental engineering, 290
    excess biochemicals, expending, 291
    excess energy, expending, 291

exercise, 291
    meditation, 293
    mind engineering, 290
    mind-over-matter, 290
    physical engineering, 291
    physiological reactivity, 291
    self-talk, 291
    stress resistance, 291
stress reaction
    alarm, 284–285
    exhaustion, 286–287
    resistance, 285–286
stress resistance, 291
stressors, 283–284
stretch reflex, 258
stretching exercises. *See also* flexibility.
    abdomen, 264
    active stretching, 259
    arm across chest, 263
    back, lower, 265–266, 271–272
    back, upper 263–264
    back scratch, 263
    ballistic stretching, 259
    butterfly, 267
    calf, 265, 267
    cat and camel, 266, 272
    chest, 263–264
    chin to chest, 262
    curl-up, 270
    double knee to chest, 265
    double-leg raises, 269
    duration, 260
    ear to shoulder, 262
    elbow-to-knee, 267
    flexibility assessment, 261
    frequency, 260
    full neck circles, 269
    full squat, 268
    gluteals, 267
    groin, 264
    guidelines, 260–261
    hamstring, 264
    hamstrings, 264–265
    handcuff stretch, 264
    hyperextension, 268
    hyperflexion, 268
    improper stretching, 268–269
    intensity, 260
    knee to chest, 271
    look right and left, 262
    low back pain, 271–272
    lower back, 265–266
    lunge, 271
    modified chest lift, 272
    modified hurdler, 264
    neck, 262
    passive stretching, 259
    plough, 269
    proprioceptive neuromuscular facilitation stretching, 259–260
    quads, 267
    rack stretch, 263
    reach up, 263
    sample program, 261–268
    scheduling, 260
    seated toe stretch, 265

    seated toe touch, 271
    shoulder, 263–264
    shoulder roll, 263
    side lunge, 267
    single bent-leg vertical, 264
    single knee to chest, 265
    single straight-leg vertical, 264
    skater stretch, 267
    slow arm circles, 263
    standing heel-to-buttock, 266
    standing lunge, 266
    standing toe touch, 269
    static stretching, 258
    thigh, 267
    trunk, 267
    upper back, 263–264
    V-sit stretch, 266
    wall chest stretch, 263
    wall lean, 267
stroke
    definition, 84
    recognizing, 384
stroke volume, 71
subarachnoid hemorrhage, 84, 85
subcutaneous fat, 176
substrates, 152
sucrose, 114–115
sugar, 114–115
sugars, dietary guidelines, 129
supersets, 248–250
Surgeon General, 81
    Report, 81
sympathetic nervous system, 154, 285–286
sympathoadrenal system, 285
syndrome X, 162
synergists, 231
syphilis, 373
systolic pressure, 68

T
T-scores, bone mass density, 220
target heart rate, calculating, 31, 73
tars, in tobacco, 322
TEA (thermic effect of activity). *See* thermic effect of activity (TEA).
TEF (thermic effect of feeding). *See* thermic effect of feeding (TEF).
temperature control, 69
tendinitis, 385
termination stage, 52
tertiary prevention, 48
testes, 357
thermic effect of activity (TEA), 152–154
thermic effect of food (TEF)
    calculation, 409
    definition, 153
    and physical activity, 157–158
thermoregulation, 69
thighs, stretching exercise, 266–267
time management
    and physical activity, 38
    relaxation technique, 294
tissue interference, 256–257
tobacco. *See also* smoking.
    carbon monoxide, 323

carcinogens in, 322
cause of death, 319
as cause of death, 319
chemical composition, 322–323
and lung cancer, 96–98
nicotine, 322–323
tars, 322
Tolerable Upper Intake Level (UL), 128
tolerance, 304
toning muscles, 232–233
torch myth, 337
trace minerals, 120
training
    muscle development. *See* muscle exercises;
        muscle training; resistance training.
training principles
    individuality, 37
    overload, 37
    reversibility, 37
trans fats, 119
transition stage, 35
Treponema pallidum, 373
tri-sets, 248–250
Trichomonas vaginalis, 370
tricuspid valve, 67
triglycerides, 116–117, 155
    and metabolic syndrome, 162
trunk, stretching exercise, 267
tumors, 96, 97
Type 1 diabetes, 95
Type 2 diabetes, 95–96
    and children, 95–96
    and physical activity, 96

U
UL (Tolerable Upper Intake Level), 127
underfat, 160
underwater weighing, 185
underweight, 160
unsaturated fats, 117
upper back, stretching exercise, 263–264

uterus
    anatomy, 355–356

V
V-sit stretch exercise, 266
vagina, 354–356
valsalva maneuver, 238
valves, heart, 67–69
vanishing acts, 338
variability, 33
vasocongestion, 358
vegan diet, 143
vegetables
    dietary guidelines, 136
vegetarian diets, 143–144
veins, 68
venous return, 69
venules, 68
vibration, 337–338
vicarious experiences, 55
vigorous activity
    definition, 26
    starting a program, 30
visceral fat, 161, 162, 177–178
visualization, 293
vitamin C and bones, 220
vitamin D and bones, 212
vitamins
    and definition, 120
    dietary recommendations, 122
    fat-soluble, 121
    function, 120
    source, 120
    water-soluble, 120
VO$_2$ max test, 70
VO$_2$ reserve, 72

W
waist circumference, 162, 178
wall chest stretch exercise, 263
wall lean exercise, 267
wall sit exercise, 245

water
    dehydration, 145
    function, 123
    nutrient value, 123
    sources, 123
water-soluble vitamins, 121
weight control. *See also* fat (body); fatness;
        obesity.
    behavioral modification, 193
    body mass index, 173–174
    burning calories, 195
    eating speed, 197
    eating style, 197
    emotional eating, 197
    energy balance equation, 157, 186–187
    focus on body fat, 197
    food intake, 196–197
    healthy weight, 173–174
    and lifestyle, 193
    meal size and frequency, 197
    myths, 336–338
    quitting smoking, 324–326
    waist circumference, 162, 178
    waist loss, 178, 195
weight-corrected-for-height measure of over-
        weight and obesity, 173
weight loss, 162–163, 193. *See also* fat (body);
        fatness; obesity; weight control.
weight room etiquette, 248
weight training. *See* resistance training.
wellness, 7
wine, 309–310
withdrawal illness, 306
women's health. *See also* osteoporosis.
    female athlete triad, 201–202
    and physical activity, 24
wrist curl, 247

Y
Yerkes-Dodson law, 287–288
You-statements, 363